WILLIAM F. MAAG LIBRARY
YOUNGSTOWN STATE UNIVERSITY

Plasma Proteins

Plasma Proteins

Edited by
Birger Blombäck *Department of Coagulation Research
Karolinska Institute, Stockholm*

Lars Å. Hanson *Institute of Medical Microbiology,
University of Gothenburg*

Coordinating Editor **Håkan Winberg** *KABI AB*

Translated from the Swedish by **Dr Desmond Hogg**

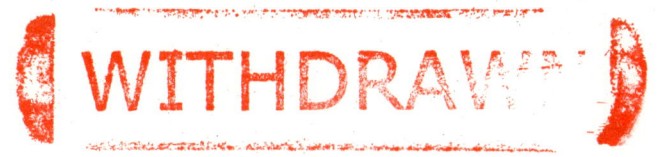

A Wiley–Interscience Publication

A KABI book

JOHN WILEY & SONS

Chichester · New York · Brisbane · Toronto

First published by AB Kabi in 1976 under the title *Plasmaproteiner*
edited by Birger Blombäch and Lars Å. Hanson

© B. Blombäck, L. Å. Hanson, L.-O. Andersson, H. Bennich, G. Birke, H. Björling, G. Cederblad, G. Claes, M. Einatsson, B. Gullbring, A. Gustafson, L. Holmberg, B. G. Johansson, S.-O. Liljedahl, R. Lundén S. Magnusson, G. Möller, H. Nihlén, K. O. Pedersen, J. A. G. Rhodin, M. Rothschild, P. Wallén
KABI AB

Copyright © 1979 by John Wiley & Sons, Ltd.
All rights reserved.

No part of this book may be reproduced by any means, nor transmitted,
nor translated into a machine language without the written
permission of the publisher.

Library of Congress Cataloging in Publication Data:

Main entry under title:

Plasma proteins.
   Translation of Plasmaproteiner.
   'A Wiley–Interscience publication.'
   Includes index.
   1. Plasma proteins. I. Blombäck, Birger.
II. Hanson, Lars A. [DNLM: 1. Blood proteins. WH400 P716]
QP99.3.P7P5713   612'.12   78-10126

ISBN 0 471 99730 7

Photoset in Malta by Interprint Limited
and printed in Great Britain by The Pitman Press, Bath, Avon.

Contributors

PRINCIPAL AUTHORS AND SCIENTIFIC EDITOR-IN-CHIEF

Birger Blombäck	Professor, Department of Coagulation Research, Karolinska Institute, Stockholm, Sweden.
Lars Å. Hanson	Professor, Senior Physician, Department of Clinical Immunology, Institute of Medical Microbiology, University of Gothenburg, Gothenburg, Sweden.

ADDITIONAL CONTRIBUTORS

Lars-Olov Andersson	Associate Professor, Department of Biochemical Research, KABI AB, Sweden.
Hans Bennich	Associate Professor, Biomedicum, University of Uppsala, Uppsala, Sweden.
Gunnar Birke	Professor, Senior Physician, Medical Clinic, Huddinge Hospital, Huddlinge, Sweden.
Henrik Björling	Research Engineer, Research Department, KABI AB, Sweden.
Gitten Cederblad	Associate Professor, Department of Clinical Chemistry, University Hospital, Linköping, Sweden.
Göran Claes	Associate Professor, Senior Physician, Surgical Clinic, Central Hospital, Borås, Sweden.
Monica Einarsson	Ph.D., Department of Biochemical Research, KABI AB, Sweden.
Bengt Guillbring	Senior Physician, Director of Stockholm Blood Center, Stockholm, Sweden.
Anders Gustafson	Professor, Senior Physician, Medical Clinic, University Hospital, Lund, Sweden.
Lars Holmberg	Associate Professor, Senior Physician, Coagulation Laboratory and Paediatric Clinic, General Hospital, Malmö, Sweden.
Bengt G. Johansson	Associate Professor, Senior Physician, Department of Clinical Chemistry, University Hospital, Lund, Sweden.
Sten-Otto Liljedahl	Professor, Senior Physician, Surgical Clinic, University Hospital, Linköping, Sweden.
Ragnar Lundén	Ph.D., Department of Biochemical Research, KABI AB, Sweden.
Staffan Magnusson	Associate Professor, Head of the Department of Molecular Biology, University of Aarhus, Århus, Denmark.
Göran Möller	Associate Professor, Department of Immunobiology, Karolinska Institute, The Wallenberg Laboratory, Lilla Frescati, Stockholm, Sweden.

vi *Contributors*

HUGO NIHLÉN (*Now deceased*)	Master of Engineering, Department of Biochemical Research, KABI AB, Stockholm, Sweden.
KAI O PEDERSEN	Associate Professor, Institute of Physical Chemistry, University of Uppsala, Sweden.
JOHANNES A G RHODIN	Professor, Department of Anatomy, Karolinska Institute, Stockholm, Sweden.
MARK ROTHSCHILD	Professor, Radio Isotope Service and Nuclear Medicine, Veterans Administration Hospital, New York, USA.
PER WALLÉN	Associate Professor, Department of Medical Chemistry, Institute of Chemistry, University of Umeå, Umeå, Sweden.

FOREWORD

JAN G WALDENSTRÖM	Emeritus Professor, General Hospital, Malmö, Sweden.

COORDINATING EDITOR

HÅKAN WINBERG	Ph. D., KABI AB, Sweden.

Contents

FOREWORD xv

PREFACE xvii

HISTORY 1

THE COMPOSITION OF HUMAN PLASMA 17

MICROCIRCULATION OF BLOOD 23

INDUSTRIAL PLASMA FRACTIONATION METHODS 29
    I. Cohn fractionation 29
    II. The Kabi fractionation methods 30
        1. AHF (Factor VIII) 31
        2. Fibrinogen 33
        3. Factor IX concentrate 34
        4. Plasminogen and plasmin 34
        5. Gamma globulin 34
        6. Transferrin, haptoglobin, and
           ceruloplasmin 36
        7. Albumin 36
        8. Glycoproteins 37
    III. Other methods for industrial plasma
       fractionation 37
        1. Ammonium sulphate precipitation
           methods 37
        2. Ether fractionation 38
        3. Rivanol precipitation 38
        4. Precipitation with synthetic
           polymers 39
        5. Chromatographic methods 39

TRANSPORT PROTEINS
    I. Serum albumin 43
       A. Biochemistry 43
          1. Purification and determination 43
          2. Physiochemical properties 43

	3. Heterogeneity	46
	4. Chemical properties	47
	5. Binding properties	51
	6. Structure and function	53
B.	Physiology and clinical aspects	54
	1. Normal values	55
	2. Synthesis, distribution, and breakdown	56
	3. Regulation of albumin metabolism	56
	4. Synthesis of albumin	56
	5. Factors affecting the synthesis of albumin	58
	6. Distribution of albumin	60
	7. Breakdown of albumin	61
	8. Albumin in illness—clinical and therapeutical points of view	63
	9. Special conditions of hypo-albuminaemia	67
	10. Treatment with albumin	69
C.	Organ storage by continuous albumin perfusion	71
II. Plasma lipoproteins		72
A.	Introduction and terminology	72
	1. Plasma lipids—the lipid components in plasma lipoproteins	73
B.	Lipid metabolism	74
C.	Lipoproteins in plasma	76
	1. Chylomicrons	76
	2. VLDL (pre-β-lipoproteins)	76
	3. LDL (β-lipoproteins)	77
	4. HDL (α-lipoproteins)	77
D.	Abnormal lipoproteins	78
	1. Lipoprotein X (LP-X)	78
	2. Sinking pre-β-LP (SPB) Lp (a+)	78
	3. Floating β-lipoproteins	79
E.	Lipoprotein families, apolipoproteins, and their polypeptides	79
F.	Methods used in the study of plasma lipoproteins	82
	1. Electrophoresis	82
	2. Preparative ultracentrifugation	82
	3. Methods of precipitation	82
	4. Nephelometry	83
	5. Immunochemical methods	83
	6. Quantification of LP	83
G.	Methods used in the study of LP families	83

H.	Methods used in the study of apolipoproteins and their peptides	84
I.	Structure of plasma lipoproteins	84
J.	Lipoprotein metabolism	84
	1. Synthesis	84
	2. Catabolism of chylomicrons	86
	3. Catabolism of VLDL	87
	4. Catabolism of LDL	87
	5. Catabolism of HDL	88
K.	Factors influencing concentration of LP in plasma	88
L.	Hyperlipidaemia and hyperlipoproteinaemia	90
M.	Hyperlipoproteinaemias and their clinical manifestations	91
N.	Reference values and frequency of hyperlipoproteinaemia	93
O.	Hypolipoproteinaemias	93
	1. Tangier's disease	93
	2. LP-A deficiency	93
	3. Lecithin-cholesterol-acyl-transferase (LCAT) deficiency	93
	4. A-β-lipoproteinaemia (Bassen–Kornzweig disease)	94
III. Plasma proteins involved in haem metabolism and in transport of metals, hormones, and vitamins		94
A.	Ceruloplasmin	96
	1. Chemical structure and biochemistry	96
	2. Biological function	97
	3. Hereditary defects in copper metabolism	99
B.	Transferrin	99
	1. Chemical structure and biochemistry	99
	2. Genetic variants	100
	3. Biological function	100
C.	Haptoglobin	102
	1. Chemical structure and biochemistry	102
	2. Genetic variants	105
	3. Biological function	106
D.	Haemopexin	106
	1. Chemical structure and biochemistry	106
	2. Biological function	107
E.	Transcobalamine	109
	1. Chemical structure and biochemistry	109
	2. Biological function	110
	3. Genetic variants	110
F.	Retinol-binding protein	111
	1. Chemical structure and biochemistry	111
	2. Biological function	112

x   Contents

  G. Proteins binding thyroid hormones 113
    1. Chemical structure and biochemistry 113
    2. Genetic variants 114
    3. Biological function. 114
  H. Transcortin 115
    1. Chemical structure and biochemistry 115
    2. Biological function. 116

IMMUNOGLOBULINS

 I. Structure and biochemistry 119
   1. Basic structure 119
   2. Classes of immunoglobulins 120
   3. Structures of heavy chains of various classes 121
   4. Variable and constant regions. 124
   5. Antigenic properties of immunoglobulins:
     isotypes, allotypes, and idiotypes 125
   6. Biosynthesis of immunoglobulins. 126

 II. Immunological mechanisms 127
   1. The lymphatic system 128
   2. Characteristics of antigens. 131
   3. Antibody formation 132
   4. Cell-mediated immunity 137
   5. Antigen–antibody reactions 140
   6. Complement 147

 III. Defence against infection 151
   1. Non-specific defence mechanisms 152
   2. Role of antibodies 156
   3. Cell-mediated immunity 163
   4. Defects in the defence mechanisms. 164

 IV. Immunological diseases: allergies,
   immune complex diseases, and
   autoimmune disease 174
   1. Mechanisms of immunological diseases 174
   2. Atopic allergies 176
   3. Drug allergies 181
   4. Contact allergies 182
   5. Immune complex diseases 182
   6. Autoimmune diseases 184

 V. Transplantation immunology 187
   1. Histocompatibility antigens 187
   2. Immune reactions against transplanted
     tissue 188
   3. The effector function 189
   4. Clinical aspects 190
   5. Immunosuppression 193

VI.	Tumour immunology		194
	1. Tumour antigens		194
	2. Immune reactions		195
	3. Immunological surveillance		195
	4. Practical applications of tumour immunology		197
VII.	Blood group serology		198
	A. Introduction		198
		1. Definitions	198
		2. Cell membrane	198
		3. Erythrocyte antigens	199
		4. Blood group antibodies	200
		5. Antiglobulin sera for the demonstration of antibodies (Coombs's test)	202
		6. Frequency of blood group antibodies	203
	B. Genetics of blood groups		204
	C. ABO and Lewis systems		205
		1. ABO system	205
		2. Antibodies within the ABO system	206
		3. Reactions towards transfusion which are caused by incompatible ABO blood	207
		4. ABO incompatibility as a cause of haemolytic diseases in the new-born	207
		5. The Lewis system	208
		6. ABH and Lewis antigens in secretion	208
		7. Chemical composition of blood group substances	210
	D. Rh system		210
		1. Nomenclature	211
		2. Frequencies of Rh types	212
		3. Rh antibodies	213
		4. The D antigen	213
		5. Special antigens within the Rh system	214
		6. Rh immunization	215
		7. Rh prophylaxis	217
	E. Certain blood group systems of clinical interest		218
		1. The Kell system	218
		2. The Duffy system	219
		3. The Kidd system	219

PROTEINS TAKING PART IN COAGULATION AND FIBRINOLYSIS

I. Factors and mechanisms involved in blood coagulation 221

II. Fibrinogen and fibrin formation 223
  1. Occurrence and role. 223
  2. Physicochemical properties 224
  3. The subunits and prosthetic groups of fibrinogen 227
  4. The primary structure of fibrinogen 230
  5. Fibrin–the ordered structure of fibrinogen 237
  6. Stabilizing the fibrin polymer 247
  7. The antigenic structure of fibrinogen and the
     location of epitopes and other structural elements 249
  8. Fibrinogen in health and disease 250
  9. Epilogue. 253

III. Thrombin and prothrombin 254
  A. Limited proteolysis as a means of regulation 254
  B. Historical outline 254
  C. Thrombin–structure and function 255
     1. Function and specificity 255
     2. Primary structure. 256
     3. Homology with serine proteases and haptoglobin 258
     4. Tentative tertiary structure 259
     5. Partial homology/analogy with angiotensin and
        with luteinizing hormone (LH) 260
  D. Prothrombin–structure and activation 261
     1. Specific cleavage by factor X_a and by thrombin.
        Nomenclature 261
     2. The primary structure of prothrombin. Internal homology.
        'Kringle' structures 262
     3. γ-Carboxylglutamic acid, Ca^{2+} and phospholipid
        binding, vitamin K 264
     4. Homology with plasminogen. 268
     5. Homology with other vitamin-K-dependent proteins . . . 268
     6. Partial homology with the pancreatic secretory
        trypsin inhibitor (Kazal's inhibitor) and with hirudin . . . 273
     7. Activation by limited proteolysis 274
     8. Activation by staphylocoagulase 275
     9. Multiple evolutionary origin of the larger serine
        protease zymogen structures 275
  E. Biosynthesis 275
  F. Inhibition of thrombin by antithrombin-III (heparin cofactor) . . 276

IV. AHF and von Willebrand's disease 276

V. Haemophilia B-factor (Factor 1X) 281

VI. Additional coagulation factors 285
  1. Factor V 285
  2. Factor VII 286
  3. Factor X 286
  4. Factor XI 287
  5. Factor XII 287

6. Factor XIII	287
VII. Plasminogen and fibrinolysis	288
1. Introduction	288
2. Plasminogen: purification and properties	289
3. Activation of the fibrinolytic system	293
4. Activators	299
5. Inhibition of fibrinolysis	303
6. Interactions between fibrin and the fibrinolytic system	304

INHIBITORS OF PROTEOLYSIS IN PLASMA

1. α_1-Antitrypsin	305
2. α_2-Protease inhibitor, antiplasmin	306
3. α_2-Macroglobulin	307
4. Antithrombin	307

PLASMA PROTEINS AS DIAGNOSTIC AIDS. METHODS AND CLINICAL APPLICATIONS

I. Introduction	309
II. Chemical methods	309
1. Determination of total protein	309
2. Determination of individual plasma proteins	311
III. Physicochemical methods	312
1. Analytical ultracentrifugation	312
2. Gel filtration	313
3. Electrophoresis	316
IV. Immunochemical methods	318
1. Introduction	318
2. Quantitative precipitation in solution	321
3. Double diffusion in agar gel	323
4. Immunoelectrophoresis	323
5. Quantitative gel immunodiffusion	324
6. Electroimmunoassay (rocket immunoelectrophoresis)	325
7. Crossed immunoelectrophoresis	329
8. Other gel immunoprecipitation techniques	330
9. Nephelometric determinations of immunoprecipitates	333
10. Radioimmunoassay	333
V. Diagnostic use of plasma protein analysis	335
1. The normal agarose electrophoresis pattern	335
2. Normal variants of the electrophoretic plasma protein pattern	337
3. Pathological variations in the electrophoretic patterns	338
4. Normal variations in the concentrations of individual plasma proteins	339

xiv *Contents*

       5. Influence of steroid hormones on the plasma protein pattern. 341

VI. Deficiency states – α_1-antitrypsin deficiency 343

VII. Immunoglobulin alterations in disease 344
       1. Decrease in the level of immunoglobulin 344
       2. Monoclonal increase of immunoglobulins 345
       3. Oligoclonal and polyclonal immunoglobulin increase 348

VIII. The plasma protein profile in inflammatory conditions 351

IX. Plasma protein changes in gastrointestinal diseases 354

X. Plasma protein alterations in liver and biliary diseases 357
       1. Hepatitis and liver cirrhosis 357
       2. Liver tumours 360
       3. Protein and lipoprotein changes in cholestasis 360

XI. Kidney disease 361

XII. Blood and bone marrow diseases 362

XIII. Analysis of proteins in body fluids other than blood 364
       1. Urinary proteins 364
       2. Cerebrospinal fluid proteins 368

REFERENCES 377

INDEX 393

Foreword

When I started in medical school some 50 years ago, we did not learn much about serum proteins. The textbook we used in physiological chemistry devoted only a few pages to this topic. We were taught that the serum contained albumin and globulins of two kinds: euglobulin and pseudoglobulin. Fibrinogen was of course regarded as an important substance but our knowledge regarding the mechanisms involved in coagulation of the blood was minimal. It is therefore fair to state that I have myself had a chance to follow practically the whole development leading to the present state of knowledge as it is described in this book. This history has been written in a superb way by Kai Pedersen in the first chapter.

I had the good fortune to enjoy collaboration with the group that was inspired by The Svedberg and Arne Tiselius. My first study with Kai Pedersen in 1937 was connected with a problem much discussed at that time. The German clinician Bennhold was a very original investigator with great imagination. He wrote some papers on the function of the plasma proteins and especially the albumin as vehicles for smaller molecules. When these were carried on the big protein molecules, they could stay in the circulation. This idea has of course been very fruitful. Bennhold attacked the problem from many aspects and his work has remained of fundamental importance. He also studied a very interesting experiment of nature, when he found two sibs, who had genetically determined almost complete lack of serum albumin but still got along fairly well. Pedersen and I were interested in the binding of bilirubin to albumin and we studied this problem in different clinical conditions with the aid of electrophoresis and ultracentrifugation.

I also had the pleasure to follow Tiselius and Pedersen when they developed new methods and discovered new facts. At this time we thought that the new names on the different serum protein fractions alpha, beta, and gamma were very special and sophisticated. They represented facts that chiefly had a theoretical, basic interest. A few years later Tiselius came back from New York and told us, laughing, that the gamma globulins had become very popular. The women in New York were parading the streets with placards inscribed: 'We want gamma globulins'. This was during a certain phase of the polio campaign.

At first glance the reader of this book will find many things that may seem very specialized. It is evident that the presentation—attempting to be complete—has to include many seemingly trivial and unimportant facts. At the same time it is quite clear that we cannot at present imagine which facts will be discussed by everybody in a few years' time. I think that it is very important to provide the kind of presentation of the facts that Kabi has given us. Earlier this company made an excellent contribution to the postgraduate education of the doctor when it edited and distributed a monograph on blood coagulation. The new volume on plasma proteins is another work with an identical aim and I think that it should be stressed that this book is not a textbook meant to be read from cover to cover. The reader who is more technically minded will be provided with recent and correct facts regarding methodology. It is probable that this does not interest the clinician who may enjoy reading other chapters that attempt to integrate basic chemistry with clinical application. In this way I feel that the book will be widely read because the individual will find presentations of subjects that interest him in a special way.

It may well be said that this is natural with a Swedish book on plasma proteins. Swedish investigators, from the times of Olof Hammarsten to The Svedberg and Arne Tiselius and the teams working with these men, have contributed decisive knowledge regarding these substances. The development of new methods in this field has been initiated by Swedish work on such subjects as electrophoresis, ultracentrifugation, and gel filtration. Swedish industry has been very active in the technical development and Kabi has been in the front line regarding preparation of different fractions in such a pure condition that they may be used in clinical medicine. The previous Swedish edition was very well accepted and it seems appropriate to print this English edition that has been revised and brought up to date on several points.

There has been a lively discussion regarding the most ideal form of therapy imaginable. Perhaps a chemotherapeutic preparation or an antibiotic that stops the further growth of a deadly bug? A cytostatic that slows down the growth of a malignant cell or under favourable circumstances causes 'eradication of the last cell', an expression that has recently become popular among oncologists? Personally I have always been of the opinion that we have only one really ideal form of therapy. That is substitution. When a deficiency of a certain kind is corrected, either a complicated vitamin molecule or the simple iron atom, we combine natural healing and natural sciences. Substitution is always physiological and carries no risks. All over the world it has become a fashion among the mass media to repeat endless stories about the many real or invented dangers of drugs. Under such circumstances it is easy to forget the millions of patients, whose lives have been saved, when we are talking about a few exceptions. This volume treats the possibilities of giving natural substitution. Kabi has for several decades been active in strengthening our therapeutical armament with a number of important preparations. Therefore, this presentation of the facts from many of the collaborators in the programme is of special interest. The importance of gamma globulin preparations as a prophylactic can hardly be overrated but also other plasma protein fractions have gained increasing importance. We do not need much imagination in order to expect that purified proteins of the blood will become valuable in new fields.

My guess is that some readers will find the content of the chapters somewhat unbalanced. Such things are unavoidable in a book with many authors representing completely different training and interests. Nevertheless I am sure that the book is very valuable as a source of information both for doctors practising in the field and for biochemists. Plasma proteins will be a subject with increasing importance during years to come.

General Hospital, JAN G. WALDENSTRÖM
Malmö, Sweden *Emeritus Professor*

Preface

The fractionation of human blood plasma has long been one of Kabi's most important fields of interest. Today Kabi can offer a wide range of plasma protein products for therapeutic use, albumin, specific immunoglobulins, fibrinogen, specific blood coagulation factors, and several other isolated proteins for research purposes.

The development of research in clinical coagulation as a new, far-reaching and important discipline together with the ever increasing understanding of the mechanism of fibrinolysis was the background to Inga Marie Nilsson's widely used book, *Haemorrhagic and Thrombotic Diseases*, which appeared in English in 1974.

The present book, *Plasma Proteins*, is complementary to Inga Marie Nilsson's book. The scientific editors-in-chief are Birger Blombäch and Lars Å. Hanson.

We wish to express our warm thanks to the editors-in-chief and to the other contributors who through their efforts have made this book possible.

It is our hope that *Plasma Proteins* will be of use as an educational textbook and as a clinical handbook.

KABI AB
Stockholm

History

KAI O. PEDERSEN

Proteins are essential in animal nutrition and they are therefore of fundamental importance for all living beings. This was the reason why Berzelius in 1838, in a correspondence with the Dutch chemist G. J. Mulder, proposed the introduction of the name protein. Mulder had studied a number of nitrogenous substances prepared from animal and plant material and had come to the conclusion that all these substances had one part in common. The difference in the material of different origin was explained by variation in the content of bound sulphur and phosphorus. The name protein was derived from a Greek word meaning 'of first rank' and should thus stress the primary importance of these substances.

Blood plasma is a solution consisting of a mixture of virtually hundreds of individual proteins, some of them in very small amounts. It is therefore not surprising that more than a century passed after the separation of the first proteins before enough information was obtained to allow the understanding of the finer molecular structure of this fascinating group of substances.

Now we know that proteins are macromolecules and are among the most complicated of organic molecules. They are built up from hundreds of α-amino acids linked together through so-called peptide bonds into one or several long chains (primary structure). Linus Pauling and co-workers have shown that the peptide chain is often folded in a spiral, the so-called α-helix. This spiral is stabilized by various bindings between amino acids which, due to the folding, have come relatively close together in space (secondary structure). The α-helix is folded further into a more compact tertiary structure kept together by, for instance, disulphide linkages between amino acids in different parts of the α-helix. These units may further be bound together to still larger units by interchain bridges.

The secondary and tertiary structures are of fundamental importance for the properties of the native proteins. If this delicate structure is changed, for instance by heating to 50–70°C or by adding some organic solvents to the protein solution, the properties of the protein may be profoundly changed—the protein becomes denatured.

In the middle of the nineteenth century it was found that a fraction of the plasma and serum proteins could be precipitated by dilution with slightly acidified water or by the addition of, for example, sodium chloride to saturation. This protein was given various names until finally it was called globulin. The protein remaining in solution was called albumin. At this time it was discovered by T. Graham that proteins would not pass through membranes permeable to ordinary salts. Protein solutions could therefore be freed from salts by dialysis. When dissolved, the proteins formed colloidal solutions having very large particles.

In the later half of the nineteenth century, many different separation methods were introduced into protein chemistry. It was found that a number of neutral salts would precipitate proteins reversibly without denaturation. Thus in 1879 Olof Hammarsten at the University of Uppsala, Sweden, succeeded in preparing fibrinogen in an amazingly pure condition. This was probably the first time a native protein had been prepared from blood plasma.

A coarse fractionation of plasma into fibrinogen, globulin, and albumin could be achieved by stepwise addition of salt followed by successive removal of the precipitate formed. By dialysing against water, a subfractionation of globulin into a euglobulin, insoluble in electrolyte-free water, and a water-soluble pseudoglobulin could be accomplished. As early as 1894 it was reported that horse serum albumin could be crystallized by precipitation with ammonium sulphate.

At the beginning of this century a most important advance in protein chemistry came through the work of the organic chemist Emil Fischer. He started a systematic study of the main breakdown products from various proteins after hydrolysis with strong solutions of hydrochloric acid, and found almost the same kinds of amino acids in the hydrolysate in all cases. However, the relative content of the different amino acids varied from protein to protein, as did the small amount of other compounds, for instance carbohydrates. Together with Emil Abderhalden he also showed that enzymes from the digestive juices broke down proteins into similar mixtures of amino acids.

From his experiments Fisher concluded that the amino acids in proteins are linked together in long polypeptide chains where the α-amino group of each amino acid is joined through an amide bond to the carboxyl group of the adjacent amino acid. The

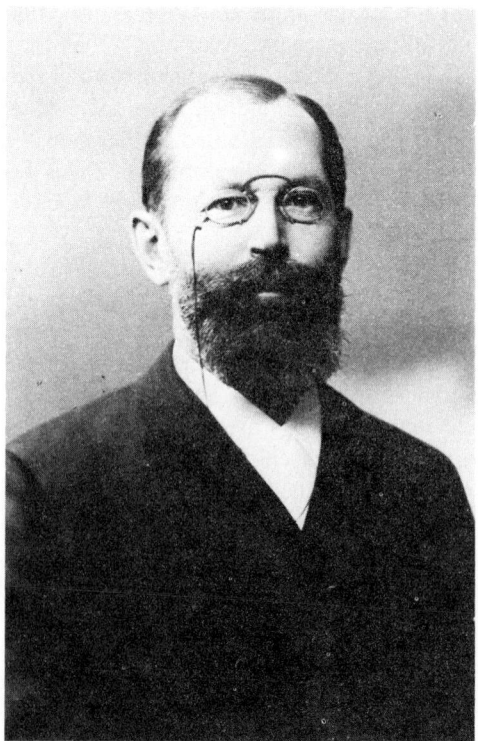

Fig. 1. Emil Fisher (1852–1919). Nobel laureate 1902

bond formed: $-CO-NH-$, the so-called peptide bond, is repeated through the length of the peptide chain. This is the characteristic feature of all protein molecules.

In the decades which followed, the protein chemists worked along different lines. Some were interested in determining the amino acid distribution and sequences in the

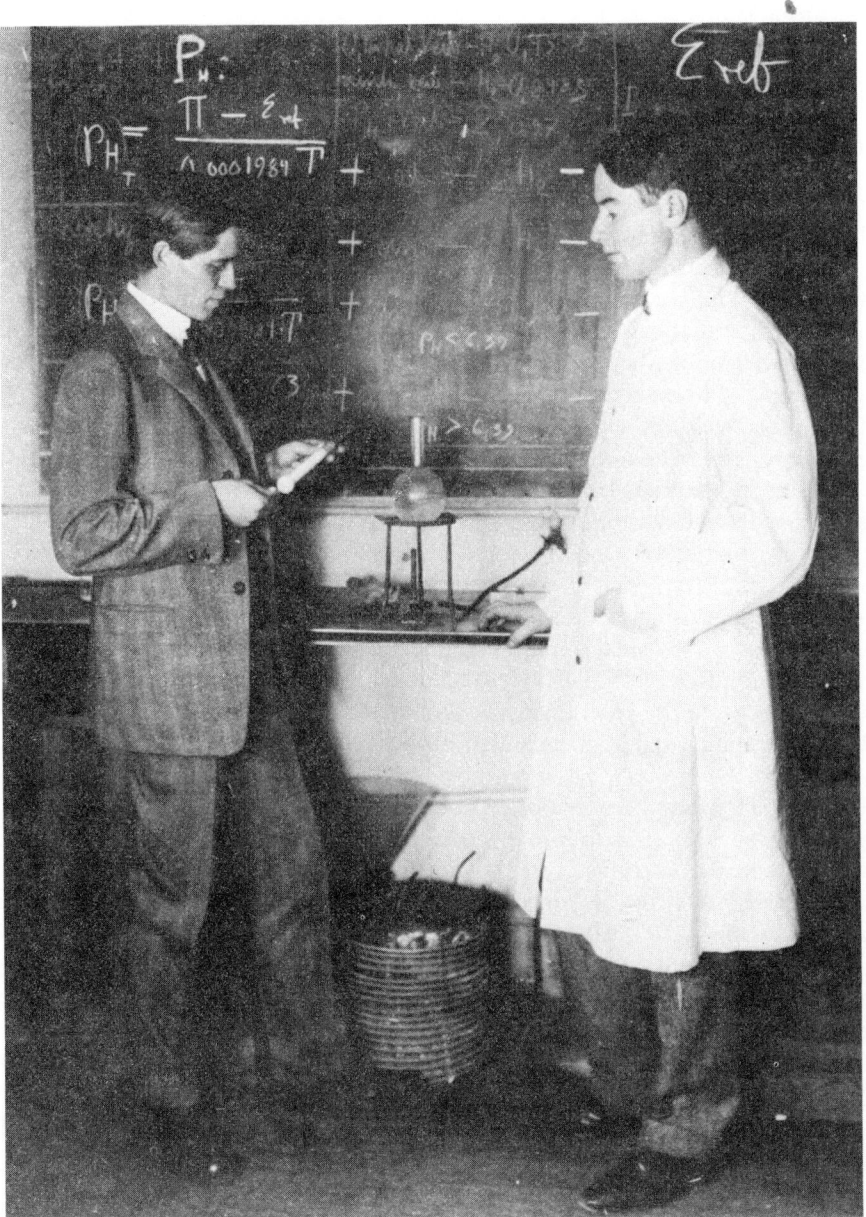

Fig. 2. The Svedberg (1884–1971), Nobel laureate 1926, with his young assistant Arne Tiselius (1902–1971), Nobel laureate 1948, in the old chemical laboratory at the University of Uppsala in 1926

various chains, others tried to elucidate problems connected with the chemical nature of the proteins.

During the first half of this century much effort was directed towards finding suitable procedures for analysing protein solutions and for preparing pure proteins. For this purpose a number of fractionation methods were developed, some of these particularly for use in the clinic.

The situation was quite difficult for the protein chemists. No criterion existed for the purity of proteins. They have no melting point, but decompose at about 150°C. Their solubility behaviour is often complicated. They were not considered as chemically well-defined molecules. Rather were they thought of as colloids whose aqueous solutions were not to be considered as true molecular solutions, but merely suspensions of micelles of varying particle size. The proteins were mainly characterized by their origin, solubility, optical rotation, elementary composition, etc.

S. P. L. Sörensen, the man who introduced the conception of pH into chemistry, published in 1917 a study on the osmotic pressure of egg albumin solutions. He came to the conclusion that egg albumin in aqueous salt solutions had an average molecular or particle weight of about 34 000. Several years later he estimated values for the particle weight of horse serum albumin and globulin, and came to 45 000 and 80 000–140 000, respectively. Sörensen was of the opinion, that proteins formed reversible, dissociable systems of components.

A new era in our knowledge of the proteins started a few years later at Uppsala. Here The Svedberg had been studying colloids for two decades. He had determined the frequency distribution of particle sizes in metal sols by measuring the rate of sedimentation of the particles in sols in the gravitational field. The smallest metal particles he could measure by this method had a diameter of about 200 nm. However, he wanted to be able to study much smaller particles, and for this purpose he constructed his first primitive ultracentrifuge 1923–24. Here he could follow the settling of the particles by optical means while the centrifuge was running. The ultracentrifuge was immediately used for determining the frequency distribution of particle sizes in a number of metal sols.

Svedberg had always been interested in biology, and it had been his dream to be able to study the particle sizes in protein solutions. As a colloid chemist, he was quite convinced that the proteins were polydisperse, and he wanted to determine the frequency distribution of the particle sizes in protein solutions. The first experiments with egg albumin were disappointing, but when he and Robin Fåhraeus tried with native casein from milk in the early autumn of 1924, it sedimented and showed a very broad frequency distribution with coarse particles of the order of 10–70 nm in diameter.

Svedberg and Fåhraeus then tried with horse haemoglobin, and it sedimented slowly. After some days, a stationary condition was reached where the haemoglobin concentration gradually increased towards the periphery (the bottom of the cell). An equilibrium had been attained between the sedimentation of the protein towards the bottom of the cell and the diffusion in the opposite direction from the higher protein concentration at the bottom of the cell. A sedimentation equilibrium had thus been established. From the concentration distribution in the cell, Svedberg and Fåhraeus calculated a molecular weight of about 67 000 for haemoglobin (November 1924). Moreover, the haemoglobin solution proved to contain particles of equal size—a monodisperse colloid produced by nature in sharp contrast to the man-made metal colloids. This was the first indication of protein molecules of uniform size. Could it be that the general concept among chemists was wrong? Were the proteins not polydisperse colloids, or did they consist of monodisperse well-defined molecules?

In order to prove that the proteins were of uniform size, it would be necessary to introduce a new method, the sedimentation velocity method, where the speed of the ultracentrifuge is so high that the sedimentation dominates over the diffusion. A larger spreading of the boundary than that which corresponded to the diffusion coefficient for the protein or the appearance of different boundaries would indicate inhomogeneity of the protein. The presence of different sized particles would thus manifest itself much more directly by this method than by the sedimentation equilibrium method where it would only appear as a drift in the values calculated between the meniscus and the bottom of the cell.

If the sedimentation velocity method should be introduced in the study of proteins, it would be necessary to increase the centrifugal force 15–20 times the one available in the sedimentation equilibrium experiments as the difference in density between protein and solution is very small. Such a new high-speed ultracentrifuge became available in 1926.

Many of the first proteins to be studied were respiratory proteins. They are usually coloured (chromoproteins) which meant that they could be studied almost directly in the ultracentrifuge, where their sedimentation could be followed directly by means of the light absorption method (Fig. 3).

After a few years of studying proteins of different origin, Svedberg proposed in 1929 a hypothesis that the molecular weights of the proteins were limited to a small number of values. His idea was that there existed some kind of 'periodic system' for the proteins, where the molecular weight of most of the higher classes could be expressed as simple multiples of those for the lower classes. In order to test this hypothesis, he worked along two different lines: (1) As many different proteins as possible and from various sources should be studied: chromoproteins, respiratory proteins, plasma proteins, seed proteins, enzymes, etc. (2) The resolving power, or the efficiency, of the ultracentrifuge should be increased.

During a first period, 1930–32, the whole ultracentrifuge machinery and system was completely reconstructed, resulting in an almost 100 per cent increase in the resolving power as compared with the 1926 model. By various technical improvements, mainly in the rotor and cell construction, during the period 1933–39, a further 50 per cent increase in the resolving power was achieved. During this period new methods of observation were also introduced, especially the so-called 'scale method' which relates the variation in the refractive index gradient (dn/dr) and therefore also the concentration gradient (dc/dr) to the position in the cell, whereas the light absorption method relates the concentration of the sedimenting substance to the position in the cell. The 'scale method' has the advantage of working equally well with uncoloured as with coloured substances. In the case where there is more than one high molecular weight component present in the solution studied, this is more easily discerned when the sedimentation diagram is a ($dc/dr, r$) diagram than when it is a (c, r) diagram (Fig. 4).

Before studying proteins in the ultracentrifuge, Svedberg had started, together with some American students, to measure the electrophoretic mobility of proteins and its variation with pH.

6 *History*

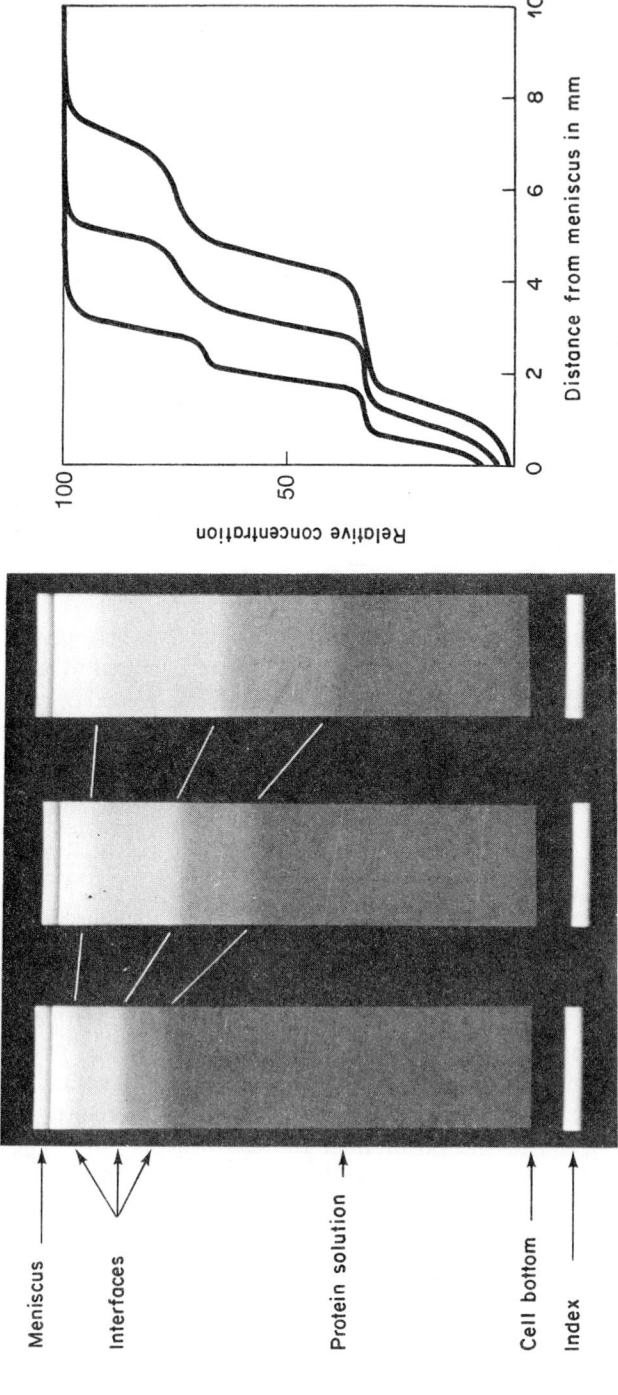

Fig. 3. Sedimentation pictures taken with the light absorption method (left) and the corresponding concentration curves (right). From a sedimentation velocity run on *Helix pomatia* haemocyanin at pH 8.2 Centrifugal force 60 000 times gravity. The three boundaries correspond to $s_{20} = 99$ S, 62 S, and 16 S, respectively. The three exposures are taken 5, 10, and 15 minutes after the centrifuge reached full speed

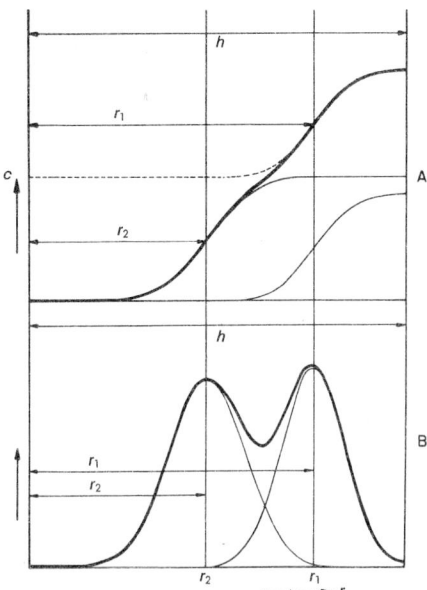

Fig. 4. Schematic drawing, showing the sedimentation diagram at the end of a run for a mixture which may just be unequivocally resolved by means of the scale method (B). With the light absorption method (A) the diagram barely indicates the presence of two components. In calculating these diagrams, it was assumed that the two components had the same initial concentration and the same light absorption, etc. The fine-lined curves show the theoretical curves for the individual components (h = height of column of solution in the cell, r_1 = distance between meniscus and the 50 per cent point for the faster sedimenting component, r_2 = the same for the slower one)

The proteins are electrically charged, and their charge depends on the pH of the solution. They are ampholytes. At the isoelectric point, IP, they have no net charge and show no mobility. On the acid side of their IP they move towards the cathode and on the basic side towards the anode. The IP and the variation of the mobility with pH depend on the amino acid composition of the protein.

In 1925 Arne Tiselius became Svedberg's research assistant and joined him in his electrophoretic studies. In 1926 they published a paper on the introduction of the light absorption method in the study of the electrophoretic mobility of proteins. Svedberg now concentrated on the problems connected with the ultracentrifuge and let Tiselius develop the electrophoresis technique and theory. In his dissertation (1930) on 'The moving boundary method of studying the electrophoresis of proteins' Tiselius treated the theoretical and experimental problems connected with this method. For simple uniform proteins the method worked well but it was usually not selective enough for mixtures, e.g. serum.

Tiselius was disappointed and abandoned the method for several years. At Uppsala, however, it was used during the following years to characterize a number of the proteins studied with the ultracentrifuge.

In the 1930s, intensive studies were carried out on all kinds of proteins. In many

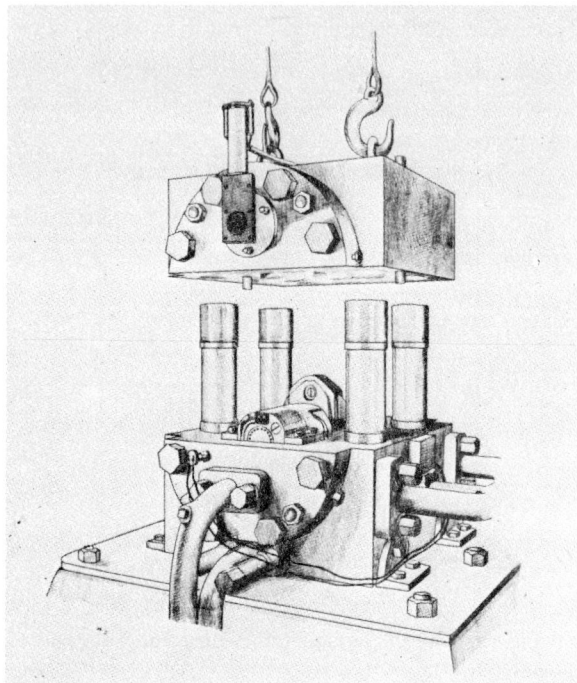

Fig. 5. Drawing of the rotor house for the Svedberg oil-turbine ultracentrifuge with the upper part of the steel casing lifted

cases only the sedimentation coefficient, s_{20}, was determined, and it was found that the s_{20}^0's were distributed on a relatively small number of values.*

Many of the proteins with identical s_{20} were also studied in electrophoresis experiments by means of the Tiselius moving boundry technique. For the respiratory proteins it was found that none of the proteins with the same s_{20} showed the same isoelectric point or the same slope on the pH-mobility curve—they were chemically different. In 1933 Svedberg expressed the matter as follows: 'The sedimentation constant and the molecular weight may be used as a group characteristic, the isoelectric point as a species characteristic'.

At this time quite a number of scientists, brought up in the tradition that proteins were very complicated substances, had difficulty in believing that the soluble proteins were so well defined with regard to size as was found by Svedberg and his group. Furthermore, when Svedberg elaborated his idea about a periodic system for proteins, the scepticism became still more pronounced. However, at about the same time investigations in other laboratories confirmed that the proteins were large, well-defined molecules. Thus J. H. Northrop had crystallized pepsin and had carried out a very thorough study on this crystalline enzyme. He concluded that it was a very well-

---

*The sedimentation coefficient is usually marked as $s_{20,w}^0$. The unit is called Svedberg (abbreviated to S). The upper index means that the solute concentration has been extrapolated to zero concentration, i.e. infinite dilution. The lower indices refer to temperature and solvent. Thus it implies that the sedimentation has been referred to a temperature of 20°C in pure water (without salt).

defined, uniform protein with a definite chemical structure. This was confirmed somewhat later in a different way when J. D. Bernal and Dorothy Crowfoot in 1933 succeeded in taking the first X-ray photographs of a globular protein. They say: 'the arrangement of atoms inside the protein molecule is also of a perfectly defined kind, although without the periodicities characterizing the fibrous proteins'.

We may now say that Svedberg was correct in regarding the proteins as being very well-defined substances; but he was wrong in assuming that his multiple systems were valid for all kinds of proteins. On the other hand, there is no doubt that within certain groups of proteins definite multiple systems exist which are based on the development of the various species from a common genetic origin.

To sum up, we may say that the introduction of the ultracentrifuge led to the discovery that the soluble proteins are well-defined chemical substances having definite molecular weights. The sedimentation velocity ultracentrifuge, and later also the Tiselius electrophoresis technique, made it possible in a much more direct way to visualize how far the isolation and purification of an individual protein had been successful. Although Svedberg's idea of a periodic system for the proteins was not of such a general nature as first assumed by him, it has been important for the development of protein chemistry, especially in the 1930s and at the beginning of the 1940s. It initiated greater interest in this group of substances and gave an impetus to new investigations. Several chemists and physicists discovered that the proteins no longer had to be considered as ill-defined lyophilic colloids, but rather as well-defined, exceedingly interesting and important substances, well worth studying. This was the first step towards the new science of molecular biology.

Attempts had been made in the early 1930s to study dilute solutions of serum in the ultracentrifuge. These were without success as long as the light absorption method was used; even the first series of experiments with the scale method were not satisfactory. It was not until A. S. McFarlane in 1934 started to work with a flexible scale projection system that a somewhat more systematic study of serum could be started. Svedberg had hoped that the ultracentrifuge would turn out to be of diagnostic value 'in the study of pathological sera'. In some cases, e.g. myelomas, new components were observed; usually, however, this was just a variation in the proportion of the different components (Fig. 6). As a whole this was a disappointment to Svedberg. For some years in the 1940s, the criteria for Waldenström's macroglobulinaemia could only be definitely settled by the ultracentrifuge.

In 1944 a new serum protein, fetuin, was discovered, first in serum from new-born calves and later in relatively large amounts in foetal sera (Fig. 7).

In 1936–37 Tiselius made a thorough reconstruction of his electrophoresis apparatus and changed the experimental technique in such a way that the resolving power for mixtures of proteins became more than 10 times better than that of his old apparatus. His earlier studies on serum globulin fractions had shown that neither pseudoglobulin nor euglobulin was homogeneous in electrophoresis. With the new, radically changed electrophoresis technique, he started to study a dialysed and diluted solution of horse serum and found four main protein components: albumin and three globulins, for which he introduced the names: α-; β-, and γ-globulin. At the end of the experiment, samples of the fastest and the slowest moving components could be separated and taken out for further analysis. It was found that serum albumin, isolated in this way, displayed a single sharp boundary in a new electrophoresis, whereas the γ-globulin,

10 *History*

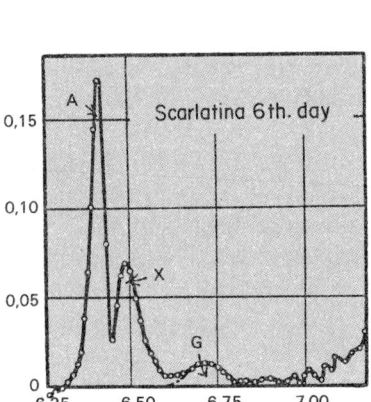
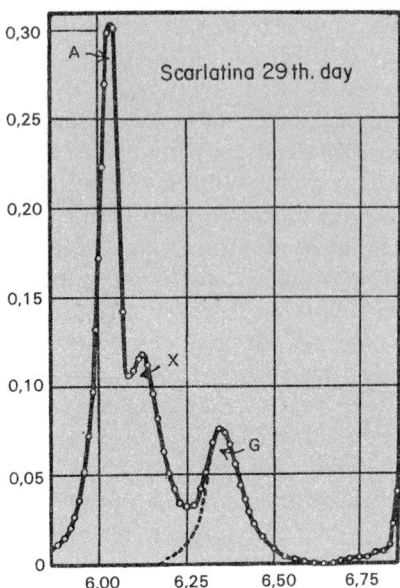

Fig. 6. Sedimentation diagrams with the scale method of two sera from a patient with scarlatina, taken the 6th and the 29th day of disease. Abscissa: distance from the axis of rotation in centimetres. Ordinate: scale line deflection in millimetres. The two exposures were taken 73 and 87 minutes after reaching full speed. Notice the marked increase in the globulin fraction (G) due to the antibody formation during the 23 days (McFarlane, 1935). This was the first time the antibodies were referred to a special component in the sedimentation diagram

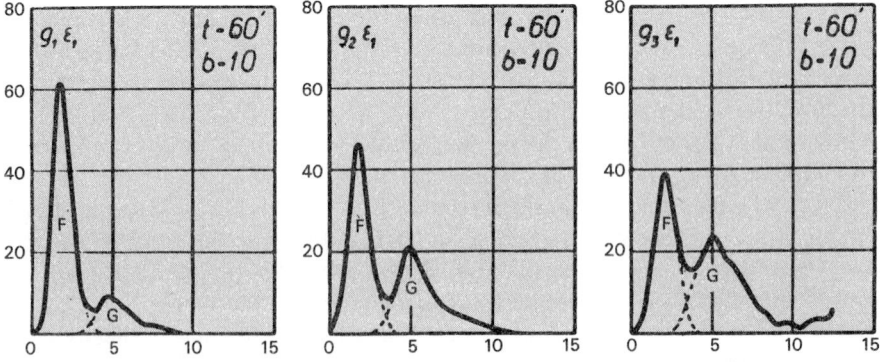

Fig. 7. Sedimentation diagrams from three successive globulin fractions from calf serum, showing the fetuin (F) and the globulin (G) peaks. The fractions were collected between the following values: 0.37–0.40, 0.40–0.45, and 0.45–0.50 concentration of saturated ammonium sulphate; pH about 6.0. Centrifugal field: 260 000 times gravity. Exposures taken 60 minutes after full speed (Pedersen, 1945). This was the first time a new plasma protein was discovered by means of the ultracentrifuge

obtained from the same experiment, gave a widespread boundary. Serum from horse, man, and rabbit gave similar electrophoresis diagrams, although with quantitative differences.

In an immune rabbit serum, the proportion of γ-globulin was much higher than in normal rabbit serum. Electrophoretic separation of the γ-globulin from this serum showed also that the antibody activity was associated exclusively with this component. For another immune serum it was found that the antibody in antipneumococcal horse serum was associated with an apparently new component having an electrophoretic mobility between that for the β- and the γ-globulin, as defined for normal horse serum.

Electrophoretic studies of serum proteins separated by salt fractionation soon disclosed the value of the electrophoresis diagrams for following purification procedures, and electrophoretic homogeneity was now introduced as a necessary, though by no means sufficient, criterion of protein purity. An entirely new vista was opened in protein investigation, and Tiselius's basic observations were quickly expanded as a consequence of the installation of 'Tiselius apparatuses' in many laboratories throughout the world. The new electrophoresis technique was now intensively used and studied in biochemical laboratories, and many modifications and improvements were introduced.

Tiselius and co-workers had previously found that the α- and β-globulins contained greater quantities of carbohydrates and lipids than did γ-globulin and albumin. The high lipid content of the β-globulin often caused trouble in the elucidation of the electrophoresis diagrams. D. A. MacInnes and L. G. Longsworth at The Rockefeller Institute introduced the use of barbital buffer of pH 8.6 which resulted in a better resolution of the electrophoresis diagrams. The α-globulin could then also be subdivided into α_1- and α_2-globulin. A further subdivision of the electrophoresis diagrams could gradually be established.

Before 1930, preparation of plasma and serum proteins was carried out mainly by salting-out with neutral salts. In the 1930s it was found that fractionation with organic solvents in many cases would be advantageous provided denaturation could be avoided by carrying out the preparation at low temperature. Various methods with different solvents were tested in many laboratories around the world. In the USA, Edwin J. Cohn (Fig. 8) and his associates made extensive investigations on the solubility behaviour of proteins in a number of different types of solutions. Based on these studies, they elaborated programmes for the fractionation of blood plasma. As precipitating agent they used ethanol and varied alcohol and salt concentrations as well as varied pH in a strictly controlled way. During the 1940s, their method underwent a number of modifications in order to improve the purity of the components and make new components available. During the first period, the fractions obtained were studied with electrophoresis and ultracentrifugation. Later on, immunochemical and immunoelectrophoretical studies were used to characterize the different fractions.

The introduction of the cold ethanol method for the fractionation of plasma was a milestone in the history of the plasma proteins and its importance can hardly be overrated. It opened possibilities for preparing plasma proteins efficiently and in a reproducible way. The Cohn method has been adapted for the industrial production of therapeutically important plasma proteins such as albumin, γ-globulin, and fibrinogen. During World War II, the main interest was concentrated on these three proteins as

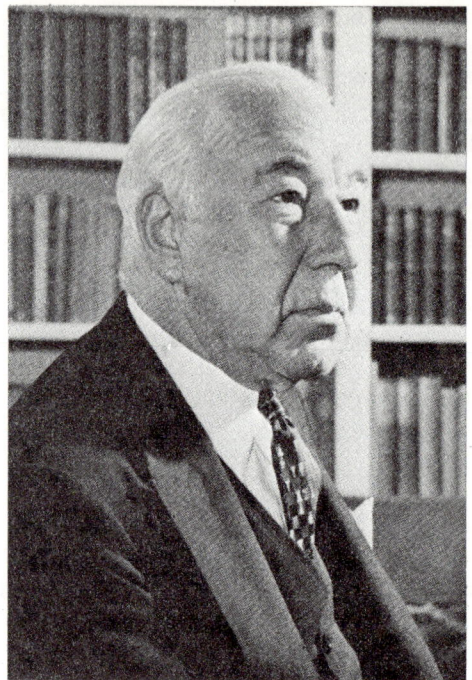

Fig. 8. Edwin J. Cohn (1892–1953)

they were of immediate interest for the military medicine and surgery. The Cohn method is now used in a number of countries all over the world, and it has been further developed (see page 29).

In the 1940s, chromatographic methods were introduced into protein chemistry. This meant a step forward for many problems connected with the analysis of amino acids, peptides, and proteins. The methods had previously been successfully used in organic chemistry to separate closely related coloured substances.

In these methods a column is packed with a suitable adsorbing substance suspended in a solvent. The coloured material to be separated is dissolved in the same solvent and is applied to the top of the column. When pure solvent is allowed to percolate through the column, different coloured zones may move down through the column at a rate that depends upon how strongly the substance in the zone is adsorbed on the packing material of the column. The materials from the zones may then be successively collected as they leave the column. Tiselius introduced optical methods for continuous determination of the concentration of the separating substances as they leave the column. He called the method adsorption analysis and showed how amino acids and peptides could be separated by this method. Furthermore, he provided the theoretical background to the various types of chromatography.

Chromatographic analysis on filter paper strips was soon introduced by A. J. P. Martin and co-workers and this led to two-dimensional chromatography on sheets of filter paper where for instance a drop of a protein hydrolysate is applied to one corner of a rectangular filter paper and the chromatogram is developed with one solvent. After drying, the filter paper is turned 90° and the chromatogram is developed with another

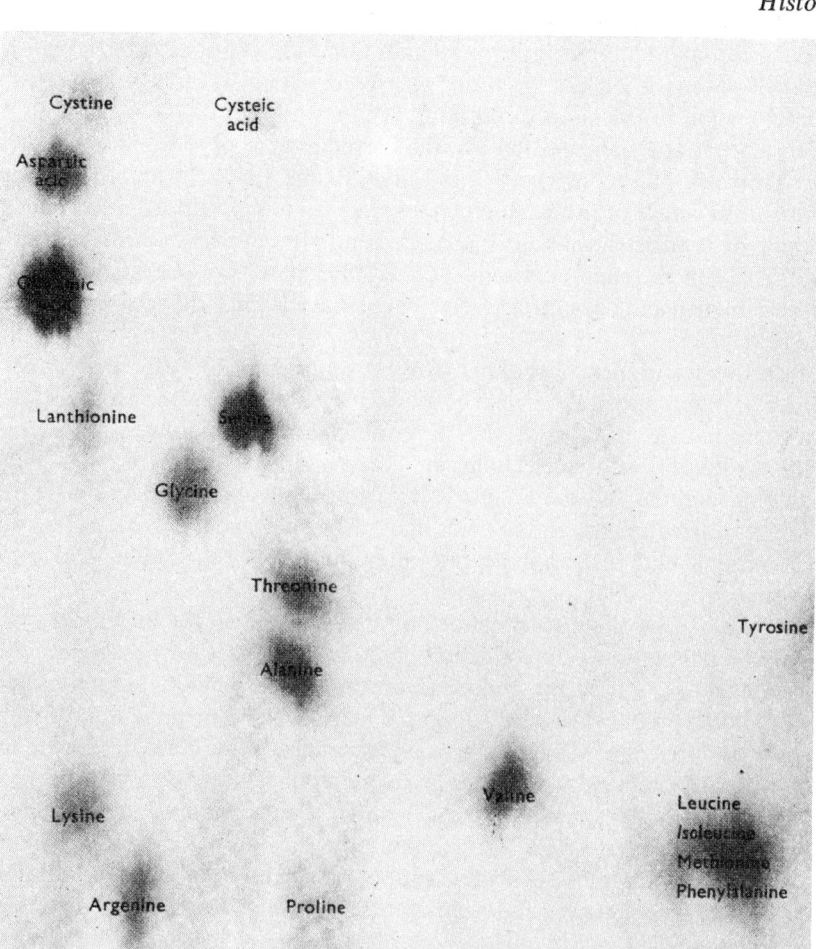

Fig. 9. Two-dimensional chromatography according to A. J. P. Martin *et al.*

solvent, resulting in a two-dimensional 'fingerprinting' of the amino acids present (Fig. 9).

W. H. Stein and S. Moore developed an amino-acid analyser based on column chromatography and continuous registration of the concentration in the effluent. The columns were first packed with starch; later various versions made use of synthetic ion exchange resins. The present amino acid analysers are now fully automated and the exact amino acid composition of a protein may be obtained overnight. Forty years ago it would perhaps have taken one year and the result was not accurate.

The great advantage of the chromatographic method is its versatility. The column can be packed with a multitude of material having different properties. It may even be possible to make packing material which is tailored for a special purpose.

Many attempts were made by Tiselius and others to separate proteins on chromatographic columns. It was, however, not until E. A. Peterson and H. A. Sober in 1956 introduced chromatography on ion exchange cellulose columns that the method was successful. The separation can be varied to a great extent by changing the pH and the salt concentration in the eluting solution.

A very important contribution to the development of protein chemistry came through the work of F. Sanger at Cambridge. In the 1940s he started a study of the building and structure of proteins. He and his associates developed a method whereby they could determine the detailed arrangement of the amino acids in the peptide chains, the so-called amino acid sequence. In 1955 they had determined the complete amino acid sequence of insulin and elucidated the detailed chemical structure of this protein.

Another important new technique was introduced in 1950 by P. Edman at the University of Lund and was further developed by him and his co-workers. By letting phenylisothiocyanate react with the N-terminal amino acid in a peptide chain, a phenylthiohydantoin is formed. Under mild acid hydrolysis the hydantoin is split from the rest of the peptide and the amino acid part of the hydantoin may be identified. By repeating the procedure, the amino acids may successively be removed, one by one, from the NH_2-terminal end of the polypeptide chain. In this way the amino acid sequence in peptides and proteins may be obtained.

During the 1950s, the use of electrophoretic methods became more and more common especially after the introduction of various methods for paper electrophoresis. They were extensively used for analytical purposes on a semiquantitative scale.

The need for preparative electrophoresis led to the introduction of zone electrophoresis in stabilizing media and gels. At Uppsala J. Porath and P. Flodin had been working with gels prepared from cross-linked dextran. The cross-linking of the dextran makes it insoluble. When suspended in water, the gel swells to different degrees depending on the extent of the cross-linking. In this way Porath and Flodin could produce gels which contained different amounts of dextran per unit volume. These gels could be packed into columns and were used successfully for zone electrophoresis. One day the electric current had by mistake not been on, and when the column was eluted it was discovered that a very marked separation had taken place. Further studies disclosed that the stronger cross-linked the dextran was, the smaller were the molecules which could be effectively separated. This is based upon the fact that the dissolved molecules cannot come closer to the dextran particles than a distance which corresponds to the radius of the dissolved molecules; they are thus excluded from a certain part of the volume of the gel. The larger the dissolved particles, the smaller the volume they can penetrate. Likewise the higher the dextran concentration in the gel (more cross-linking), the larger is the part of the gel from which the dissolved particles are excluded. If a solution containing different sizes of molecules is applied on the top of such a gel column and if it is eluted with the solvent, the larger molecules will appear first in the eluate and the smaller ones later. Thus a fractionation according to size is obtained and a principally new physical separation method has been introduced into protein chemistry. The cross-linked dextran was given the commercial name Sephadex.

A number of other gels or substances packed on columns may show similar separating effects. It has also been possible to couple enzymes and other active groups to the gel matrix. In this way columns with very specific properties have been obtained.

Much earlier, in the 1930s, the very specific protein reactions between antigens and antibodies had been studied by M. Heidelberger, J. R. Marrack, and others.

Heidelberger and F. E. Kendall had also introduced the quantitative precipitin technique, and great progress had been made in the new science of immunochemistry.

In 1948–49 Ö. Ouchterlony introduced an immunochemical two-dimensional double diffusion technique. The method offers a very sensitive test of protein purity. The test may be performed in the following way: An agar gel is cast in a Petri dish, and a number of holes are cut in the gel, one in the centre and the others in a ring at equal distances from the centre. If a certain antiserum is to be studied, a tiny amount of it is placed in the central hole. Various antigen solutions are placed in the outer holes. The antiserum and the antigens are now allowed to diffuse under standard conditions for a day or more. Precipitates will then appear in the places where equivalent proportions of antibody and antigens have met (see Fig. 58B). The type and shape of the precipitin curves may give valuable information concerning the identity or the non-identity of the antigens or concerning the question whether they contain common antigens. The test is very sensitive, and the method may even be used for quantitative measurements. It has been followed by a number of modifications. One may say that it has opened the way for many new methods in analytical protein chemistry.

One of these is the immunoelectrophoretic method introduced in 1953 by P. Grabar and C. A. Williams. Here an antigen solution (e.g. normal serum) is applied to an agar gel and is subjected to electrophoresis. At the end of the electrophoresis, an antiserum solution is applied to a trough in the agar gel which is cut out parallel to the direction of the electrophoretic migration and at a suitable distance from this. The different antigens separated by the electrophoresis will now diffuse in all directions and they will meet the antibodies diffusing perpendicularly out from the trough. Where corresponding antigens and antibodies meet in equivalent concentrations, precipitates are formed. These appear as a series of arcs parallel to the trough and each corresponding to one antigen.

An important improvement in the immunoelectrophoretic method was introduced in the middle of the 1960s by C.-B. Laurell. He made an antigen–antibody crossed electrophoresis where the antigen solution is first subjected to electrophoresis in agar in the usual way. Afterwards, the agar strip is placed in contact with agar impregnated with antibody and a second electrophoresis is made in a direction at right angle to the first run. After staining, the precipitation curves appear as peaks or 'rockets' on the plate (see Fig. 58E). The area under the peak is proportional to the antigen/antibody ratio for the individual proteins. A number of modifications to this technique were later introduced.

The composition of human plasma

LÅRS-OLOV ANDERSSON and RAGNAR LUNDEN

Blood plasma is an extraordinarily complex aqueous solution of proteins, lipids, carbohydrates, amino acids, salts, etc. This complexity must be viewed in relation to the diversity in the function of blood. Blood is the body's most important transport system. Proteins essential for the body's defence against infection are to be found in blood. Furthermore, a variety of processes are regulated by substances which are released into the blood.

Proteins constitute the major part of the soluble material in blood, where their concentration is usually 70–80 g/l. The total number of different proteins in blood is probably greater than 150, of which about 70 have so far been isolated in pure form.

The plasma proteins can be classified according to their electrophoretic mobility. This is the classical method of Tiselius where the proteins are arranged in decreasing order of mobility: α-globulin, β-globulin, γ-globulin. In Fig. 10 the electrophoretic mobility and sedimentation pattern of some important human plasma proteins have been illustrated.

The plasma proteins can be classified also according to their function (Table 1). First listed are the various transport proteins, of which albumin is quantitatively the most important component, followed by the lipoproteins which constitute a special group of transport proteins. Next follow plasma proteins which take part in the turnover of haem and the transport of metals, hormones, and vitamins. The immunoglobulins constitute an essential part of the body's apparatus for the defence against infection. Some of the complement factors are also listed. These proteins also play an important role in the defence mechanism. The protease inhibitors have an essential regulatory function e.g. in the maintenance of the haemostatic balance.

Blood coagulation is a mechanism of fundamental importance for protection against leakages in the blood vessels. This system consists of a variety of different components, some of which are listed in Table 1. The most important protein in the fibrinolytic system, plasminogen, is included in this group. Finally, a few proteins are listed which are difficult to attribute to a particular group.

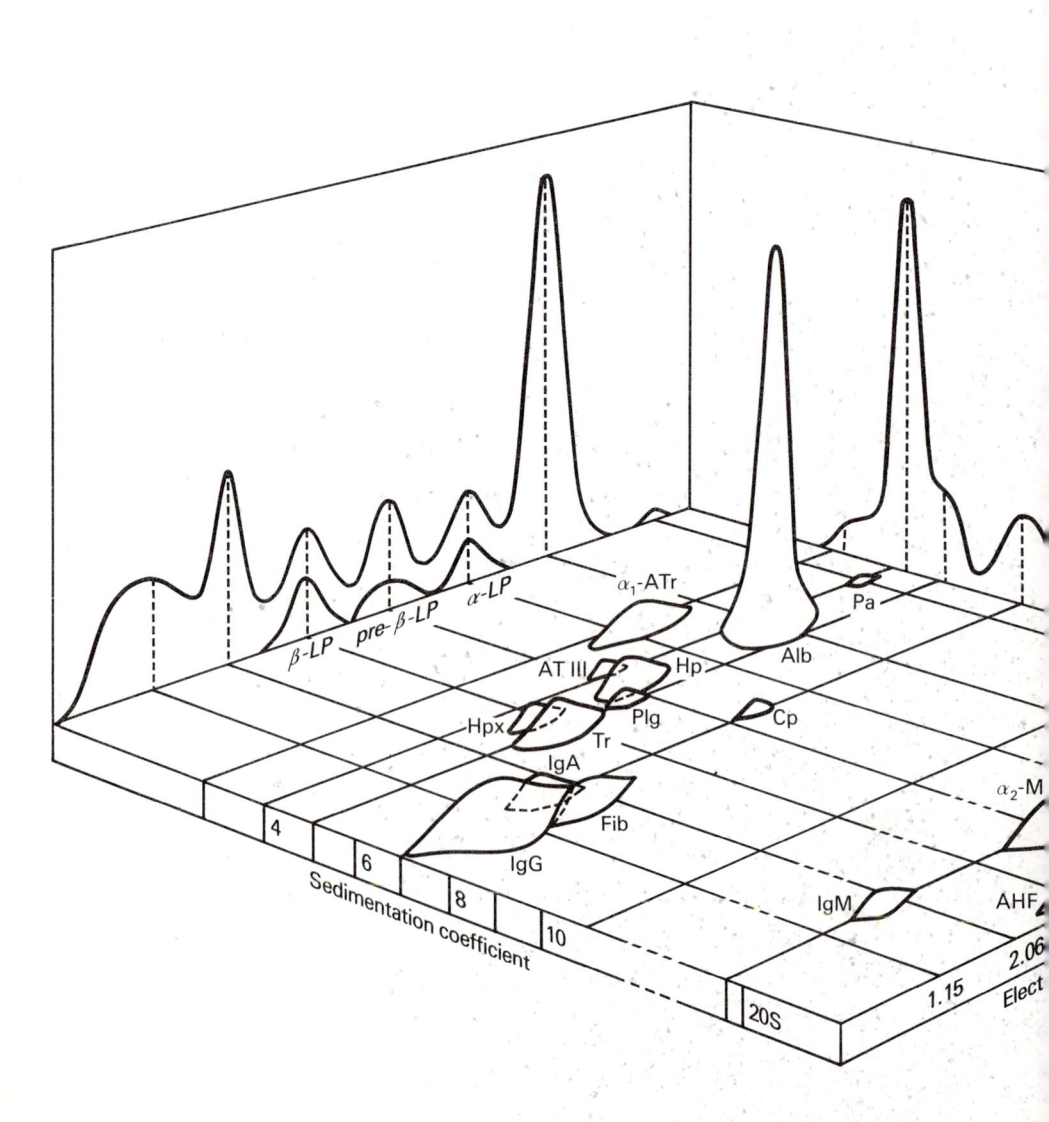

18   *The composition of human plasma*

Fig. 10. A three-dimensional representation of the electrophoretic and ultracentrifugation pattern of human plasma proteins. The various plasma proteins are depicted in the form of three-dimensional bodies. The volume of each body is an approximate measure of the amount of the corresponding protein in relation to the total amount of the proteins depicted in the diagram. The plasma proteins which are isolated by Kabi are described below

Also shown in the diagram are: α-lipoprotein (α-LP), β-lipoprotein (β-LP), pre-β-lipo-protein (pre-β-LP), Pa = prealbumin, αATr = antitrypsin, Hpx = haemopexin, $\alpha_2 M = \alpha_2$-macroglobulin

As the lipoproteins float during ultracentrifugation, they are represented only in the electrophoretic diagram. Fractions for clinical use are indicated by an asterisk.

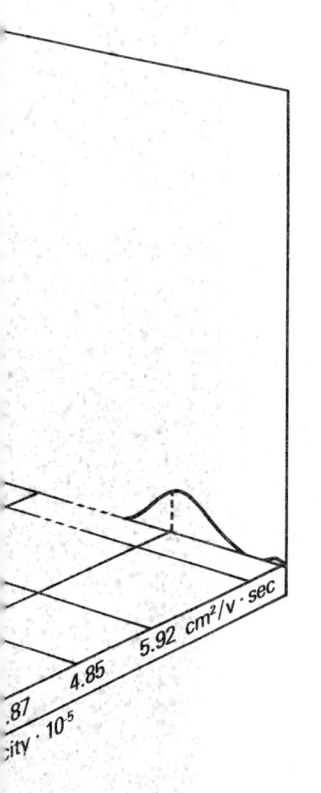

Alb: Albumin* has a relatively low molecular weight of approximately 66 000 and constitutes 50–60 per cent of the plasma proteins. It acts as an important plasma expander and as a carrier of vitamins, hormones etc.

IgG, IgA, IgM: Gamma globulins* immunoglobulins, a group of proteins which are classified into 5 classes (IgG, IgA, IgM, IgD, IgE). Only IgG, IgA, and IgM are shown in the diagram. Gamma Globulin Kabi consists almost entirely of IgG

AHF: Antihaemophilic factor,* Factor VIII, a component which is necessary for normal coagulation which is deficient in type A haemophilia. It is supplied as a concentrate

Fib: Fibrinogen*, a rod-shaped plasma protein with a molecular weight of approximately 340 000 making it one of the plasma proteins of highest molecular weight. Fibrinogen is the precursor of fibrin

Plg: Plasminogen, the inactive precursor plasmin

Cp: Ceruloplasmin, a copper-containing protein which in solution has a deep blue colour. Its physiological function is unknown. Low concentrations are found in Wilson's disease.

Antithrombin III(AT III) is a proteas inhibitor and the main coagulation inhibitor in blood. It is of great importance for maintaining the haemostatic balance.

Hp: Haptoglobin, a heterogeneous group of glycoproteins with a polysaccharide content of approximately 20%. It forms a complex with haemoglobin.

Tr: Transferrin, a metal-binding protein which acts as a carrier of iron in the body. The estimation of the iron-binding capacity of serum is of diagnostic importance.

The composition of human plasma

Table 1. Some of the important protein components of human plasma

Component	Molecular weight	Concentration g/l	μmol/l	Electrophoretic mobility
Transport proteins				
Serum albumin	66 000	40	600	α
Lipoproteins				
α-lipoprotein (HDL$_2$)	360 000	0.5	1.4	α$_1$
α-lipoprotein (HDL$_3$)	170 000	3	18	α$_1^-$
Pre-β-lipoproteins	6·10^6	1.5	0.3	β
β-lipoproteins	2·10^6	4.0	2	β
Other transport proteins				
Ceruloplasmin	124 000–134 000	0.22	1.7	α$_2$
Transferrin	77 000	2.3	30	β$_1$
Haptoglobin 1-1	99 000	2.0	20	α$_2$
Haptoglobin 2-1	200 000	1.6–3	8–15	α$_2$
Haptoglobin 2-2	400 000	1.2–2.6	3–6.6	α$_2$
Haemopexin	57 000	0.85	15	β$_1$
Transcobalamine I	120 000	—	—	—
Transcobalamine II	60 000	—	—	—
Retinol binding proteins	21 000	0.045	2	—
Prealbumin	50 000–66 000	0.25	4	pre-α
Thyroxin binding globulin	36 000–64 000	0.01	0.2	—
Transcortin	53 000	0.03	0.6	—
Immunoglobulins				
IgG	150 000	8–17	53–113	α$_2$-γ$_3$
IgA (serum)	150 000	1–4	7–27	α$_2$-γ$_3$
IgM	900 000	0.05–2	0.06–2	β$_2$-γ$_3$
IgD	170 000	(3–200)·10^{-3}	0.02–1,2	γ$_1$
IgE (serum)	190 000	(1–100)·10^{-6}	(5–500)·10^{-6}	γ$_1$
β-microglobulin	11 600	(1–2)·10^{-3}	0.1–0.2	β
Complement factors				
C1q	400 000	0.18	0.5	γ$_2$
C1r	180 000	—	—	β
C1s	86 000	0.11	1.3	α
C2	117 000	0.025	0.2	β$_1$
C3	180 000	1.6	9	β$_2$
C4	206 000	0.64	3	β$_1$
C5	180 000	0.08	0.4	β$_1$
C6	95 000	0.075	0.8	β$_2$
C7	110 000	0.055	0.5	β$_2$
C8	163 000	0.080	0.5	γ$_1$
C9	79 000	0.23	3	α
Properdin	184 000	0.025	0.14	γ$_2$
Proteins of coagulation and fibrinolysis				
Factor I, fibrinogen	340 000	2–3	6–9	β$_2$
Factor II, prothrombin	68 700	0.15	2.2	α$_2$
Factor V, proaccelerin	410 000	0.01	0.025	—
Factor VII, proconvertin	63 000	0.001	0.016	β

Table 1 (continued)

Component	Molecular weight	Concentration g/l	Concentration μmol/l	Electrophoretic mobility
Factor VIII, antihaemophilic globulin	1 100 000	0.01	0.009	β
Factor IX, haemophilic factor B	67 000	0.01	0.14	α
Factor X, Stuart factor	55 000	0.05	0.9	α
Factor XI, haemophilic factor C	160 000	0.01	0.06	β
Factor XII, Hageman factor	90 000	0.1	1	β_2
Factor XIII, fibrin stabilizing factor	320 000	0.01–0.02	0.03–0.06	β
Plasminogen	93 000	0.2–0.3	2–3	β
Protease inhibitors				
α_1-antitrypsin	54 000	2	40	α_1
α_1-antichymotrypsin	69 000	0.5	7.2	α_1
Inter-α-trypsin inhib.	160 000	0.5	3.1	α_1–α_2
Antithrombin III	62 000	0.2	3.1	α_2
α_2-macroglobulin	820 000	2.7	3.3	α_2
α_2-plasmin inhibitor (antiplasmin)	70 000	0.07	1.0	α_2
Other plasma proteins				
Gc-globulin	51 000	0.2	4.0	α_2
α_1 acid glycoprotein (orosomucoid)	44 000	1	23	α_1
Cold insoluble globulin	450 000	0.2–0.4	0.4–0.9	β

Microcirculation of blood

JOHANNES A. G. RHODIN

In the mammalian body, oxygen is required to sustain all life processes. The exchange of oxygen and metabolic end products between the various tissues of the body and the bloodstream occurs across the extremely delicate capillary membrane. The physiological processes which constitute the basis for this exchange have been extensively explored for many decades, but the structure of the capillary membrane has only recently been analysed in some detail. Improvements in methodologies employed in the exploration of the architecture and ultrastructure of the capillary network now make it possible to investigate not only the capillary membrane, but also the arterioles which feed into the capillary, as well as the venules draining the area. Primarily, the major breakthrough came by combining the methods of observing and recording by high speed cinemicrophotography (5 000–10 000 frames per second) the microvascular bed *in vivo*, and of fixing the identical area for electron microscopy, making it possible to enlarge gradually the same vascular segment from the magnification levels of the light microscope ($\times 10 - \times 1 000$) to those of the electron microscope ($\times 1 000 - \times 100 000$).*

As a result of these explorations, it has been found that the arterioles, which deliver the blood to the capillary network, are provided with smooth muscle cells arranged concentrically around the inner tube of delicate endothelial cells. The contraction of the smooth muscle cells is probably controlled in two ways. Perivascular autonomic nerve endings exert a peripheral influence, and the myoendothelial junctions, short foot-like processes of the endothelial cells, establish contacts between the endothelial cells and the smooth muscle cells via cell membrane gap-junctions. Through this arrangement, contraction impulses may be initiated, not only from the perivascular nerve endings, but also from the endothelial cells to the smooth muscle cells via blood-borne neurotransmitter substances such as adrenaline and noradrenaline.

The combination of *in vivo*, light microscope observations and electron microscope analyses of a variety of capillary beds has led to a better understanding of the structural basis which may be responsible for the known variation in capillary permeability. The capillaries of the liver, often referred to as hepatic sinusoids, have a high permeability. The capillary membrane, formed by the endothelial cells, is provided with a large number of openings, ranging from 0.1 μm to 1 μm in diameter, permitting the passage of plasma proteins and other substances of high molecular weight. The capillaries of the skeletal muscle tissue have a relatively low permeability and are completely devoid of the perforations found in liver capillaries. In the central nervous system, the majority of the capillaries have a very low permeability. They lack endothelial cell perforations, and in contrast to capillaries elsewhere, the intercellular contacts are established by tight junctions of opposing cell membranes, which block

---

*Illustrations from Rhodin: 'The ultrastructure of mammalian arterioles and precapillary sphincters'. *J. Ultrastruct. Res.*, **18** (1967) p. 181.

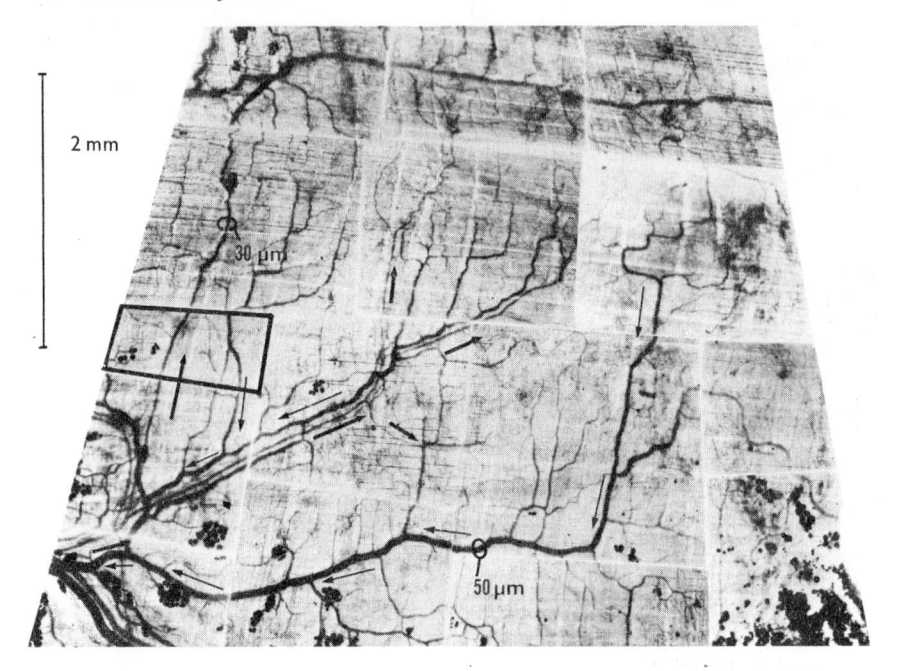

Fig. 11. Microcirculatory bed of the dermis in the rabbit. The small blood vessels extend mainly in a two-dimensional plane and can be observed *in vivo* after removal of the epidermis. The capillaries emerge as a very fine network between the arterioles (direction of blood flow indicated by heavy arrows) and the venules (thin arrows). This micrograph was taken following the arrest of the blood flow by the administration of osmic acid as a fixative, and the subsequent embedding of the specimen in epoxy resin. The outlined area is enlarged for detailed analysis in Figs. 12–15. Magnification × 26

the passage of molecules between the endothelial cells. This structural arrangement is believed to be responsible for the physiological blood–brain barrier. Through the combination of light and electron microscope research methods, it has also been possible to localize the arterial part of a capillary loop in the skin and intestines, and to compare its fine structure with the venous part of the same loop. Accordingly, the venous part contains a large number of round, evenly distributed fenestrations, averaging 0.06 μm in diameter, all bridged by a thin diaphragm. These fenestrations do not exist in the arterial part of the capillary loop, a fact which seems to support the assumption, based on physiological experiments, that the venous capillaries have a higher permeability than their arterial counterparts.

The exploration of the physiology and architecture of capillary networks which was pioneered by the Nobel prizewinner August Krogh around 1920, and continued by Landis, Pappenheimer, Zweifach, and many others, made it clear that the venules which drain the capillary bed are very sensitive to mechanical, chemical, and thermal factors, quite contrary to the situation in the arterioles and capillaries. The method of identifying specific segments of the microvascular bed by combining *in vivo* observations with electron microscope analyses has made it possible to explore the nature of the susceptibility of the venules. Mechanical, chemical, and thermal factors make the perivascular mast cells release histamine and serotonin, vasoactive agents, which

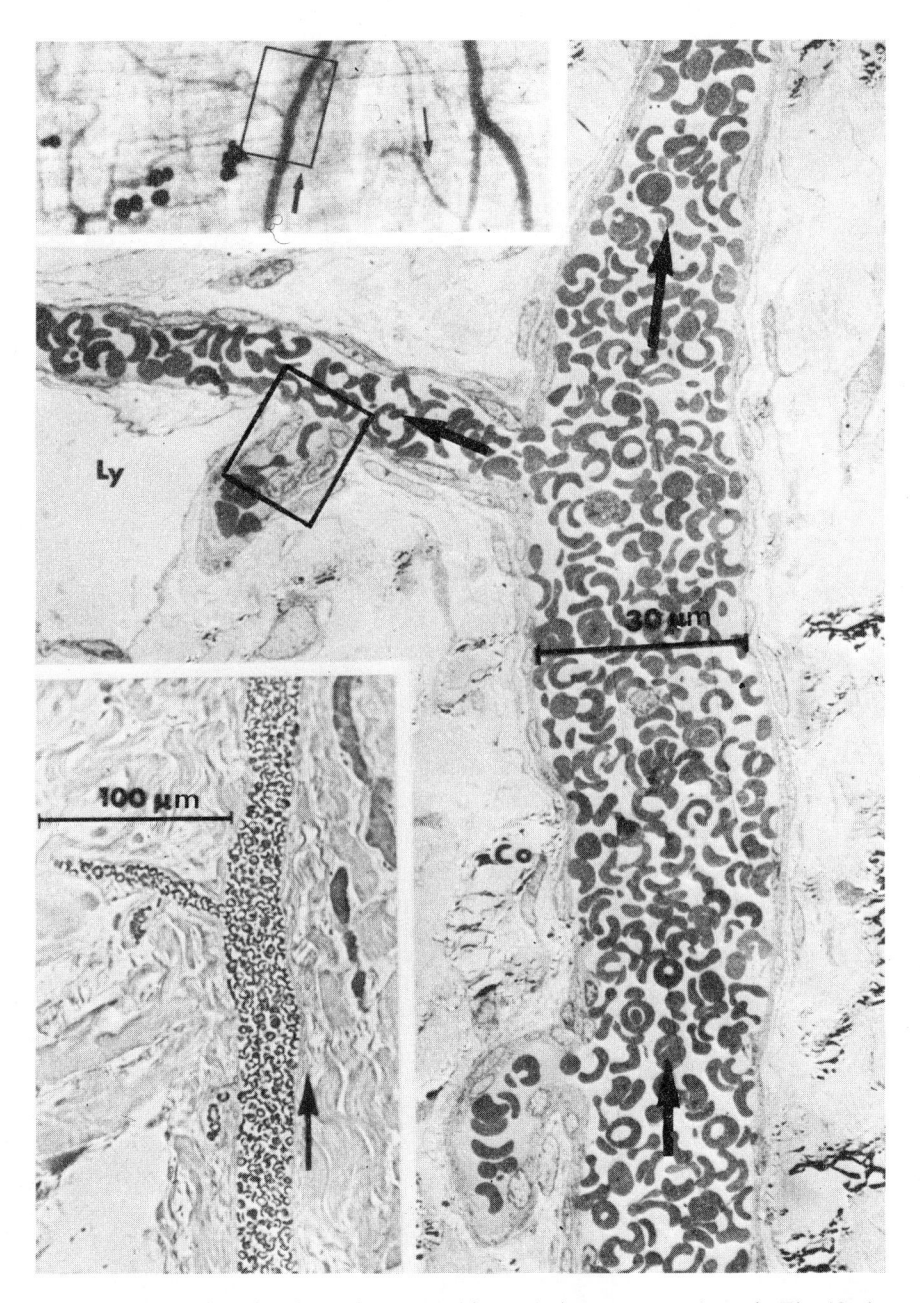

Figs. 12–14. Area outlined in Fig. 11 is recorded in a whole-mount specimen in Fig. 12; the area outlined in Fig. 12 is sectioned and photographed in the light microscope in Fig. 13 and in the electron microscope in Fig. 14. Through this procedure, all vascular segments in Fig. 11 can be analysed. This series illustrates the terminal of an arteriole which averages 30 μm in diameter. The precapillary sphincter area is marked by a rectangle in Fig. 14 and can be seen at greater enlargement in Fig. 15. Magnification: Fig. 12: ×35; Fig. 13: ×75; Fig. 14; ×1 000

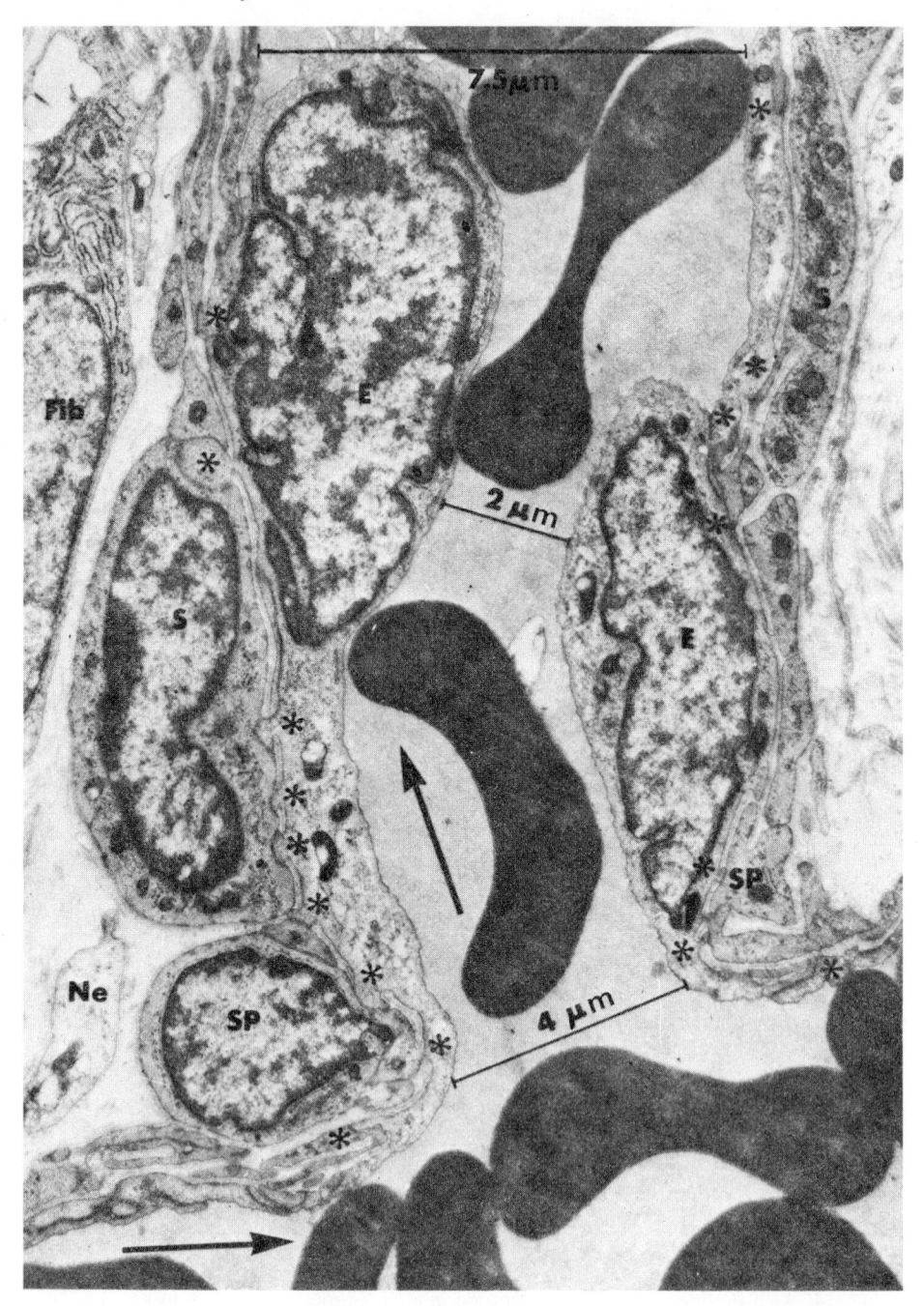

Fig. 15. Precapillary sphincter area. Enlargement of area outlined by rectangle in Fig. 14. Direction of blood flow is indicated by the arrows, and the variation in vascular diameter by the bars and μm-markers. Nuclei of endothelial cells (E). Nuclei of smooth muscle cells (S and SP). Asterisks (*) indicate myoendothelial junctions and endothelial foot processes. Autonomic nerve endings (Ne). Nucleus (Fib) of fibroblast in the perivascular connective tissue. Magnification: × 30 000

reduce the degree of junctional adhesion between adjoining endothelial cells of the venules. As a result, intercellular gaps arise through which both blood plasma and formed elements of the blood may escape. This is the structural basis for diapedisis (blood cells 'walking' across the wall of blood vessels), petechiae (small haemorrhages), and inflammatory reactions by the venules.

Light microscope observations of live tissues and organs, combined with electron microscope observations of the same areas, have resulted in many interesting observations of the normal fine architecture of the microvascular bed. Future research in this field will focus on the experimental effects of a variety of pharmacological agents on the different segments of the microvascular bed. This field of research has great potential if the recording of vascular responses to the pharmacological agents in terms of smooth muscle reactivity, capillary permeability, and alterations in venular sensitivity to physical, chemical, and thermal factors is followed by electron microscope analyses and search for possible structural changes. This particular approach is also well suited for explorations of the pathogenesis and development of vascular lesions leading to arteriosclerosis and hypertension.

Industrial plasma fractionation methods

I. Cohn fractionation
HENRIK BJÖRLING

Of all the proteins in human plasma, albumin accounts for a little more than 50 per cent. However, due to its relatively low molecular weight it is responsible for about 80 per cent of the colloid osmotic pressure of the blood and in this way is the main regulator of the plasma volume. The second main function of albumin is to transport low molecular weight substances and to function as an acceptor for fatty acids in lipid metabolism. A third function is to act as a storage form of protein and amino acids.

Naturally, it has been of great interest for a long time to be able to produce albumin on an industrial scale. This was particularly true during World War II, when the difficulties of transporting and storage of whole human blood was of great concern. However, concentrated albumin solution can be transported without refrigeration and can be stored at low temperatures for years. The very good results of albumin therapy, which were obtained during the war years on the battlefields and at military hospitals, soon brought about its use in civilian hospitals.

The man who first solved the problem of producing human albumin on an industrial scale was Professor Edwin Joseph Cohn at Harvard Medical School in Boston, USA. The method which usually is called the Cohn 5-variable system or the Cohn cold ethanol method is based on the principle of using ethanol as a precipitating agent at low temperatures. By varying the ethanol concentration and temperature, the different plasma proteins can be precipitated in different fractions. However, in order to obtain reproducible results it is also necessary in each precipitation step to keep the other three variables constant, namely the ionic strength, pH, and the protein concentration.

To adjust the ionic strength and pH in the Cohn system an acetate or phosphate buffer is used to lower the pH and when raising the pH usually a sodium bicarbonate buffer is used. Sodium chloride is used when only the ionic strength requires adjustment.

The first publication concerning alcohol fractionation from Cohn and collaborators came in 1946. Six different modifications of the cold ethanol method were described in this paper. The plasma proteins are precipitated into five main fractions (I–V). However, these main fractions have to be refractionated under strict conditions in the 5-variable system in order to obtain pure proteins. In the above mentioned publication all details are given of the last modification of the method known as the Cohn method 6. This method was very soon applied for large-scale production of albumin for clinical use and is still the main plasma fractionation method used in the USA and elsewhere.

During more recent years the Cohn method 6 has been replaced more and more by a modified Cohn method 5. In this method four main fractions are precipitated instead of the five in method 6. Fractions IV-1 and IV-4, are precipitated together. Further, in the modified method 5 an undiluted ethanol solution is used and in this way the final volumes in the precipitating steps have been reduced quite considerably. The disadvantage is a somewhat reduced albumin yield but the main advantage is a considerably increased total capacity of the whole fractionation unit.

The next publication from Cohn and co-workers described the first industrial method to isolate gamma globulin from fraction II + III. This method which usually is called the Oncley method 9, was published in 1949. It was very soon accepted as an industrial method and it is still the most common method for the production of human gamma globulin for clinical use.

The third plasma protein produced on an industrial scale was fibrinogen. This protein together with some of the other clotting factors is concentrated in Cohn fraction I. This fraction was used clinically for many years as a fibrinogen concentrate and as an antihaemophilic globulin concentrate, as Factor VIII is also concentrated in this fraction. During the years very many methods have been published to isolate more or less pure fibrinogen and Factor VIII concentrate using Cohn fraction I as starting material.

The most serious disadvantage with the Cohn fractionation method is that the precipitation steps must be carried out at low temperatures, 0 to $-5°C$, to prevent the alcohol denaturation of the plasma proteins. The plasma solution must first be cooled to $0°C$ before the precooled (usually $-30°C$) ethanol solution is added during constant cooling. During addition of alcohol to a water solution chemical heat is produced and this heat must be compensated for during the whole alcohol addition by cooling to prevent the temperature from rising above $0°C$.

Another risk factor in the Cohn method is the rather low pH values in some of the precipitation steps, 4.6–4.8. To eliminate the risk of too low pH values and too high alcohol concentrations, Cohn realized very early that the alcohol method should be combined with other methods of protein precipitation. The first method by Cohn and collaborators which was based on this principle was published in 1950. In this method, some of the alcohol is replaced by a zinc salt which under special conditions has the advantage of selectively precipitating some proteins. In this method, which is usually known as Cohn method 10, another important principle of protein isolation was introduced. The plasma proteins are first separated in only two main fractions. From these main fractions the proteins to be isolated are extracted by using selective extraction methods. The risk of denaturing precipitated proteins in an extraction step is much less compared to a selective precipitation of proteins from a solution of a mixture of proteins.

However, the Cohn method 10 never reached industrial application mainly because of difficulties in selective removal of the zinc ions in large-scale production.

II. The Kabi fractionation methods
HENRIK BJÖRLING

Kabi was one of the first institutions in Europe to apply the Cohn cold ethanol fractionation technique for human plasma fractionation on an industrial scale. This production started in 1949.

At this time, a military stockpile of human dried plasma from the World War II had been built up in Sweden. This dried plasma had been prepared during 1941–44 on a contract between Kabi and the Swedish military medical authorities. The method used for drying this plasma was a spray drying technique in the presence of sucrose. This plasma was the first starting material for the industrial production of albumin and gamma globulin in Sweden.

However, one complication with this dried plasma was that the Cohn method 6 could not be used due to the presence of sucrose. A modification of the Cohn method 10 was successfully worked out. It was possible to use the Cohn method 10 with some modifications to isolate albumin in a very good yield from this sucrose containing dried plasma.

This stockpile of dried plasma was finished in 1951 and the major problem then was how to get human plasma for the continuation of the fractionation work. At that time we had only about 10 established blood banks in Sweden and no one had any surplus of plasma to spare. This problem was solved by collecting retroplacental blood at maternity hospitals all over Sweden.

The man who first suggested this blood as a possible source for albumin and gamma globulin production was Dr Clarence Malmnäs at the South Hospital in Stockholm.

The main problem with this blood, however, was that it became quite haemolysed during collection. Further it could not be prevented from clotting by adding citrate solution during collection. Thus, this blood had to be separated into serum and blood clot.

Due to the high haemoglobulin content in this retroplacental serum the Cohn method 6 could not be used and the fractionation method had to be modified again. This work gave rise to a new modification of the Cohn technique. By combining the cold ethanol method with chromatography purification steps it was possible to isolate both albumin and gamma globulin from retroplacental serum with good purity and high yields.

The method now in use at Kabi for the large-scale fractionation of human plasma is schematically illustrated as a flow diagram in Fig. 16. The starting material is frozen plasma or retroplacental serum. The method can be described as a further development of the original Cohn methods by using chromatography methods both in the gamma globulin and the albumin purification. It has been possible to reduce the alcohol precipitation steps and also to increase the yields quite considerably compared to the Cohn method 6. New in this method is the first separation of the cryoprecipitate containing the Factor VIII activity and the following chromatographic steps. The Factor IX complex is adsorbed firstly on DEAE–Sephadex and in a second adsorption step plasminogen is adsorbed on lycine–Sepharose. The following description will give a short summary of the further purification of the different plasma proteins isolated according to this method.

1. AHF (Factor VIII)

The so-called Blombäck's fraction I-0 (1958) is obtained by washing Cohn fraction I twice in a glycine–citrate buffer.

The fraction I-0 is dissolved in citrate buffer at room temperature, sterile filtered, dispensed in final bottles and lyophilized (AHF concentrate Kabi).

In 1962 the first collection of resh frozen human plasma was started at Kabi. When thawing this plasma at 0°C a small precipitate was noticed which did not go into solution until the temperature was raised to about 8°C. This insoluble fraction was found to contain almost all of the factor VIII activity in the original plasma. It was thus shown that it was not necessary to add ethanol to 8 per cent as in earlier methods to precipitate the Factor VIII together with fibrinogen in Cohn fraction I. By using the cryoprecipitate instead of the fraction I, the fibrinogen could be reduced to about one-third in the AHF concentrate. Fraction I, after first removing the cold insoluble globulin, gave an almost pure fibrinogen fraction.

However, at the time of this discovery Blombäck's fraction I-0 made from fresh not

32 Industrial plasma fractionation methods

```
Frozen plasma
    │
[Thawing at 0°C]
    │
Thawed plasma or           ╌╌> Cryoprecipitate
cryocentrifugate                      │
    ▼                                 ▼
[Ethanol to 8%]                [Factor VIII concentrate]
    │
Centrifugate I             ╌╌> Fraction I
    ▼                             │
[DEAE-Sephadex adsorption]        ▼
    │                         [Fibrinogen]
Filtrate                   ╌╌> DEAE-Sephadex gel
    ▼                             │
[Lysine-Sepharose                 ▼
 adsorption]                 [Factor IX concentrate]
Centrifugate I or          ╌╌> Lysine-Sepharose gel
Sepharose filtrate                │
    ▼                             ▼
[Ethanol to 25%]             Plasminogen (activates
    │                         to plasmin)
Centrifugate II+III        ──> Fraction II + III
    ▼
[Ethanol to 35%]              [Gamma globulin]
    │
Centrifugate IV            ──> Fraction IV
    ▼                             │
[Ethanol to 40%]                  ▼
    │                         Transferrin
                              Ceruloplasmin
Centrifugate V             ──> Fraction V
    ▼
[DEAE-Sephadex adsorption]    [Albumin]
    │
Filtrate                   ╌╌> DEAE-Sephadex gel
    ▼                             │
[Ethanol recovery]                ▼
                              Glycoproteins
```

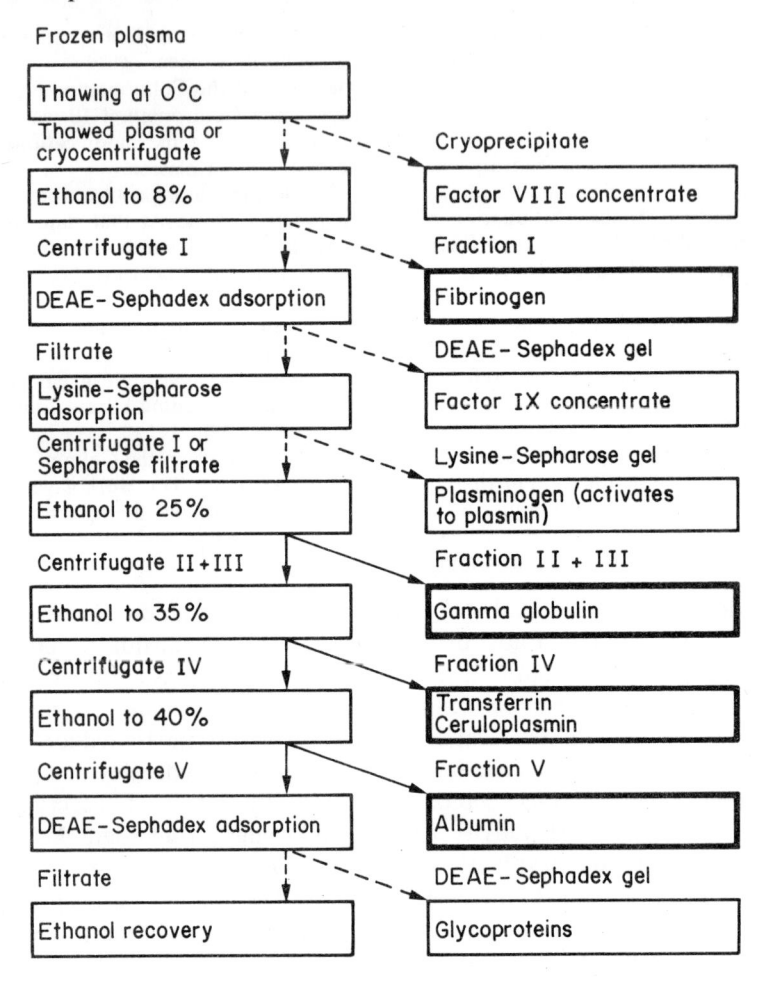

Fig. 16. Flow diagram for the Kabi plasma fractionation method. Starting material is frozen blood plasma or frozen retroplacental serum. The method is a further development of the Cohn methods. The main fractions I, II+III, IV, and V correspond fairly closely to the classical Cohn fractions I–V (in the figure marked with heavier lines). The subfractionation of the main fractions is described in the text. The dashed lines indicate that these preparation steps are not always carried out in ordinary plasma fractionation

frozen plasma had been used clinically since 1956 with great success. It was therefore considered not realistic to introduce a new AHF preparation on the market in 1962.

At the 3rd International Haematological Congress in Stockholm in 1964 Pool presented a cryoprecipitation method for the preparation of a Factor VIII concentrate. This method corresponded almost exactly to the Kabi method described above. At the same time, Pool presented very good clinical results which were achieved with this AHF concentrate. This method has been used very extensively in many different countries and is now the most widely used method for isolating AHF concentrate for clinical use.

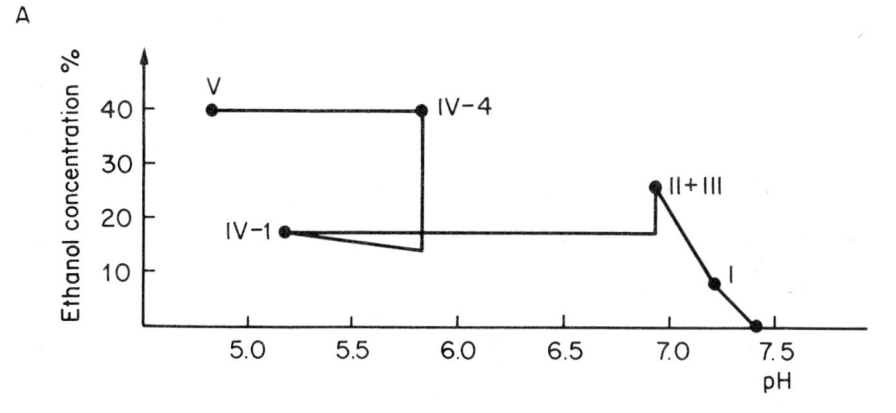

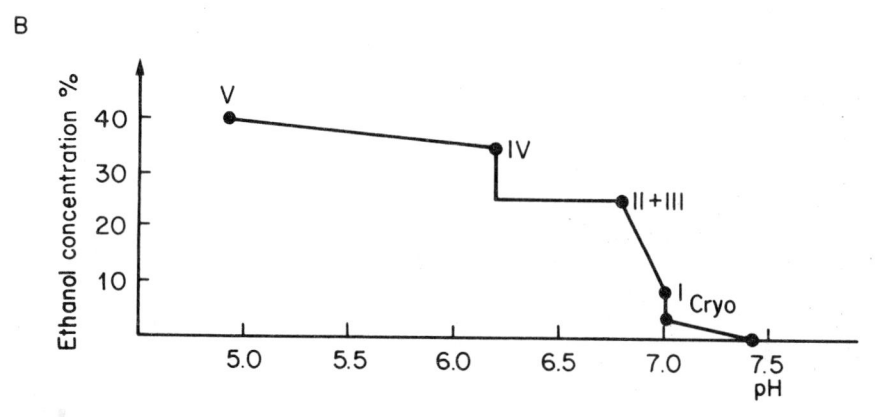

Fig. 17. Variation of pH and alcohol concentration when isolating plasma protein fractions:
A. According to Cohn method 6. The roman numerals denote the numbers of the different fractions according to the classical Cohn method
B. According to the Kabi method. The precipitation conditions are similar to the Cohn method and the fractions have corresponding numerals

2. Fibrinogen

The method for fibrinogen production which is currently in use at Kabi is based on a combination of alcohol precipitation, cryoprecipitation, barium sulphate adsorption, glycine extraction, and acetone precipitation at low temperature. This method was ready for large-scale production in 1956. At that time the only plasma available for fibrinogen production was outdated plasma containing more or less denatured fibrinogen and cryoglobulin. Published methods for fibrinogen isolation at that time were not applicable to outdated plasma but only on fresh frozen plasma or liquid plasma (Blombäck and Blombäck, 1956).

The final precipitation step with acetone was added to the technique in 1968 in order to reduce the risk of transmitting serum hepatitis with this blood fraction. (Andrassy et al., 1970; Berg et al., 1972).

3. Factor IX-concentrate

For the isolation of the Factor IX complex a chromatographic method is used. To the supernatant I of Cohn, a DEAE–Sephadex gel is added which adsorbs all the vitamin-K-dependent clotting factors (Factor II, prothrombin, Factor VII, proconvertin, Factor IX, haemophilia B factor, and Factor X, Stuart factor). The Sephadex gel is eluted in a salt solution and the eluate is sterile filtered and lyophilized to get a stable product for storage.

4. Plasminogen and plasmin

The isolation of plasminogen is based on affinity chromatography. The plasminogen is specificly bound to a lysine–Sepharose 4B gel, eluted, and the eluate sterile filtered and lyophilized. This method, which is a modified Deutsch–Mertz method (1970), was introduced into production in 1972.

To activate plasminogen to plasmin, urokinase bound to a gel matrix is used (Wiman and Wallen, 1973). The plasmin solution is lyophilized to get a stable product for storage.

5. Gamma globulin

The Kabi method for gamma globulin production is a modified Deutsch procedure (1946) combined with a chromatography step. The gamma globulin is first extracted directly from Cohn fractions II + III and from the extract fraction II is precipitated at 25 per cent ethanol concentration and pH 7.2. The fraction II paste is dissolved in ice water and to this solution is added enough DEAE–Sephadex A50 gel to adsorb all proteins except the IgG gamma globulin. This amounts to about 85 per cent of the proteins in fraction II. Using this method, the IgA gamma globulin is also adsorbed on the gel almost quantitatively. The gel is removed by filtration and glycine is added to the filtrate to prevent dimerization and polymerization of the IgG molecules during freezing and lyophilization.

One problem with the gamma globulin isolated according to the Cohn cold ethanol technique is that this gamma globulin can not be given intravenously due to anticomplementary activity. However, several methods have been published describing how to modify this gamma globulin for intravenous use. In 1962 Barandun described a method for reducing the anticomplementary activity by acid treatment of a gamma globulin solution at pH 4.0 and 37°C. In this way treated gamma globulin solutions have been given intravenously even to agammaglobulinaemic patients without side reactions.

In 1962, Schultze and Schwick described a method for the elimination of the anticomplementary activity in gamma globulin by pepsin digestion of aggregates. Since then, other proteolytic enzymes have replaced pepsin.

Another method for the treatment of gamma globulin with plasmin was described in 1967 by Sgouris, who could break up dimer and polymer units of gamma globulin into monomer units. But he found also some breakdown of the monomer molecules into subunits. However, this could be kept within 15–20 per cent. The native gamma globulin molecules were broken down to molecular weight of 50 000–55 000. Good

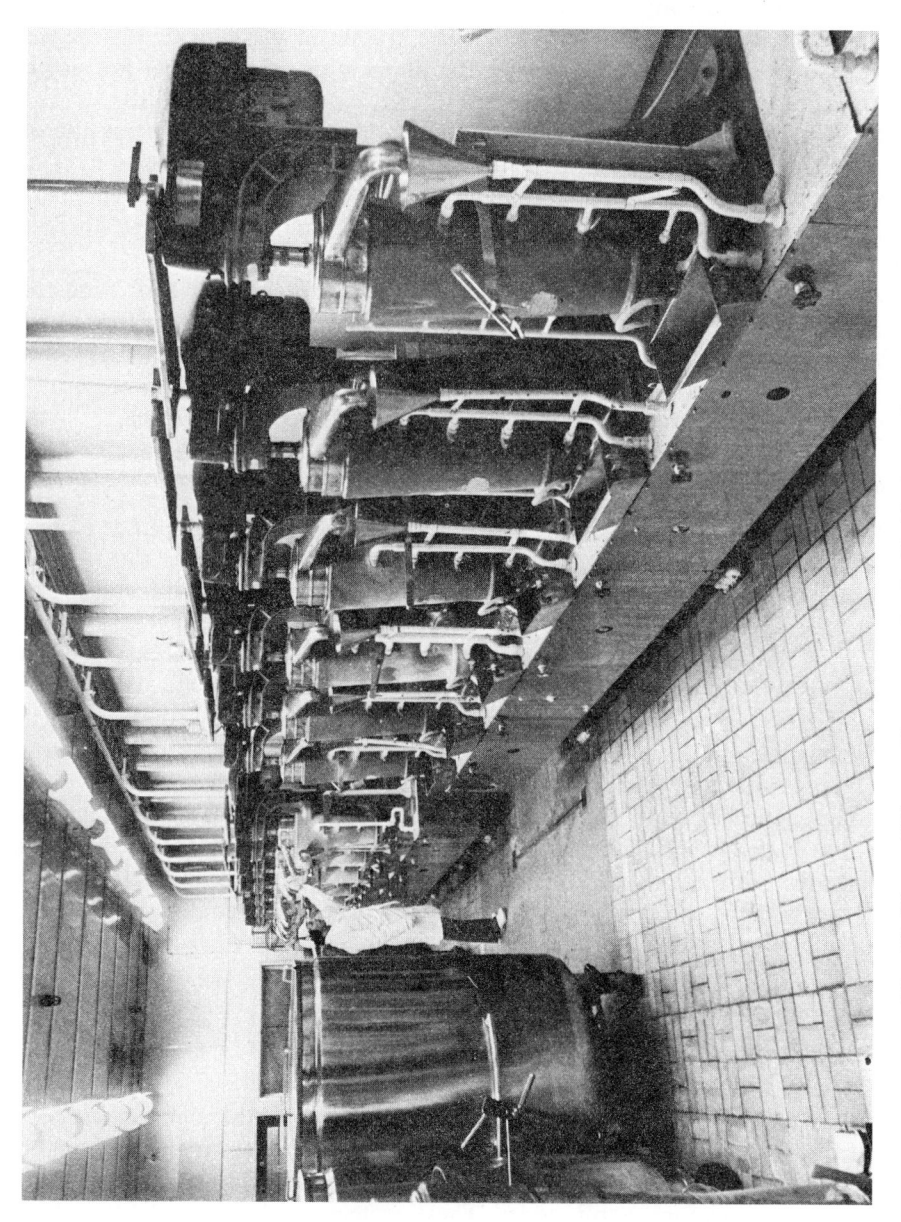

Fig. 18. The −5°C centrifuge room in the Kabi plasma fractionation plant

clinical results have been reported with these plasmin treated gamma globulin preparations.

In 1964 we also worked out a method at Kabi for the plasmin treatment of gamma globulin. These preparations were free from anticomplementary activity. However, in a study by Hanson and Johansson (1967) it was concluded that the fragmentation of the monomer is too high even in a very low concentration of plasmin. It was therefore considered not to be an ideal method for the preparation of a polymer-free gamma globulin that does not fix complements.

Further work to obtain a non-degraded gamma globulin for intravenous use was more successful. By using fresh frozen plasma and a slight modification of the fractionation procedure a monomer gamma globulin could be prepared. This native gamma globulin could further be stabilized by adding albumin for long time storage as a 5 per cent solution for intravenous use.

Since 1969 this preparation has been used clinically. Stefansson and Lundström (1974) reported on 17 patients having acute severe infections, who were treated with intravenous gamma globulin and in most cases conventional antibiotic therapy. About half of these patients showed immediate improvement after infusion of this preparation. The authors find the results encouraging and clinical testing is proceeding.

6. Transferrin, haptoglobin, and ceruloplasmin

Using fraction IV as starting material, new methods have been developed at Kabi for the isolation of transferrin, haptoglobin, and ceruloplasmin from this fraction. All these methods are based on chromatography with the use of DEAE–Sephadex in a batch system.

Transferrin and haptoglobin are prepared from non-haemolysed plasma. The separation of haptoglobin from transferrin is carried out under such conditions that the haptoglobin but not the transferrin is bound to the Sephadex gel. After elution the haptoglobin is precipitated at low temperature with ethanol. The transferrin is also further purified by precipitation with ethanol in the Cohn 5-variable system.

The earlier published method for the isolation of ceruloplasmin from different Cohn fractions has been further simplified. From a fraction IV solution the ceruloplasmin can be adsorbed directly on a DEAE–Sephadex gel at high ionic strength and then eluted as described in the earlier published method. The eluate containing 5 per cent ceruloplasmin of at least 90 per cent purity is sterile filtered and stored as a solution in the dark. The ceruloplasmin solution should be protected from ultraviolet light. Freezing and lyophilization cause it to lose copper.

7. Albumin

After fraction IV is separated by centrifugation and filtration the albumin fraction is precipitated according to Cohn method 5. The fraction IV filtrate is adjusted to 40 per cent ethanol at pH 4.8 and $-5°C$. To remove trace impurities and haemoglobin-bound proteins, a chromatography step is added. These proteins are bound to CM–Sephadex under strict conditions of pH and ionic strength. After removing the gel by filtration the albumin is again precipitated at 40 per cent ethanol at pH 5.1. The precipitate is separated by Sharples centrifugation and the paste is dissolved in ice-water for lyophilization and removal of the alcohol. The dried powder is dissolved in water, the pH is adjusted to 6.8 with sodium bicarbonate and acetyl tryptophane and sodium caprylate are added as stabilizers.

8. Glycoproteins

When albumin is precipitated in fraction V, about 1 per cent of the total plasma proteins are left in supernatant V. These proteins which are the most soluble proteins in the plasma are mainly glycoproteins. So far these proteins have not found any clinical use but are only isolated for research and experimental use. The Kabi method for concentrating these proteins also makes use of chromatography. After diluting the supernatant V with two volumes of ice-water, the proteins are bound to DEAE–Sephadex or CM–Sephadex after adjusting the pH to the right value depending on the Sephadex used.

III. Other methods for industrial plasma fractionation
HUGO NIHLÉN

1. Ammonium sulphate precipitation methods

The first tentative attempts to separate blood plasma into components were carried out at the beginning of the nineteenth century. The only method which was known at that time was precipitation with neutral salts such as sodium chloride or sodium sulphate. Considerable improvement came with the finding of a French physician, P-S Denis in 1847, that the clotting factor of blood was precipitated when plasma became saturated with sodium chloride. This precipitate could be redissolved with a return of the clotability when the salt was removed by dialysis. Denis suggested that this factor be called *fibrinogène*. The method was refined by Olaf Hammarsten who in 1879 published a procedure for the isolation of a fibrinogen which was practically pure.

Quite some time before this development, several workers had been of the opinion that the liquid which remained after the removal of fibrinogen from plasma, i.e. blood serum, was not homogeneous, but different methods which were used to separate the components gave different results. First through the work of Paul Hofmeister and co-workers at the German University of Prague a generally accepted method was developed for the isolation of the two main groups of proteins in serum, albumin and globulin. These two fractions could be separated by the addition of ammonium sulphate to half saturation, resulting in the precipitation of the globulins while albumin remained in solution. It was later discovered that the globulins could be further fractionated into three different subfractions by employing a successive increase in added amounts of ammonium sulphate, i.e. fractional precipitation.

The work of the Hofmeister school has been of fundamental importance for our understanding of proteins isolated from plasma as well as those isolated from other sources. Ammonium sulphate precipitation soon became the most widely used method for the separation of proteins in solution, on both a preparative as well as on an analytical scale.

38 Industrial plasma fractionation methods

When E. J. Cohn began his work to develop a method for the industrial isolation of plasma fractions, his starting point was the use of ammonium sulphate precipitation with practically the same precipitation limits as used by the Hofmeister school. Using this technique, Cohn was able to isolate a reasonably pure albumin in high yield and an almost pure γ-globulin in a lower yield. Particularly in large-scale preparations, the method has one obvious disadvantage, namely that the precipitating agent must be removed by, for example, dialysis. This was a considerable complication and Cohn began to develop methods for alcohol precipitation instead.

Nevertheless methods using ammonium sulphate have had considerable use for plasma fractionation, often in combination with rivanol precipitation. By a combined rivanol–ammonium sulphate method it is possible to obtain a γ-globulin which is practically undenatured and albumin of high purity in a high yield. The method is employed on an industrial scale in West Germany (Behringwerke) and in several East European states for the isolation of plasma proteins for clinical use.

2. Ether fractionation

At about the same time as Cohn and co-workers were developing the alcohol precipitation methods for the industrial preparation of plasma fractions, a group of workers at The Lister Institute of Preventive Medicine in England were experimenting with diethylether as a precipitating agent. Ether has a limited solubility in water and it is impossible to achieve a sufficiently high concentration of it in the system so that a precipitation of albumin results. Another serious drawback with the use of ether is the high explosion risk.

In spite of these obstacles much time was devoted to the development of the ether method for large-scale preparations, probably due to the fact that this method produced a high quality fibrinogen and a prothrombin concentrate which could easily be activated to thrombin. The method was further developed so that also γ-globulin could be obtained in satisfactory yield. On the other hand, attempts to isolate albumin or to develop a method for the recovery of other proteins were not successful.

After World War II, the ether method was used in a few fractionation plants in Western Europe but was abandoned after a few years except at The Lister Institute, where the method was in use until the beginning of the 1960s. At that time the method was replaced by Cohn fractionation as the difficulties inherent in ether fractionation proved to be practically insurmountable.

3. Rivanol precipitation

In 1956, Horejsi and Smetana published a method for the isolation of plasma proteins which employed Rivanol, 2-ethyl-6-9-diaminoacridine lactate, as a precipitating agent. They found that in alkaline media (pH = 8.0) albumin and fibrinogen were precipitated quantitatively with 0.4 per cent Rivanol. The α- and β-globulins were largely precipitated while the γ-globulins were not at all precipitated. The γ-globulins could be precipitated with ammonium sulphate and after disolving, adsorption of impurities, and dialysis a very pure preparation (98 per cent pure) was obtained.

Precipitation with Rivanol was developed originally as a simple and rapid laboratory method for the isolation of gamma globulin from serum or plasma. The procedure was soon being used in combination with ammonium sulphate precipitation in different parts of Europe as a useful method for the fractionation of plasma on an industrial scale. The Rivanol must be removed from all fractions which are to be used for clinical purposes. This was achieved inherently in the procedure as the Rivanol base-sulphate is highly insoluble. This method provides an equally efficient alternative to the alcohol fractionation method of Cohn. As has been mentioned previously, the Rivanol–ammonium sulphate method is in present day use in several European countries.

In several places, such as Centre National de Transfusion Sanguine in Paris, the Rivanol method has been used for the isolation of by-products from Cohn fractions e.g. α_{-2}-macroglobulin from fraction III.

4. Precipitation with synthetic polymers

Water-soluble highly polymerized substances precipitate proteins in a manner which is similar to that produced by neutral salts. In the early 1960s, Polson and co-workers at the University of Capetown experimented with several water-soluble linear polymers and found that most of these caused denaturation or were unsuitable for other reasons. The only agent which was found to be suitable was polyethylene glycol (PEG). According to Polson, the mechanism of precipitation by PEG is completely different from that of all precipitating agents which had hitherto been used. In contrast to the course of events when precipitation is achieved by using neutral salts or alcohol, PEG causes a protection of labile proteins. Such is the effect of PEG that precipitation can be carried out at room temperature or even at 30°C, and the sharpness of separation is very good. According to Polson, albumin can be obtained free of Au-antigen and γ-globulin and can be purified free of complement activity by using polyethylene glycol precipitation.

Fractionation with PEG has had a certain industrial use as a comparatively simple and safe method for the production of highly pure AHF from cryoprecipitate or Cohn fraction I. The precipitating agent must be removed completely after separation and purification of AHF. This can be achieved by reprecipitation or by chromatography.

5. Chromatographic methods

Three chromatographic procedures have been used in the preparation of plasma fractions: gel filtration, ion exchange chromatography, and affinity chromatography. In each of these methods, the solution containing the various protein components is allowed to flow through a bed of insoluble chromatographic material which is packed in a column. Depending on the properties of the chromatic material, the protein components are bound or retarded to various degrees to give rise to separation in the outflow.

Gel filtration

Gel filtration or molecular sieving is carried out by using a chromatographic bed of round granules which have a well defined upper limit of porosity. With the passage of the solution through the bed, molecules which are smaller than the average cross-section of the pores diffuse to a certain extent into the pores of the bed. In this way, the smaller molecules are retarded to a greater extent than the larger ones, the result being a fractionation of the molecules according to their size. In order to obtain the best separation, it is essential that the rate of flow through the column is adequately low so that the smaller molecules can be optimally retarded by the diffusion effect. In addition, the column bed must consist of a material which is inert to the solution. Sephadex, polyacrylamide, and agarose are the most commonly used materials but even porous glass beads have been used in more recent years. However, the surface of glass has a tendency to activate the coagulation system in plasma, but this complication can be circumvented by prior siliconizing of the glass surface. Gel filtration for separation covers a wide variety of compounds, ranging from amino acids to the largest protein molecules and several species of virus. Generally, it can be said that the sharpness of separation in favourable cases is sufficient to permit the separation of two components whose molecular size differs by 20 per cent.

Ion exchange chromatography

This technique consists of the passage of a protein solution through a column which contains an ion exchange substance which has been previously equilibrated with a buffer solution having a low ionic strength and a suitable pH. Under these conditions adsorption of protein is obtained. Elution is effected by subsequent increase in ionic strength. This can be achieved stepwise or continually with the help of a so-called gradient mixer. The ions of the eluting buffer compete with the adsorbed protein for binding sites on the ion exchange surface. The protein is released when the ionic strength of the buffer is sufficiently high. The ionic strength required to bring about this situation is a characteristic feature of each protein and buffer system. Elution can be effected even by altering the pH of the buffer which results in changes in the dissociation of charged groups on both the ion exchange surface and the protein. Systems exploying a combined ionic strength and pH gradient have also been used.

Ion exchange chromatography has proved useful for certain purposes in plasma fractionation. In particular, mention should be made of the recovery of B-factor concentrate from the supernatant obtained on the alcohol precipitation of fibrinogen from plasma.

Affinity chromatography or biospecific adsorption

This method implies that a preparation containing the substance to be purified must be passed through a column which is filled with a solid inert carrier, for example, cross-linked agarose, to which has been coupled a ligand which displays a high affinity for the substance in question. The adsorption takes place on the passage of the solution through the column. Following washing of the column, the adsorbed substance is eluted by changing the pH or increasing the ionic strength of the buffer. In this way, the substance can be isolated in a high yield with a purification factor of up to 1 000. Such an elution can be achieved often by altering either the pH or the ionic strength of the buffer. A much more selective technique is the use of specific elution, i.e. elution using a solution of the ligand. Typical ligand–protein pairs which are used for biospecific adsorption are antigen–antibody (so-called immunoadsorption), substrate–enzyme, coenzyme–apoenzyme and hormone–receptor.

In the case of the techniques used in the fractionation of plasma, one such specific adsorption is that involving the recovery of plasminogen from Cohn fraction III by using lysine–agarose. According to Deutsch and Mertz, the plasminogen can be eluted after adsorption by using a buffer which contains ε-aminocaproic acid.

It is likely that the technique of biospecific adsorption will become of great importance in the future for the recovery of valuable active substances in blood plasma. On the other hand, on account of the high price of the adsorbents it is not likely that this technique will become an alternative to precipitation procedures when applied to the isolation of proteins which are present in high concentration in blood.

Transport proteins

I. Serum albumin

A. Biochemistry

LARS-OLOV ANDERSSON

Serum albumin occupies a special position among the plasma proteins. It is the protein that is present in the largest amount in plasma where approximately one-half of the protein is albumin. Furthermore, it is one of the most intensely studied proteins. This is probably due to the fact that it was isolated early on in the pure form and that large amounts were easily prepared. Albumin has been used as a general protein model in a great number of studies such as amphoteric properties, denaturation processes, conformational changes, and ion binding properties.

Despite the fact that so much effort has been devoted to the study of albumin, many questions remain unanswered. The primary structure is known but we so far only have a rough idea about the tertiary structure. Albumin is thought to have three main functions. These are, the colloidosmotic regulation, the function as an easily accessible protein reserve, and the function as transport protein. However, it can not be excluded that albumin has functions in addition to these. The important question of the relation between the structure and the function remains unanswered.

Albumin-like protein is present in all mammals which have been studied as well as in birds, reptiles, and most fish. This article is concerned primarily with human serum albumin but in those cases where there is a lack of experimental data on human serum albumin, data on other albumins, mostly bovine albumin, will be given. In certain aspects, bovine serum albumin has been studied considerably more than human serum albumin.

A number of review articles on albumin are available (Foster, 1960; Putnam, 1965; Peters Jr, 1970).

1. Purification and determination

Methods for the preparation of albumin in a pure form have long been available. These are based on solubility fractionation with salt, most commonly ammonium sulphate. Albumin could be obtained in 90–95 per cent purity by the precipitation of the globulins at 50 per cent saturation of ammonium sulphate followed by lowering the pH to 4.4 and dialysing the precipitate obtained against water. Today the method most commonly used is still the ethanol precipitation method developed by Cohn and co-workers during the 1940s. In this method (Cohn method 6) the albumin is precipitated at pH 5 and $-5°C$ by the addition of ethanol to 40 per cent. The albumin obtained usually has a purity of 95–98 per cent. Recently, affinity chromatography has been applied successfully for the purification of albumin (Peters Jr, 1970 Wichman and Andersson, 1974). The affinity adsorbents used contained hydrophobic or fatty acid like ligands.

The determination of albumin can be performed in several different ways. If the sample is pure, some of the common methods for protein determination such as determination of nitrogen, the biuret reaction, U.V. absorption at 280 nm can be used. If other proteins are present in the sample, such as in blood, use is normally made of the following properties of albumin: (1) the high solubility; (2) the electrophoretic mobility; (3) the ability to bind dye; and (4) the immunological properties.

The high solubility of albumin makes the use of various types of precipitation techniques advantageous. One assay method for albumin is based on precipitation of the globulins at 1.8 mol/l sodium sulphate (Watson, 1965) followed by determination of the albumin remaining in solution by U.V. absorption measurements or the biuret reaction. Ethanol in combination with various acids has also been used as a precipitation agent. A classical method for the determination of albumin is moving boundary electrophoresis according to Tiselius. This method is not used any longer as it requires special equipment and is painstaking. It has been replaced by zone electrophoresis on paper, cellulose acetate strips, or agarose gel.

Different types of dye-binding techniques have been used quite frequently for the routine determination of albumin in plasma or serum. This type of technique is based on the finding that the dye is bound to albumin and that this binding induces a change in the visible absorption spectrum of the dye. By making measurements at some suitably chosen wavelength it is possible to determine the fraction of the dye which is bound to albumin and hence to calculate the albumin concentration. The dyes which are most commonly used are bromocresol green, methyl orange, and 2-(4-hydroxyazobenzene) benzoic acid (HABA).

Bromocresol green has certain advantages and has become the most popular dye (Rodkey, 1965; Doumas et al., 1971). The dye-binding methods have the advantage that they are easy to automate.

Immunological methods have become increasingly popular for the determination of albumin as well as for other plasma proteins. The two methods most commonly used are the radial immunodiffusion according to Mancini and the 'rocket' electroimmuno assay according to Laurell. Both those methods have good specificity and accuracy. A disadvantage with the immunodiffusion technique is that it takes a fairly long time to complete.

The bromocresol green dye-binding method is probably the best rapid routine method for albumin determination. If high accuracy is required and the time required to complete the analysis is not so important, immunological methods are probably the best. Most of the methods mentioned above require the use of a standard. One such suitable standard is human albumin which has a high purity.

2. Physicochemical properties

The molecular weight of albumin is less than that of most of the other proteins of plasma. The previously used value of 69 000 is now known to be too high. From the amino acid sequence, a value around 66 000 can be calculated. The higher values were due to the

Table 2. Physical chemical data for human serum albumin

Molecular weight		66 000
Sedimentation coefficient	$s^o_{20,w}$	4.5×10^{-13} S
Diffusion coefficient	$D^o_{20,w}$	5.9×10^{-7} cm^2/s
Partial specific volume	V	0.734 cm^3/g
The radius of gyration	R_G	2.98 nm
Isoelectric point	IP	4.7–5.5
Electrophoretic mobility in barbital buffer pH 8.6		5.92×10^{-5} cm^2/v.s
Light absorption	$A^{1\%}_{279}$	5.3

presence of small amounts of dimer and polymer and the fact that the techniques such as sedimentation equilibrium produce average values for the molecular weight. The aggregates that can be found in almost all albumin preparations are probably not present in the circulating blood (Andersson, 1966) but are formed during the preparation and storage. Large amounts of various aggregates can be found in old samples of albumin (Pedersen, 1962).

The hydrodynamic properties of albumin have been studied in detail. Sedimentation, diffusion, viscosity, light scattering, and several other methods have been used in these studies. Some data are given in Table 2. The data obtained indicate that the molecule is fairly asymmetric. An ellipsoid of rotation with a large axis of 14 nm and a short axis of 4 nm has been suggested as a model for albumin (Squire et al., 1968).

Albumin is one of the most soluble plasma proteins. Solutions containing up to 30 per cent of albumin can be prepared. The high solubility of albumin is probably connected with the large number of ionizable groups present in the molecule. At neutral pH the number of charged groups is roughly 200. Since the number of carboxyl groups is somewhat larger than the number of basic groups, the isoelectric point is lower than 7. Several different methods has been used for the determination of the isoelectric point of the protein but somewhat varied results have been obtained. Measurements of the electrophoretic mobility at different pH values have provided values between 4.9 and 5.2. Isoelectric focusing of native human serum albumin gives a distribution of material with isoelectric points between 4.7 and 5.5 (Valmet, 1969; Rosseneu-Motreff et al., 1970). However, it has been shown that this distribution of isoelectric points is related to the fact that different albumin molecules contain different amounts of bound fatty acids (Valmet, 1969; Rosseneu-Motreff et al., 1970).

Isoelectric focusing of bovine serum albumin in 8 mol/l urea gives a rather surprising value for the isoelectric point of 5.9–6.0. Even here a certain degree of heterogeneity could be detected (Salaman and Williamson, 1971). These results may be explained by supposing that serum albumin, probably both human and bovine, contains basic groups which are normally not protonated, e.g. amino groups which are situated in the interior of the molecule and which are not accessible to the solvent when the molecule assumes the native conformation. These groups would then be in the uncharged form in the native conformation of the molecule but would become protonated in the presence of 8 mol/l urea which unfolds the albumin molecule.

The size and shape of the molecule of albumin is somewhat dependent on pH. When the pH of an albumin solution is lowered from 4.5 to 3.5 there is a reversible expansion of the molecule. This expansion depends on the fact that the carboxyl groups are successively transformed into the uncharged form, leaving the positively charged groups in excess and increasing the repulsion between various segments of the peptide chains. This conformational change is usually called the N–F transformation (Foster, 1960). A similar conformation change takes place in the alkaline pH region where the alteration in size and shape begins to occur at pH 10.3 (Tanford et al., 1955). Furthermore there are indications from measurements of optical rotation that a small conformational change occurs in the pH interval 7–8 (Leonard et al., 1963; Harmsen et al., 1971).

The ultraviolet absorption spectrum of human serum albumin is of the normal protein type showing a maximum at 279 nm and a minimum around 255 nm. However, solutions of albumin often show additional absorption in the visible region. The colour of concentrated albumin solutions usually varies between yellow and reddish brown. This colour is caused by the presence of coloured substances such as bilirubin and haemin which bind to the protein.

3. Heterogeneity

While serum albumin is usually regarded as a homogeneous protein, it is quite clear that the protein is heterogeneous in several respects. It was discovered quite early that albumin is heterogeneous with respect to the SH content. Values for the SH content of 0.6–0.7 SH/mole were obtained. This was taken as evidence for the existence of two types of albumin, one containing one SH group and the other without SH. Those two fractions are usually called mercaptalbumin and non-mercaptalbumin respectively. Several methods have been used to separate these components. An early method employed the addition of Hg^{2+} to form a mercury dimer of the mercaptalbumin. This dimer crystallized easily and the crystals could be separated from the rest of the solution. The mercaptalbumin could then be regenerated by splitting of the dimer by treatment with some suitable thiol, e.g. cysteine. An improved method for the separation of mercaptalbumin and non-mercaptalbumin makes use of ion exchange chromatography of DEAE–Sephadex. This separation method has also demonstrated that the non-mercaptalbumin fraction is not homogeneous but consists of several components (Janatova et al., 1968; Spencer and King 1971; Fuller-Noel and Hunter, 1972). Studies on the non-mercaptalbumin fraction have shown that small amounts of cysteine and glutathione are released on reduction or oxidation of the disulphide bonds (Andersson, 1966; King, 1961). This is not the case with the mercaptalbumin fraction. This has been interpreted to mean that the SH group in the non-mercaptalbumin fraction forms a mixed disulphide with cysteine and glutathione. However, there are indications that there is also a non-mercaptalbumin component where the SH group has been oxidized to the sulphinic or sulphonic stage (Fuller-Noel and Hunter, 1972). In conclusion, regarding the SH heterogeneity of albumin it can be said that albumin is composed of three or four components which differ only slightly.

A second type of heterogeneity observed in serum albumin is the so-called 'microheterogeneity'. This was discovered in connection with electrophoretic studies on albumin which were performed in the pH range 4–5 (Foster, et al., 1965) and has further been demonstrated in pH solubility studies (Petersen and Foster, 1965a). This type of heterogeneity has been shown to be dependent on several factors. The SH heterogeneity which was described earlier is of importance together with the fact that most albumin preparations contain varying amounts of aggregated molecules (Petersen and Foster, 1965b). Furthermore, it is clear that the content of bound fatty acids affects the behaviour of albumin (McMenamy and Lee, 1967; Andersson, 1969). However, even mercaptalbumin which is free from fatty acids still showed signs of heterogeneity. Additional studies have shown that disulphide exchange reactions take place at alkaline pH causing the formation of a 'new' albumin molecule which has a different pairing of some of the disulphide bridges (Nikkel and Foster, 1971). These two forms of albumin could be separated by ion exchange chromatography on SE–Sephadex. The process was reversible and the equilibrium constant was found to be 1 at pH 9.5. Recently, it was shown that bovine serum albumin components having different pairings of the disulphide bonds could be separated by isoelectric focusing (Wallevik, 1976a). The rate of catabolism was shown to be different for the various components indicating that disulphide bond interchange may be a determinant is the normal catabolism (Wallevik, 1976b).

4. Chemical properties

Most plasma proteins contain carbohydrate, i.e. they are glycoproteins. This is not the case with serum albumin which is devoid of carbohydrate. Small amounts of carbohydrate have been detected occasionally in albumin preparations but this is probably due to contamination of the albumin by small amounts of other plasma proteins which contain carbohydrate. The presence of lipids, mainly long chain fatty acids, can almost always be demonstrated in albumin preparations. Albumin contains a number of binding sites for long chain fatty acid anions and has strong affinity for these. Different studies have shown that various preparations of albumin contain between 1–3 moles of fatty acid per mole of albumin. This corresponds to a lipid content in albumin of 0.3–1.0 per cent. The fatty acids present in albumin are mainly stearic acid, palmitic acid, and oleic acid.

The content of nitrogen in human serum albumin has been studied by a number of research groups. One such study was performed by Watson (1967) who reported a nitrogen content of 15.7–15.8 per cent. The nitrogen factor, i.e. the number of grams of protein per gram of nitrogen, corresponding to this is 6.4. However, if the nitrogen factor is calculated from the amino acid composition a slightly lower value of 6.2 is obtained. This difference can be explained by the fact that native albumin contains small amounts of fatty acids and probably also some tightly bound water molecules. Thus, it is possible to use two different nitrogen factors depending on how one would like to define the serum albumin molecule. If albumin is defined as a 'naked' peptide chain without fatty acids and without water the value is 6.2. If albumin is defined as the native molecule containing fatty acids and some water, this value is around 6.4. The value which is most commonly used is 6.25.

The amino acid composition, is shown in Table 3. The total number of amino acid residues is 585 and the molecular weight is approximately 66 300. It is worth noting that there is only one tryptophane and six methionine residues. The molecule contains

Table 3. The amino acid composition of human serum albumin

Amino acid	Number of amino acid residues
Asparell acid	53
Treonine	27
Serine	23
Glutamil acid	83
Proline	25
Glycine	12
Alanine	64
Half-cystine	35
Valine	42
Methionine	6
Isoleucine	8
Leucine	61
Tyrosine	17
Phenylalanine	30
Lysine	59
Histidine	16
Arginine	23
Tryptophan	1
Amide–NH$_3$	35

Total 585

a large number of polar amino acid residues which account for the high solubility of albumin.

Human serum albumin consists of one peptide chain cross-linked by 17 disulphide bridges. This is evident from the finding of only one amino-terminal amino acid residue, aspartic acid, and one carboxyl-terminal amino acid, leucine, and that the molecular weight is not changed upon reduction of the disulphide bridges in 8 mol/l urea solution.

Recently the complete amino acid sequences of human and bovine serum albumin have been elucidated (Behrens et al., 1975; Meloun et al., 1975). The sequence of human serum albumin is shown in Fig. 19. It is immediately obvious that a kind of repeating structure is present. The entire molecule can be viewed as being composed of three repeating units or domains (1–191, 192–384, 385–585). This is in good agreement with the model of the albumin molecule provided in Fig. 20. Many sequence homologies are found between the three domains indicating that gene duplication has occurred twice in the evolution of serum albumin. Even within the domains, the pairing of the disulphide bridges follows a certain pattern. Each domain contains six peptide loops formed by the disulphide bridges. Sequence similarities can also be detected between the two large loops within each domain. On examination it can be seen that there is a small degree of sequence homology between the large loop structures in albumin and the G–H helix regions in myoglobin and haemoglobin. Comparison shows that albumin is as similar to the globins as they are to each other.

The sequence of bovine serum albumin is very similar to that of the corresponding human protein. The general structure in domains and loops is the same and 78 per cent of the residues are the same.

There are certain residues in serum albumin which are of special importance.

I. Serum albumin   49

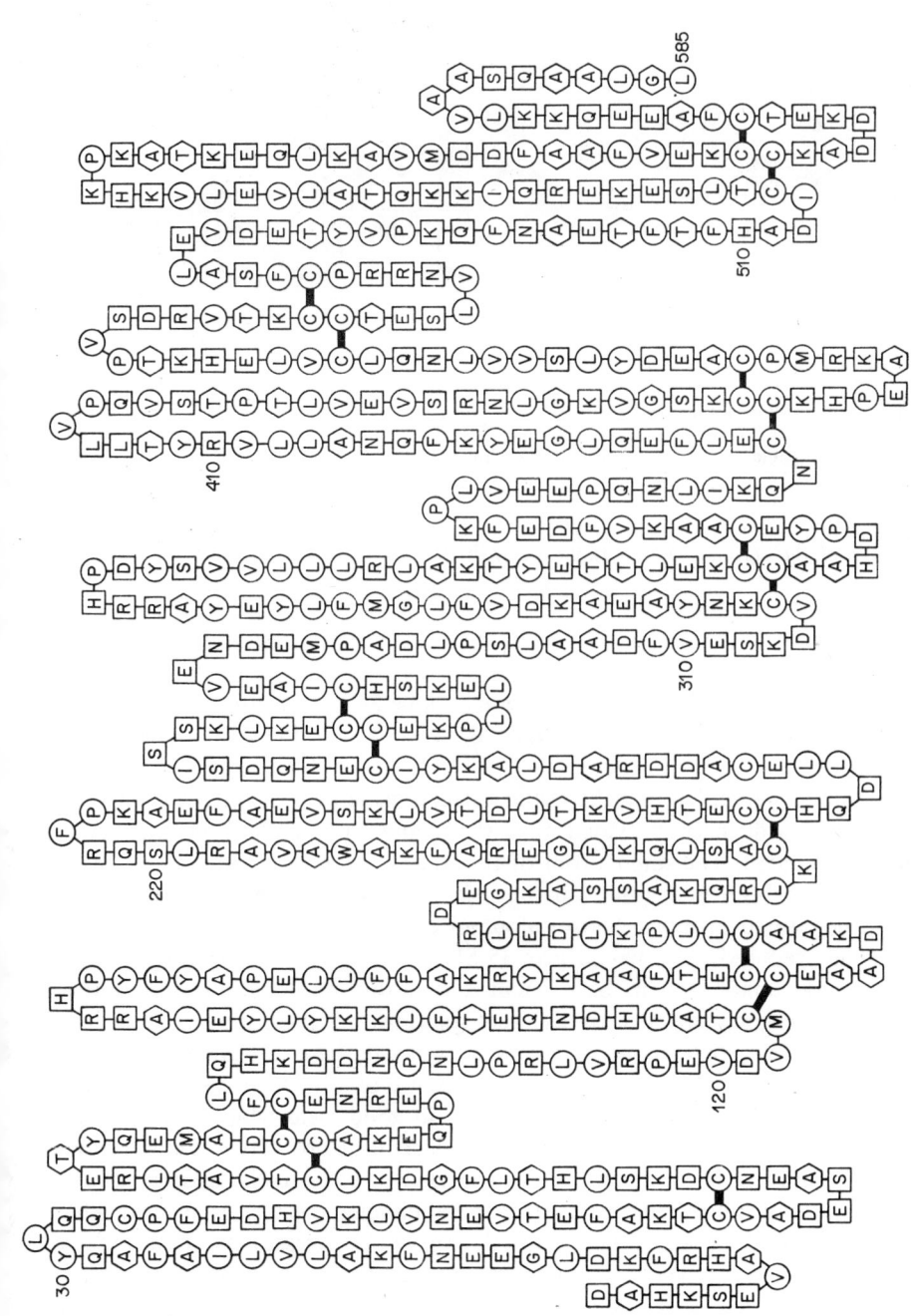

Fig. 19. Amino acid sequence of human serum albumin. Hydrophilic amino acid residues □, hydrophobic amino acid residues ○, amino acid residues of intermediate hydrophobicity ◇

A = Ala, C = Cys, D = Asp, E = Glu, F = Phe, G = Gly, H = His, I = Ile, K = Lys, L = Leu, M = Met, N = Asn, P = Pro, Q = Gln, R = Arg, S = Ser, T = Thr, V = Val, W = Trp, Y = Tyr

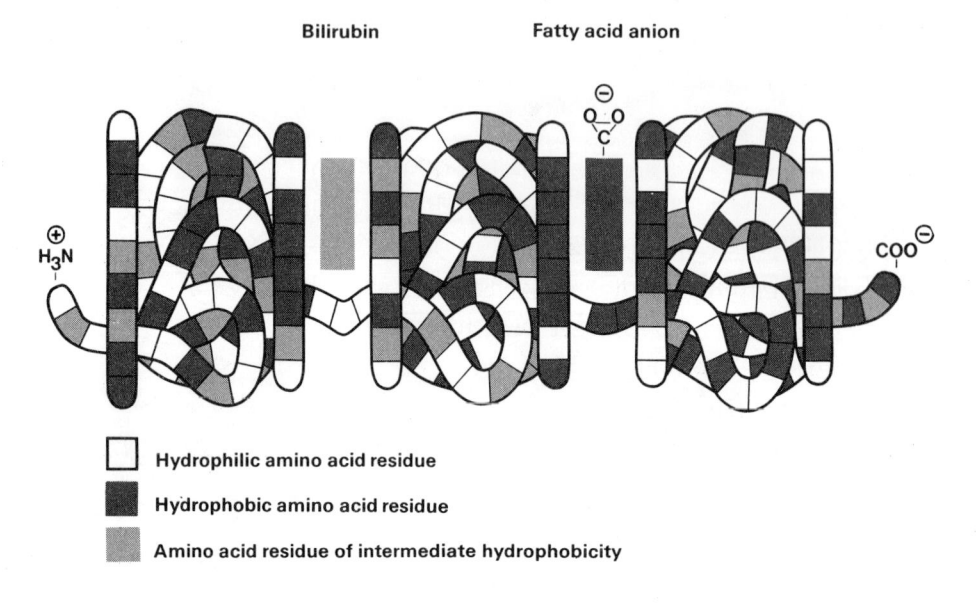

Fig. 20. Model of the serum albumin molecule with binding sites for bilirubin and fatty acid anions

The SH group present in albumin is situated at residue 34 close to the amino-terminal end of the molecule. The lone tryptophane is found at residue 214 in the middle domain.

It is now generally accepted that the tertiary structures of proteins are determined by their amino acid sequences provided that the folding takes place in the natural biological environment. The main proof of this thesis has come from the numerous studies which have been performed on the refolding and reoxidation of completely reduced and denatured proteins. Serum albumin contains 17 disulphide bridges and when completely reduced these would give 35 SH groups accessible for the formation of new disulphide bonds. It can be calculated that this would allow formation of 2.2×10^{10} different conformers with different pairings of these disulphide bonds. However, when completely reduced bovine serum albumin is allowed to slowly reoxidize at neutral or weakly basic pH in the presence of a low concentration of long chain fatty acids there is formation of a product in good yield which is identical to native albumin with regard to number of physicochemical properties. Thus it would appear the albumin has become renatured (Andersson, 1969). In the absence of fatty acids, a considerably more heterogeneous population of molecules is formed where solubility, optical rotation, and other properties vary. This stresses the importance of environmental factors in the folding of protein. Recent studies on reduction and refolding of the separated domains, prepared by proteolytic cleavage, have shown that the domains fold to give immunologically active structures even in the isolated form. This indicates that the folding of the domains to some degree takes place independent of each other.

5. Binding properties

A characteristic feature of serum albumin is its ability to bind a large number of different substances. Biological substances such as long chain fatty acids and steroids as well as synthetic substances such as dyes and drugs become bound to the protein. The binding data for a number of different types of substances are given in Table 4.

The binding studies have usually been performed in order to obtain information concerning the transport of the substance by albumin or as a means of studying the properties and structure of albumin.

The binding and transport of long chain fatty acids is probably one of the main physiological functions of serum albumin. These fatty acids, i.e. stearic acid, oleic acid, palmitic acid, and others, have very low solubility in water and would not dissolve in the blood if they were not solubilized by binding to protein. An albumin solution is capable of solubilizing considerable amounts of long chain fatty acids. The mechanism of the solubilizing process is based on the tiny amount of fatty acid which dissolves in water being immediately bound to albumin. This allows more fatty acid to dissolve and the process continues until the maximal binding capacity of albumin is reached.

The binding of long chain fatty acids to albumin has been studied by several research groups. The number of binding sites and the binding constants are best studied by examining the distribution of labelled fatty acid between an albumin solution and an organic solvent, usually heptane, at different fatty acid concentrations. The values obtained in the early studies indicated the presence of two very strong binding sites ($K_A=10^8$), five strong binding sites ($K_A=10^5$), and about twenty weak binding sites ($K_A=10^3$) for long chain fatty acids of the stearic acid type (Goodman, 1958). Recent studies have given rise to slightly different data and other interpretations (Fletcher et al., 1970). It is possible to assign separate binding constants for each binding site. However, irrespective of the manner of treating the data it is quite clear that the

Table 4. *Association constants for binding of some different types of substances to albumin at neutral pH.* (HSA, human serum albumin; BSA, bovine serum albumin)

Substance	Number of binding sites	Association constant K_A	Type of albumin
Stearic acid	2 very strong	1.1×10^8	
	5 strong	4.0×10^6	(HSA)
Bilirubin	1 strong	1.5×10^6	
	1 weak	2.5×10^4	(HSA)
Chloride ion	1 weak	2.4×10^3	
	8 very weak	$\times 10^2$	(HSA)
Testosterone	3 weak	3.2×10^4	(HSA)
Tyrosine	1 strong	2.5×10^6	
	5 weak	6×10^4	(HSA)
Phenoxymethyl-penicillin	1 weak	2.3×10^3	(BSA)
Salicylic acid	1 strong	2×10^5	
	5 weak	1.7×10^3	(BSA)
Fluorescein	3 weak	2.8×10^4	(BSA)

binding of long chain fatty acids to albumin is very strong. It is not possible to remove long chain fatty acids from albumin by using dialysis or some of the conventional separation methods. One way of obtaining albumin which is free of fatty acids is to treat the albumin solution with charcoal powder at pH 3 (Chen, 1967). The binding of fatty acids affects the structure of albumin. The U.V. spectrum and the tryptophane fluorescence is changed on the binding of fatty acids to the protein. The digestibility by proteolytic enzymes is decreased as well as the sensitivity to heat denaturation. This has been utilized in the inactivation of possible hepatitis virus contamination by heat treatment of albumin solutions prior to clinical use. In this process the albumin solution is kept at 60°C for 10 hours. In order to withstand this treatment and avoid heat denaturation the albumin is stabilized by the addition of sodium caprylate or acetyl tryptophane. These stabilizers have been chosen because of their fairly good solubility and the ease with which they can be worked. This is not the case with stearic acid and the other naturally occurring long chain fatty acids.

Detergents such as alkylsulphonates and alkylsulphates are similar to the fatty acids. The binding of those detergents to albumin has been studied by Steinhart and co-workers and the results show that there are many similarities between the binding of these two types of substances.

The binding of bilirubin to serum albumin is important. This substance has toxic effects when present in the free state but binding to albumin renders it non-toxic. Bilirubin is transported by albumin to the liver where it is conjugated and excreted. Albumin has one very strong binding site for bilirubin and probably a second binding site which has low affinity. The amount of bilirubin normally present in plasma is very small. Approximately one molecule of albumin in 15 contains bound bilirubin. Haemin is also bound to albumin, explaining the finding that albumin prepared from haemolysed blood is reddish brown in colour.

Several different types of hormones are bound to serum albumin. However, most of these hormones have other special transport proteins and albumin acts merely as a second-hand transport protein in cases where the concentration of the hormone in question is raised above the binding capacity of its specific carrier protein. Examples of hormones of this type are thyroxine and the steroid hormones.

Various metal ions bind to serum albumin; Cu^{2+} is strongly bound to several sites and the mechanism for the binding to one of these sites has been elucidated (Bradshaw et al., 1968). Certain anions such as the chloride ion are also bound; although with low affinity.

The binding of dyes to serum albumin has been studied rather extensively. When a dye is bound to albumin the visible spectrum of the dye is usually changed. The character and magnitude of this change or shift has been utilized to obtain information concerning the nature of the binding site. The dyes most commonly studied are methyl red, phenol red, bromocresol green, and congo red. These dyes are usually bound with considerably lower affinity than the long chain fatty acids and bilirubin. Synthetic dyes are not natural ligands of serum albumin and it is to be expected that the binding sites do not generally fit the dyes very well, explaining the comparatively low binding constants for these ligands. The binding of various fluorescent compounds to albumin has been studied. When anilinonaphthalenesulphonic acid (ANS) is bound to albumin it becomes strongly fluorescent, indicating that the binding sites are hydrophobic in nature. ANS is almost non-fluorescent in water solution but becomes strongly fluorescent, when dissolved in non-polar solvents. In contrast, the fluorescence of fluorescein is quenched when the molecules become bound to albumin.

The binding of various drugs such as salicylates, sulphonamides, barbiturates, penicillin, phenylbutazon, and warfarin to albumin is of great pharmacological importance. This binding is usually fairly weak but exceptionally strong binding is known, e.g. phenylbutazon. The binding of drugs to serum albumin results in only a fraction of the given dose being immediately effective. The magnitude of this fraction is dependent not only on the strength of the binding to albumin but also on the strength of the binding to the receptors for the drug. The solubilizing properties of serum albumin are probably important for the transport of certain drugs.

6. Structure and functional relations

As we mentioned previously, serum albumin has several different functions. The structure of albumin is designed to enable the protein to function primarily in the binding and transport of different substances. The two other main functions of albumin, the regulation of the colloid osmotic pressure and the function as a reserve protein, do not require any special structure characteristics but merely that the molecular weight be appropriate and the amino acid composition be normal.

Despite the fact that many studies have been performed on the binding of long chain fatty acids and similar substances to albumin, comparatively little is known concerning the structures responsible for the binding. It has been shown that the tryptophane fluorescence of serum albumin is affected by the binding of long chain fatty acids. Thus it has been suggested that one of the binding sites for fatty acids should be close to the lone tryptophane at position 214 in human serum albumin. However, it may be argued that this effect on the tryptophane fluoresence is produced by a general conformational change in the albumin molecule and that this is induced by the binding of fatty acid at a site which is remote from this tryptophane residue. In fact there is evidence indicating that the entire structure of albumin is affected to some degree by the binding of fatty acids. Studies on the binding of long chain fatty acids to various fragments of bovine serum albumin (Reed et al., 1975) indicate that the three strongest binding sites are situated in the carboxy-terminal two-thirds of the molecule. The strongest palmitate binding site $K_A = 2 \times 10^7$ M^{-1}) has been suggested to be situated within the sequence 377–503, the second strongest site ($K_A = 8 \times 10^6$ M^{-1}) within the sequence 239–306, and the third strongest site ($K^a = 2 \times 10^6$ M^{-1}) within the sequence 307–377. Affinity labelling of the binding sites in bovine serum albumin for long chain fatty acid anions has been studied using special reactive compound, trinitrobenzene sulphonic acid (TNBS), which forms covalent bonds with amino groups (Andersson, et al., 1971). This compound is also bound to albumin and experiments have shown that this takes place in some of the binding sites for fatty acid anions. Following the affinity labelling, a labelled pentapeptide was isolated and sequenced. Its position corresponds to residues 347–351 in bovine serum albumin which is in agreement with the position of the third palmitate binding site found by Reed et al. As a general model for the character of the binding sites, it was suggested some time ago that this is a hydrophobic pocket containing one or more positively charged groups. Support for this hypothesis has been obtained from several different studies. Investigations into the binding of various dyes and fluorescent molecules such as anilinonaphthalenesulphonic acid indicate strongly that the binding sites are hydrophobic in character. However, electrostatic interactions are also important as is evident in the observations (Arvidsson *et al.*, 1971) that long chain fatty acid anions are bound more strongly than the corresponding ester or alcohol (Reynolds *et al.*, 1961).

Using the model of serum albumin which was given earlier (Fig. 20) a hypothesis for the binding of fatty acid anions and other substances to serum albumin can be suggested. In this system the binding sites are situated between the globular segments. The inner parts of these clefts or pockets should be hydrophobic and positive charged lysyl or arginyl residues could be situated in the outer parts of these clefts. The binding would then be dependent on hydrophobic and electrostatic interactions in agreement with experimental results. As a consequence of this model, it is probable that the binding of fatty acid anions or other substances would diminish the mobility of the globular segments in the albumin molecule. This, this would to some extent 'freeze' the molecule. This is in agreement with the observation that the binding of fatty acid anions increases the stability of the molecule in several respects.

Certain data regarding binding sites and mechanisms of binding have been obtained from studies using other compounds such as bilirubin and tryptophane. Affinity labelling studies using a tryptophane derivative (Gamghir *et al.*, 1975) indicate that this binding site is situated in the aminoterminal part of the molecule, residues 1–86. This is in contrast to the binding sites for fatty acid anions which appear to be situated in the middle and carboxy-terminal portions of the molecule. Studies which have been performed on the binding properties of fragments of human serum albumin indicate that the bilirubin binding site is located somewhere in the region between residues 182 and 298.

Many metal ions are bound to serum albumin and the site and mechanism of the binding have been elucidated for a few of these. Copper ions, Cu^{2+}, are bound to several sites in albumin but the strongest site with a K_A-value of approximately 10^7 M^{-1} is found in the amino-terminal tripeptide sequence H_2N-Asp-Ala-His-. The amino-terminal amino group, the nitrogens of the first two peptide bonds, and one nitrogen in the imidazole group of histidine participate in the binding of Cu^{2+} in a planar square conformation (Bradshaw *et al.*, 1968). The binding of copper can be regarded as one of the detoxification functions of serum albumin. Another detoxification function is the binding of Hg^{2+} and various mercury compounds. This binding involves the SH groups in albumin and is very strong. Silver and cadmium also bind to the thiol groups of albumin.

B. Physiology and clinical aspects

GUNNAR BIRKE, STEN-OTTO LILJEDAHL, and MARK ROTHSCHILD

Albumin constitutes 50–60 per cent of the total protein in blood and has several important functions. Perhaps the most significant of these is its high colloid osmotic effect. Albumin is responsible for 80 per cent of the colloid osmosis in blood, this being determined by the low molecular weight (66 000) of the protein. Thus, albumin is vital for the suspension stability of blood.

The function of albumin as an important transport protein is well known, especially the part played by it in the transport of long chain fatty acids, calcium, sex hormones, steroid, and thyroid hormones as well as catecholamines. In addition, a great number of drugs bind to albumin which is crucial for their function. Much work is at present being devoted to the study of this interaction between albumin and drugs. Furthermore, albumin serves as an easily available reserve protein. In this connection, the protein does not enter the cell. There is first a breakdown to form peptides and amino acids which are used later in the synthesis of protein.

However, it should be realized that all of the functions of albumin which have been mentioned above are replaceable. A few cases have been described of patients having analbuminaemia. In this condition, the patient's plasma shows a high level of globulins and the only discomfort is mild oedema of the legs. Apart from this, the patient leads a practically normal life.

1. Normal values

In clinical work involving albumin, the values of this protein which are most commonly given are its concentration in serum and its distribution within the various globulin fractions of serum. It is generally accepted that the normal concentration in serum is 35–45 g/l and that it comprises 50–60 per cent of the total serum protein (Fig. 21).

The concentration of albumin in serum is merely a reflection of a finished product of synthesis distribution, and breakdown of protein. Additional information concerning the synthesis, breakdown, and distribution of albumin in the intra- and extracellular space has been obtained by using albumin and amino acids which were labelled with isotope. The improved methodology of recent years has provided reliable data on the metabolism of albumin. Labelling with radionuclides can be carried out without causing any denaturation of the protein and the introduction of immunochemical methods has permitted a more efficient determination of this protein. The technique of assay has improved and the use of whole body counters and new methods of mathematical calculation have provided more reliable results. Studies of the synthesis of albumin have been made possible by using isotope-labelled amino acids which

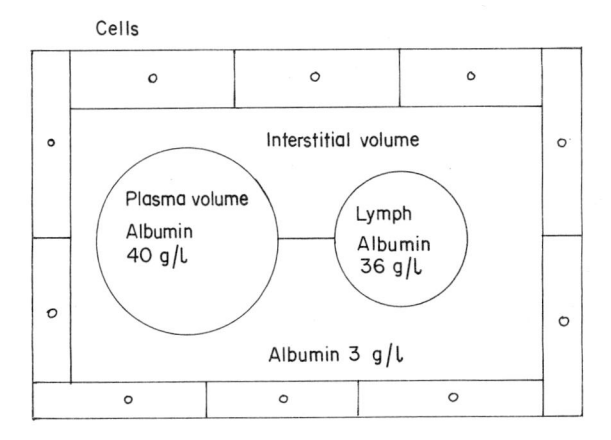

Fig. 21. Distribution of albumin within the interstitial fluid space, plasma, and lymph

56 Transport proteins

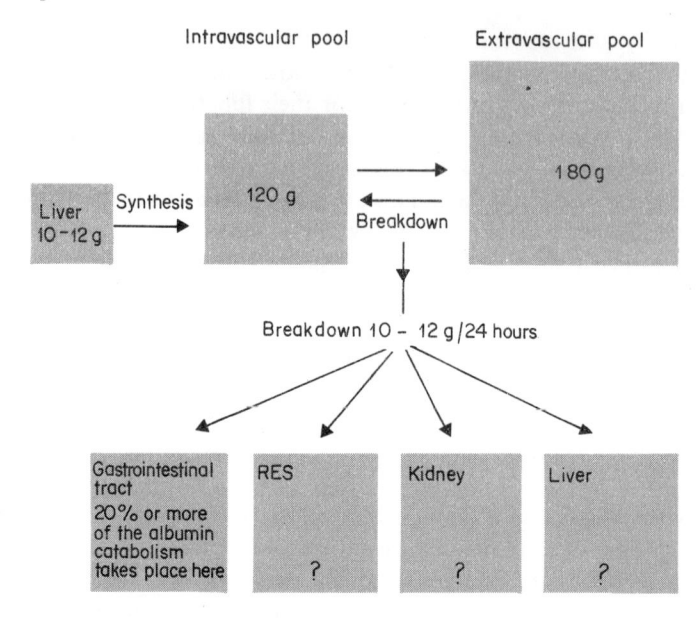

Fig. 22. The synthesis, distribution, and breakdown of albumin

become incorporated into the protein. Experimental liver perfusion has expanded further our knowledge of the various factors which affect this synthesis.

2. Synthesis, distribution, and breakdown

The synthesis of albumin takes place in the liver and is greatest during the first few years following birth, to produce 180–300 mg/kg body weight daily. For adults and children over the age of three years, the corresponding figure is 120–200 mg/kg body weight daily. The synthesis is somewhat lower in women, 120–150 mg/kg body weight daily. The total pool of albumin in women and men has been determined to be 4 and 4–5 g/kg body weight, respectively. Between 38 per cent and 45 per cent of the total pool is to be found intravascularly. The breakdown has been estimated to be 6–10 per cent of the intravascular albumin daily.

The normal values for the turnover of albumin in a 70 kg healthy individual are provided in Fig. 22.

3. Regulation of albumin metabolism

Organisms strive to maintain a normal concentration of albumin, i.e. a normal colloid osmotic pressure in plasma. This is achieved by a balance between synthesis, distribution, and breakdown of albumin. It is not fully understood how this balance is regulated. Several factors which are known to take part in the synthesis, distribution, and breakdown of albumin are discussed in what follows.

4. Synthesis of albumin

Using the technique of liver perfusion, Miller and co-workers (1954) showed that the synthesis of albumin takes place in the liver. Kukral and co-workers (1961) demonstrated that the administration of ^{35}S-labelled amino acids to dogs, the livers of which had been removed, did not result in the incorporation of these amino acids in albumin but resulted in their normal imcorporation into the immunoglobulins.

The various stages in the synthesis of albumin in the liver have not been clearly defined. The hepatocytes contain separate systems for the synthesis of different proteins (Fig. 23). The ribosomes, consisting of 60 S and 40 S subunits, appear partially bound to the endoplasmatic reticulum and partially free from this structure. The most active form of m-RNA in the synthesis contains a number of ribosomes. Proteins synthesized on the endoplasmic reticulum are not necessarily destined to be secreted. Reticulum recognition of secretory proteins may require a label in the form of a signal peptide. A major fraction of newly synthesized albumin by hepatic polysomes is a proalbumin, which accounts for much of the 200–500 μg of the intrahepatic albumin. At present, much attention is being paid to the intracellular albumin synthetic pathway with its many interrelated steps. This attention will result most probably in defining the synthesis of albumin within the not-too-distant future.

Munro has demonstrated that there is a species-dependent relationship between the distribution of albumin and the amount of m-RNA found in the liver of full-grown animals. The half-life of albumin is 1.2 days in mouse and 20.7 days in the cow. On the other hand, the absolute amount of albumin (mg/kg body weight) which is synthesized daily is relatively constant in all species including man. The normal daily synthesis is 150–250 mg/kg body weight. While the albumin which is produced in the cell is eliminated to plasma within 30 minutes, it appears in the microsomes within 1–2 minutes and remains in the endoplasmic reticulum during a period of 15 minutes. As the total amount of albumin found in the normal liver is less than 1 g, an exchange of this albumin must take place 15–20 times per day. It appears, that under normal circumstances, the liver cell delivers its newly synthesized albumin directly into hepatic plasma; and that fraction of the newly synthesized albumin which reaches hepatic lymph directly is related primarily to the ratio of hepatic lymph flow to plasma flow, (0.0005/0.9

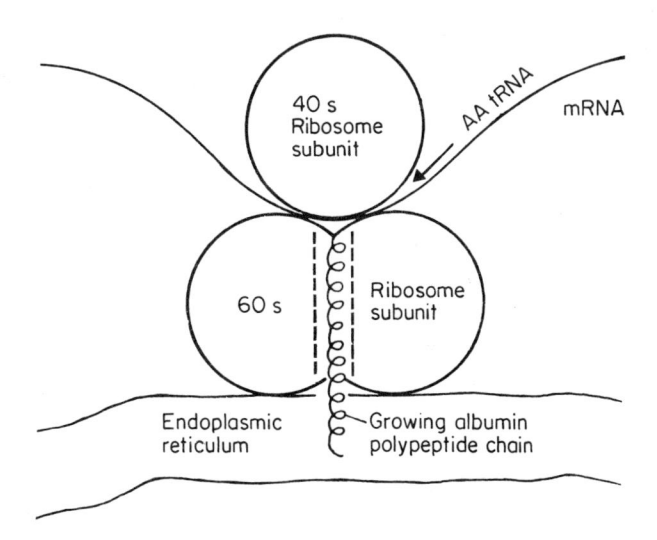

Fig. 23. The various stages in the synthesis of albumin in the liver

ml/g/min) or about 0.05 per cent. The lymph returns extravascular albumin to the plasma pool via the thoracic duct.

5. Factors affecting the synthesis of albumin

The factors which regulate the synthesis of albumin are not completely understood. However, it is known that the state of nutrition, the hormone balance, the colloid osmotic pressure in the plasma, and the general condition of the liver influence the synthesis of this protein (Fig. 22).

Nutrition

By using liver perfusion techniques, it has been shown that fasting or an insufficient diet can decrease the rate of production of albumin. It has been shown that this low level of albumin is caused by impaired synthesis and not by reduced elimination. The nucleolus of the cell, where the synthesis of ribosomal RNA takes place, is extremely sensitive to any changes in the nutrition. In fasting, the size of the nucleolus can decrease and if the animal is provided with sufficient nutrition the size can double within 3 hours. A deficiency of amino acids, especially tryptophane, will permit ribosomal disaggregation, while on the other hand, excess tryptophane, arginine, as well as ornithine, result in a reaggregation of the polysome and a stimulus to albumin synthesis in liver perfusion experiments, where livers from fasted donors are studied.

The level of albumin drops in clinical conditions of poor nutrition and starvation. In the case of kwashiorkor, this level drops to under 100 mg/kg body weight daily. In children who have been poorly nourished and who have a low intake of protein, values of albumin synthesis of 100–148 mg/kg body weight have been recorded as opposed to values of 200–223 mg/kg body weight in well nourished children.

If the diet is deficient in protein, addition of arginine and lysine produce no marked effects on the growth. However, this becomes normal if a balanced diet is provided.

Our understanding of the role played by nutrition in the synthesis of albumin is still incomplete and, as such, requires further clinical and experimental work.

Hormone balance

Hormones, particularly thyroid hormones and those originating in the cortex of the adrenal gland, have a specific effect on the protein metabolism of the cell. Removal of the hypophysis or the thyroid glands causes a decrease in the concentration of ribosomal RNA, indicating that such operations affect the synthesis of this RNA. In patients having myxoedema, low levels of the relative and absolute synthesis of albumin, corresponding to 1.9 per cent of the total pool of this protein, have been observed. An increase in the relative and absolute rates of breakdown and synthesis of albumin have been recorded in Cushing's syndrome as well as in conditions of stress where there is a high production of endogenic cortisol. The administration of cortisol has been shown to produce an increase in the synthesis of albumin by 50 per cent.

Changes in the colloid osmotic pressure of plasma

Several reports have appeared suggesting that there exists a connection between the colloid osmosis in plasma and the synthesis of albumin. It would appear that hypoalbuminaemia is of less importance in this connection. The rate of synthesis and breakdown was decreased in patients showing hypoalbuminaemia but this effect was secondary to the increased loss of this protein via the kidneys. Björneboe and co-workers have observed that the concentration of albumin decreased after administration of dextran or after hyperimmunization or globulin infusion, suggesting that the production of albumin is sensitive to changes in the colloid osmotic pressure. In these experiments, no change was observed in this osmotic pressure in plasma, but the changes in the synthesis of albumin were shown to be inversely proportional to the extravascular albumin as opposed to the intravascular albumin. The concentration of extravascular albumin was found to be very low (110 mg/kg of liver) in rats showing an extremely high rate of synthesis of albumin. On the other hand, the infusion of dextran into rabbits gave rise to very high levels of extravascular albumin, 520 mg/kg in liver, while the synthesis of the protein was drastically reduced.

Under normal conditions, the concentration of extravascular albumin is very low, providing a very sensitive means of regulating the synthesis of this protein. In addition, experiments using plasma electrophoresis have shown the presence of increased synthesis when the extravascular pool was reduced. The above experiments, when taken together, indicate that if the production of albumin is steered by the osmotic activity, then this mechanism is localized by and large to the extravascular pool. However, no direct correlation has been demonstrated to exist between the synthesis and the breakdown of albumin.

Temperature

It is believed that changes in the surrounding temperature can even play a role in the synthesis. A reduction in the level of albumin and a corresponding increase in the immunoglobulin fraction can appear in individuals who live for a considerable period in tropical climates. A 62 per cent decrease in the synthesis of albumin was observed in rabbits which were exposed to high temperatures for a shorter period of time. This reduction in synthesis can be explained as being due partially to a reduction in the activity of the thyroid gland and partially to a lower intake of food. Changes in albumin synthesis due to exposure to the cold have not been demonstrated.

Stress and trauma

Stress caused by a variety of factors results in changes in albumin synthesis. A doubling of the synthesis has been measured in connection with removal of part of the liver or injection of toxins. Such an injection of endotoxin causes a 60 per cent increase in this synthesis. An increased breakdown and distribution of albumin arise in connection with burns. Just how this increase is brought about is not completely understood. While the cause of the increased synthesis in connection with stress is not known, it is probable that corticosteroids are a contributing factor. The effect can be caused by increased mobilization of extrahepatic amino acids, stimulation of the production of

RNA in the liver, and changes in the ribosomal function of the cell. No specific factor affecting the synthesis of albumin has been shown.

6. Distribution of albumin

The flow of fluid through the capillaries is related in part to the intra- and extravascular distribution of albumin. Following the intravenous injection of albumin, a period of 10–15 minutes is required for a complete intravenous distribution of the protein. During the first 3 minutes following the injection of ^{131}I-albumin, the plasma in the spleen, liver, and heart has a higher concentration of this protein than does the blood plasma after complete distribution has been attained. The concentration in the plasma in the arms and legs is lower even after the elapse of 6 minutes. Thus, the distribution is determined by the blood flow to the different organs.

The space available to the albumin molecule in blood is 1–3 per cent higher than for other large molecules. The latter molecules display also a slower rate of exchange across the capillaries. Larger molecules have an excluding volume, i.e. they can be bound to a liquid environment which is available to other large molecules. It is possible that fibrinogen and albumin do not have the same space available for distribution within the water content of plasma.

During the first few minutes following an injection of albumin, only a minute portion of this protein travels over to the extravascular pool.

According to Reeve and Chen (1970), the extravascular distribution of albumin and other proteins is related primarily to the inflow and outflow from the extravascular plasma pool. A remarkably constant concentration of interstitial albumin exists despite the fact that the capillary transport increases drastically and the flow of lymph is changed 10 or more times.

Two-thirds of the plasma pool of protein can be lost daily via the *ductus thoracicus*. Thus, lymph is the most important factor determining the retransport of protein from the interstitial space to blood. Only a very small quantity can pass between the endothelial cells of the capillaries as these are normally packed tightly together. The endothelium contains small vesicles (maximum size 10 μm) which can transport fluid by pinocytosis. These vesicles, which can vary in size, are normally completely or partially enclosed in a thin membrane. It is probable that the pores contain a complex gel of macromolecules which can exclude even other larger molecules.

Variations in the size of the pores and the composition of the interstitial matrix may constitute a mechanism for the regulation of albumin distribution. The extravascular distribution of different proteins is dependent on the size of these molecules. Fibrinogen and IgG, 10–20 per cent and 50 per cent respectively, are localized extravascularly. The distribution of still larger molecules is even more restricted.

Because of its high colloid osmotic pressure, albumin is of considerable importance in regulating the volume of the interstitial fluid.

Following the intravenous administration of ^{131}I-albumin to an individual, an equilibrium is set up between the intra- and extravascular pool within a period of one week. Most of the injected protein reaches a state of equilibrium very quickly, but a slow exchange takes place in certain tissue such as skin and muscle. Two days is required for an exchange of 80–90 per cent of the albumin, while the remainder is exchanged at a slower rate. When a state of complete equilibration has been attained,

35–40 per cent of the protein is to be found in the intravascular pool while the remainder is present in the extravascular space of the various tissues. The exchange of albumin takes place at different rates; visceral albumin is in equilibrium with plasma within a period of a few hours, while skin and muscle require days before an equilibrium is attained.

The concentration of albumin in the lymph varies according to which area is drained. The amount of albumin found in the lymph in *ductus thoracicus* is 40–80 per cent of that found in plasma. The corresponding value for the lymph which comes direct from the liver is 80–95 per cent. It has been shown that the sinusoids of the liver are almost independent of molecules having molecular weights up to 250 000. The exchange between lymph, sinusoids of the liver, and plasma is very quick. On the other hand, the concentration of albumin in the interstitial space of the liver is less than 3 g/l.

Even the lungs have a high specific requirement for albumin, but the extravascular space which is available to albumin in this organ is small.

If the plasma space is expressed in wet weight, then the lungs and liver have the largest plasma space while the brain and skin have the smallest volume. The distribution of albumin in the plasma of the kidney is approximately 10 per cent of the wet weight.

The skin has a very high concentration of extracellular albumin and contains more than half of the extravascular pool of albumin. The reason for this high value is unknown but it may be that the high level of albumin is correlated to the function of skin in the transport of water.

Albumin is the most important protein component of oedema fluid. This protein can appear in concentrations lower than 5–10 g/l in oedema fluid from patients suffering from heart insufficience, malfunction of the kidney, liver cirrhosis, pericarditis, and venous stasis. In oedema due to burns or following allergic manifestations, values greater than 20 g/l can be detected.

In ascites fluid caused by heart insufficiency, liver cirrhosis, or nephrosis, the concentration of albumin can often be greater than 10 g/l while in that arising from infection or chemical irritation considerably higher values appear, especially when the level of albumin in the plasma is normal.

Exudate in pleura contains substantial amounts of albumin. Albumin occurs also normally in smaller amounts in bronchial secretion. In oedema of the lungs, these levels of albumin increase dramatically.

Albumin exists even in gastric juice, perspiration, and amnion fluid. In humans, albumin is transferred directly to the foetus and this process begins three months after conception.

7. Breakdown of albumin

Neither the site of breakdown nor the factors affecting it are particularly well understood.

The breakdown of ^{131}I-albumin which is injected into the interstitial fluid of muscle or skin does not take place until an equilibrium has been established between it and the plasma space.

Those serum proteins which are completely distributed within the intravascular pool have a high rate of breakdown. This breakdown takes place in close connection to the intravascular pool. It is unlikely that a specific organ exists for the breakdown of all plasma proteins. There is experimental evidence indicating that the breakdown does not take place in either the plasma pool or the extravascular pool.

It is important to distinguish between the absolute and relative breakdown when measuring the breakdown of albumin.

In cases of low serum concentration, after infusion of dextran or an increase in the concentration of globulins, the relative breakdown is unchanged while the absolute breakdown is drastically reduced. In malnutrition, nephrosis, and liver cirrhosis, where the level of albumin in serum is greatly reduced, the absolute breakdown of albumin is also greatly reduced while the relative breakdown is often increased. The low absolute breakdown of albumin appears to be correlated to the low plasma level. This arises later than the reduction of synthesis. In cases of normal levels of albumin, infusion of this protein results in an increase in both the relative and absolute breakdown.

The site of breakdown of albumin has not been precisely located (Fig. 25). It has not been possible to register any significant breakdown in the liver. On the other hand, it has been shown that albumin can be catabolized by mitochondria preparations from liver, indicating that there may exist a certain potential catabolic reaction in liver.

The importance of the reticuloendothelial system in the breakdown of albumin is uncertain. One interesting observation is that an injection of a colloidal suspension of carbon into rats caused a rapid drop in the concentration of albumin in the serum while the breakdown of albumin increased.

Just as in liver, no normal catabolism of albumin has been detected in the kidney. On the other hand, large quantities of this protein can leak from the interstitial space to the tubules in nephrosis. In this condition, an increased breakdown of albumin takes place in the kidney. This effect has been demonstrated in rats. The catabolism increases when the albumin in the urine exceeds 40–50 mg/h/kg body weight.

It has been concluded by several authors that the gastrointestinal tract is that system of organs where the major part of the normal catabolism takes place. Certain difficulties have stood in the way of attempts to obtain quantitative results. Serum proteins are found normally in the intestines and stomach, thus, after the intravenous injection of radioactive albumin, radioactivity can be found after a few minutes localized in the mucosal layer. However, no great loss of radioactivity via faeces could be detected after injection with ^{51}Cr-albumin, ^{59}Fe-dextran or ^{131}I-PVP. These experiments have shown that a part of the breakdown of albumin can take place in the stomach and intestines. The validity of these methods has been discussed critically by Wetterfors.

Most workers in the field are in agreement with the proposal that the gastrointestinal tract plays a part in the breakdown of albumin. However, there is disagreement as to the magnitude of this breakdown. By simultaneously using ^{125}I- and ^{51}Cr-albumin, it has been established that at least 25 per cent of the daily absolute endogenous catabolism is caused by these organs to give rise to a loss of radioactivity via the faeces. The group of workers in Stockholm believe that the major part of the breakdown follows this course. In certain malfunctions of the gastrointestinal tract, there appears to be a drastic increase in the leakage of albumin. This is discussed later.

In connection with the breakdown in the case of altered capillaries and an altered lymphatic circulation, there is every reason to suppose that the normal barrier has been altered. In such cases, loss via the faeces is increased. The loss of albumin is also increased in situations where the drainage of lymph is partially blocked.

It is not impossible that a certain amount of the catabolism takes place in different parts of the organism, but the large surface area presented by the intestines would lead one to believe that this is the region where a large portion of the breakdown takes place. So that the protein can be broken down, it must come into contact with proteolytic enzymes in the cell or in the intestines. This implies that newly synthesized protein, which exists within the cell, is protected against the action of enzymes. The relationship between the breakdown of albumin and its concentration indicates that the system which regulates this breakdown can react very quickly to changes in its environment. The factors which start this system are, as yet, unknown.

8. Albumin in illness—clinical and therapeutical points of view

Hyperalbuminaemia appears only in cases of acute dehydration. The causes of hypoalbuminaemia are listed in Table 5. These can be grouped under the following headings:

1. Reduced synthesis.
2. Increased catabolism.
3. Abnormal loss.
4. Pathological distribution.

Table 5. Causes of hypoalbuminaemia

Reduced synthesis
Insufficient supply
Defective digestion
Impaired absorption
Liver lesions
Hereditary albuminaemia

Abnormal losses
Shock
Bleeding
Losses through the kidneys
Losses through the gastrointestinal tract
Losses through the skin
Exudate–transudate

Increased catabolism
Hypercortisonism
Hyperthyroidism
Infections
Malignant tumours
Trauma

Pathological distribution
Peritoneal carcinosis
Burns
Postoperatively
After high therapeutic doses of ionizing radiation to the abdomen.

Reduced synthesis

a. Cirrhosis of the liver. Low levels of albumin in serum appears in patients having cirrhosis of the liver (with or without ascites). However, the total pool of albumin remains unchanged in one-third to one-half of the cases. Thus, the low level of albumin is more a reflection of a change in the distribution. Patients having ascites show a very large extra pool of albumin in the ascites fluid. This albumin is exchanged only very slowly with plasma. A continuous loss of albumin to the ascitic pool takes place in patients showing advanced ascites. It has been shown that the synthesis of albumin can become normal and may even exceed the normal of patients having liver cirrhosis who abstain from alcohol and are provided with adequate nutrition. Such a treatment of 19 patients, several of whom had marked ascites and signs of portalhypertension, resulted in an increased or normal synthesis of albumin in 13 of the cases. While hypoalbuminaemia is common in cirrhosis, the synthesis can be normal, low, or even increased. However, the relative synthesis is low in cirrhosis of the liver, in agreement with the low level of albumin. The increased synthesis and the reduced catabolism tend to increase the level of albumin in such conditions. The onset of an infection can lead often to a reduced synthesis, which can effect the hypoalbuminaemia.

b. Malnutrition. A second important cause of a reduced synthesis is insufficient intake of amino acids via the food. This can arise in malnutrition or in various kinds of malabsorption. The extravascular albumin and the proteins in muscle are used primarily as a source of protein. This gives rise to loss of weight and repeated hypoalbuminaemia. In poorly nourished children, the relative breakdown is reduced and the synthesis of albumin is lower than normal. The reduction in breakdown arises only after a reduction in the level of albumin. The level of albumin in serum is maintained by a redistribution of the protein from the extravascular pool to the intravascular pool. The enzymes responsible for the activation of amino acids in the liver are increased, while the enzymes of the urea cycle are reduced in malnutrition but not in starvation. In the latter condition, irrespective of the aetiology, another homeostatic factor is at play. This factor has the potential to alter the *in vivo* synthesis of albumin. The level of corticosteroids can be increased, possibly as a consequence of the reduced breakdown, and the level of thyroid hormone drops. While there is no detailed information available concerning the level of growth hormone, it is not unlikely that this is also affected. It is probable that the reduction in the synthesis of albumin is regulated by several of those factors which have been discussed previously.

Increased catabolism

This implies that the catabolism exceeds the value of 7–9 percent for the intravascular pool. This can of course give rise to hypoalbuminaemia in the case where the catabolism exceeds the liver's capacity for synthesis. It is known that this capacity of the liver can increase 2–3 times. A combination of increased catabolism with reduced synthesis can arise in, for example, malabsorption. As can be seen in Table 5, an increased catabolism of albumin can appear in a variety of illnesses such as infection, trauma, and in certain endocrinic conditions such as hypercortisonism, Cushing's syndrome, and hyperthyroidism.

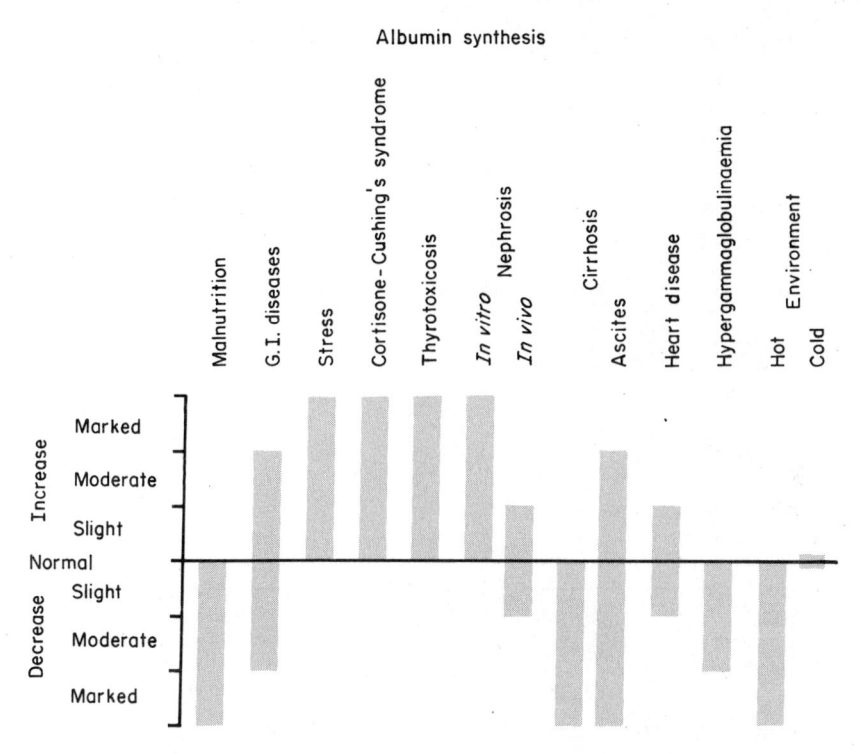

Fig. 24. The synthesis of albumin in some clinical conditions showing hypoalbuminaemia

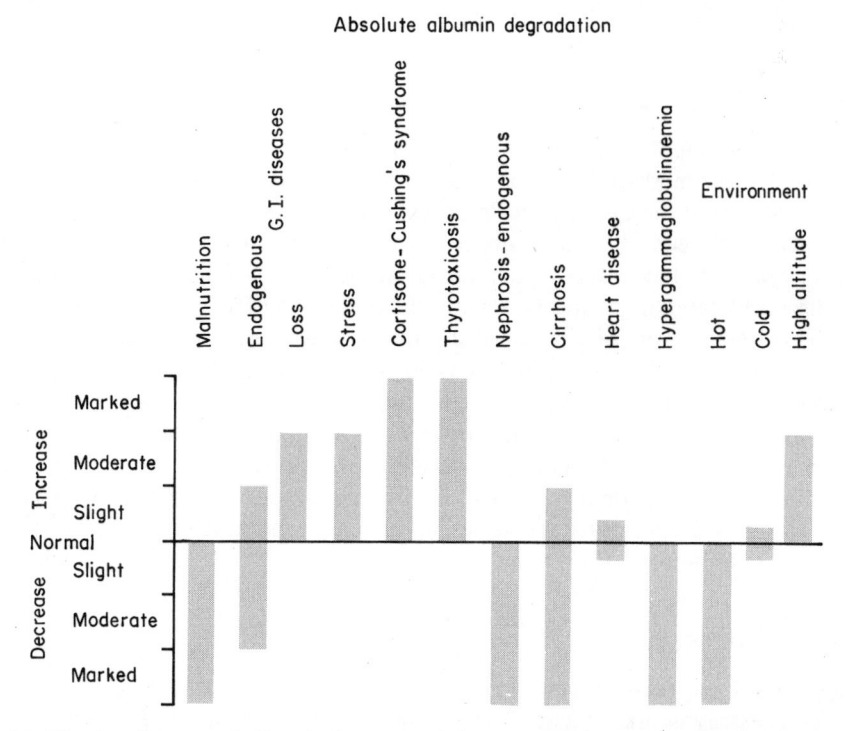

Fig. 25. The breakdown of albumin in some clinical conditions showing hypoalbuminaemia

66 *Transport proteins*

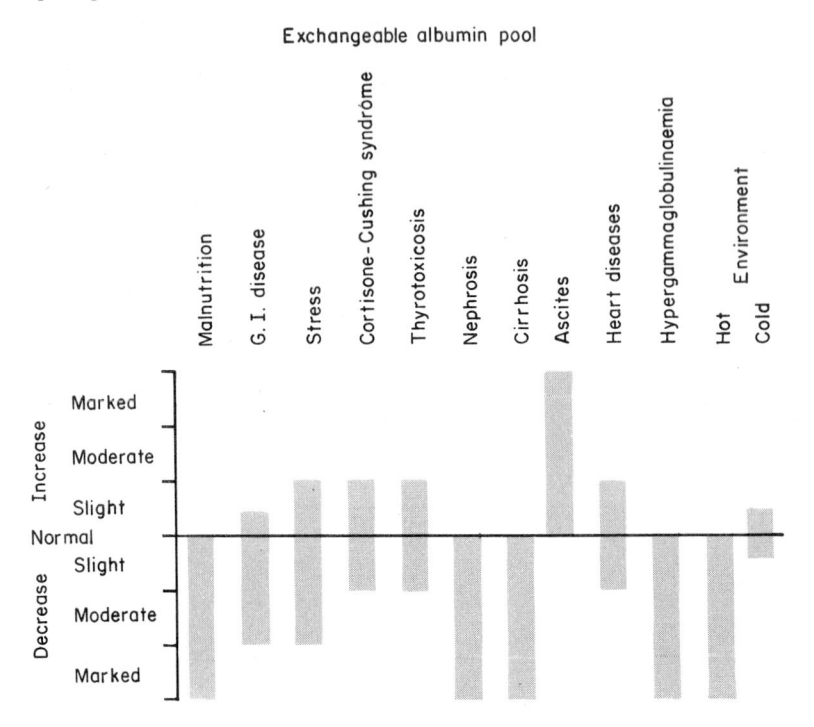

Fig. 26. Comparison of the extravascular and intravascular quota of albumin in some clinical conditions

Abnormal loss

Abnormal loss of albumin can arise in various conditions and from various organs. In several illnesses, an increased loss via the gastrointestinal tract has been observed. If the leakage occurs in the upper portion of this canal, the protein is broken down into amino acids which can then be reabsorbed. Despite the fact that the endogenous catabolism can be reduced, this can result in an increased total loss of albumin. This will be discussed later in connection with gastroenteropathy which shows a loss of protein. Increased leakage of albumin distal in the intestine gives rise to direct loss of albumin via the faeces. This loss can take place in a variety of other ways. A very small loss of albumin from the kidneys can arise but in certain renal conditions, especially the nephrotic symdrome, these losses can be large. This often gives rise to hypovolaemic oedema. Significant losses of albumin in severe nephrosis have also been observed via the intestines. This is probably caused by interstitial oedema of the walls of the intestine. Exfoliative dermatitis and especially extensive burns cause very large losses of albumin via the injured skin.

Pathological distribution

In many conditions, there arises a redistribution of albumin from the intravascular space to the extravascular space. This is characterized primarily by increased permeability of the capillaries. This can appear for example in peritoneal carcinosis with ascites, extensive burns, postoperative in the region of a wound, and following excessive treatment with ionized radiation, especially if the intestines have been exposed to the treatment. Using isotopic methods, it has been shown that at least one plasma pool of albumin is redistributed extravascularly during the first 48 hours following adequate treatment of extensive burns.

9. Special conditions of hypoalbuminaemia

Heart diseases

The part played by albumin in the appearance of cardial oedema has been a subject of study for a long time. In ten cases of heart insufficiency, both the synthesis and breakdown of albumin were unchanged when compared with a control group. The total pool in both groups was approximately 200–300 mg/kg body weight per day. Furthermore, the total pool of exchangeable albumin was not reduced and the small changes observed in the level of albumin were caused probably by alterations in the distribution of protein between the intra- and extravascular pools.

In five patients suffering from constrictive pericarditis, the level and breakdown of albumin were seen to vary between 13–50 g/l and 139–356 mg/kg body weight per day, respectively. A pronounced loss of albumin via the intestines was observed in these cases. No decrease in the synthesis could be observed and the pool of albumin was found to have increased in three of the five cases which were studied. While no effects on the metabolism of albumin have been observed to be produced by heart conditions as such, it is clear that these can act as complicating factors.

Gastroenteropathies with loss of protein

Gastrointestinal illnesses showing a loss of albumin have been studied intensively during the last ten years. These illnesses can be connected eventually with loss of immunoglobulin. The various conditions which can give rise to a loss of protein via the gastrointestinal tract are presented in Tables 6 and 7.

a. The stomach. It is known that a moderate leakage of albumin does not necessarily cause hypoalbuminaemia if the liver is intact and capable of increasing its normal synthesis by a factor of at least two.

While the various illnesses involving increased leakage will not be discussed in detail, some characteristic features are described below. *Hypertrophic gastritis* can give rise to a leakage of both albumin and IgG. A moderate treatment is usually sufficient but in exceptional cases subtotal gastrectomy must be considered. It is unclear if polyposis in the stomach, where individual polyps occur, can give rise to loss of albumin. This is especially unclear in the case of solitary polyps. In the only published case of such a leakage, the patient had also areas of malignant degeneration. Thus, it is not clear if the hypoalbuminaemia in this case was caused by an increased leakage.

Cancer of the stomach is often connected with hypoalbuminaemia. It is obvious that the most important cause of this is the increased leakage which occurs most probably from the malignant tumour. It is possible that a certain amount of toxic effect from the

Table 6. Diseases attended with gastrointestinal leakage of protein. Birke et al., 1968

Stomach
Hypertrophic gastritis
Menetrier's disease
Atrophic gastritis
Eosinophilic granuloma
Distal stenosis of the stomach
Cancer of the stomach
Postgastrectomy syndrome
Postoperative gastric retention

Small intestine
Sprue (gluten-induced or idiopathic)
Jejuno-ileitis
Idiopathic exudative enteropathy
Whipple's disease
Intestinal lymphangiectasis
Lymphogranulomatosis and lymphosarcoma of the intestine
Eosinophilic granuloma
Amyloidosis
Jejunal deverticulitis
Intestinal stenosis (blind-loop syndrome)
Regional ileitis (Crohn's disease)
Some parasitic diseases
Some vascular malformations
Lympho-intestinal fistulas.

Large intestine
Ulcerative colitis
Cancer of the colon
Hirschsprung's disease

liver can contribute to a reduced synthesis which, in addition, intensifies the hypoalbuminaemia and increases the extravascular distribution of albumin.

Distal stenosis in the stomach gives rise to hypoalbuminaemia because of increased leakage in this organ.

Postgastrectomy syndrome, which gives rise to anorexia, steatorrhoea, malabsorption, and hypoproteinaemia (especially hypoalbuminaemia), has been shown to be caused by both reduced synthesis in the liver and increased leakage of albumin.

b. *The small intestine.* In gluten induced sprue, where gliadin has been eliminated from the diet, there appears most often a dramatic remission with reduced leakage and increased concentration of albumin.

Table 7. Other conditions attended with gastrointestinal leakage of protein. Birke et al., 1968

Agammaglobulinaemia
Constrictive pericarditis
Nephrotic syndrome
Ionizing radiation to the abdomen

Jejuno ileitis which has sufficiently long duration, is connected with hypoalbuminaemia. In such cases, we have a two to three fold increase in the intestinal leakage above the normal.

Hypoalbuminaemia together with agammaglobulinaemia is not infrequently linked to increased leakage of albumin and IgG in the small intestine. In the case of the diverticula of the jejunum, it is not clear if a true leakage of protein takes place from the diverticula. Only a few cases of this have been studied. Chronic intestinal stenosis including 'the blind-loop syndrome', gives rise to hypoproteinaemia which is dependent on both malabsorption and a pathological leakage of albumin. A series of factors, which can cause pathological intestinal flora, can result in increased leakage. These conditions can often be improved and normalized by surgical correction.

Regional ileitis, irrespective of the location, is not infrequently linked to hypoalbuminaemia. This is due to the increased leakage of albumin from the affected region of the intestine.

c. The large intestine. In patients having ulcerative colitis, albumin leaks through the pathologically changed wall in the large intestine and is lost via the faeces. This loss of protein increases if the condition becomes acute. It is recommended that the hypoalbuminaemia be corrected before surgical intervention is used in these cases. In some cases, the leakage of IgG is also considerable and necessitates treatment with satisfactory protein.

Exposure of the abdomen to ionized radiation can cause a leakage of protein, which is accentuated with increasing doses. In this connection, the small intestine is particularly sensitive. This leakage can be so profound that hypoalbuminaemia arises during the treatment. It can also happen that the leakage of IgG is so widespread that hypogammaglobulinaemia can arise.

10. Treatment with albumin

The indications for albumin therapy are given in Table 8, grouped under three headings: clear indications, relative, and doubtful. Without discussing the individual illnesses or syndromes, we wish to state that those patients who show signs of any of the conditions listed under 'clear indications', should be given albumin therapy. Albumin therapy can be of use in the group, 'relative indications', but is not absolutely indicated. Many of these conditions of deficiency respond satisfactorily to other forms of treatment.

In the case of cirrhosis of the liver, for example, the best results are obtained by treating with duretics. Under the heading, 'doubtful indications', we have collected together the conditions where previous authors have suggested albumin therapy to be valuable, but which we doubt to be of use. However, this does not mean that albumin therapy may prove helpful in any particular case. Better results are quite often obtained by using another form of treatment. In amino acid deficiency caused by, for example, defective digestion, amino acid therapy is of course indicated for several reasons.

This treatment is much preferred to albumin therapy. Treatment with a high protein and caloric diet is usually sufficient in malnutrition. It should be stressed that albumin is no substitute for adequate nutrition and should not be used to replace adequate parental nutrition.

Table 8. Indications for albumin therapy, Birke et al., 1968

Clear
Nephrotic syndrome (exacerbation with hypovolaemia)
Hypovolaemic shock
Burns and exfoliative dermatitis
Acute phase of gastrointestinal leakage of protein
Extracorporal circulation

Relative
Uncompensated liver cirrhosis
Chronic phase of gastrointestinal leakage of protein in sprue; postgastrectomy syndrome
Preoperatively in hypoalbuminaemia
Pathological distribution
After high therapeutic doses of ionizing radiation to the abdomen
Hypoalbuminaemia in acute postoperative phase

Doubtful
Coma and hepatic pre-coma
Nephrotic syndrome (chronic phase)
Chronic internal-medical diseases attended with hypoalbuminaemia; malabsorption, malnutrition, hypercatabolism
Pancreatic insufficiency
Starvation, late postoperative phase

Many clinical conditions are linked to moderate hypoalbuminaemia which can sometimes appear in conjunction with an increase in IgG. Most of these conditions do not require any special treatment to correct the hypoalbuminaemia. This is particularly true of the more advanced common chronic conditions.

Other chronic and postoperative illnesses can be linked with a pronounced hypoalbuminaemia which is often caused by inadequate administration of protein and calories. This usually leads to a defective synthesis rather than to an increased metabolism or increased loss. The deficiency of calories and amino acids is the most essential factor. On the administration of albumin, plasma, or whole blood, the protein must first be broken down to polypeptides and amino acids before it can be used again in the general synthesis of protein.

This is an indication of the need to supply the body with ample amino acids and calories in order to build up its store of protein. However, it should be kept in mind that even if administration of amino acids is warranted, the liver can not always carry out its synthesis of albumin sufficiently rapidly. The maximum rate of synthesis can be taken as 20–30 g/day. In acute conditions where the intravascular pool is low, it is important that the patient is provided initially with sufficient albumin. Such a situation is that prior to operation. In a less serious phase, the patient should be provided with amino acids and calories.

Burns are a typical example of a complex situation where the synthesis, breakdown, and distribution are affected. Here, there is an initial loss of protein and no matter how adequate the treatment with amino acids, the protein concentration is initially very low. Such patients should be given large doses of plasma and albumin after the first 24 hours and, thereafter, various measures should be taken to build up the patients' protein depots.

During certain phases of conditions showing a loss of albumin, the use of albumin therapy over different lengths of time can be necessary. Such conditions are gastroenteropathy involving loss of protein, the nephrotic syndrome, and in certain selected cases of reduced synthesis, e.g. in cirrhosis of the liver.

It should be emphasized that direct measures should be taken against the primary illness. Certain illnesses are suited to surgical treatment while others are best treated by internal medicine. Unfortunately, there does not exist any causal therapy for those cases showing leakage of albumin. With this in mind, one of the most important lines of research should be the study of factors affecting the permeability of the capillaries in both acute conditions and chronic alterations.

C. Organ storage by continuous albumin perfusion
GÖRAN CLAES

One of the most important factors within transplantation surgery is the preservation of viability in a removed organ until transplantation is possible. A high degree of viability is a prerequisite for a successful transplantation. In this matter the greatest problems are those concerning kidneys removed from cadavers where the matching of tissues, the selection of a suitable recipient, and also the transportation and preparation of the recipient often take a great deal of time. The method which has produced the best results in the matter of long-term (24–48 hours) storage of kidneys for transplantation purposes is continuous hypothermal perfusion. This method involves the perfusion, via the artery, of the kidney with a fluid which is chilled to approximately 8°C. The fluid is oxygenated by direct surface oxygenation: by this means the oxygen pressure appropriate in the fluid is PO_2 300 mm Hg. The perfusion fluid is buffered to a PH between 7.0 and 7.2 measured at 37°C. The perfusion liquid is pumped into the kidney with a pulsatory flow at a systolic pressure of 60 mm Hg. There is a special type of apparatus commercially available for this kind of organ storage (Gambro P F 3 A). The apparatus runs on batteries and can be transported between different transplantation centres.

The fluid which has shown itself to be most suitable for continuous hypothermal perfusion is albumin at a concentration of 4.5 per cent: 500 ml of fluid which will circulate in the apparatus, is used for each perfusion. Potassium, magnesium, glucose, cortisone, and penicillin are added to the albumin. The perfusion fluid serves partly as an oxygen transporter, and partly as a substrate for the kidney's metabolism. Of the albumin preparations commercially available the best perfusion results have been obtained with Kabi albumin. The reasons for this have not, as yet, been fully explained but it is assumed that they are due to the Kabi albumin's high concentration of short chain fatty acids, particularly caprylic acid which is consumed during perfusion.

With experiments carried out on dogs this method permits the storage of the kidney for up to 96 hours. After this time the kidney then immediately resumes its function after transplantation. With this technology it has been possible to store a pancreas for 24 hours. Nowadays this method is the routine storage method at a number of transplantation centres and it permits human kidneys to be stored for at least 48 hours. This makes possible the thorough examination and pretreatment of the intended recipient prior to operation, and it also means that the transplantation operation can be scheduled in the normal programme of operations during the day.

II. Plasma lipoproteins
ANDERS GUSTAFSON

A. Introduction and terminology

The lipids which are found in plasma—cholesterol, triglycerides, and phospholipids—are insoluble in water. In plasma, these lipids are transported together with specific proteins (apolipoproteins) as micellular or macromolecular *lipoproteins* (LP). It is generally accepted that LP are spherical particles (Fig. 27) which have a surface consisting of phospholipids, 'free' cholesterol, and protein (apolipoprotein), which encloses a 'nucleus' consisting of triglycerides and esters of cholesterol (page 74). Each component of LP has a characteristic density: triglyceride 0.9, cholesterol 1.0, phospholipid 1.0, and protein 1.3 g/ml. Internal variations in the relative amounts of the components of LP give rise to particles which have various densities and sizes. LP found in plasma can have a density of 0.92–1.21 g/ml. This variation in density gives rise to a spectrum of lipoprotein as depicted in Fig. 28. In this representation there are four classes of density, 'high density lipoproteins' (HDL), 'low density lipoproteins' (LDL), 'very low density lipoproteins' (VLDL), and the chylomicrons. Advantage can be taken of this difference in density when separating and isolating LP via ultracentrifugation (page 82).

The presence of protein on the surface of LP provides them with their electrical charge. A second terminology for LP is based on their electrophoretic mobility. In this system, HDL corresponds to α-LP (LP which migrates together with the α-globulins), LDL corresponds to β-LP (LP which migrates together with the β-globulins), and VLDL corresponds to pre-β-LP (LP having a greater mobility than the β-globulins). The chylomicrons remain at the origin. The three quantitatively dominating apolipo-

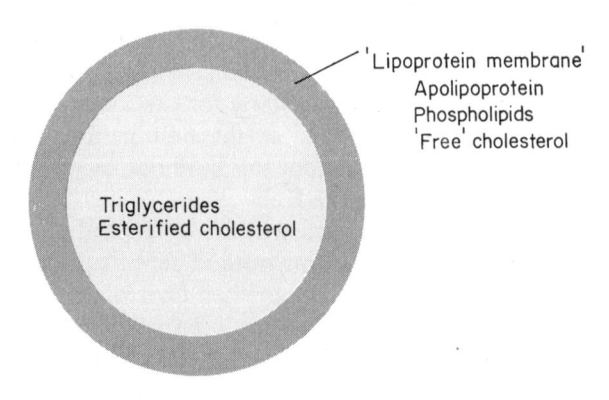

Fig. 27. Simplified picture of a plasma lipoprotein

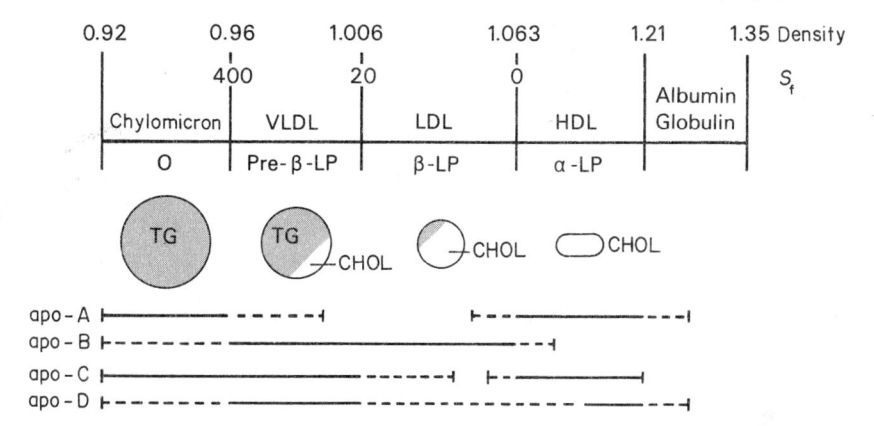

Fig. 28. The 'lipoprotein spectrum' showing the two terminologies for the plasma lipoproteins, the intervals of density, and S_f-values. The relationship between the density classes and the distribution of four apolipoproteins, apoA, apoB, apoC, and apoD is also shown. CHOL = cholesterol, TG = triglyceride

proteins, apoA, apoB, and apoC (page 80) determine the electrophoretic mobility of α-LP, β-LP, and pre-β-LP, respectively.

1. Plasma lipids—the lipid components in plasma lipoproteins. The lipids, cholesterol, triglycerides, and phospholipids, are always transported by plasma LP.

The triglycerides in plasma (normally 0.5–1.5 g/l) are transported primarily (60–70 per cent) by VLDL (pre-β-LP, Table 9). VLDL originates in the liver (page 84). The chylomicrons, which appear after a meal, contain triglycerides from the food and are formed in the mucous membrane of the intestine.

The normal level of cholesterol in plasma is 1.0–2.5 g/l and this is made up of 70 per cent LDL (β-LP), 25 per cent HDL (α-LP), and the remainder is VLDL (pre-β-LP). The plasma phospholipids, 0.75–1.1 g/l, are distributed equally between HDL and LDL with a small amount present in VLDL (Table 9).

Fatty acids, free fatty acids (FFA), and triglycerides. Fatty acids are present in cholesterol esters, triglycerides, phopholipids, and free fatty acids (FFA). Palmitic acid (16:0) and stearic acid (18:0) are saturated fatty acids, oleic acid (18:1, n-9) is monounsaturated and linoleic acid (18:2 n-6), linolenic acid (18:3, n-3), and arachidonic acid (20:4, n-6) are poly unsaturated fatty acids.

FFA are transported by albumin and to a lesser extent by plasma LP. The free fatty acids, FFA (depending on the earlier composition of the diet) are composed of palmitic acid (25 per cent), oleic acid (25 per cent), and variable amounts (15–25 per cent) of linoleic acid. FFA are released primarily on the hydrolysis of the triglycerides of adipose tissue and also on metabolism of chylomicrons and VLDL (page 87). The plasma level of FFA is normally 0.2–1.0 g/l and the half-life is 2 minutes.

Triglycerides are esters of glycerol. The triglycerides in human plasma form esters primarily with palmitic acid (25 per cent), oleic acid (37 per cent), and linoleic acid (16 per cent) and have an average molecular weight of 860.

Cholesterol in plasma exists in the free form (30 per cent) and as esters of cholesterol

Table 9. Approximate distribution of cholesterol (CHOL), phospholipid (PL), triglyceride (TG), and apolipoprotein (PR) in the various fractions of LP, during fasting with the level of cholesterol and triglycerides in plasma corresponding to 2.5 g/l and 1.0 g/l, respectively

LP-fraction (density class)	Electrophoretic synonym	S_f	Distribution (mg/l)			
			CHOL	PL	TG	PR
Chylomicrons	Origin	$S_f > 400$	≈0	≈0	≈0	≈0
VLDL	Pre-β-LP	S_f 20–400	2	2	6	1
LDL	β-LP	S_f 0–20	17	10	2.5	6
HDL	α-LP	—	6	9	1.5	8
Total			25	21	10	15

(70 per cent). In some cases e.g. LDL, the cholesterol is esterified with palmitic acid (12 per cent), oleic acid (20 per cent) but mostly with linoleic acid (50 per cent). Free cholesterol has a molecular weight of 387 and the average molecular weight of cholesterol esters in plasma is 648. The greater part of the formation of esters of cholesterol in plasma takes place in HDL via the enzyme lecithin-cholesterol-acyl-transferase (LCAT, page 88).

Like the phospholipids, cholesterol is an important constituent of the cells of different tissues. Cholesterol is the precursor of gonadotropic hormones and the hormones of the adrenal cortex. However, the transport of cholesterol is an expression of the continual exchange of this substance from various tissues. One prerequisite for this exchange is the capability of cholesterol to exist in free and esterified forms which have different properties.

The phospholipids of plasma LP are phosphoglycerides (80 per cent) and sphingomyelin (20 per cent). Lecithin (phosphatidyl-choline) constitutes 69 per cent of the phospholipids and of the remainder, 11 per cent is composed of cephalin (phosphatidyl-ethanolamine) and lysolecithin (lysol-phosphatidyl-choline). Sphingomyelin (26 per cent) is found characteristically in LDL while lysolecithin is found primarily in HDL–VHDL ($D > 1.063$ g/ml). The phospholipid in LP is bound more tightly to the protein portion of the molecule (apolipoprotein) than are the other lipids. It is usually found that the concentration of phospholipid is directly proportional to the level of cholesterol in plasma. Lecithin normally forms an ester with a saturated fatty acid (palmitic acid 30 per cent, stearic acid 14 per cent) in the 1-position and an unsaturated fatty acid (oleic acid 14 per cent, linoleic acid 29 per cent, arachidonic acid 7 per cent) in the 2-position.

B. Lipid metabolism

Free fatty acids (*FFA*). FFA are transported to the various tissues by albumin. Among other things, muscle and the heart can make use of FFA. Free fatty acids are metabolized in the peripheral tissues to provide energy. In the liver, FFA can form triglycerides as well as ketone bodies.

Triglycerides can be synthesized in the mucous membrane of the intestine from the triglycerides which are obtained from the food and are hydrolysed in the intestine. Synthesis can also take place in the liver (endogenic triglycerides) and in adipose tissue. The presence of fatty acids e.g. FFA and glycerol formed via the production of glycerophosphate from glucose, is a prerequisite for the synthesis of triglycerides.

In vivo experiments (Cahlin et al., 1973) have shown that administration of sugar to patients having hypertriglyceridaemia caused an increase in the synthesis of triglycerides in the liver.

Cholesterol is synthesized in the liver from acetyl–CoA via, among other things, mevalonate and squalene (Fig. 29). The steps in this synthesis which precede mevalonate are reversible. The rate of synthesis of cholesterol appears to be regulated by the enzyme, HMG-CoA-reductase. This enzyme catalyses a rate-determining step in the production of mevalonate from acetyl-CoA. The enzyme is controlled by hormonal, dietary, and heriditary factors.

A considerable amount of cholesterol is broken down in the liver to form bile acids which are then excreted with the bile. The primary bile acids, cholic acid and chenodeoxycholic acid, are reabsorbed by and large in the intestines after being conjugated and hydroxylated to form secondary bile acids. A smaller amount of bile acid leaves the body in the faeces. The bile acids return to the liver via *vena porta* in the so-called enterohepatic circulation (EHC).

The enzyme which catalyses the rate-limiting step in the breakdown of cholesterol, cholesterol-7-α-hydroxylase, is inhibited by bile acids which return to the liver via the EHC.

Phospholipids in plasma are synthesized in the liver as well as in the mucous cells of the intestine. The phospholipids which are synthesized in the liver can be divided into two pools, one which is in equilibrium with the phospholipids in bile and the other which is in equilibrium with the phospholipids in plasma LP.

Lecithin is synthesized in the liver, especially via two pathways. One of these, Kennedy's pathway, is quantitatively dominant and gives rise to lecithin with palmitic acid in the 1-position and either oleic acid or linoleic acid in the 2-position. The second

Acetyl-CoA
↓
HMG-CoA ← HMG-CoA-Reductase
↓
Mevalonate
↓
↓
Squalene
↓
Cholesterol
↓
7-α-Hydroxycholesterol ← 7-α-Hydroxylase
↓
Bile acids
Cholic acid
Chenodeoxycholic acid

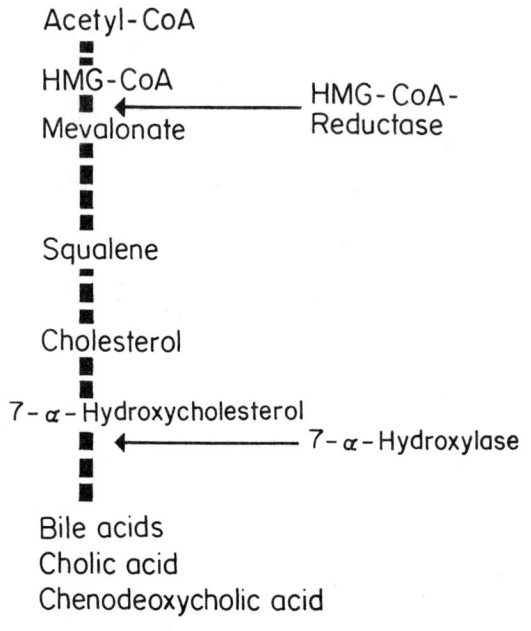

Fig. 29. Schematic representation of the synthesis and breakdown of cholesterol, showing the rate-determining step. HMG = β-Hydroxy-β-methyl-glutamic acid

pathway, that suggested by Greenberg, is quantitatively less significant and implies a methylation of ethanolamine in phosphatidyl-ethanolamine (cephalin). The lecithin which is synthesized by the second pathway has stearic acid in the 1-position and arachidonic acid in the 2-position. Both of these pathways for the synthesis of lecithin in liver are probably affected reciprocally.

Using slices of human liver, it has been shown *in vivo* that the administration of a diet having increased amounts of sugar caused a reduction in the synthesis of lecithin in patients having hypertriglyceridaemia (Cahlin *et al.*, 1973).

C. Lipoproteins in plasma

1. Chylomicrons

The name, chylomicrons, was suggested by Gage in 1920 for those blood particles which were observed via the dark-field microscope in persons who had been given a meal containing a high fat content. The word, chylomicron, signifies 'the microscopic blood corpuscle of lymph'. Chylomicrons are triglyceride-rich particles in lymph or plasma which have a flotation greater than S_f 400 and a diameter of 75 nm. These particles do not migrate when subjected to electrophoresis on paper or agarose, but can be separated by using starch gel electrophoresis where they migrate as primary and secondary particles with the same mobility as the α- and β-globulins. The fatty acid composition of the triglycerides obtained from plasma chylomicrons is the same as the fatty acid composition of the fat in the diet. Prior to reabsorption in the intestine, the triglycerides are cleaved primarily at the ester bond in the 1-position while the monoglyceride in the 2-position is left intact to become re-esterified in the mucous cells.

The amount of cholesterol in the chylomicrons varies between 6 per cent and 10 per cent. The chylomicrons of lymph contain esters of cholesterol. The proportion of cholesterol esters increases with increased cholesterol in the food. The amount of phospholipid in the chylimicrons varies between 4 per cent and 7 per cent. Just as with lecithin which is obtained from other sources, the lecithin obtained from the chylomicrons is esterified primarily with a saturated fatty acid (e.g. stearic acid) in the 1-position and an unsaturated fatty acid (e.g. linoleic acid) in the 2-position. In rats, up to 40 per cent of the lecithin in the chylomicrons originates from the dietary phospholipid.

The protein content of the chylomicrons varies between 1 per cent and 2 per cent where the chylomicrons in plasma have a higher content of protein than those of lymph. The chylomicrons of lymph take up protein from other LP on entering the bloodstream.

2. VLDL (pre-β-lipoproteins)

VLDL exists as a spectrum of particles having various sizes. The heterogeneity can be demonstrated by stepwise separation using ultracentrifugation. The molecular weights range from 6×10^6 to 27×10^6. As seen in the electron microscope, the particles are slightly flattened spheres having an average diameter of 32–80 nm.

As the size of the VLDL particles decreases, the triglyceride content decreases and the protein content increases from 5 per cent to 12 per cent. Under normal conditions, the major portion of VLDL exists as the subfraction VLDL-III (S_f 20–50) while in cases of hypertriglyceridaemia (hyperlipoproteinaemia types IV and II B), the relative proportions of subfractions VLDL-I and VLDL-II (S_f 50–400) increase (see Table 10). The proportion of free cholesterol is higher in VLDL than in LDL.

3. LDL (β-lipoproteins)

LDL is also heterogeneous and is usually divided into two subfractions, LDL_1 (S_f 18.8) and LDL_2 (S_f 7.0) at a density of 1.019 g/ml. As is the case with VLDL, as the S_f-value and LP-size decrease in LDL, the content of triglyceride decreases and the protein content increases from 16 per cent to 28 per cent (Table 10).

LDL is sensitive to freezing and looses its solubility on freezing and thawing. The addition of saccharose, glucose, and glycerol can partially prevent this occurrence. Auto-oxidation of LDL can also take place causing a change in its composition and solubility. This oxidation can be reduced by the addition of EDTA. LDL easily forms aggregates, explaining the variation in the earlier determinations of the particle weight.

An increased level of LDL and VLDL in plasma has been shown statistically to be connected to the appearance of atherosclerosis (Gofman et al., 1954) and in particular to the appearance of coronary heart disease (CHD) in men less than 55 years old (page 92).

4. HDL (α-lipoproteins)

Two density classes of LP are denoted by HDL. These are HDL_2 and HDL_3 which are separated at a density of 1.125 g/ml. The latter is quantitatively dominant and has a lower particle weight and a higher protein content than HDL_2. The particles of HDL take the form of an ellipsoid.

Table 10. Physical characteristics, density, S_f-value (or $S^0_{20,w}$-value), particle weight, and composition (in weight per cent) in 13 subfractions of the LP spectrum; chylomicrons (Gustafson et al., 1965), VLDL (Gustafson et al., 1965), LDL (Lee and Alaupovic, 1970) and HDL (Scanu et al., 1969)

LP	Density (g/ml)	$S^0_f (s^0_{20,w})$	Particle weight ($\times 10^6$)	CHOL	FL	TG	PR
Chylomicron I	0.93	>5 000	5 000	6	4	89	1
Chylomicron II	0.94	570	230	10	7	81	2
VLDL-I	0.96	112	27	15	12	68	5
VLDL-II	0.98	61.4	15	18	14	59	9
VLDL-III	0.99	29.7	6	18	13	57	12
LDL-I	1.006–1.009	18.8		31	22	31	16
LDL-II	1.009–1.019			38	23	20	19
LDL-III	1.019–1.030			45	23	10	22
LDL-IV	1.030–1.040	7.0	2.0–3.0	48	23	5	23
LDL-V	1.040–1.053			47	23	5	25
LDL-VI	1.053–1.063	—		45	22	5	28
HDL_2	1.063–1.125	4.8 ($s^0_{20,w}$)	0.36	27	29	11	33
HDL_3	1.125–1.21	5.0 ($s^0_{20,w}$)	0.17	15	20	8	57

HDL appears to be stable when stored at +4°C at an LP concentration of 5–10 mg/ml. The reciprocal relationship between the lipid components of the isolated HDL is very constant. Storing for a longer time at −10°C or over +60°C causes a destruction of the structure and a breakdown of the lipid–protein complex.

It has been shown statistically that the plasma of one person in every five contains sinking pre-β-LP (page 78) at a concentration of 0.2–0.8 g/l in the HDL which is isolated by ultracentrifugation at a density of 1.063–1.21 g/ml.

D. Abnormal lipoproteins (Table 11)

1. Lipoprotein X (LP-X)

These lipoproteins are in the density class 1.040–1.045 g/ml and migrate together with β-LP when subjected to electrophoresis. Their compositions are characterized by a low protein content, a high phospholipid content, and the presence of free cholesterol. When viewed in the electron microscope, the particles have a laminar structure. The apolipoprotein in LP-X consists of albumin (40 per cent), apoC (60 per cent), and traces of apoD (page 80).

The presence of LP-X in plasma has been demonstrated in cholestasis as well as in LCAT deficiency (page 93).

2. Sinking pre-β-LP, (SPB) Lp(a+)

The lipoprotein, Lp(a+), was shown by Berg (1963) to be a genetic variant of β-LP (LDL) and is found in the HDL class having density 1.050–1.080 g/ml. Lp(a+) reacts immunologically with monospecific antisera against β-Lp and Lp(a+). When subjected to electrophoresis, Lp(a+) migrates between pre-β-and β-LP. It has been shown recently that Lp(a+) is synonymous with the LP fraction which is called 'pre-β-1-LP' (Gustafson et al., 1975) and also with the LP fraction which is called sinking pre-β-LP (pre-β-HDL) (Ellefson et al., 1971; Rider et al., 1970).

SPB has a lipid–protein composition which is similar to that of LDL$_2$. The fatty acid composition of lecithin and the esters of cholesterol in SPB is identical with that in LDL (β-LP) (Gustafson et al., 1975).

The protein component of Lp(a+) consists of 'normal' apoB and a specific peptide fragment.

Table 11. Pathological LP. Physical characteristics and lipid–protein composition (in weight %) of LP-X, LP (a+), and 'floating β-LP'. Abbreviations as in Table 9

LP	Density g/ml	CHOL	PL	TG	RR	Ref
LP-X	1.040–1.045	25	66	3	6	Seidel, Alaupovic and Furman, 1969;
Pre-β-1-LP(Lp(a+))	1.050–1.080	48	21	6	25	Gustafson et al., 1975
Floating-β-LP	< 1.006	33	19	39	9	Quarfordt, Levy and Fredrickson, 1971

Depending on the technique used, the phenotype Lp(a+), preβ-1-LP and SPB can be demonstrated respectively by electrophoresis and immunological techniques in 20–80 per cent of the male white population. 'Pre-β-1-LP', identified by the technique of electrophoresis, appears more often in men who have experienced early coronary heart disease (Dahlen and Ericson, 1971).

3. Floating β-lipoproteins

Floating β-LP belongs to the VLDL class which has a density of less than 1.006 g/ml but which has an electrophoretic mobility which is the same as that of β-LP. The lipid-protein composition in floating β-LP is similar to that of a cholesterol-rich VLDL. When compared with 'normal' VLDL, floating β-LP contains a relatively high proportion of apoC and apoE.

The presence of floating β-LP can be detected in cases of hyperlipoproteinaemia type III but can also be found in individuals who show 'normal' levels of lipid in their plasma. Type III hyperlipoproteinaemia is present in the male population at a level of less than 1 per cent and is connected with the early appearance of atherosclerosis. For references in this connection, see Stanbury et al., 1972.

E. Lipoprotein families, apolipoproteins, and their polypeptides

All lipoprotein fractions belonging to the density classes VLDL, LDL, and HDL show heterogeneity. Subfractions within each class can be isolated and these show various lipid–protein compositions. The heterogeneity is caused by the presence of several *families of lipoproteins* within each density class. To date, five such families are known: LP-A, LP-B, LP-C, LP-D, and LP-E. (Alaupovic, 1972; Gustafson et al., 1974; Kostner and Holasek, 1972).

Each lipoprotein family is characterized by a specific protein, *apolipoprotein*. Thus, there are five apolipoproteins, one for each lipoprotein family: apolipoprotein A (apoA), apolipoprotein B (apoB), apolipoprotein C (apoC), apolipoprotein D (apoD), and apolipoprotein E (apoE).

In HDL (α-LP), apoA is dominant and determines the electrophoretic mobility of this LP. ApoB is the principal protein in LDL (β-LP). ApoC is found mainly in VLDL (pre-β-LP) and is believed to determine the electrophoretic mobility of this class (Fig. 28) LP-D and LP-E are less abundant. An apolipoprotein can be isolated by removing the lipid from an isolated LP family or by removing the lipid from a density class which contains several LP families and then separating the apolipoproteins.

Apolipoproteins consist of two or more *polypeptides*. These polypeptides are often designated by their carboxy-terminal (C-terminal) amino acid or by the numbering system: A-I, A-II, C-I, C-II, and C-III (Table 12). ApoD contains one characteristic polypeptide which is called, 'thin-line peptide' (Gustafson et al., 1974; Lee and Alaupovic, 1970) and apoE three separable by iso-electrofocusing.

ApoA consists of the polypeptides A-I (R-gln-I) and A-II (R-gln-II) which have molecular weights of 22 000 and 13 000 respectively. To date, only one common antigenic determinant has been found to exist on A-I and A-II. The amino acid composition of both of these polypeptides is known (Scanu, 1972). The amino acid

Transport proteins

Table 12. Physicochemical characteristics of the polypeptides of the apolipoproteins. Data taken from Alaupovic (1972), Kostner (1974), and Brown et al. (1970) among others

Apolipo-protein	Polypeptides	C-terminal	N-terminal	Molecular weight (approx.)	Function
ApoA	A-I	Glutamine	Aspartic acid	23 000	Activates LCAT
	A-II	Glutamine	'Blocked'	13 000	Inhibits LCAT
ApoD	'thin-line', A-III	Serine	—	20 000	
ApoB	B[a]	Serine	Glutamic acid	27 000	
ApoC	C-I	Serine[b]	Threonine	7 000	Activates liver LP-lipase
	C-II	Glutamic acid	Threonine	10 000	Activates adipose tissue LP-lipase
	C-III	Alanine	Serine	14 000	
ApoE	arginine-rich				

[a] Not isolated.   [b] Earlier given as valine.

sequence of A-II (Fig. 30) and C-III have been determined (Brewer et al., 1972a,b). The polypeptide, A-II, consists of two identical peptides which have 77 amino acid residues and are joined by a disulphide bridge at residue 6.

The polypeptides, A-I and A-II, are present primarily as the dominant polypeptides in HDL where their relative abundance is 3:1. They exist also in smaller amounts in the chylomicrons where they are present in equal amounts (Kostner and Holasek, 1972). Conditions have been described which display a change in this ratio in HDL (see 'Tangier's disease) and a deficiency of polypeptide A-I (see 'LP-A deficiency').

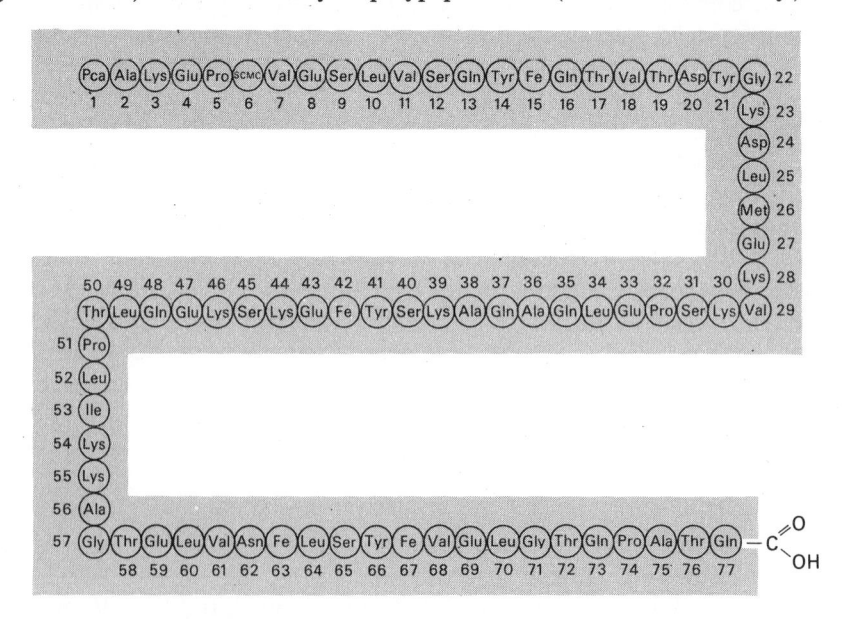

Pca = pyrrolidonecarboxylic acid

Fig. 30. The primary structure of reduced and carboxymethylated apoA-II (apo-Gln-II) (Brewer et al., 1972a)

II. Plasma lipoproteins

The polypeptide, A-I, is believed to have an important function in the activation of the enzyme, lecithin-cholesterol-acyl-transferase (LCAT) (Fielding, et al., 1972). ApoA is thought to function in the retransport of cholesterol from the 'periphery' to the liver (page 88).

LP-A was shown to possess two antigenic determinants. One of these, 'thick-line', is believed to arise from the common antigenic determinant of A-I and A-II. The other antigenic determinant of LP-A has been attributed to the fourth apolipoprotein, apoD (thin-line peptide). Because of its close relationship to A-I and A-II, apoD has also been designated as A-III (Kostner, 1974). This apolipoprotein has been isolated recently and its molecular weight, C-terminal amino acid (Table 12) and amino acid composition are known (Kostner, 1974). This apolipoprotein has been isolated in its lipoprotein form, LP-D, and has been shown then to contain high amounts of lysolocithin (Gustafson et al., 1974). It is believed that LP-D plays some role in the LCAT reaction.

LP-B and thus apoB is the dominating lipoprotein in LDL_2 (density 1.019–1.063) where it constitutes 90–95 per cent of the total amount of protein. Between 50 per cent and 60 per cent of the protein in VLDL and LDL_1 is LP-B (Alaupovic, 1972). ApoB constitutes 20 per cent of the protein in chylomicrons of lymph (Kostner and Holasek, 1972).

ApoB consists of two or more non-identical polypeptides. Lipid-free apoB and its polypeptides are highly insoluble in all solvents which have hitherto been investigated. For this reason, apoB has been studied in a modified form, e.g. in the presence of SDS (sodium dodecylsulphate).

LP-C is characteristic of the chylomicron family of lipoproteins and constitutes 65 per cent of the total protein in the chylomicrons of lymph and 35–40 per cent in plasma VLDL. It is also present in LDL (5–10 per cent of the apoprotein in LDL_2) and constitutes 8–14 per cent of the total protein in HDL (Alaupovic, 1972; Kostner and Holasek, 1972).

ApoC consists of three polypeptides, C-I (R-Ser), C-II (R-Glu), and C-III (R-Ala). These, like the other polypeptides, have been studied mainly after total removal of lipid, by using polyacrylamide electrophoresis in the presence of 8 mol/l urea. Two or three forms of C-III, C-III-0, C-III-1, and C-III-2, can be separated by this procedure. Each form has a characteristic sialic acid content but apart from this, all three forms are identical (Brown, et al., 1970).

The three polypeptides of apoC have been isolated and their molecular weights have been determined (Table 12). The C- and N-terminal amino acids have been identified (Table 12) and total amino acid composition is known (Brown, et al., 1970). Each of the polypeptide chains contains one antigenic determinant.

The polypeptides, C-I and C-II, are activators of their respective lipoprotein lipase (Ganesan et al., 1971). With the help of liver-LP lipase, C-I activates the substrate in the final stage of the hydrolysis of triglycerides in chylomicrons and VLDL. The polypeptide, C-II, functions in the hydrolysis of triglycerides which is mediated by the lipoprotein lipase of adipose tissue.

As yet, no conditions have been described where there is a deficiency of apoC or its polypeptides.*

Recently, apoE, 'arginine-rich polypeptide', was described. This was isolated from

---

* *Added in proof*: Cotto A.M. Jr: Apo-C-II deficiency: a new mutant. *N.Engl.J.Med.*, **298**, 1978, p. 1308.

VLDL obtained from patients who showed type III hyperlipoproteinaemia. Total amino acid composition of apoE has been reported (Havel and Kane, 1973).

F. Methods used in the study of plasma lipoproteins

1. Electrophoresis

Electrophoresis of lipoproteins is usually carried out on paper, agarose gel, or cellulose acetate and albumin is normally present in the electrophoresis buffer. The relative rates of migration of the four LP bands are the same in all of these media. It is worth mentioning here that the chylomicrons do not remain at the origin when cellulose acetate obtained from certain manufacturers is used. In all media and when large amounts of VLDL are present, tailing is obtained from pre-β-LP to the origin. When polyacrylamide gel is used, the order of migration of LP is different from that obtained when other media are used.

It is possible to quantitate the LP bands by using densitometry or by eluting the stained bands. Without a simultaneous quantitative determination of VLDL and LDL, the technique of electrophoresis is of little use. For practical purposes, it can be assumed that the triglycerides in plasma reflect directly the concentration of VLDL during periods of fasting (when there are no chylomicrons). This being the case, an increase in the plasma level of triglycerides implies an increased level of VLDL. The level of LDL in plasma can then be calculated if the level of cholesterol and triglyceride in plasma is known as well as the HDL cholesterol.

The technique of LP-electrophoresis is not sufficient to verify the presence of type III hyperlipoproteinaemia (floating β-LP).

2. Preparative ultracentrifugation

Plasma has a density of 1.006 g/ml. By subjecting plasma to ultracentrifugation for a short period of time, the chylomicrons can be made to accumulate at the surface of the sample of plasma. The same effect can be achieved by allowing the plasma to stand overnight in the cold. A longer time of ultracentrifugation at the density of plasma permits the isolation of VLDL. Various classes of lipoprotein can be isolated by adding salt (NaCl and KBr) to increase the density of the medium to a desirable level. LDL can be isolated at a density of 1.006–1.063 g/ml and HDL at a density of 1.063–1.21 g/ml (Fig. 28).

The LP isolated by preparative ultracentrifugation can be determined quantitatively by assaying one or more of the lipid components. This is most usually done by assaying cholesterol.

3. Methods of precipitation

In the presence of certain cations such as Mg^{++} and Mn^{++}, several sulphonated polymers such as heparin and dextran sulphate form complexes with LDL, VLDL, and chylomicrons. Such precipitation procedures give a sharp separation of these LP from HDL. By determining the amount of cholesterol in the supernatant obtained on precipitating with for example manganese chloride and heparin, the level of HDL can be determined. A separation of chylomicrons, VLDL, and LDL can be obtained by using other polymers in a variety of concentrations. One such polymer is polyvinylpyrrolidone (PVP).

4. Nephelometry

A rough estimation of the plasma level of triglyceride can be obtained by measuring the light scattering produced by the large triglyceride-rich LP, chylomicrons, and VLDL. Attempts have been made to determine the individual fraction quantitatively by using filters which have various pore size.

5. Immunochemical methods

Immunodiffusion (Mancini technique) and immunoelectrophoresis (rocket method) using monospecific antisera provide means of quantitatively determining the lipoprotein families in plasma and in the various density classes.

6. Quantification of LP

Monogram has been used to identify the various types of hyperlipoproteinaemia from a knowledge of the levels of cholesterol (CHOL) and triglyceride (TE) in plasma. The level of LDL can be determined more precisely if the amount of cholesterol in HDL is known: LDL-CHOL = plasma-CHOL−(plasma-TG/5 + HDL-CHOL).

This formula can be used in those cases where the level of triglyceride in plasma is less than 2.0 g/l and where the presence of type III hyperlipoproteinaemia has been ruled out.

G. Methods used in the study of LP families

The lipoprotein families, LP-A and LP-C, can be isolated from HDL. The HDL is first freed of all LDL and albumin by repeated ultracentrifugation. Any LP-B which remains in the preparation can be removed by immunoabsorption. Separation of LP-A and LP-C can be achieved by chromatography on hydroxyapatite or by fractionally precipitating the LP-A with 33 per cent polyethyleneglycol (Alaupovic, 1972). More recent studies* (Gustafson et al., 1974) have shown that the yields of LP-A and LP-C obtained on using this technique are dependent on the conditions used in the isolation of HDL. No 'release' of LP-A or LP-C is observed in the presence of a SH-blocking reagent such as DTNB. This suggests that the subdividing of HDL into lipoprotein families might be brought about by an enzymic reaction.

Attempts to isolate LP-A and LP-C in the pure form from VLDL and LDL by using similar chromatographic and precipitation techniques have not been successful (Alaupovic, 1972). This suggests that the association between the lipoprotein families in VLDL and LDL is different from that in HDL.

The B family of lipoprotein, LP-B, can be isolated with great difficulty in the pure

---

*These studies have in addition described a method for the purification of the lipoprotein family LP-D.

form. When present in high concentrations, LP-B aggregates and gives rise eventually to a precipitation of LP. LP-B can be isolated free or almost free of LP-C by using the technique of preparative ultracentrifugation at a density of 1.040–1.050 g/ml (Lee and Alaupovic, 1970; Fig. 28).

H. Methods used in the study of apolipoproteins and their peptides

Following the complete removal of lipid from a lipoprotein fraction which contains several lipoprotein families, the protein material (apolipoprotein) can be redissolved and fractionated by chromatography.

To dissolve and elute the lipoproteins obtained from HDL, urea solution (6 mol/l or 8 mol/l) is usually used while for VLDL a buffer containing tris-HCl is suitable.

The first chromatography is usually gel filtration on Sephadex G 75, G 100, G 200, or Sepharose 4 B. A complete separation of the polypeptides of the apolipoprotein can not be obtained by using this method, even if the columns are as long as 100 cm. For this reason, the gel filtration is usually complemented by chromatography on DEAE-cellulose. The buffers used for disolving HDL and VLDL are the same as those mentioned above. Elution is performed by using a gradient of sodium chloride. Further details are given elsewhere for HDL (Rudman *et al.*, 1970; Scanu *et al.*, 1969) and VLDL (Brown *et al.*, 1970).

I. Structure of plasma lipoproteins

LDL. A model of the structure of LDL_2 (density 1.019–1.063 g/ml) has been suggested by Pollard *et al.* (1969). This is shown in Fig. 31 and is based on electron microscope studies (Scanu, 1972) and physicochemical data (Table 10). The particle is spherical in shape and has a characteristic size (*c.* 20 nm) and weight (2.2×10^6). The structure contains 20 units of apoB, each having a molecular weight of 25 000–30 000, placed in the corners of a dodecahedron (a geometric figure having 20 corners and 12 surfaces). The surfaces between the protein units are occupied by phospholipid and probably even free cholesterol. The inside of the particle is occupied by the water-insoluble neutral lipids (esters of cholesterol and triglycerides).

J. Lipoprotein metabolism

1. Synthesis

The chylomicrons, some VLDL and HDL are synthesized in the mucosal membrane of the intestine. The major part of VLDL and possibly some HDL is synthesized in the liver. LDL is probably formed exclusively via the catabolism of VLDL.

Of protein synthesis it can be generally said that it takes place on the ribosomes when they are bound to the endoplasmic reticulum. In the case of the lipoprotein, *in vitro* studies have demonstrated that the peptide part is indeed built in this system but that the lipid part is attached afterwards. In liver homogenates, it has been shown that the protein portion (apolipoprotein) of VLDL and HDL is present in the microsomes. Newly synthesized VLDL and HDL have been demonstrated by the electron microscope within the liver of the rat and guinea-pig. These lipoproteins have been isolated

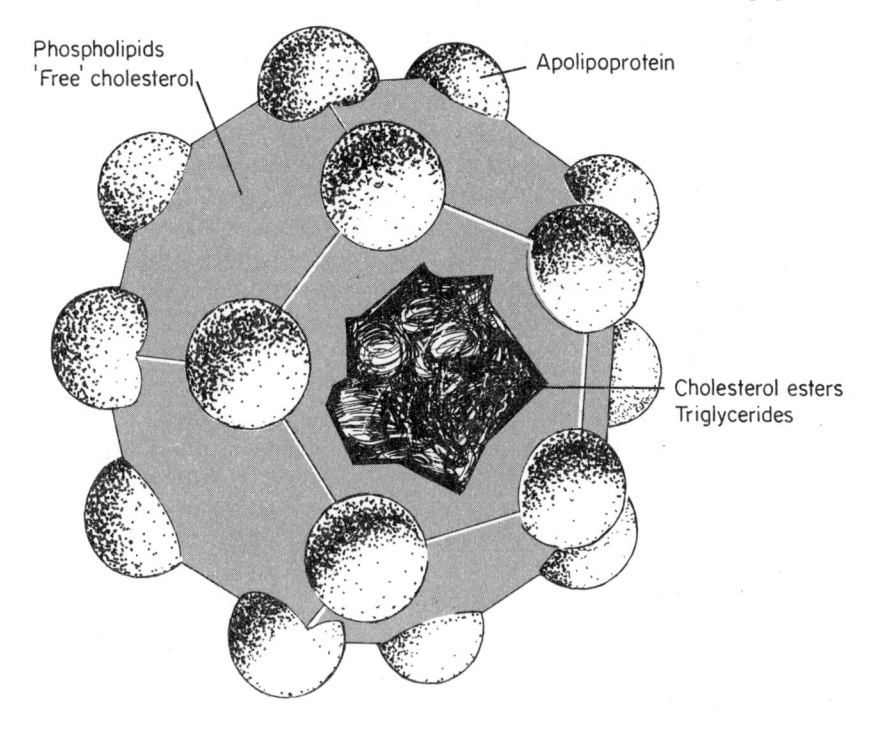

Fig. 31. Model of the plasma lipoprotein, LDL$_2$ (Pollard, Scanu, and Taylor, 1969)

from the Golgi apparatus of the liver cells by a specific fractionation (Hamilton et al., 1967). The VLDL isolated from the Golgi apparatus contains relatively more free cholesterol and less apolipoprotein than the VLDL isolated from plasma. In the rat, all the apolipoproteins which are characteristic of the VLDL of plasma are found also in the VLDL isolated from the Golgi apparatus.

In the case of the chylomicrons, it would appear that the entire particle, including portions of the apolipoprotein, is synthesized in the mucous cells of the intestine. The inhibition of protein synthesis in the mucous cells prevents the resorption of fat and brings the production of chylomicrons to a halt.

The half-life of VLDL in plasma is approximately 2 hours. If the plasma pool of VLDL-triglycerides is taken to be 1.5 g, the secretion of triglyceride from the liver must amount to 18 g of VLDL-triglyceride per day, i.e. 500 µg per hour for each gram of liver. Nilsson (1970) using the liver slice technique on material take during human biopsy, obtained a value of 300 µg per hour for each gram of liver. Liver perfusion experiments performed on non-fasting rats produced a corresponding value of 3 000 µg per hour for each gram of liver (Scanu et al., 1969). The discrepancy in the last results may indicate that only a fraction of the triglycerides which are synthesized in liver are used in the production of VLDL.

The corresponding calculated rate of synthesis of apolipoprotein which is required for the formation of VLDL is 70 µg per hour for each gram of liver. This is in good agreement with the experimental value (80 µg per hour for each gram of liver) found by perfusing rat liver (Scanu et al., 1969).

The secretion of VLDL from liver is determined by (a) the amount of available lipid,

(b) the amount of available protein, (c) the capacity of liver to combine lipid and protein, and (d) the ability of the liver to release the newly formed VLDL.

FFA in plasma (page 73) supplies the liver with fatty acids. This FFA is used by the liver via oxidation and via ester formation to produce triglycerides. The synthesis in the liver of new fatty acids from carbohydrate is limited. In cases of hypertriglyceridaemia, the level of FFA in plasma is increased as a result of an increased release of FFA from adipose tissue. In cases of hypertriglyceridaemia which is linked to overweight (large fat cells), the increase in the release of FFA is due to the simultaneous occurrence of hyperinsulinaemia. Recently published data (Smith, 1974) indicate that under conditions of increased levels of insulin, large fat cells as distinct from normal fat cells undergo increased lipolysis.

In the synthesis of VLDL, insulin can also give rise to an increase in the amount of available lipid (triglyceride) in liver by influencing the endogenic pool of triglyceride in this organ. Insulin can cause a reduction in the level of cyclic AMP in the liver and therby dampen the effect of the lipase in liver which is sensitive to hormone. The result is a diminished lipolysis and increased availabiliy of the triglycerides in the liver (Topping and Mayes, 1972).

2. Catabolism of chylomicrons

The chylomicrons which are synthesized in the mucous cells of the intestine are transported via lymph to *ductus thoracicus* and eventually reach the bloodstream at *vena jugularis*. During their transport in plasma, the chylomicrons take up protein from other LP and eventually become 'bound' to the cells of the endothelium when they reach the capillaries (Fig. 32). The triglyceride parts of the chylomicrons are 'devoured' by these cells and are hydrolysed by the action of the LP-lipase of adipose tissue to produce fatty acid and diglyceride. While the fatty acid is released into the bloodstream as FFA, the diglyceride is taken up in a vacuole in the cells of the endothelium. The continued hydrolysis of diglyceride and monoglyceride takes place during the transport

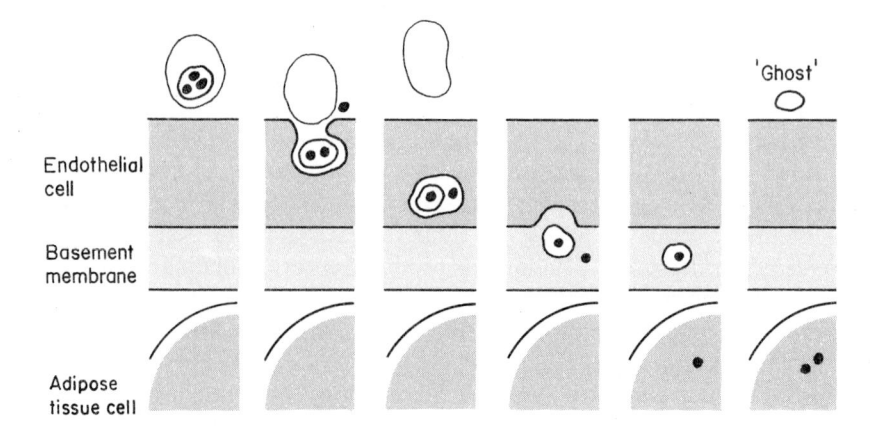

Fig. 32. Schematic representation of the transport of the fatty acids of the chylomicrons through the walls of the capillaries to the adipose tissue. Triglycerides are represented by three points, diglycerides as two points, and monoglycerides as one point within a spherical particle

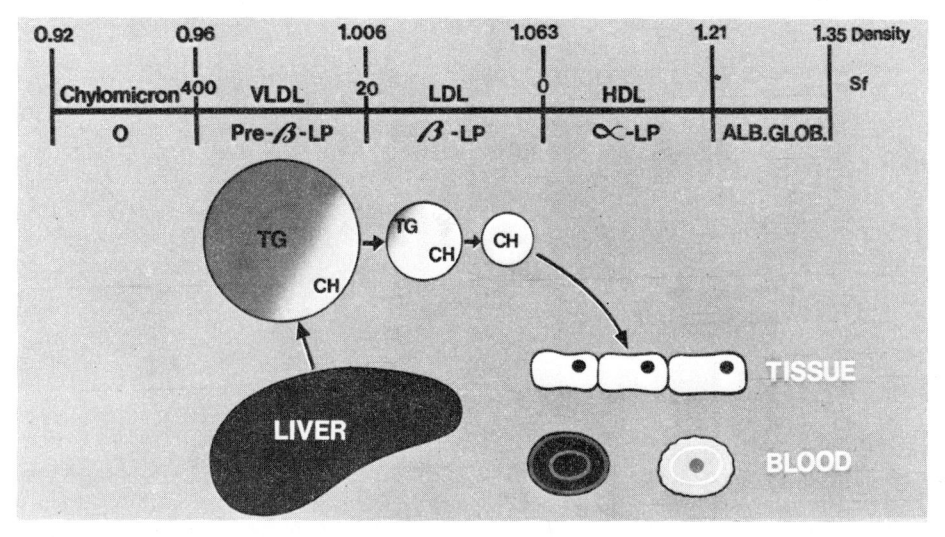

Fig. 33. Schematic representation of the metabolism of pre-β-LP and β-LP. An explanation is provided in the text

through the endothelium. The fatty acid which is released becomes esterified by adipose tissue while the final product of released glycerol is transported via the blood to the liver (Scow et al., 1972). The residue of the chylomicron, 'ghost', is released into the bloodstream and is taken up by the liver. This latter step is catalysed probably by liver LP-lipase.

3. Catabolism of VLDL (Fig. 33)

The half-life of VLDL is approximately two hours. VLDL is transformed into LDL by the hydrolysis of the triglyceride portion. This hydrolysis is catalysed by adipose tissue LP-lipase. For the enzyme to be capable of exercising its function, the presence of the polypeptide, C-II is required. ApoB is transferred from VLDL to LDL by the transformation while polypeptides CII and CIII (of apoC) most likely exchange among VLDL and HDL (Bilheimer et al., 1972).

The hydrolysis of the triglycerides causes a reduction in both the size and the surface area of the lipoprotein. The material of the membrane, free cholesterol and phospholipid, is carried over (probably by the polypeptides, C-II and C-III from VLDL to HDL). At the same time, the cholesterol ester content of the metabolizing lipoprotein increases (Schumaker and Adams, 1969). There is much evidence to support the theory that these esters of cholesterol are provided by HDL. A continuous esterification of the cholesterol in HDL, catalysed by lecithin-cholesterol-acyl-transferase (LCAT), is required so that this exchange can take place (Fig. 34).

4. Catabolism of LDL (Fig. 33)

The half-life of LDL is three and a half days. The elimination of LDL takes place by internalization into body cells, e.g. fibroblasts and smooth muscles cells, and possibly also through an active process by macrophages of the reticuloendothelial system (RES).

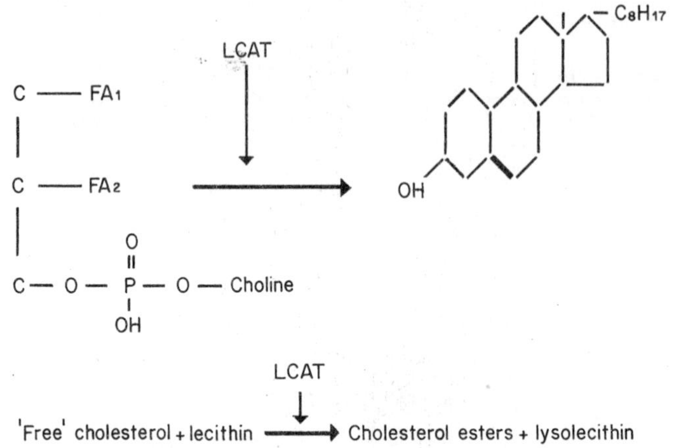

88 Transport proteins

$$C - FA_1$$
$$|$$
$$C - FA_2$$
$$|$$
$$\underset{OH}{C - O - \overset{O}{\underset{\|}{P}} - O - Choline}$$

$$\xrightarrow{LCAT}$$

cholesterol (OH, C_8H_{17} side chain)

'Free' cholesterol + lecithin $\xrightarrow{LCAT}$ Cholesterol esters + lysolecithin

Fig. 34. The lecithin-cholesterol-acyl-transferase (LCAT) reaction. Esterification of free cholesterol in serum, catalysed by LCAT which is responsible for the removal of a fatty acid from the 2-position of lecithin (phosphatidyl choline) and its attachment to the 3-position of cholesterol

This internalization is regulated by specific cell surface receptors, synthesized by the cells themselves, in proportion to plasma LDL concentration. LDL is degraded by the cell lysosomes and cholesterol esters hydrolysed to free cholesterol to exchange for cholesterol in the cell membrane. Excess cholesterol leaves the cells through uptake by HDL. In HDL, cholesterol becomes esterified under the influence of LCAT (see above).

In vivo studies, using isotope-labelled LDL, have demonstrated the presence of a reduced catabolism of LDL in patients suffering from hypercholesterolaemia, i. e. type II A hyperlipoproteinaemia (Langer *et al.*, 1972) and in heterozygotes and homozygotes of familial type II, deficiency of LDL cell receptor mediated internalization has recently been shown.

5. Catabolism of HDL

HDL are formed in the liver and in the intestine. The quantitatively dominating apolipoprotein of HDL, apolipoprotein-A (containing polypeptides A I and A II) might originate with the chylomicrons in the intestinal mucosa. Through the catabolism of chylomicrons in plasma, apolipoprotein-A is transferred to HDL to compose its major protein moiety. Free cholesterol is esterified in HDL by the action of LCAT. This reaction involves the transfer of a fatty acid on the 2-position of lecithin to the free cholesterol during the formation of lysolecithin and cholesterol ester (Glomset, 1968; Fig. 34). Preliminary investigations have suggested that the production of HDL_2 in the LCAT reaction causes HDL_3 to release the polypeptides which 'carry' the newly formed cholesterol esters (Gustafson *et al.*, 1974) presumably to VLDL.

K. Factors influencing concentration of LP in plasma

In both normolipidaemic and hypertriglyceridaemic persons, an increased level of triglycerides and VLDL in plasma can be caused by carbohydrate-rich food which contains more than 65 per cent of the calories in the form of refined carbohydrate, saccharose, glucose, or fructose. While this increase in persons having normolipidaemia is reversed at the end of two weeks' administration of sugar, those persons having hypertriglyceridaemia show a further increase in the level of triglycerides in their plasma (Cahlin et al., 1973).

A reduction in the level of triglycerides and VLDL can be obtained by slimming which is induced by a reduced caloric diet or by increased physical activity (Gustafson, 1971). This also causes a drop in the level of insulin in the plasma.

The level of LDL can be reduced by putting the patient on a diet which contains an increased amount of polyunsaturated fat. However in the case of patients showing hypertriglyceridaemia, such a diet can also cause a reduction in the level of VLDL. The effect of polyunsaturated fat on LDL is brought about most likely by an increased catabolism of LDL.

An increased level of VLDL and/or LDL can be reduced by medication with clofibrate. This treatment also causes an increase in the level of HDL. Substances such as cholestyramine which sequestrate bile acids, cause a reduction of an increased level of LDL but can accentuate an existing high level of VLDL.

Generally speaking, both oestrogen and androgen have an effect on LP which is opposite to that described above. Oestrogen produces a simultaneous increase in the level of VLDL and HDL and may cause a reduction in the level of LDL.

A characteristic of hypothyroidism is the occurrence of hypercholesterolaemia with an increased level of LDL. Treatment involving the use of thyroid hormone, especially in the case of hypothyroidism, can quite often produce hypertriglyceridaemia (increased VLDL).

Recent studies on juvenile *diabetes mellitus* have shown that patients treated with insulin have an increase in the lipid content of HDL (Gustafson et al., unpublished

Table 13. The effect of various diets, drugs, hormones, and diseases on the amounts of lipoprotein in each density class

	Agent	VLD	LDL	HDL
Diet	Polyunsaturated fat (>5% of calories)	↓	↓	
	Rich in sugar (>65% of calories)	↑		
Medication	Clofibrate	↓	↓	↑
	Nicotinic acid derivative	↓	↓	
	Bile sequesting substance	↑	↓	
Hormone	Oestrogen	↑	↓	↓
	Androgen	↓	↑	↑
	Corticosteroids	↑ [a]		
	Thyroxine	↑	↓	
Illness	Biliary stasis		↑ [b]	↓
	Hypothyreosis		↑	
	Juvenile diabetes			↑
	Adult diabetes	↑ [a]		↓

[a] Non obligatory finding.
[b] As LP-X.

data). The mechanism of this has not been studied in more detail. The occurrence of hypertriglyceridaemia (increased VLDL) is rather common in adult diabetics treated with sulphonyl urea (Gustafson et al., unpublished data).

L. Hyperlipidaemia and hyperlipoproteinaemia

Any terminology which describes merely an increase in a lipid fraction in plasma, e.g. hypertriglyceridaemia or hypercholesterolaemia, is not sufficiently precise to characterize an underlying primary LP disorder. Identification of the type and classification of hyperlipoproteinaemia, originally suggested by Fredrickson and Lees, enables a better evaluation and understanding of the term, hyperlipidaemia. The six types of hyperlipoproteinaemia and their relation to the spectrum of LP are depicted in Fig. 35. Of these, types II A, II B, and IV are the most common.

Type II A is characterized by an increase in β-LP (LDL) and gives rise to an increased level of cholesterol in plasma—hypercholesterolaemia.

Types II B and III show an increase in the level of pre-β-LP as well as β-LP. Type III is characterized by the presence of a pathological β-lipoprotein, 'floating β-LP' (page 79).

In types II B and III, there is an increased level of cholesterol and triglycerides. This has been described earlier as 'mixed' hyperlipidaemia.

Type IV is characterized by an increase in pre-β-LP (VLDL) which produces an enhanced level of triglycerides and moderate increase in the level of cholesterol in the plasma.

Types I and V are relatively rare. The former is characterized by an increase in the chylomicrons while the latter is characterized by an increase in both chylomicrons and pre-β-LP.

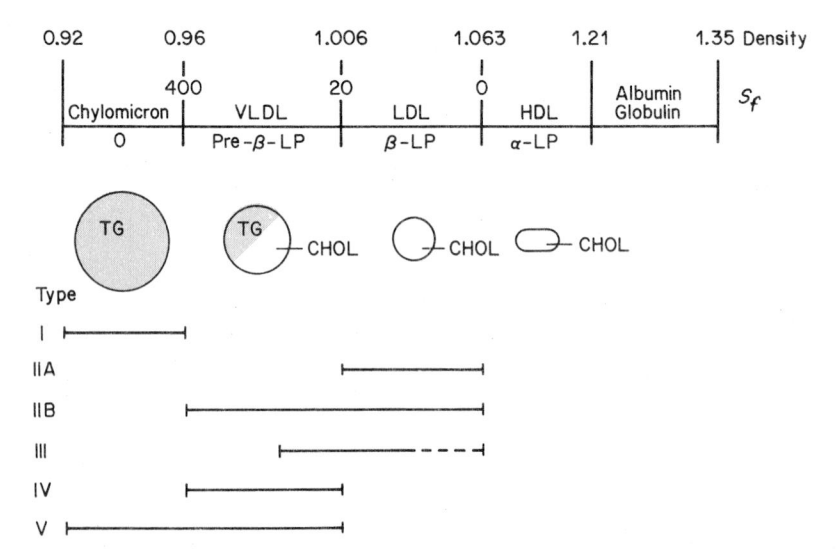

Fig. 35. The spectrum of lipoprotein showing the two terminologies, the intervals of density, and S_f-value. The distribution of the six types of hyperlipoproteinaemia as classified by Fredrickson and Lees (1965) is also given. CHOL = cholesterol, TG = triglycerides

It was originally thought that each individual type of hyperlipoproteinaemia was an expression of an hereditary disorder, *hereditary form*. Today, it is clear that different types of hyperlipoproteinaemia can appear in the same family (Hazzard et al., 1973).

Secondary hyperlipoproteinaemia appears in diseases such as *diabetes mellitus*, hepatopathy, and nephropathy. Population studies have shown that between 1 per cent and 2 per cent of the cases of hyperlipoproteinaemia are of this secondary type.

A third type of hyperlipoproteinaemia is the *acquired* type. In males who are moderately overweight, type IV is characterized by the presence of enlarged fat cells in adipose tissue (Björntorp et al., 1971). This form is believed to be an acquired form of hyperlipoproteinaemia.

M. Hyperlipoproteinaemias and their clinical manifestations

Type I, chylomicronaemia is rare and is usually hereditary, having been described in only approximately 40 cases. Chylomicronaemia appears first during childhood where the usual primary symptom is abdominal pains. Hepatosplenomegaly appears in later years.

Chylomicronaemia causes the plasma to take on a milky appearance and gives rise to a marked increase in the level of triglycerides. The level of cholesterol in the plasma is usually normal. The presence of chylomicronaemia can be ascertained by allowing a sample of plasma to stand in the cold overnight.

Chylomicronaemia is caused by a deficiency of a lipoprotein lipase (LP-lipase of adipose tissue, see page 86). The presence of fat in the food gives rise to a marked increase in the level of chylomicrons in plasma.

Type II A, hyper-β-lipoproteinaemia, hypercholesterolaemia. Type II A exists in a *hereditary form* (Muller–Harbitz disease) which has a dominant penetration. Patients suffering from hereditary type II A often have xanthomata in the extensor tendons of the back of the hand and in the Achilles' tendons. The presence of xantelasma is also common. Clinical manifestations of atherosclerosis appear often. In teenagers, cases of myocardial infarction have been described in homozygotes.

The most common form of type II A, hyper-β-lipoproteinaemia, is the *acquired form*. There is much evidence in favour of the fact that also patients suffering from acquired type II A run the risk of atherosclerosis, especially in the coronary arteries. This type is characterized by an increased level of cholesterol in plasma. In cases of the hereditary form, levels of up to 10 g/l can be detected. The level of triglycerides is normal.

Type II B, mixed hyperlipidaemia. Just as with type II A, this type appears in the *hereditary* and *acquired* form. A high incidence of occlusive vascular disease has been demonstrated to exist among patients who suffer from type II B. These appear in both coronary arteries and in the peripheral arteries (Table 14).

On subjecting the lipoproteins to electrophoresis, an increased amount of β-LP and pre-β-LP can be seen. The level of cholesterol and triglycerides in the plasma is increased.

A pathological LP, 'floating β-LP', is present in *type III* (page 79). This type is

Table 14. Distribution (in %) of the occurrence of hyperlipoproteinaemia in randomized material obtained from (a) 55-year-old men (born 1913) and (b) 50-year-old men who survived their myocardial infarction and who were examined three months after the acute stage. Upper 'limiting value' for LDL-(β-LP) cholesterol and VLDL-(pre-β-LP) cholesterol is 2.0 g/l and 350 mg/l, respectively (Gustafson et al., 1972)

	Number	Normal plasma-lipids %	Type II A %	Type II B-III %	Type IV %	Type V %
55-year-old healthy men	76	77	12	1	8	3
50-year-old men (27–55 years) with a sustained myocardial infarction	229	53	19	10	18	0

thought to be relatively rare. Skin xanthomata are present in the *hereditary form* and appear characteristically in the palms of the hands. The occurrence of type III has also been reported as a secondary effect of hypothyroidism. In cases of type III there is an overrepresentation of occlusive vascular disease (Stanbury et al., 1972).

On electrophoresis, the abnormal lipoprotein (floating β-LP) appears as a characteristic broad band between β-LP and pre-β-LP. The presence of this type can be diagnosed by performing ultracentrifugation. In type III there can even be increased levels of chylomicrons in plasma. Type III is characterized by the presence of increased levels of cholesterol and triglycerides where the quota is greater than 0.42 (Quarfordt et al., 1971).

Type IV, pre-β-hyperlipoproteinaemia, hypertriglyceridaemia. This type is common in Scandinavia (Table 14). It is thought that this type can exist in a hereditary form. Skin xanthomata are present on rare occasions. Type IV appears often in conjunction with moderate overweight where it is characterized by enlarged fat cells in the adipose tissue (Björntorp et al., 1971). Patients suffering from this type have often a hereditary tendency to *diabetes mellitus*.

Secondary hyperlipoproteinaemia of type IV appears in adult diabetes. A reversible, acquired form of this type is present in patients who drink excessive amounts of alcohol. Type IV is often present in conjunction with myocardial infarction in men who are younger than 55 (Table 14).

When the lipoproteins of type IV are subjected to electrophoresis, an increased level of pre-β-LP is seen. The level of triglycerides is increased, the level of cholesterol is slightly increased, and the plasma can be opalescent. An increased level of plasma insulin is often present in patients having type IV.

Type V is uncommon. The misuse of alcohol is one cause of this type. The hyperlipoproteinaemia thus produced is reversible. It is believed that a hereditary form of this type may exist. A *secondary* form of type V is seen in cases of *diabetes mellitus*, chronic pancreatitis, hepatopathy, nephropathy, and the nephrotic syndrome.

In type V a characteristic increase in the level of chylomicrons and pre-β-LP can be seen on subjecting the lipoproteins to electrophoresis. In general, the level of triglycerides in the plasma is markedly increased ($>$5 g/l) while that of cholesterol is only moderately increased and the plasma appears milky.

N. Reference values and frequency of hyperlipoproteinaemia

Types II A and IV are believed to be the most common types of hyperlipoproteinaemia in Sweden (Table 14). The absolute frequency is dependent on the chosen limiting values, 'cut-off-points'. An ideal *'biological reference value'* should constitute a limiting value, *under* which levels of plasma lipid do not imply an increased risk for the development of vascular atherosclerosis. However, in practice one is forced to use *'statistical reference values'*. These values should be determined for each population which is under consideration. Sex, age, eating habits, and geographical location are factors which can determine these 'cut-off-points'.

O. Hypolipoproteinaemias

1. Tangier's disease

Deficiency of α (high-density)-lipoprotein, Tangier's disease, is rare. The disease is autosomal recessive and is inherited. It is characterized by an almost complete lack of HDL and the storage of cholesterol esters in the foam cells of various tissues. The disease was reported for the first time on the island of Tangier, off the east coast of USA. The clinical features are: enlarged yellowish coloured tonsils, splenomegaly, and peripheral neuropathy. Hepatomegaly, clouding of the cornea, skin manifestations, and atherosclerosis were detected in 12 patients suffering from this disease (Stanbury et al., 1972). The disease is characterized by the presence of cholesterol esters in the foam cells in the skin. These esters may even exist extracellularly.

The level of cholesterol in the plasma is low and that of triglycerides is slightly enhanced. The proportion of apolipoprotein in HDL is between 1 per cent and 5 per cent of the normal value and the ratio of the polypeptides, A–I and A–II is 1:11 (Lux et al., 1972).

2. LP-A deficiency

A case of a 45-year-old woman having extensive skin xanthoma was reported recently (Lindeskog et al., 1972). Splenomegaly, hepatomegaly, discrete clouding of the cornea, neuropathy, and atherosclerosis were among the observed clinical manifestations. The tonsils appeared normal.

Histochemical features included extracellular accumulation of cholesterol, in both the free form and the form of esters, in the skin and the mucous membrane of the rectum.

The level of cholesterol in the plasma was low, that of triglycerides was moderately increased and the proportion of apolipoprotein in HDL was approximately 1 per cent of the normal value. The polypeptide, A-I, was not present in the plasma and the level of A-II was markedly reduced (Gustafson et al., 1976).

3. Lecithincholesterol-acyl-transferase (LCAT) deficiency

The rare occurrence of a deficiency of the enzyme, lecithin-cholesterol-acyl-transferase (LCAT) was described for the first time in Norway. In Scandinavia, four families having this deficiency have been described. Characteristic features of the illness are:

anaemia, proteinuria, and clouding of the cornea. The patients develop lesions of the kidneys which lead eventually to renal insufficiency (Stanbury, et al., 1972).

The histochemical features are the presence of free cholesterol in foam cells of the bone marrow and the glomeruli.

The level of free cholesterol and lecithin in the plasma are increased while that of cholesterol esters and lysolecithin are reduced. An electrophoresis of the lipoproteins is devoid of α-LP and pre-β-LP. The plasma shows the presence of 'large' LDL in addition to 'normal' LDL, a reduced level of HDL with a high proportion of free cholesterol and lecithin as well as the presence of immunologically 'normal' apoA (Norum et al., 1971). LP-X is present in cases of LCAT deficiency.

4. A-β-lipoproteinaemia (Bassen–Kornzweig disease)

A-β-LP-aemia is a hereditary disorder where the most important manifestations are: cerebral ataxia, *retinitis pigmentosa*, acanthosis, defective resorption of fat, and pronounced hypolipidaemia (Stanbury et al., 1972). The disease appears exclusively in children. The condition has been detected, in a milder form, in adults.

A-β-LP-aemia is characterized by the lack of chylomicrons, VLDL, and LDL. ApoB is missing completely while the presence of the polypeptides, C-I, C-II, and C-III as well as A-I and A-II can be verified. The presence of apoD in cases of a-β-LP-aemia has recently been ascertained (Gustafson et al.). The level of LCAT is reduced.

III. Plasma proteins involved in haem metabolism and in transport of metals, hormones, and vitamins

GITTEN CEDERBLAD

Formerly, research in the area of the plasma proteins could be divided into two different fields of interest; characterization of the physiocochemical properties of the proteins on one hand, and the study of their function on the other. More recent research has brought together information obtained in the two areas. However, there are still proteins for which the physiocochemical properties are well defined but to which no function has been attributed. Similarly, certain observed functions can not as yet be attributed to particular proteins.

According to Freeman (1968), the following properties of a plasma protein must be known before that protein can be classified as fully characterized:

1. Physiocochemical properties such as molecular weight, isoelectric point, amino acid content, and carbohydrate content, etc.
2. Biological function.
3. Synthesis: tissue responsible for production and the factors which control the rate of synthesis.
4. Catabolism: both basic and specific catabolism, the tissue and controlling factors.
5. Distribution: the size of the pools and the exchange between them. In the cases of proteins involved in transport, this list should be complemented with the asso-

ciation constant of the ligand–protein interaction as well as the nature of the binding. Also of interest is the rate constant for the dissociation. Knowledge of those substances which interfere with the binding is of value in understanding the nature of this binding and can be sometimes of significance in clinical work.

The *distribution and metabolism* of plasma proteins is investigated usually with the help of isotope-labelled proteins. The experimental difficulties encountered in such studies are often great. It is desirable that the isolation and labelling procedures do not change the nature of the proteins to such an extent that their metabolism becomes different from those of the native proteins. A variety of compartment models can be set up. A complete description of the kinetics implies that information must be made available concerning the rate constants (per unit of time) for synthesis and elimination as well as knowledge of the size of the protein pools and the exchange between them. The magnitude of the body's pool of a given protein at any particular time is determined by the balance between synthesis and catabolism. In healthy individuals this is controlled by the existence of an equilibrium between synthesis and catabolism. In the cases of proteins which are involved in transport, additional studies are usually performed to provide information about the half-lives and the distribution of the transported substances. The metabolic data of many proteins are far from being complete. Different plasma proteins have different rates of synthesis and breakdown. It appears that a common mechanism for breakdown does not exist. In several cases, the production of a complex, e.g. that between α_2-macroglobulin and plasmin, is followed by a rapid elimination of this complex. In the majority of cases, the catabolism of low molecular weight proteins takes place in the kidney. Recently, it has been demonstrated that several glycoproteins disappear rapidly from the circulation when their terminal residues of sialic acid have been removed to reveal at least two residues of galactose. The serum glycoprotein, transferrin, is a notable exception in this respect. The hepatocytes possess receptors which have pronounced selectivity for such modified proteins. The presence of covalently linked sialic acid residues on the receptor sites is required for successful binding by a solubilized receptor complex of hepatic plasma membranes. The principal subcellular site of catabolism has been shown to be lysosomal. However, more experimental evidence is needed before the biological significance of this mechanism can be evaluated (Ashwell and Morell, 1974).

Freeman (1968) has suggested that plasma proteins should be classified as either 'biophilic' or 'suicidal' proteins. The latter are characterized by the fact that they are broken down after mediating their function. Most of the proteins of the coagulation and complement systems belong to this group. In certain situations, activation of either of these two systems can constitute a potential threat to the life of the organism. To counteract this possibility, these systems are comprised of complex sequences of reactions which are limited either in themselves or by the short life of the inherent active factors. In contrast to these systems, those involved in the transport of various substances by plasma proteins can not constitute any threat to the organism. Complex chain reactions do not arise but instead the transport is mediated by a single protein, e.g. transferrin in the transport of iron. Consequently, biophilic proteins can take part in several 'transport cycles' before they eventually become catabolized.

Haptoglobin is a suicidal protein, the function of which is the disposal of material and not the maintenance of cells. It would appear therefore that Freeman's hypothesis is not applicable to all transport proteins.

96   Transport proteins

The transport proteins which are described in the following sections, take part in the turnover of metals and haem and function in the transport of vitamins and hormones:

Transport of metal: ceruloplasmin and transferrin.
Metabolism of haemoglobin and haem: haptoglobin and haemopexin.
Vitamin-transporting proteins: transcobalamine and retinol-binding protein.
Hormone-transporting proteins: thyroxine-binding globulin, thyroxine-binding prealbumin, and transcortin.

Generally accepted data do not exist for the physicochemical properties of all proteins. Those values which are given in the tables which follow can be taken as estimates. The values given for the concentrations in plasma of several proteins have been taken from the thesis by Weeke (1973) and are the average values for men between the ages of 15 and 44. The half-lives in plasma of the proteins have been taken in many cases from a compilation by Bocci (1970).

A. Ceruloplasmin

1. Chemical structure and biochemistry

Ceruloplasmin is a copper-containing glycoprotein which possesses oxidase activity and which is of importance in the copper metabolism of organisms. It was isolated and characterized by Holmberg and Laurell (1948). Because of experimental difficulties a generally accepted picture of the molecular structure has not been obtained. Ceruloplasmin is extremely sensitive to enzymic proteolysis. In recent publications, the molecular weight has been indicated to lie between 124 000 and 134 000. Information concerning the structure is even more uncertain. Simons and Bearn (1969) believed that the molecule was composed of two polypeptide chains, the molecular weights of which differed considerably. Ryden (1972) proposed a single polypeptide chain and that the appearance of subunits was probably caused by the presence of proteolytic enzymes in the starting material. In addition, he found that the N-terminal amino acid was valine. The results published by Freeman and Daniel (1973) agreed largely with those of Simons and co-workers. In these studies, ceruloplasmin (molecular weight 124 000) was treated with several agents which promote dissociation of polypeptide chains. Three fragments were obtained, having molecular weights of 16 000 (L), 53 000 (H), and 69 000 (HL). A return of oxidase activity was obtained on the removal of the dissociating agents. Thus, Freeman and Daniel suggested the structure to be an L_2H_2 tetramer with the N-terminal amino acids valine and lysine. Lövenstein (1975) proposed a single polypeptide chain structure and the existence of at least one very labile

Table 15. Ceruloplasmin

Molecular weight	124 000–134 000
$E^{1\%}_{280\,nm}$	14.7
$E^{1\%}_{610\,nm}$	0.66
Carbohydrate content, %	7
Copper content, atoms	7–8
Number of polypeptide chains	1?, 4?
Concentration in plasma, g/l	0.22
Half-life in plasma, days	5–7

peptide bond. The heterogeneities, known for many years, he attributed to differences in the carbohydrate content only. The amino acid composition has been determined. Ryden and Eaker (1974) report the amino acid sequences of three glycopeptides. The carbohydrate content is reported to be 7 per cent: 9 moles of sialic acid, 18 moles of N-acetylglucosamine, 2 moles of fucose and 36 moles of hexose per mole of protein. The ratio of mannose to galactose was 3:2 (Jamieson 1965).

Enzymic function of ceruloplasmin. Ceruloplasmin contains 6–8 atoms of copper. This copper is present in the form of 'blue', 'non-blue', and a form which cannot be detected by electron paramagnetic resonance. The enzymes containing the blue form of copper represent a small group of oxidases capable of catalysing the reduction of molecular oxygen to water. The presence of all three forms of copper in ceruloplasmin seems to be essential for its catalytic function. The 'blue' Cu^{2+} ions have a high oxidation–reduction potential and the oxidation of substrates is believed to be mediated by this ion. 'Non-blue' Cu^{2+} ions show a great affinity for anions. The third form, diamagnetic Cu^{2+}–Cu^{2+} pair, is considered to function as a two-electron acceptor.

Ceruloplasmin can oxidize Fe^{2+}, various aromatic phenols, and polyamines. The oxidation of some substrates is inhibited more or less completely by iron-chelating agents.

$$\begin{array}{c} Fe^{2+} \\ \text{Aromatic diamines} \end{array} \searrow \nearrow \text{Ferroxidase}-(Cu^{2+})_4 \searrow \nearrow 2H_2O$$
$$\begin{array}{c} Fe^{3+} \\ \text{Oxidized products} \end{array} \nearrow \searrow \text{Ferroxidase}-(Cu^{+})_4 \nearrow \searrow O_2, 4H^+$$

$$\begin{array}{c} \text{Reducing agents} \\ \text{Aromatic diamines} \end{array} \searrow \nearrow Fe^{3+} \searrow \nearrow \text{Ferroxidase}-(Cu^{+})_4 \searrow \nearrow O_2, 4H^+$$
$$\text{Oxidized products} \nearrow \searrow Fe^{2+} \nearrow \searrow \text{Ferroxidase}-(Cu^{2+})_4 \nearrow \searrow 2H_2O$$

Ceruloplasmin has even been called ferroxidase; iron (II): oxygen oxidoreductase EC 1.16.3.1. The existence in plasma of an additional ferroxidase has been reported.

2. Biological function

Ceruoplasmin is of importance in the body's turnover of copper. The distribution of copper in an organism is given in Fig. 36. When radioactive copper was given orally to an individual, the radioactivity soon appeared in the plasma and was bound to albumin and to some extent to amino acids. The radioactivity in the plasma decreased thereafter and was accumulated in the liver. The radioactive copper was then released from liver into plasma as ceruloplasmin. In steady state, ceruloplasmin carries 93 per cent of the copper content of plasma while albumin and amino acids are responsible for the remainder. Copper is stored in the liver and the major pathway for removal of hepatic copper is biliary excretion. Both albumin and ceruloplasmin give off copper to various organs. Using isotopic methods, it was shown that the copper which was donated to tissue by albumin was easily exchanged with the copper in plasma, in contrast to the copper which was donated by ceruloplasmin (Marceau and Aspin,

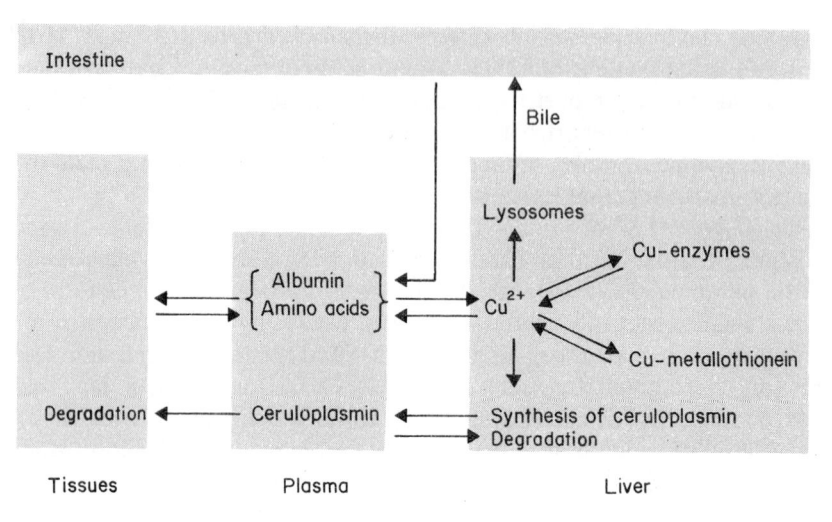

Fig. 36. Schematic representation of the most important metabolic pathways for copper

1972). There is experimental evidence that ceruloplasmin transfers copper to copper-containing enzymes, which suggests that ceruloplasmin is a transport protein for copper (Hsieh and Frieden, 1975).

Ceruloplasmin is synthesized in the liver. Being an acute phase reactant, the concentration in plasma increases as a response to inflammatory conditions. The plasma ceruloplasmin level is also altered by a variety of hormones. *In vivo* and *in vitro* experiments using human liver tissue have shown that copper can induce this synthesis. The studies which are described below demonstrate that several mechanisms, in addition to that involving copper, exist for the regulation of the synthesis. Holtzman and Gaumnitz (1970) found that the oxidase activity in the plasma of copper-deficient rats was not measurable. When measured by an immunological technique, employing anti-rat ceruloplasmin, the apoceruloplasmin concentration was 25 per cent of that found in normal rats. In addition, this study showed that ceruloplasmin and apoceruloplasmin were synthesized at the same rate in the liver. However, apoceruloplasmin seemed to be the more unstable of the two and was eliminated more quickly from the circulation. In most mammals, the level of copper in the liver is highest around the time of birth. Evans (1973) has shown that new-born rats appear to have a limited ability to dispose of copper from the liver. On the administration of copper to such animals, the level of copper in the liver rose while the level of ceruloplasmin in the plasma remained unchanged. Quite a different result was obtained if adult rats were injected with copper. In these cases, the increase in the concentration of copper in the liver was transient and the level of ceruloplasmin in the plasma was doubled. The new-born human has a low concentration of ceruloplasmin in the plasma and a high level of copper in the liver. These values change during the first two years of life to become comparable with the corresponding values for adults.

In spite of the considerable amount of detailed information available for ceruloplasmin, it is not yet possible to fully answer the question: What is the biological function of ceruloplasmin? The suggested functions discussed are: ceruloplasmin acts as a copper transporting protein and is involved in the maintenance of hepatic copper homeostasis. In addition, the ferroxidase activity of ceruloplasmin is believed to be of significance in the mobilizing of iron (see under transferrin).

3. Hereditary defects in copper metabolism

Wilson's disease or hepatolenticular degeneration is characterized by neurological symptoms, cirrhosis of the liver, and Kayser–Fleischer ring around the cornea. The genetic defect is unknown. The defect causes an inability to remove copper from the liver. It is caused most probably by a failure in a metabolic step which precedes the release of copper into bile and the subsequent incorporation of this copper into ceruloplasmin. One hypothesis which has been put forward is the existence of abnormal protein which has a high affinity for copper (Evans, 1973). Most patients (90–95 per cent) suffering from Wilson's disease show a low concentration of ceruloplasmin in their plasma.

Menke's 'kinky hair' syndrome is characterized by a slow rate of growth, hypothermia, progressing cerebral degeneration, and fair 'metal-wool-like' hair. The illness is recessively inherent. The level of copper and the copper-oxidase activity in plasma is low. The cause of the syndrome is unkown but may be a defect in the intestinal absorption of copper which gives rise to stores of not-available copper in the intestinal mucosa cells (Möllekaer and Reske Nielsen, 1974).

B. Transferrin

1. Chemical structure and biochemistry

Transferrin is a glycoprotein which takes part in the transport of iron. The protein was discovered and named in the 1940s by Laurell. The molecular weight is approximately 77 000 and the amino acid composition is known. Recently, the amino acid sequence analysis has been reported for several fragments obtained on cyanogen bromide cleavage (Sutton et al., 1975). Human transferrin is composed of one polypeptide chain which has two specific binding sites for iron. In addition, the molecule has two carbohydrate chains (Mann et al., 1970) and the N-terminal amino acid is valine. The structure suggests that a gene duplication may have taken place during its evolution. However, examination of transferrin obtained from several higher and lower vertebrates has shown that the molecule is not identical in all species (Palmour and Sutton, 1971). Transferrin isolated from the hagfish has a molecular weight of 44 000 and contains only one binding site for iron. A comparison of the amino acid compositions of transferrin obtained from humans and hagfish did not suggest that an exact gene duplication had taken place. Nevertheless, it is possible that a partial gene duplication

Table 16. Transferrin

Molecular weight	77 000
$E^{1\%}_{280nm}$ (Fe-)	13.8
$E^{1\%}_{280nm}$ (Apo-)	11.2
Carbohydrate content, %	6
Number of polypeptide chains	1
Concentration in plasma, g/l	2.3
Half-life in plasma, days	8–9

has occurred as a result of multiple point mutations. Complete amino acid sequence analyses are required before a definite standpoint can be taken in this interesting question.

The carbohydrate content of transferrin is approximately 6 per cent. Sialic acid, coupled to galactose, occupies the terminal position on each branch of the two heterosaccharides. Different complete carbohydrate sequences have been reported (Jamieson et al., 1971; Spik et al., 1975). The two heterosaccharides are attached to the polypeptide chain at asparagines, probably situated at two different parts of the polypeptide chains as the adjacent amino acid is not the same.

Binding between iron and transferrin. Each molecule of transferrin binds two Fe^{3+} ions. Tyrosine residues are believed to take part in this binding. The two iron-binding sites have identical or almost identical thermodynamic and spectroscopic properties There is no evidence to suggest that exchange can take place between two iron atoms within the same molecule. At physiological pH, the association constant for the Fe^{3+}–transferrin complex is greater than 10^{24} M^{-1}, explaining the finding that the spontaneous dissociation of this complex is negligible. An anion must be bound simultaneously with the binding of an atom of iron and it is possible that there is interaction between the two anion-binding sites (Aisen et al., 1973a). It is not clear whether this anion is carbonate or bicarbonate under physiological conditions. Additional physicochemical evidence for non-equivalence of the two metal binding sites is now gathering. The sites have been shown to differ slightly, e.g. in the mode of interaction with several metal ions and with perchlorate. They also differ in their pH-dependence and on anion exchange chromatography. These observations are interesting as a hypothesis has been put forward that the two binding sites are also physiologically different, cf. below.

2. Genetic variants

Transferrin can exist in several forms which can be separated on starch gel electrophoresis. The most significant of these is called C. Those variants which have a greater mobility than those of C belong to a group called B. So far, eight members of this group have been described. The variants having a lower mobility than those of C belong to group D, of which nine have been described. It is thought that several variable mutations have occurred in the gene locus for transferrin in different populations. Caucasians have a relatively high frequency of unusual transferrin molecules. None of the transferrin variants has been associated with any clinical abnormality.

One report has appeared of a patient having a hereditary deficiency of transferrin (Heilmeyer et al., 1961). The patient was a seven-year-old girl suffering from severe hypochromic anaemia which was diagnosed when she was three and a half months old. Other symptoms were repeated infections and impaired growth.

3. Biological function

In humans, transferrin is synthesized in the liver. The rate of synthesis increases with iron deficiency, during pregnancy, and after administration of oestrogen. The chief function is the transport of iron to the bone marrow and tissue storage organs. Under normal conditions transferrin is saturated only to one-third of its iron-binding capacity. Almost two-thirds of the iron which is used by blood producing cells for the synthesis of haemoglobin is supplied by transferrin. This amounts to 30–40 mg daily and is 6–10 times greater than the amount of transferrin-bound iron in plasma. Thus, this iron has a high rate of turnover. It has been estimated that each molecule of transferrin transports approximately 15 atoms of iron during its lifetime.

Erythroblasts and reticulocytes have specific receptors for transferrin which are lost when the synthesis of haemoglobin ceases. In general, homologue transferrins have a higher affinity for the corresponding reticulocytes than do the heterologue transferrins. The utilization of iron within the cell is independent of the homology of the iron-donating transferrin. Human apotransferrin differs from ferritransferrin in its lower affinity for reticulocytes and in its chromatographic behaviour. On the other hand, the two corresponding proteins obtained from rabbit displayed the same affinity for reticulocytes (Lane, 1972). The exact fate of the iron-saturated transferrin after binding to its receptor is not yet known. Different results have been obtained in experiments where the distribution of iron in various subcellular fractions was studied after incubation with transferrin. Isotope-labelled transferrin has been detected intracellularly by using a variety of techniques. Other evidence is also consistent with the idea that transferrin penetrates the reticulocyte cell wall. Endocytosis may be the mechanism (Sullivan et al., 1976). As the transferrin molecule remains intact, there must exist a specific mechanism whereby the iron is released from the protein. It is believed that the anion-binding sites play a significant role in this connection (Aisen et al., 1973b). When the bicarbonate was destroyed experimentally, transferrin showed no great affinity for ferric iron. The binding of anion to transferrin and the uptake of the Fe^{3+}–transferrin complex by reticulocytes did not change appreciably when the bicarbonate was replaced by oxalate. However, the transferrin–oxalate complex proved to be less effective in the synthesis of haemoglobin. Apparently, the disruption of the binding between oxalate and transferrin was performed less easily by the reticulocyte than was the disruption of the binding between bicarbonate and transferrin.

The transition from Fe^{2+} to Fe^{3+} occurs in almost every stage of iron metabolism. The iron in ferritin is present as hydroxy iron polymer, $(Fe^{3+})_n$–ferritin, and is released probably via a reductive mechanism. Spontaneous oxidation of Fe^{2+} is not sufficient to satisfy the iron requirements of Fe^{3+}–transferrin. Ceruloplasmin is believed to be a link between the metabolism of copper and that of iron, where it acts as a catalyst for this oxidation (Frieden, 1973). Ceruloplasmin induced a fast and specific mobilizing of iron from the liver of laboratory animals. It should be kept in mind that only one-tenth of the normal concentration of ceruloplasmin in plasma was required to produce the maximum effect.

Iron differs from other metals in that its haemostasis is regulated by absorption and not by excretion. In certain situations, the degree of saturation of transferrin is without doubt of significance in this absorption. Using in vitro experiments, Levine et al. (1972) showed that serum obtained from rats which had iron deficiency caused the release of more iron from mucous cells than was caused by serum from normal rats. The effect was independent of the source of the mucous cells, i.e. the same result was obtained by using mucous cells from either rat.

Fletcher and Huehns (1968) presented the interesting hypothesis that the two iron-binding sites have different functional roles in iron transport. This would imply that the plasma pool of transferrin-bound iron was heterogeneous. According to Fletcher and Huehns' hypothesis four forms of the transferrin molecule are possible.

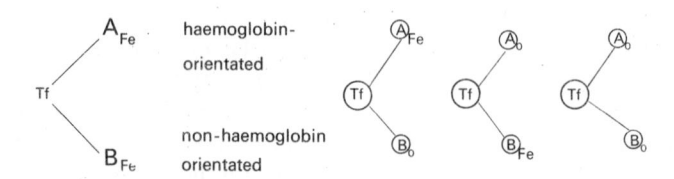

```
         A_Fe     haemoglobin-          A_Fe        A_0          A_0
        /         orientated           /           /            /
    Tf <                             (Tf)        (Tf)         (Tf)
        \         non-haemoglobin      \           \            \
         B_Fe     orientated            B_0         B_Fe         B_0
```

On the addition of iron, transferrin in plasma combines at random with the iron to give complexes containing no, one, or two atoms of iron. The relative proportion of these molecules is dependent on the degree of saturation. At a high saturation level, most molecules of transferrin had one or two atoms of iron. When radioactive iron was added to a solution of transferrin which had a high degree of saturation, the isotope bound preferentially to those molecules which had already one atom of iron. Under conditions of low saturation, the isotope bound largely to those molecules which were devoid of iron. Under *in vitro* conditions, half-saturated and saturated molecules of transferrin had different affinities for cell receptors. Saturated transferrin was more efficient in donating iron to reticulocytes. Receptors in the small intestine are believed also to have a high affinity for saturated transferrin. Fletcher (1970) is of the opinion that the proportion of half-saturated and saturated molecules may be a factor determining the rate of absorption and, hence, may be a factor contributing to the formation of iron-depots in the body and to erythropoiesis. Various studies have been published, some which are consistent with this hypothesis and some which are contradictory. This holds for both *in vivo* and *in vtiro* experiments (Hahn and Ganzoni, 1975; Brown *et al.*, 1975; Harris and Aisen, 1975).

Bacteria require iron for their growth. The growth of bacteria is inhibited in serum by unsaturated transferrin and in milk by unsaturated lactoferrin. Sometimes the presence of an antibody is required (Bullen *et al.*, 1972). Lactoferrin is a protein having iron-binding properties which are the same as those of transferrin. Saturating the iron-binding capacities of these proteins abolishes the bacteriostatic action.

C. Haptoglobin

1. Chemical structure and biochemistry

Haptoglobin is a glycoprotein present in plasma which has the capacity to bind haemoglobin specifically and stoichiometrically. In 1938, Polonowski and Jayle demonstrated the existence in serum of a protein which had the ability to bind haemoglobin and to cause an increase in its peroxidase activity. They called the protein haptoglobin.

Haptoglobin occurs in three forms; haptoglobin 1–1, haptoglobin 2–1, and haptoglobin 2–2. It has been shown by starch gel electrophoresis that haptoglobin 1–1 exists as a monomer while the other two forms are polymers. The molecule of haptoglobin 1–1 is a four-chain monomer consisting of two small α-chains and two large β-chains. A representation of the proposed structure is given in Fig. 37 (Malchy *et al.*, 1973). The smaller α-chains are responsible for the genetic polymorphism which is displayed by the molecule. These chains are of two main types, α1 and α2, where α1 can exist in two forms, α1F and α1S. Haptoglobin 1–1 contains α1-chains, haptoglobin 1–2 contains α1- and α2-chains while haptoglobin 2–2 contains α2-chains. The larger β-chain is identical

Table 17. Haptoglobin 1–1

Molecular weight	99 000
$E^{1\%}_{280nm}$	12.0
Carbohydrate content, %	19.3
Number of polypeptide chains	4
Concentration in plasma, g/l	2.0
Half-life in plasma, days	2–4

in all three molecules. A schematic representation of the three common forms and the six common phenotypes of haptoglobin is given in Fig. 38.

Haptoglobin 2–1 and 2–2 exist in the form of stable polymers. Fuller et al. (1973) determined the molecular weights of six haptoglobin 2–2 molecules. It was observed that the difference in molecular weight between each polymer and its next member could be accounted for by the addition of an α2- and a β-chain. The polymers of haptoglobin are held together by disulphide bonds. On treating the isolated polymers with relatively low concentrations of β-mercaptoethanol, the dissociation of the polymers increased in proportion to the concentration of reducing agent to give rise to polymeric forms of lower molecular weight. However, as no monomeric forms were obtained, it would appear that the disulphide bonds which link the α2/β-subunits in the polymers are more susceptible to reduction than those linking the α2- and β-chains. This may indicate that the disulphides in the former cases are orientated more towards the surface of the molecule and are consequently attacked more easily by the reducing agent. It is not known whether the polymers are joined together during synthesis or at a later stage.

The structure of the polypeptide chains of haptoglobin is known almost completely. The molecular weight of the α1-chain is 9 100 and its amino acid sequence has been determined (Black and Dixon, 1968). The N- and C-terminal amino acids are valine

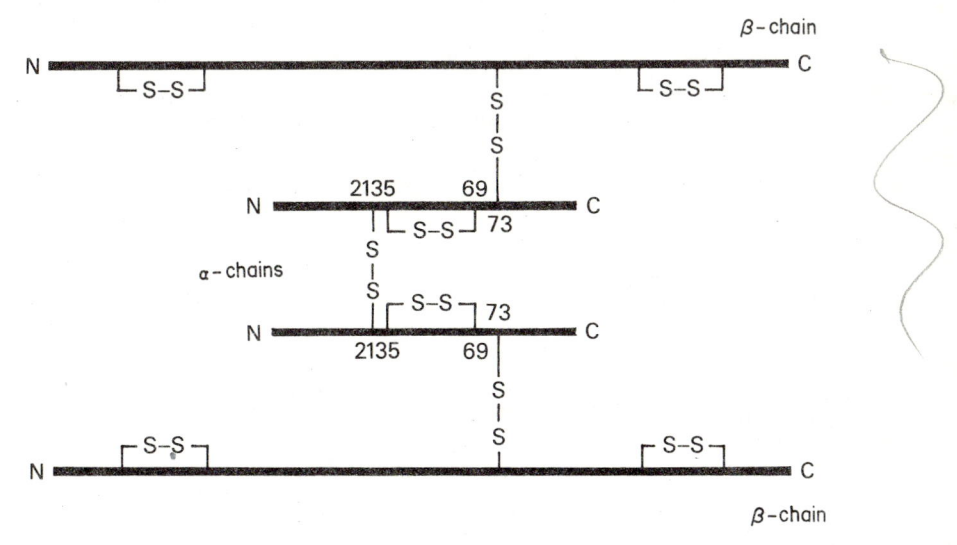

Fig. 37. Tentative structure of a molecule of haptoglobin 1–1 showing the disulphide bonds. By kind permission of B. Malchy et al., Can. J. Biochem., **51** (1973) p. 266

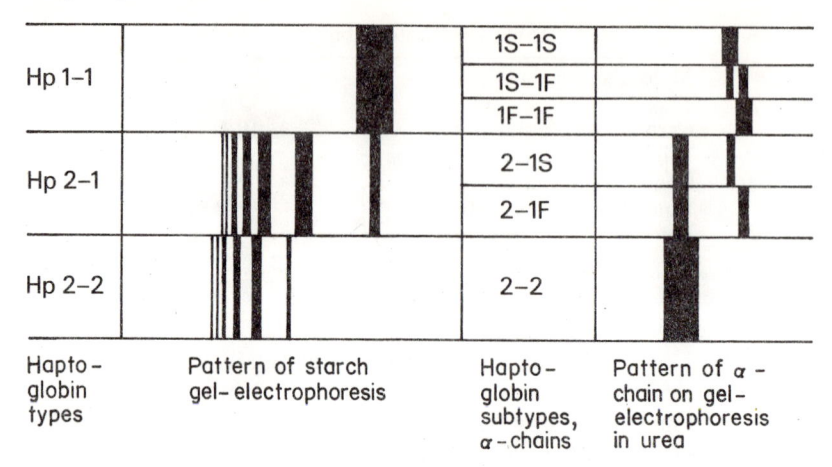

Fig. 38. Schematic representation of the types and subtypes of haptoglobin. By kind permission of E. R. Giblett, *Genetic Markers in Human Blood* (1969) p. 74

and glutamine, respectively. The two α1-chains differ only in the substitution of a single amino acid. The molecular weight of the α2-chain is 16 000, i.e. almost twice that of the α1-chain. Judging by its amino acid sequence, it appears that this chain is composed of two incomplete α1-chains. Even before the amino acid sequence of the α2-chain became known, it was suggested by Smithies et al. (1966) that this chain resulted from a partial gene duplication. A tentative mechanism for such an event is provided in Fig. 39. The β-chains of all genetic types of haptoglobin are identical. The molecular weight is 40 000 and the amino acid sequences of the N- and C-terminal portions are known. The N- and C-terminal amino acids are isoleucine and tryptophan, respectively (Barnett et al., 1972).

When Black and Dixon (1968) determined the amino acid sequence of the α-chains, they pointed out similarities between haptoglobin and immunoglobin G. Both molecules consist of two light and two heavy chains and they both display the ability to bind other proteins in a bivalent manner. Furthermore, certain regions of the α-chains showed amino acid sequence homology with regions of the light chains of immunoglobulin. However, no detectable homology has been found between the β-chain and immunoglobulins. Instead, recent partial determination of the amino acid sequence of

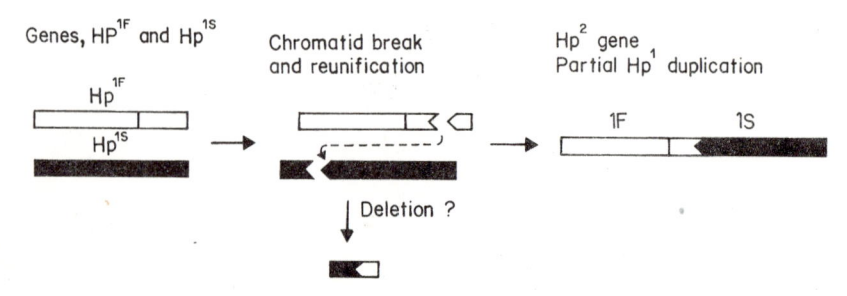

Fig. 39. Schematic representation of a possible mechanism for the appearance of the Hp² gene. By kind permission of E. R. Giblett, *Genetic Markers in Human Blood* (1969) p. 75

the β-chain has shown that there are significant similarities between this chain and corresponding regions in the bovine serine proteinases (Barnett et al., 1972).

The carbohydrate portion of haptoglobin is located in the β-chain. The carbohydrate composition of haptoglobin 2–1 and 2–2 is known. The presence of hexose (galactose and mannose), N-glucosamine, and sialic acid has been shown (Gerbeck et al., 1967).

Haptoglobin–haemoglobin complex. Much attention has been paid to the complex formed between haptoglobin and haemoglobin because it provides an example of interaction between protein surfaces. One molecule of haptoglobin 1–1 binds one molecule of haemoglobin to form a saturated complex. An intermediate form can exist in which one molecule of haptoglobin binds half a molecule of haemoglobin; possible alternative forms of the subunits of haemoglobin are $\alpha\alpha$, $\beta\beta$, and $\alpha\beta$. Laurell and Grönvall suggested the alternative $(\alpha\beta)^{Hb}$, which has now been confirmed. Before binding can take place between haptoglobin and haemoglobin, the haemoglobin tetramers, $(\alpha_2\beta_2)^{Hb}$, must dissociate to give the dimeric form, $(\alpha\beta)^{Hb}$ (Nagel and Gibson, 1971), The α- and β-subunits of haemoglobin have separate binding sites for haptoglobin. The α-subunit binds first, thereby inducing the binding of the β-subunit. Thus, a molecule of haptoglobin is capable of binding two haemoglobin dimers in such a way that the two regions of binding are independent of each other. Using a variety of spectroscopic methods, Makinen et al. (1972) demonstrated that the two dimeric molecules of haemoglobin bind symmetrically to the molecule of haptoglobin to produce a complex which is longer than the molecule of haptoglobin. The authors have proposed two alternative models for such a complex which could not be distinguished under the conditions used (Fig. 40). The nature of the bond between haptoglobin and haemoglobin is still not clear. Using affinity chromatography with immobilized haemoglobin, Javid and Liang (1973) have studied the conditions of dissociation. Proper configuration of the two proteins and the formation of hydrophobic bonds seemed to be essential, whereas any covalent bond did not appear to be involved. In another study, tyrosyl groups of haptoglobin have been proposed to be involved in the binding (Chiao and Bezkorovainy, 1972).

2. Genetic variants

Apart from those mentioned above, there exist other more uncommon variants of haptoglobin. One of these shows certain similarities with haptoglobin 2–1 and is therefore called, modified 2–1 or 2–1 M. In this variant, the normal ratio of α1-chains to α2-chains is changed by a relative decrease of the latter. This variant is present in

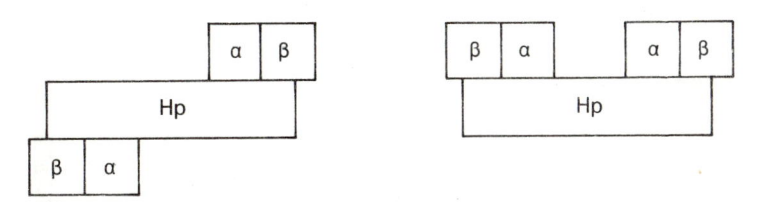

Fig. 40. Tentative models for the binding to haptoglobin (Hp) of the α- and β-subunits of haemoglobin. Under the experimental conditions used, the alternatives could not be distinguished. By kind permission of M. W. Makinen et al., Biochem., 11 (1972) p. 3858. Copyright, the American Chemical Society

about 10 per cent of Negroes. Another phenotype, haptoglobin 0, is devoid of haptoglobin. This is also most common in Negroes, especially in families where haptoglobin 2–1 M is present. The genetic control of these variants is unknown. Several variants which are even less common have been described (Kirk, 1968).

3. Biological function

The synthesis of haptoglobin takes place in the liver. The factors controlling this synthesis are not completely known. It would appear that the presence of a low level of haptoglobin is not in itself sufficient to stimulate an increase in the synthesis. Patients with haemolytic anaemia have a low concentration of haptoglobin in their plasma. The rate of synthesis in a small group of such patients was of the same order of magnitude as that in normal individuals (Freeman, 1965). The synthesis increases in conditions which are combined with an inflammatory reaction.

The role of the reticuloendothelial system in removing non-viable red blood cells from the circulation is well documented. Under normal conditions, the pathway via haemoglobin in plasma is not believed to be the major one for the degradation of haemoglobin. Measurements have shown that haptoglobin can not play a quantitatively dominating role in the normal catabolism of haemoglobin. Thus, it has been suggested that the function of haptoglobin is to remove haemoglobin when the latter is released in pathological processes (Freeman, 1965). Under haemolytic conditions, considerable amounts of free haemoglobin can reach the circulation where it quickly becomes bound to haptoglobin. According to different authors, the half-life of haptoglobin in plasma of normal individuals varies between two and four days. The half-life of the haptoglobin haemoglobin-complex is considerably less, varying between 10 and 20 minutes. In experiments performed on rats, it has been shown that the catabolism of the complex takes place in the hepatocytes and not in the Kupffer cells (Hershko et al., 1972).

In haemolytic conditions and conditions connected with an ineffective erythropoiesis a decline in the concentration of haptoglobin in plasma is seen due to an increased elimination. Haptoglobin is not usually detected in plasma when the half-life of ^{51}Cr-labelled red blood cells is less than approximately 17 days. In this connection, it is interesting to note that individuals who, for genetic reasons, have no haptoglobin do not appear to show any metabolic disorders. Even today, the physiological or adaptive function of haptoglobin must be considered as unclear (cf. below 'The fate of circulating haemoglobin').

D. Haemopexin

1. Chemical structure and biochemistry

Haemopexin is a glycoprotein which binds haem. Towards the end of the 1950s experiments were performed using sera obtained from patients who suffered from intravascular haemolysis. After separation of the serum proteins by electrophoresis, it was observed that peroxidase activity was present in the β-region. This led to the discovery of a specific haem-binding glycoprotein, haemopexin. Schultze et al. (1961) purified this protein which proved to bind haem in equimolar amounts. The molecular weight of haemopexin is 57 000; earlier determinations gave values which were

Table 18. Haemopexin

Molecular weight	57 000
$E_{280\ nm}^{1\%}$	16.9
Carbohydrate content, %	20
Number of polypeptide chains	1
Concentration in plasma, g/l	0.85

somewhat higher than this. The amino acid composition is known and shows the presence of unusually high amounts of tyrosine and tryptophan. The molecule probably consists of a single chain, as no subunits appeared on treating the protein with disulphide-reducing agents (Müller-Eberhard, 1970). The N-terminal residue of human haemopexin has not been unequivocally identified, both serine and threonine have been reported.

The carbohydrate content is approximately 20 per cent and is composed of sialic acid, mannose, galactose, and glucosamine.

2. Biological function

Haemopexin is synthesized in the liver. It is thought that haem is capable of inducing this synthesis. Rabbits injected with a small amount of haem showed an initial drop in the concentration of haemopexin in plasma. This was soon replaced by a doubling of the haemopexin concentration during a period of two days. Pentabarbital and other polycyclic hydrocarbons have also been shown to be capable of inducing the synthesis (Smibert et al., 1972).

Haem-haemopexin complex. There exist two plasma proteins, haemopexin and albumin, which bind haem. Each molecule of haemopexin binds one molecule of haem. The participation of two histidine residues in the binding of haem by haemopexin is indicated by the use of different experimental techniques. The haem–haemopexin complex is eliminated very quickly from plasma by the hepatocytes. When normal individuals were injected with a dose of haem which was sufficient to exceed the binding-capacity of haemopexin, the concentration of haem in plasma decreased exponentially with a half-life of 7–8 hours (Sears, 1970). The haem in this case was bound to both haemopexin and albumin. When the experiment was repeated using patients suffering from haemolysis and showing subnormal concentrations of haemopexin in their plasma, a biphasic curve was obtained where the half-lives were approximately 4 hours and 22 hours, respectively. In this case, the haem was found to be bound only to albumin. Thus, the haem–albumin complex was removed from the circulation at a considerably slower rate than the haem–haemopexin complex.

Several functions have been suggested for haemopexin. It has been stated that haemopexin functions specifically in forming a complex with haem. Only this complex and not the haem–albumin complex enters the liver cells. It has been suggested that the rate of synthesis of haemopexin is a controlling factor in the elimination of haem from rabbits which have low levels of haemopexin (Lane et al., 1973). Thus, albumin, which is present in a higher concentration than haemopexin, may represent a reservoir for haem. It has also been suggested that haemopexin takes part in the catabolism of precursors of haem, e.g. protoporphyrin IX. The binding of porphyrins to haemopexin

108 *Transport proteins*

has been studied more closely by several workers, e.g. Seery and Müller–Eberhard (1973) who used rabbit haemopexin to demonstrate that this protein has an affinity for deuterated haem (the structure of which is very like that of haem) which is 60 times greater than that for albumin. On the other hand, the two proteins showed identical and considerably lower affinities for protoporphyrin IX. An accelerated breakdown of haemopexin has been observed in patients with aberrations of porphyrin metabolism. Further information is required before these proposals can be taken as valid.

The fate of circulating haemoglobin

A possible sequence of events leading to the removal of haemoglobin from plasma after an increased intravascular supply of the protein is depicted in Fig. 41. Following intravascular release, haemoglobin dissociates into $\alpha\beta$-dimers and binding occurs between haemoglobin and haptoglobin. This complex is eliminated quickly from the blood system. Free haemoglobin appears when the binding capacity of circulating haptoglobin has been exceeded. The free haemoglobin is easily oxidized and dissociates into ferrihaem and globin. Haemopexin has a higher affinity for ferrihaem than albumin and a haem–haemopexin complex is formed. Like the haptoglobin–haemoglobin complex, this complex is also rapidly cleared from the circulation by the hepatic parenchymal cells. Haem not bound to haemopexin is trapped by albumin. Metalbumin is not cleared from plasma and it is suggested that metalbumin delivers its haem to apohaemopexin. A portion of the circulating haemoglobin, dissociated into $\alpha\beta$-dimers, is filtered by the renal glomeruli and is either reabsorbed or catabolized in the tubules. If the reabsorption capacity of the tubules is exceeded, subunits of haemoglobin appear in the urine.

The haptoglobin level in serum is low in conditions which are connected with haemolysis and ineffective erythropoiesis and thus, it can be difficult to estimate the degree of haemolysis. The determination of haemopexin in plasma may be of value in these situations. A high level of haem in plasma is the major factor responsible for a reduced level of haemopexin. Thus, the concentration of haemopexin can be taken as

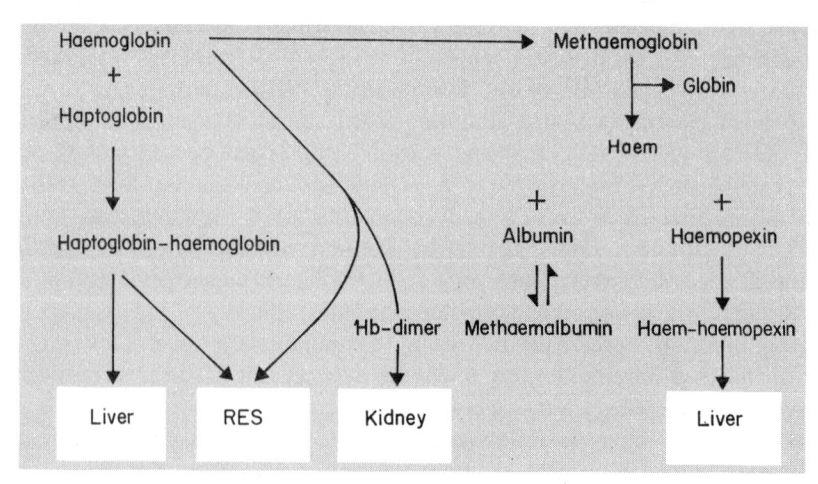

Fig. 41. Possible sequence of events in the catabolism of an increased level of intravascular haemoglobin

an indication of the accumulation of haem in plasma. Removal of red blood cells under normal conditions occurs in the reticuloendothelial system. This pathway of haemoglobin catabolism is thought to be the major one. A haem-oxygenase has been reported as being capable of transforming haem into biliverdin, which is subsequently reduced to bilirubin. This enzyme, which has been demonstrated in several organs, requires the presence of NADPH and molecular oxygen for its catalytic function. Ferrihaem proved to be the best of the substrates tested. Haem proteins such as oxyhaemoglobin and the haptoglobin–haemoglobin complex, where the haem is tightly bound, were shown to be almost inactive as substrates while haem bound to haemopexin was active.

E. Transcobalamin

1. Chemical structure and biochemistry

The proteins present in body fluids which bind vitamin B_{12} are of at least three types: intrinsic factor in gastric juice, transcobalamin II in plasma, and the proteins present in plasma, gastric juice, saliva, cerebrospinal fluid, and milk which are called R-proteins (Gräsbeck, 1969). The R-proteins are immunologically related vitamin B_{12}-binding proteins observed in a number of human body fluids. There are at least two vitamin B_{12}-binding proteins in plasma. These have been named transcobalamin I and II by Hall and Finkler. The former belongs to the group of R-proteins.

Transcobalamin I

Granulocytes contain a vitamin B_{12}-binding protein which may even be synthesized within these cells. According to ultracentrifugation analysis, this protein has a molecular weight of 56 000. The carbohydrate content is 33 per cent which implies that molecular weight determinations by gelfiltration are less reliable. A hypothesis has been put forward suggesting that the protein is released from granulocytes into plasma where it exists as transcobalamin I. Support for this hypothesis is found in the following observations: incubation of granulocytes causes a release of vitamin B_{12} binding activity into the incubation medium; antibodies raised against the vitamin B_{12} binding protein of granulocytes cross-react with transcobalamin I: it would appear that the level of transcobalamin I in plasma is correlated to the pool of granulocytes in the body. Burger *et al.* (1975) have isolated highly purified transcobalamin I and the vitamin B_{12}-binding protein in granulocytes. The proteins were indistinguishable from each other when studied by immunodiffusion with antiserum to milk vitamin B_{12}-binding protein. On the other hand, differences in the carbohydrate compositions were found and they therefore suggested that transcobalamin I may not be derived from granulocytes. A third transcobalamin, belonging to R-proteins, was also purified and this showed several similarities with the granulocyte vitamin B_{12}-binding protein. They suggested that this protein is released *in vitro* from granulocytes.

Transcobalamin I is a glycoprotein having a molecular weight of 120 000 as determined by gel filtration. Transcobalamin I and the vitamin B_{12}-binding protein obtained from granulocytes have different electrophoretic mobilities. This is believed to arise as a consequence of the difference in the sialic acid contents of these two proteins. teins.

Transcobalamin II

Transcobalamin II has been purified by Allen and Majerus (1972) by using a combination of conventional methods and affinity chromatography. In the latter case, the ligand used was vitamin B_{12}. Unlike the material obtained by other workers, the final preparation obtained by Allen and co-workers was homogeneous. The molecular weight was determined as approximately 60 000. In other studies values in the region of 37 000 were obtained. The protein is devoid of carbohydrate and free sulphydryl groups. The amino acid composition has been determined. Each molecule has one binding site for vitamin B_{12}.

2. Biological function

The concept that transcobalamin I originates from granulocytes is questioned in recent studies. Transcobalamin II can be synthesized in the liver of rats. However, the synthesis of the protein in dogs was unaffected by the removal of the liver. The known functions of the transcobalamins are (a) to combat the loss of vitamin B_{12} via urine, perspiration, sputum, and intestinal fluid and (b) to facilitate the transport of vitamin B_{12} across cell membranes. The molecular weight of transcobalamin II is such that the molecule could be filtered through the glomeruli. However, it is thought that the protein exists in plasma in the form of a complex with an unknown protein.

The concentration of transcobalamin I and II in plasma is very low, about 33 and 45 µg/l respectively. Most of the endogenic vitamin B_{12} is bound to transcobalamin I while 10–30 per cent is bound to transcobalamin II. Transcobalamin II is responsible for approximately 80 per cent of the binding capacity of plasma for exogenic vitamin B_{12}.

Radioactive-labelled vitamin B_{12}, when administered orally or intravenously, appeared initially bound to transcobalamin II and the half-life of the vitamin in plasma was approximately 12 hours. The radioactivity reappeared later bound to transcobalamin I where the half-life of the vitamin was approximately 6 days (Hom and Oleson, 1969). Transcobalamin II is believed to be of great importance in the transport of vitamin B_{12}. When vitamin B_{12} was bound to transcobalamin I, or intrinsic factor, or was in the free form, its uptake by reticulocytes and HeLa-cells was much lower than when it was bound to transcobalamin II (Hall and Finkler, 1971). The study of patients having a genetically determined deficiency of transcobalamin II has contributed much to our understanding of the function of this protein (see later). Transcobalamin II is required for the absorption and transport of vitamin B_{12}. The complex formed between transcobalamin II and vitamin B_{12} is essential for the normal maturation of haematopoietic cells. On the other hand, it is not thought that the protein is required by the two enzymes which are known to specifically require vitamin B_{12}, i.e. N-methyltetrahydrofolate-homocysteinmethyl-transferase and methylmalonyl-CoA-mutase. In the case of the patient who was mentioned above, no disorders in the functions of these enzymes could be demonstrated (Scott *et al.*, 1972).

3. Genetic variants

Carmel and Herbert (1969) have described two members of a family who were shown to be without transcobalamine I. Furthermore, the presence of this protein could not be detected in either granulocytes or saliva. The level of vitamin B_{12} in serum was low and there were no metabolic signs of a deficiency of vitamin B_{12}.

The clinical picture is completely different in the case of two members of a family who showed a deficiency of transcobalamin II (Hakami et al., 1971). Extreme symptoms of diarrhoea, vomiting, increasing anaemia, and megaloblastic changes in the bone marrow appear already during the first weeks after birth. Frequent administration of massive doses of vitamin B_{12} were required for haematologic remission and normal development. On examining the family relations, an autosomal recessive inheritance was indicated.

F. Retinol-binding protein

1. Chemical structure and biochemistry

Following resorption in the small intestine, vitamin A (retinol) is transported as fatty acid esters by the chylomicron fraction via the lymph to the liver. A specific carrier protein, retinol-binding protein, is responsible for the continuous transport in plasma from the liver. Under physiological conditions, one molecule of vitamin A binds to one molecule of the protein. In plasma, this complex is bound non-covalently to another protein, prealbumin.

Retinol-binding protein was isolated first in the late 1960s by Kanai and co-workers. It is a small protein, molecular weight 21 000. The amino acid composition and a partial sequence of the N-terminal portion is known (Morgan et al., 1971). The N-terminal amino acid is glutamic acid. Under physiological conditions the protein exists in two forms, one having arginine as the C-terminal amino acid and the other having lysine in this position. This difference results in the two forms having different conformations and, consequently, different immunological, chemical, and optical properties. The form having arginine as C-terminal amino acid has the capacity to bind retinol and to be bound to prealbumin. The other form does not have these properties.

Thyroxine-binding prealbumin was isolated first in the early 1960s by Schultze and co-workers. As the protein has two physiological ligands; retinol-binding protein and thyroxine, it is thought to exhibit an interesting 'double function'. Recent molecular weight determinations (Morgan et al., 1971) have suggested values from 50 000 to over 60 000. Preparations of prealbumin isolated by different workers have been shown to have considerable differences in their amino acid compositions, carbohydrate contents, and association constants for the binding of thyroid hormones. The protein contains unusually high quantities of tryptophane and tyrosine. The N-terminal amino acid is glycine. When incubated with high concentrations of guanidine hydrochloride, the protein dissociates into apparently identical subunits, each with a molecular weight of approximately 16 000, showing a tetrameric structure of the protein. The three-

Table 19. Retinol-binding protein

Molecular weight	21 000
$E_{280nm}^{1\%}$	19.4
Carbohydrate content, %	0
Number of polypeptide chains	1
Concentration in plasma, g/l	0.045

Table 20. Prealbumin

Molecular weight	50 000–66 000
$E^{1\%}_{280nm}$	14.1
Carbohydrate content, %	?
Number of polypeptide chains	4
Concentration in plasma, g/l	0.25
Half-life in plasma, days	2–3

dimensional structure of prealbumin consists of a tetrahedral arrangement of the subunits with a channel through the centre of the molecule.

Complex formed between prealbumin and retinol-binding protein

In recent years, much attention has been paid to the complex which is formed between prealbumin and retinol-binding protein. The interaction between these two proteins is highly dependent on the pH. The maximum binding takes place under conditions which are close to physiological pH. Furthermore, this binding is very sensitive to ionic strength, being greatest at moderately high ionic strengths. Vitamin A is bound only to retinol-binding protein and its presence does not affect the interaction between this protein and prealbumin. Van Jaarsveld *et al* (1973) suggest that four molecules of retinol-binding protein bind to one molecule of prealbumin. The four binding sites are independent of each other. In plasma, the molar concentration of retinol-binding protein is slightly less than that of prealbumin and, under physiological conditions, one molecule of retinol-binding protein binds to one molecule of prealbumin. Several investigations have demonstrated that the binding of retinol-binding protein and thyroxine to prealbumin are independent of each other.

2. Biological function

Retinol-binding protein is synthesized in the liver. The work of Peterson *et al.* (1973), who used both normal and vitamin-A-deficient rats, has contributed much to our understanding of the synthesis of the protein and its relation to vitamin A. In the case of vitamin A deficiency, there was first a drop in the amount of vitamin A stored in the liver. This was followed by a drop in the level of this vitamin in plasma and an eventual drop in the level of retinol-binding protein in plasma. At the same time, the concentration of retinol-binding protein in the liver increased. Following an injection of vitamin A, the level of retinol-binding protein in the plasma increased. It can be concluded from this that a deficiency of vitamin A did not affect the synthesis of retinol-binding protein but did affect its secretion. Newly synthesized retinol-binding protein seems to require retinol for its release from the liver. It has been suggested that the form of the protein which has lysine as C-terminal amino acid, and which does not have the capacity to bind retinol, is a catabolite. If this is the case, then the C-terminal residue of arginine is lost by the protein after it has carried out its function.

Retinol-binding protein appears in several forms in plasma. The major portion exists in a complex with prealbumin. The molecular weight of this complex normally prevents a rapid excretion of retinol-binding protein in the kidneys. A small fraction exists in the free form. The major portion of this form is composed of the form of the molecule which does not have arginine as the C-terminal amino acid. As mentioned above, this form can not bind retinol nor can it be bound to prealbumin. Another portion of the free fraction is composed of retinol-binding protein which exists in an equilibrium with the complex formed between this protein and prealbumin. Vahlquist et al. (1973) have studied the metabolism of the various forms in both normal individuals and patients with reduced kidney function. The complex formed between prealbumin and retinol-binding protein had a half-life which was considerably less than that of the free retinol-binding protein. It is thought that almost all of the free retinol-binding protein is catabolized in the kidney where, along with several other low molecular weight proteins, it passes through the glomeruli to become reabsorbed and catabolized in the cells of the kidney proximal tubules. Consequently, patients showing a reduced filtration through the glomeruli were found to have an increased concentration of free retinol-binding protein in their plasma. In these patients, the half-life of the protein was increased ten- to fifteenfold compared to the normal individuals. It is believed that approximately one-third of the amount of vitamin A in the plasma eventually reaches the kidney. It is not known if vitamin A has a specific function in this organ or if it can be recirculated.

G. Proteins binding thyroid hormones

1. Chemical structure and biochemistry

The thyroid hormones, thyroxine (T_4) and triiodothyronine (T_3), are transported by several proteins: thyroxine-binding globulin, thyroxine-binding prealbumin, and albumin. Several groups of workers have purified thyroxine-binding globulin and reported its physical and chemical properties. The reports do not agree on several points, thus these must be taken as tentative. More recently isolation techniques employing affinity chromatography on thyroxine-substituted matrix have been used. The protein has been obtained in higher yield and with a higher degree of purity than with conventional techniques. Several laboratories have reported a molecular weight in the range of 54 000–65 000 (Marshall and Pensky, 1971; Nilsson and Peterson, 1975). The amino acid composition is reported.

The carbohydrate content varies in different reports between 8–30 per cent. Discrepancies are found in the quantities reported of sialic acid, which might be explained by differences in the methodologies employed.

Marshall et al (1972) have described an additional thyroxine-binding globulin which has a slow rate of electrophoretic mobility. They are not of the opinion that this protein is an artefact.

Table 21. Thyroxine-binding globulin

Molecular weight	54 000–65 000
$E^{1\%}_{280nm}$	6.9–8.4
Carbohydrate content, %	15–30
Concentration in plasma, g/l	0.01

Binding between thyroid hormones and protein

The results obtained in most investigations suggest that each molecule of thyroxine-binding globulin binds one molecule of T_4. The binding is dependent on the pH and diminishes below pH 6.4. The protein has a higher binding affinity for T_4 than it has for T_3. This may be a consequence of the fact that T_3 has only one atom of iodine in the β-ring, giving rise to two possible configurations. Thyroxine-binding globulin shows a higher binding affinity for one of these configurations and thyroxine always exists in the suitable configuration (Schussler, 1972). Thyroxine-binding prealbumin is described in more detail in the section dealing with those proteins which transport vitamin A. Prealbumin contains one binding site for T_4 and under normal conditions, a few per cent of the prealbumin present in plasma form a complex with this hormone. Recent work has shown that even T_3 binds to prealbumin and that both hormones appear to bind in the phenolate form (Pages *et al.*, 1973). The binding to prealbumin of each of the two ligands, T_4 and retinol-binding protein, is independent of each other. Among other substances, several pharmaceuticals can interfere with the binding of thyroid hormone to thyroxine-binding globulin. Examples of these are diphenylhydantoin, chloropropamide, heparin, and tolbutamide. Acetyl salicylic acid interferes with the binding to prealbumin.

2. Genetic variants

In man, neither thyroxine-binding globulin nor thyroxine-binding prealbumin display polymorphism (Robbins, 1973). On the other hand, the occurrence of genetic variants which give rise to an altered level of thyroxine-binding globulin is relatively common. In general, the method used in these studies was a determination of the binding capacity of thyroxine-binding globulin for thyroxine. In patients showing an increased binding capacity, a good correlation has been shown to exist between this binding capacity and the level of thyroxine-binding globulin. Related studies suggest the occurrence of a dominant inheritance which is connected with an X-chromosome. From a clinical point of view, an understanding of these abnormalities is important as they can affect the results of those thyroid function analyses which are based on the level and binding of hormone in blood. Furthermore, the genetic variants are interesting from a point of view of human genetics where they affect the X-chromosome as well as being one of the few abnormalities which give rise to an increased level of protein.

3. Biological function

Only a very small fraction of the thyroid hormones in blood appears in the free state. The fraction of free T_4 and T_3 comprises merely a few parts per 10 000 and a few parts per 1 000, respectively, of the total concentration of these hormones in plasma. The remainder is bound to the three hormone-carrying proteins in plasma. Of these proteins, thyroxine-binding globulin binds between one-half and three-quarters of the relative distribution of both T_3 and T_4. In the case of T_3, Dussault *et al.* (1973) have shown that there exists an inverse relationship between dialysable hormone and the thyroxine-binding globulin when the concentration of the latter is varied. The concentration was increased by the administration of oestrogen and was decreased by the

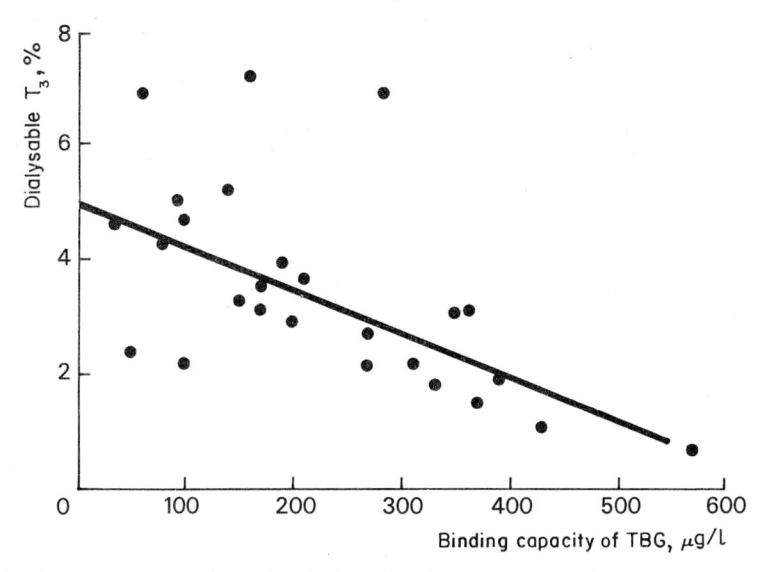

Fig. 42. The fraction of dialysable triiodothyronine (free hormone) is inversely proportional to the thyroxine-binding capacity of thyroxin-binding globulin in serum. By kind permission of J. H. Dussault *et al.*, *Acta Endocrin.*, **72** (1973) p. 269

administration of androgen. Alternatively the increase or decrease was caused by genetic factors (Fig. 42). Thus, the fractions of free T_4 and T_3 are related to the concentration of thyroxine-binding globulin. The inverse relationship between the dialysable fraction, i.e. free hormone, and the total concentration of hormone constitutes a means whereby the absolute amount of free hormone can be held stable. The hormone mediates its effect in its free form.

H. Transcortin

1. Chemical structure and biochemistry

Steroid hormones bind to plasma proteins to form dissociable complexes. Apart from albumin, there are specific glycoproteins which are present in low concentrations: corticosteroid-binding protein or transcortin, sex hormone-binding protein, and even a progesterone-binding protein which is present in the guinea-pig.

In the mid-1950s, different groups of workers under the direction of Daughaday, Bush and Sandberg described a protein which was present at low concentration in human plasma and which showed a high affinity for cortisol. This protein is now called corticosteroid-binding globulin or transcortin. The glycoprotein has a molecular

Table 22. Transcortin

Molecular weight	53 000
$E^{1\%}_{280\,nm}$	6.5
Carbohydrate content, %	16–26
Number of polypeptide chains	1
Concentration in plasma, g/l	0.03

weight of approximately 52 000. Recent reports of the amino acid composition are in good agreement, in contrast to those concerning the N-terminal amino acid, arginine (Rosner, 1972) and methionine (Le Gaillard et al., 1972). The C-terminal amino acid is leucine. The protein consists of a single polypeptide chain. Human transcortin tends to polymerize rapidly.

Different values for the carbohydrate content ranging from 16 per cent to 26 per cent have been reported; hexose, hexosamine, and sialic acid are present (Burton and Westphal, 1972).

Binding of steroids to protein. Hydrophobic interactions and hydrogen bonds exist in the complex formed between steroid hormone and plasma proteins. The study of the binding of steroid to albumin has led to the proposal of a rule of polarity which states that the affinity decreases as the number of polar groups increases: oestradiol > progesterone > testosterone > deoxycorticosterone > corticosterone > cortisol.

The degree of fit of the specific proteins is very good and it is believed that steric factors are also of importance in this binding. Corticosteroid-binding globulins isolated from man and various other species display differences in their specificity of steroid binding. The rule of polarity applies roughly to human transcortin and the molecule has one site of binding for cortisol. The sulphydryl reagent, paramercuribenzoate, decreased considerably the association constant for the binding of cortisol to rabbit transcortin. Cortisol protected the protein against this reagent. The amino acids taking part in the binding have not been identified. In contrast to the situation with albumin, the binding constants for the reaction of steroid and the specific proteins have been shown to be dependent on temperature. Furthermore the rate of association between cortisol and human transcortin is significantly dependent on temperature (Paterson, 1973).

2. Biological function

The synthesis of transcortin is affected by several hormones. The level of transcortin increases after the administration of oestrogen and during pregnancy. Even thyroxine is capable of stimulating the synthesis.

Under physiological conditions, approximately 92–97 per cent of the corticosteroids are bound to protein and most of this fraction is bound to transcortin. The steroids are thought to exert their effect in the free form, which is 3–8 per cent of the total fraction. The relationship between the protein-bound and the non-protein-bound fractions has been studied in healthy individuals (Uete and Tsuchikura 1972). When the level of steroid is less than that required to saturate the maximum binding capacity of the proteins, the free and bound fractions are in equilibrium. This is depicted in Fig. 43. When the level of steroid increases, the greatest relative increase occurs in the unbound fraction, even if the absolute increase in steroid is small. It is well known that following infusion of cortisol into humans, the fraction of free hormone decreases much more rapidly than the fraction of protein-bound hormone. Thus, it has been suggested that there exists an autoregulation mechanism for the metabolism of corticosteroid in liver (Uete and Tsuchikura, 1972). This implies that the inactivation of corticosteroid is regulated primarily by steroid hydrogenase activity in the liver when the maximum capacity of the plasma proteins for the binding of steroid has been exceeded.

It is generally believed, although not proven, that transcortin-bound cortisol is

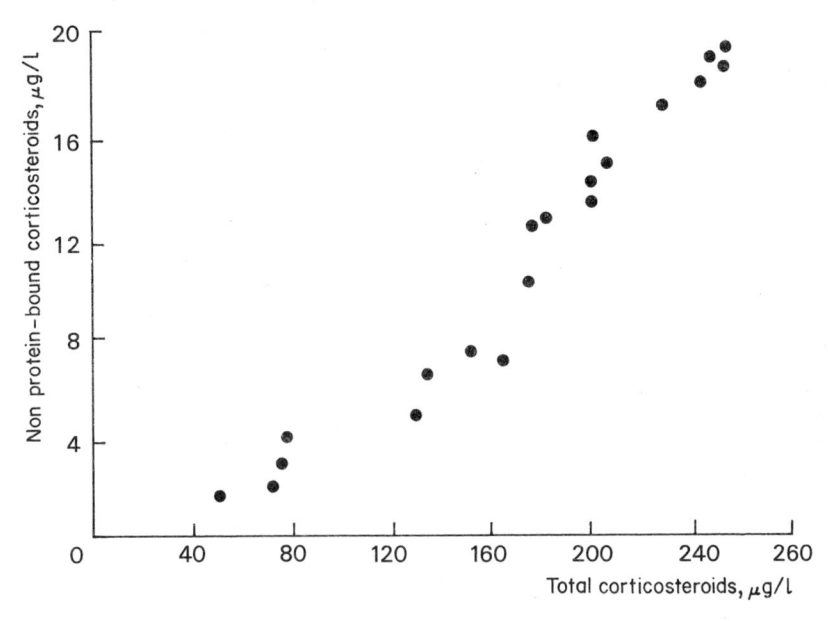

Fig. 43. Relation between free and protein-bound corticosteroids in serum from normal individuals. By kind permission of T. Ucte and H. Tsuchikura, *Metabolism*, **21** (1972) p. 80

biologically inactive, i.e. that transcortin functions in an organism to maintain a plasma pool of inert hormone which can act as a buffer against changes in the hormone concentration and can make available free hormone via dissociation. However, the function of this protein is still unclear and there is some evidence which suggests that transcortin complexes have a biological function in the regulation of the genetic activity observed subsequent to the administration of cortisol. The existence of a transcortin-like molecule within the nucleus of the human liver cell has been demonstrated (Amaral et al., 1974). At present, its origin and significance is not known.

Immunoglobulins

I. Structure and biochemistry
HANS BENNICH

The term 'immunoglobulin' is used as a collective designation of a chemically related group of proteins having an antibody function and whose synthesis and excretion in the blood and body fluids is a result of specific antigen-activating processes in the lymphoid organs. Each immunoglobulin having antibody activity can be characterized by its ability to bind specifically a particular antigen. By 'antigen', is meant a substance which is seen by the individual's immune system as foreign, having endo- or exogenic origin. Thus, it follows that immunoglobulins possessing different antibody specificities have different chemical structures within that part of the antibody which is responsible for binding the antigen. Furthermore, it has been found that the immunoglobulins can be divided into a relatively limited number of classes and subgroups, depending on those properties which are independent of their antibody specificity.

Intensive research over the past 10–15 years, notably in the field of immunochemistry, has provided us with an explanation of the complex nature of the immunoglobulins and an understanding of their wide variety of biological specificity.

1. Basic structure

All immunoglobulins, irrespective of specificity or class, can be described by using a common basic structure. This structure consists of two types of polypeptide chains which are linked in pairs to form a symmetrical four-chain molecule (Fig. 44A). The polypeptide chains, *light* (L) and *heavy* (H), are linked together by covalent and non-covalent bonds. The former, disulphide bonds, are sensitive to mercaptan (an SH-reagent) and can be cleaved without affecting the individual structures of the chains by mild reduction (Fig. 44B). As this reaction is reversible, the free SH-groups must be blocked by alkylation with, for example, iodoacetamide. Mild reduction and alkylation of an antibody does not affect its ability to bind antigen, nor does it change its physiochemical properties, as non-covalent forces of various types and strengths, cooperate in holding the antibody molecule together under physiological conditions (Fig. 44B). On the other hand, if the environment of the molecule is changed, such as dropping the pH or increasing the ionic strength of the solution, the non-covalent bonds can be weakened causing the molecule to fall apart and giving rise to 'free' light and heavy chains (Fig. 44C). The same result is obtained if the partially reduced and alkylated antibody comes into contact with high concentrations of denaturating or dissociating agents such as urea or guanidine (6–8 mol/l). Thus, isolation or analysis of the polypeptide chains of immunoglobulins must be carried out in dissociating media (Fig. 44D).

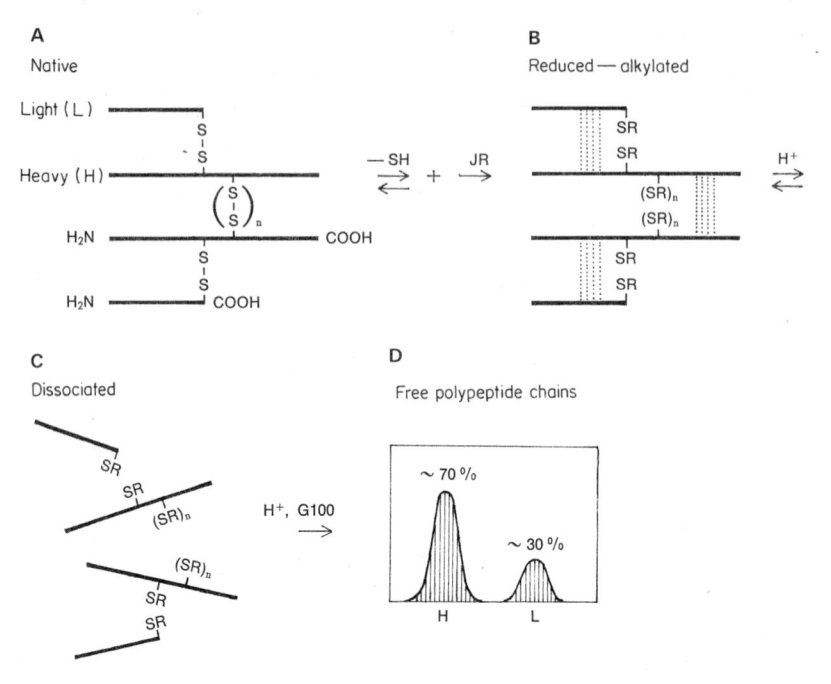

Fig. 44. A. The basic structure of a molecule of immunoglobulin consisting of a symmetrical four-chain structure having two light (L) and two heavy (H) polypeptide chains linked via disulphide bridges (—S—S—) and non-covalent bonds
B. Despite reduction and alkylation (R) of the disulphide bridges, the four-chain structure remains intact at neutral pH because of the presence of the non-covalent bonds ( )
C. At acid pH or in the presence of dissociating agents such as urea, the force of attraction between the chains decreases and gives rise to free chains
D. Following reduction and alkylation, the isolation of the light and heavy chains is best carried out by using molecular sieving material (e.g. Sephadex gels) in acid media

Isolated light or heavy chains no longer exhibit the antigen-binding properties displayed by the native molecule. However, these properties can be recovered if the chains are allowed to be recombined in a certain way at slightly acid pH (5.5).

Enzymes which produce limited degradation of the immunoglobulins have been useful tools for the location of various functional regions within the antibody molecules. On digesting a 7 S antibody with proteolytic enzymes such as papain and trypsin, three fragments which are approximately equal in size are produced. Of these, the two Fab-fragments are antibody active while the Fc-fragment is responsible for other important biological functions (Fig. 45 and Table 23). As the basic structure is symmetrical, the molecule contains two antigen-binding surfaces. This is a prerequisite for such *secondary* effects of antigen-antibody reaction, such as *agglutination* of particle antigens (cells, bacteria, etc.) and *precipitation* of soluble antigen. These effects have long been exploited in the *in vitro* determination of antigen–antibody reactions.

2. Classes of immunoglobulins

Circulating immunoglobulins (Ig) can be divided into five main classes: G, A, M, D, and E (Table 23). Antibodies in the classes IgG, IgD, and IgE exist normally as monomers having the unit structure, H_2L_2, while those belonging to IgM are com-

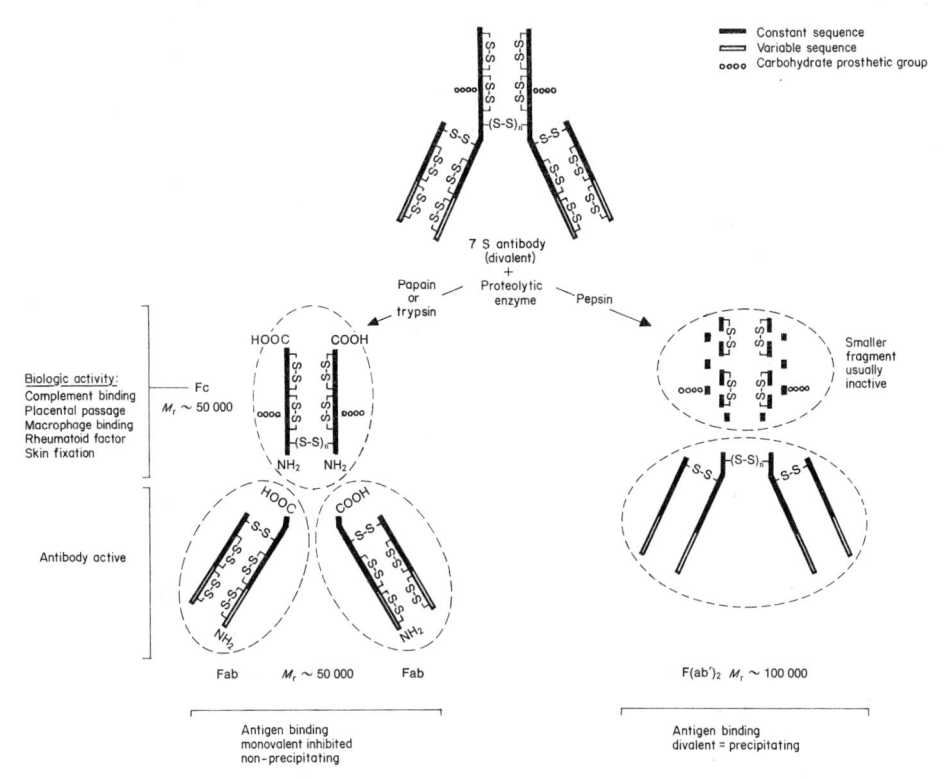

Fig. 45. Schematic representation of the fragmentation of an antibody produced on treatment with proteolytic enzymes such as papain or pepsin. Note the distribution of the various biological functions between the different portions of the molecule and how the secondary effects of the antigen–antibody reaction are dependent on the position of cleavage

posed of five units which are linked by disulphide bridges to form pentamers $(H_2L_2)_5$ having a molecular weight of 900 000. In serum, IgA exists normally as a monomer of the type H_2L_2 but can frequently give rise to dimers $(H_2L_2)_2$ and oligomers $(H_2L_2)_n$ J-chain (J=join). A more complex form exists in secretion (Table 23, Fig. 46) where IgA exists as a dimer which is covalently bound both to a protein of epithelial origin which is called secretory component and to J-chain. Immunoglobulins are characterized sometimes by stating their sedimentation coefficients $(S_{20,w}^0)$. The s-values of monomeric immunoglobins (Ig, IgA, IgD, and IgE are around 7–8, while that of IgM is approximately 19. A schematic representation of the various classes of immunoglobulins is given in Fig. 46.

3. Structures of heavy chains of various classes

Since the features of the heavy polypeptide chains are characteristic of each class, the immunoglobulins can be identified by determining their antigenic and chemical properties. As can be seen in Table 23 the heavy chains of different classes vary in size (molecular weight) and in carbohydrate content. Furthermore, there can exist several types of heavy chains within a given class. This is evident in the γ- and α-chains. The α-chains are of two types, α1 and α2, which differ in the way in which the light chain

Table 23. Some of the properties of the human immunoglobulins

	IgG	IgA serum	IgA secretion	IgM	IgD	IgE serum	IgE secretion
Molecular weight	150 000	150 000	370 000[a]	900 000	170 000	190 000	—
Sedimentation coefficient ($s^o_{20,w}$)	6.6–7 S	7 S	11 S	19 S	7 S	8 S	8 S
Carbohydrate %[b]	3	9	11	12	12	12	—
Polypeptide chains							
Heavy:							
Molecular weight including CHO	50 000	54 000		68 000	60 000	72 000	
Molecular weight excluding CHO	46 000	48 000		60 000	—	62 000	
Class	γ	α		μ	δ	ε	
Types (number)	4[c]	2[c]		?	?	?	
Allotypes (number)	Gm(24)	Am(2)					
Light:							
Types	κ, λ	κ, λ		κ, λ	κ, λ	κ, λ	
Allotypes (number)	Km(3)[d]	Km(3)		Km(3)	Km(3)	Km(3)	
Biological properties							
Level in serum (g/l)	8–17	1–4	—	0.05–2	0.003–0.2	0.000001–0.0001	
Complement binding	+[e]	0	0	+	0	0	
Placental passage	+	0	0	0	0	+	
Release from serous membrane	0	0	+	0	0	+	
Binding to homologous tissue	0	0	0	0	0		

[a] Dimeric form of IgA bound in part to a special peptide, secretory component, having a molecular weight of 50 000 daltons, and in part to another polypeptide chain, called J-chain, which has a molecular weight of 15 000 daltons.
[b] Covalently bound to the heavy chain: the number of carbohydrate prosthetic groups varies with class. Thus, the γ-chain has one and the μ-chain has five carbohydrate chains.
[c] See Table 24.
[d] Applies to the κ-chain. Allotypes of the λ-chain are not known.
[e] Complement binding properties of the γ-chain vary with the γ-type. See Table 24.

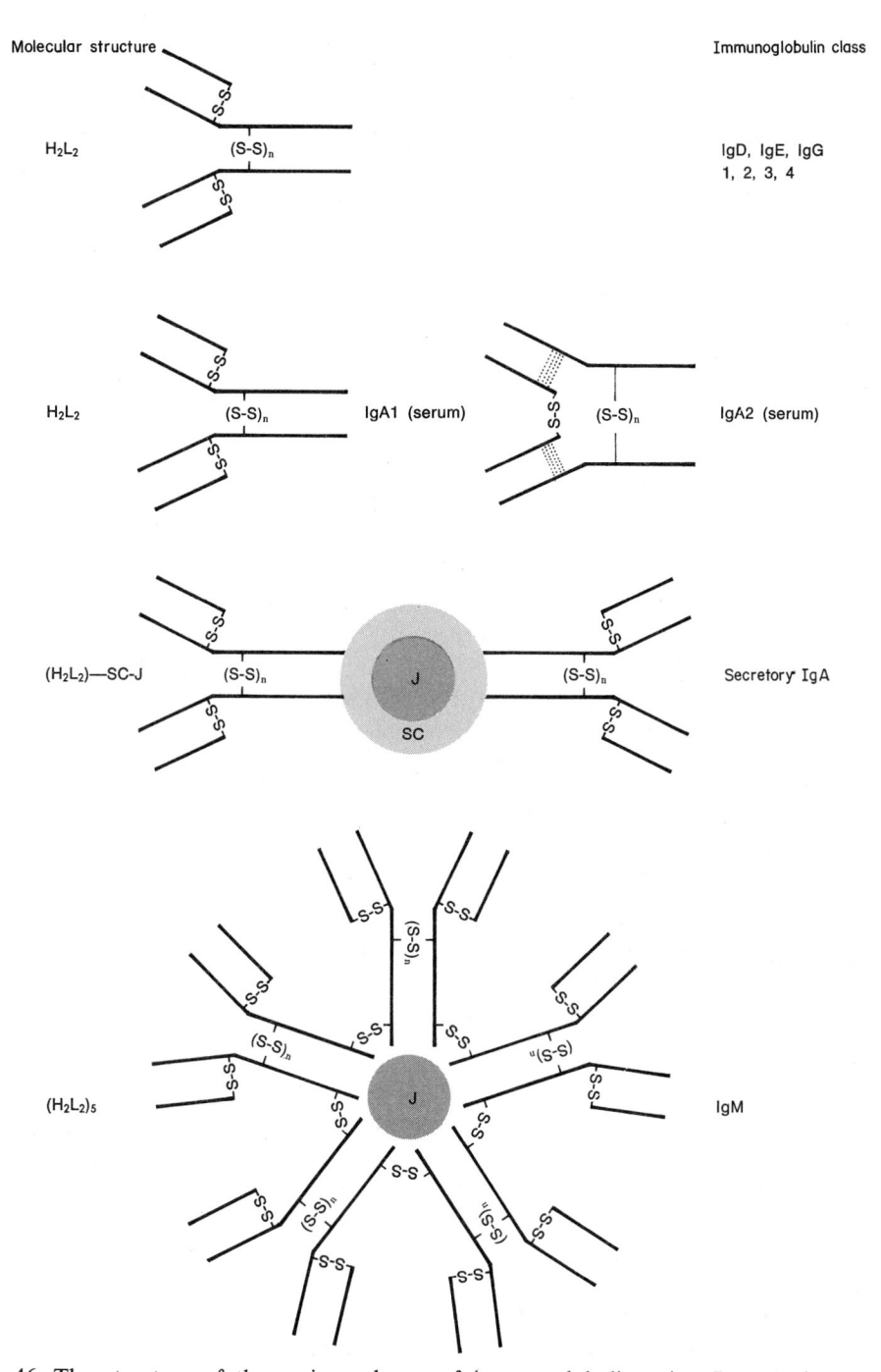

Fig. 46. The structure of the various classes of immunoglobulin using Porter's four-chain structure as a basic. Note that the light chains of IgA2 are present as a disulphide-bonded dimer which is associated to the α-chains via non-covalent bonds. The number of disulphide bonds in the heavy chains varies according to the class and type of the immunoglobulin (see Table 24). SC = secretory component—a polypeptide of epithelial, origin having a molecular weight of 50 000 daltons. J = 'join'-chain—a polypeptide which is synthesized in plasma cells and has a molecular weight of approximately 15 000 daltons

binds to them. In the case of α1, this binding is via disulphide bonds and in the case of α2, it is caused by non-covalent forces (Fig. 46). There are four types of γ-chain, γ1, γ2, γ3, and γ4, which differ in the number of disulphide bridges existing between the two heavy chains (Table 24). The light chains exist in two forms, kappa (κ) and lambda (λ), which can occur in combination with the heavy chains of any class or subclass. However, both types never occur with one and the same molecule. Consequently, there can exist *at least* 18 different basic combinations of the immunoglobulins in each healthy individual.

4. Variable and constant regions

There exist two structural regions in both the light and heavy chains, one having a *variable* and the other having a *constant* amino acid sequence. Such an arrangement, which appears to be unique for the polypeptide chains of the immunoglobulins, explains how antibodies having different specificities can belong to the same class or subclass and can contain the same type of light chain. The amino acid sequence of the constant region is characteristic of each class and subgroup of heavy chain, and the same is true for the light chains.

The variable region (V-region, Fig. 47A) in both the light and the heavy chains is strictly limited to the amino-terminal portions of the polypeptide chains and consists of 106–120 amino acids. By comparing the variable regions of different types and classes of light and heavy chains, it can be seen that the sequence of amino acids within a limited segment varies according to a set pattern. This permits a classification of the V-regions into *subgroups*. Furthermore, in other segments which are limited in number (three per chain) and length (six to eleven amino acid residues), it has been found that the variability is total. Such *hypervariable* regions from each heavy-light chain pair contribute to the formation of an antigen binding cavity having a particular specificity.

As can be seen in Fig. 47B, the various subgroups of the variable regions of the light chains are discretely connected with the properties of the constant regions. This is not the case in the subgroups of the variable regions of the heavy chains.

Table 24. Biological and chemical properties of the subgroups of IgG

Type	γ1	γ2	γ3	γ4
Relative concentration (%)	70	10	15	5
Number of disulphide bridges (γ-SS-γ)	2	5	5	2
Gm-allotypes	1, 2, 4, 17, 22	24	3, 5, 6, 13, 14, 15, 16, 21	—[a]
Complement binding	+	(±)	+	0
Binding to heterologous tissue	+	0	+	+

[a] As yet, no allotypes have been shown to exist.

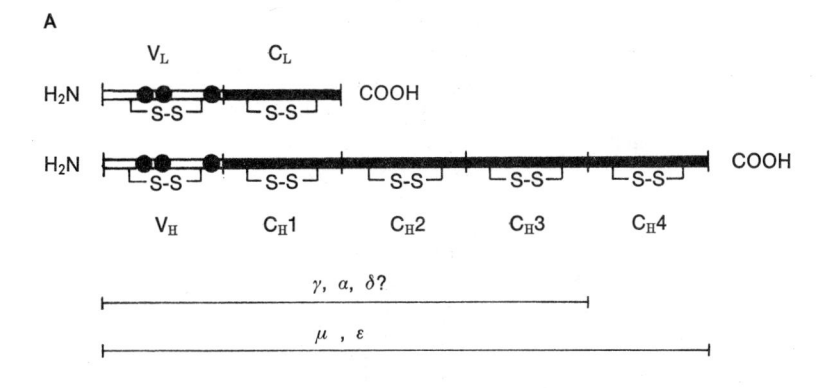

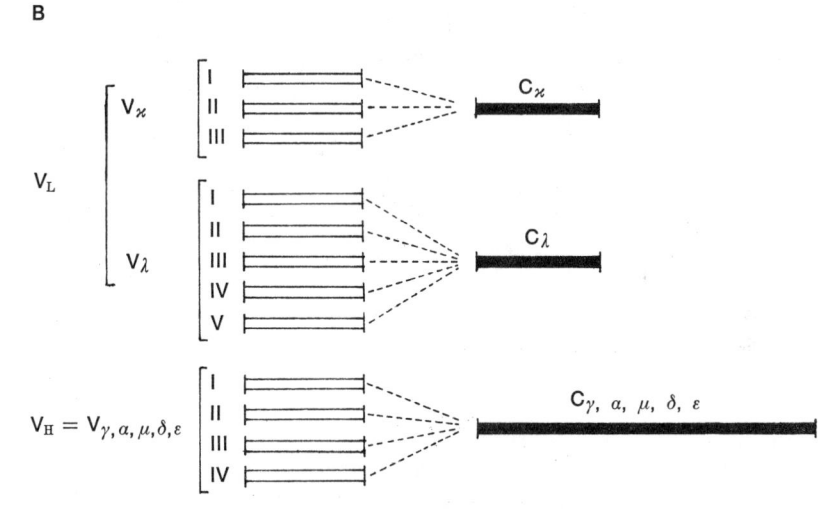

Fig. 4.7. A. Distribution of the variable (V) and constant (C) regions of amino acid sequence within the light (L) and leavy (H) chains. There are approximately 60 amino acid residues between each halfcystine residue of any one disulphide bridge (−S−S−). Note the existence of an extra C-region within the ε- and μ-chains
B. Subgroups of the variable region exist in both light and heavy chains. Subgroups of the type, V_L, are coupled to chains of the type α and λ, while those of the type, V_H, may combine with C_H-regions of any of the classes of immunoglobulin

5. Antigenic properties of immunoglobulins: isotypes, allotypes, and idiotypes

The antigenic properties of a molecule are dependent on the structure of the molecule. In the case of proteins, which consist of approximately 20 different amino acids which can be arranged into an almost indefinite variety of structures, various portions of the molecules can display different antigenic properties. This is usually manifested in the several different *antigenic determinants* of the molecule.

As the structure of the constant region within a heavy chains is unique for a given class (or subclass), the immunoglobulins can be classified according to the antigenic properties of the heavy chain. However, immunoglobulins belonging to different classes can cross-react if they contain the same type of light chain. In all normal individuals, such antigenic determinants which are present within the constant portions of the light and heavy chains and which are present in all molecules of the same class, subgroup, or type from every individual are called, *isotypic* determinants.

Both the light and the heavy chains can exist in poly-forms which are determined by *allelic* genes. The allotypes of a given class differ in the position of a few amino acids within the constant region. This can give rise to additional antigenic determinants which are called *allotypic antigenic determinants* or *allotype markers*. To date, 24 allotypes (Gm factors) of the γ-chain are known and some of these are characteristic of a particular subclass (Table 24). The frequency of allotype specificities varies according to population and race. So far, two allotypes (Am) of the α-chains have been identified. In the case of the light chains, the κ-chains have three allotypes (Km-factors), two of which arise as a result of the substitution of a single amino acid within the constant portion. Each individual can be antigenically homozygous or heterozygous with respect to the Km-genes. In the former case, only one allotype specificity can be detected in the serum while in the latter, two of the three known specificities can be present.

The light chains of the lambda type occur in two forms (Oz) depending on a single amino acid substitution within the constant region. In this case, the term allotype is not applicable since both forms are present in all individuals.

The clinical importance of the human allotypes is determined by their antigenicity. If a given type of immunoglobulin is introduced to the circulation of an individual which is lacking in this specificity, the recipient can become immunized against this allotype and consequently can produce antibodies which react with all immunoglobulins carrying the allotype in question. Such an immunization can arise during pregnancy; the mother can be immunized against the allotype of the embryo and, conversely, the embryo or new-born can produce antibodies against the allotype of the mother which are transfused to the circulation of the embryo during pregnancy. Immunization against immunoglobulin allotypes can also be caused by blood transfusion. Sera from immunized individuals are used as a source of antiallotype antibodies in the determination of the allotype of an unknown serum.

Individuals suffering from rheumatic arthritis very often produce antibodies against immunoglobulin allotypes, even if they have not been given a transfusion or have not been exposed in any other way to the immunoglobulins of other individuals. Furthermore, sera from such individuals very often contain additional antibodies which are directed against various antigenic determinants of human or even animal immunoglobulins.

Immunoglobulins possess even antigenic qualities which are characteristic of each individual. These so-called, *idiotype* determinants reflect the individual structure of the antigen-binding portions of the variable regions.

6. Biosynthesis of immunoglobulins

The biosynthesis of light and heavy polypeptide chains and the joining of these to form a disulphide linked four-chain structure takes place in plasma cells. The plasma cell represents one of the final stages of the lymphocyte differentiation initiated by the contact of antigen with antigen-specific sites on the surface of B-lymphocytes (see later). Generally speaking, a plasma cell at any given moment is capable of synthesizing only one kind of immunoglobulin.

The biosynthesis of light and heavy chains is controlled by separate, independent genes which transcribe to produce individual molecules of mRNA. The synthesis of a chain takes place on a polysome, a structure which consists of a complex of a molecule of mRNA and several ribosomes. The number of ribosomes varies according to the length of the mRNA which, in its turn, is proportional to the length of the polypeptide chain for which it codes. In normal cells, the synthesis of the light and heavy chains is in close balance. The time required for the synthesis of a light chain is approximately 30 seconds while that for a heavy chain is 60–70 seconds. The combining of the two types of chains to form a four-chain structure takes place during or shortly after the release of the chains from the polyribosomes.

The release of the completed molecule into the extracellular space takes place approximately 30 minutes after the completion of the synthesis. During this time, membrane-bound enzymes (glycosyl transferases) attach successively covalently bound prosthetic groups of carbohydrate to the heavy chain.

The compositions of the sugar chains (hexosamine, mannose, galactose, fructose, and sialic acid) vary according to the type of the polypeptide chain. This is also true of the number of sugar chains per molecule.

II. Immunological mechanisms

LARS Å. HANSON

In order to understand fully the formation and function of the antibody-active serum proteins, an outline of the basic immunological mechanisms must be provided. The existence of antibodies and other immunological phenomena can be attributed to a primary cell reaction, namely, that which involves the interaction of special cells belonging to the lymphatic system and foreign material which is recognized as 'non-self'. This ability to differentiate between 'self' and 'non-self' can be found at various levels in plants and animals. One example of this is the ability of the amoeba to digest foreign material but not its own cell structure. In the case of higher animals, this mechanism of recognition has developed into a highly differentiated system of lymphoid cells. These cells have receptors on their surfaces which recognize 'non-self' or foreign material called antigen. According to present-day understanding, the human body contains lymphoid cells equipped with receptors which fit a large number of substances (probably several tens of thousands) which are foreign to the body. One of the important tasks of immunology is to explain the presence in the body of such lymphoid cells. One must assume that either each individual is born with cells which contain the genetic information which is necessary for the production of these many different receptors on the surface of the lymphoid cells, or that this enormous variety is

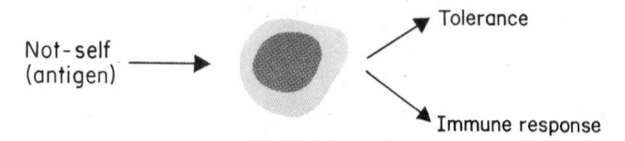

Fig. 48. The phenomena of immunology are based on the ability of lymphoid cells to recognize foreign material, 'non-self' (antigen), as opposed to 'self'. Lymphoid cells, which react with antigen via their specific receptors, can develop tolerance or an immune response. Tolerance implies specific non-reactivity while an immune response entails the development of two effector mechanism: (a) stimulated B-lymphocytes which produce circulating antibodies, (b) stimulated T-lymphocytes which becomes cytotoxic and produce lymphokines

caused by mutations which take place in the lymphoid cells during the embryo period or following birth. As yet, this question remains unanswered but there is evidence to suggest that the mechanism is a combination of these two possibilities.

When a foreign substance in an organism comes into contact with lymphoid cells which have receptors matching the foreign substance or antigen, one of two alternative events can be brought into play. The first of these results in *tolerance* or immunological unresponsiveness. This implies that a reaction against just that particular antigen fails to arise—specific immunological tolerance (Fig. 48).

The second alternative entails specific stimulation of cells having receptors which match the antigen in question. This causes the development of an *immune response*. A more detailed understanding of the mechanism of immune response demands a prior understanding of those cells which belong to the lymphoid system and which are responsible for the mechanism of recognition.

1. The lymphoid system

The lymphoid system consists of cells which are believed to originate as stem cells in the bone marrow (Fig. 49). In addition, such cells must mature and become equipped with necessary receptors so that they can take part in the recognition mechanism. One population of cells can attain this state through the help of the thymus, a central immunological organ. The function of this organ has long been a mystery. Less than two decades have passed since Miller (in Australia) and Good (in the USA) demonstrated the important role of this organ in immunological function. Whether the thymus influences the lymphoid cells directly or through some form of humoral substance or both is not clear. Those cells which are helped by the thymus to become *immunologically competent*, i.e. become immunologically reactive because of the receptors which enable them to recognize foreign material, are called *T-lymphocytes*. Such cells are present in the circulation where they constitute 70–80 per cent of the pool of lymphocytes. These T-lymphocytes are also found in the so-called thymus-dependent parts of the spleen and the lymph glands and circulate between these tissues and the blood (Fig. 50). They can be identified by their property of spontaneously binding sheep erythrocytes to produce so-called, rosettes. Most of them also stain specifically with the enzyme d-naphthyl acetate esterase (ANAE). A second population of bone marrow cells are provided with their immunological competence by another central immunological organ. The identity of this organ in man is as yet unknown. **However**.

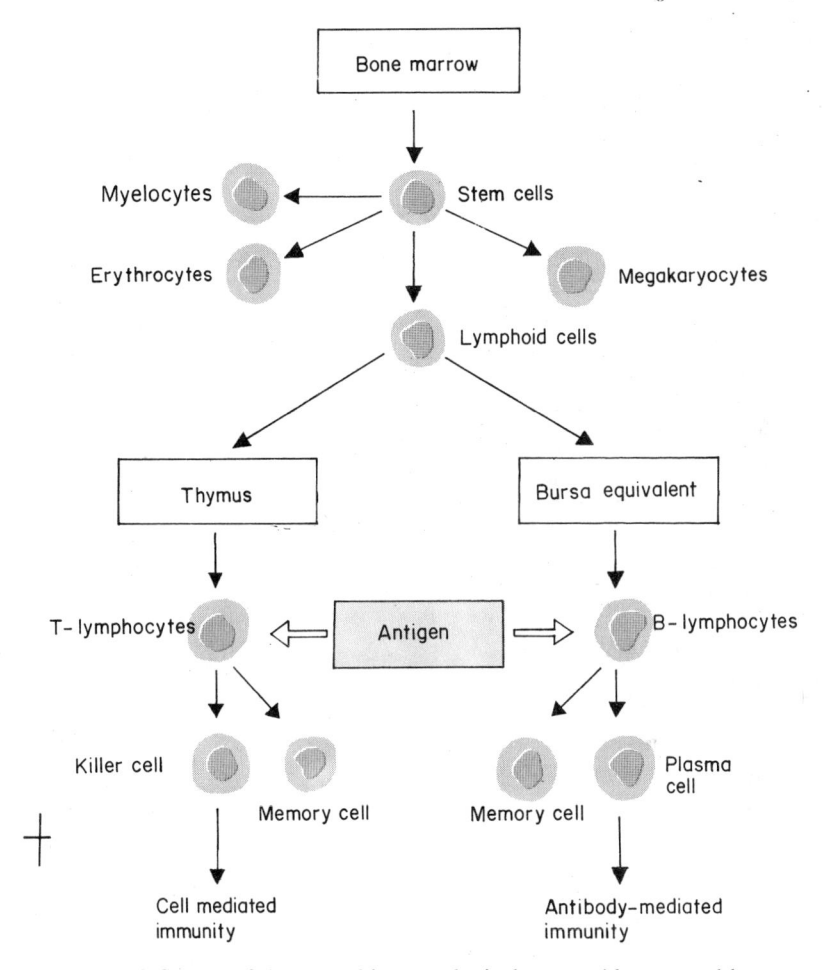

Fig. 49. Under the influence of the central immunological organs (thymus and bursa equivalent), the lymphoid system develops by differentiation of stem cells from the bone marrow into T- and B-lymphocytes which are immunologically competent. The T-lymphocytes react via their specific receptors with the antigen which fits these receptors, becoming cytotoxic killer cells and producing lymphokines. They are responsible for cell-mediated immune reactions. Similarly, B-lymphocytes (usually in cooperation with T-lymphocytes) begin to produce antibodies after they have reacted with the antigen fitting its immunoglobulin receptor. The B-lymphocytes are responsible for antibody-mediated immunity

there have been some suggestions that the function may be located in the mucous membrane of the intestine. In birds, a special organ (*bursa Fabricii*) having this central immunological function has developed from the back-most portion of the intenstine. The functional counterpart in man is called the bursa equivalent. The lymphoid cells which obtain their immunological competence via the bursa equivalent are called, *B-lymphocytes*.

The antigenic receptors on the B-lymphocytes consist of immunoglobulin structures which contain light and heavy chains of the various classes of immunoglobulin. Approximately 50 000–100 000 such receptors for antigen can be found on each B-

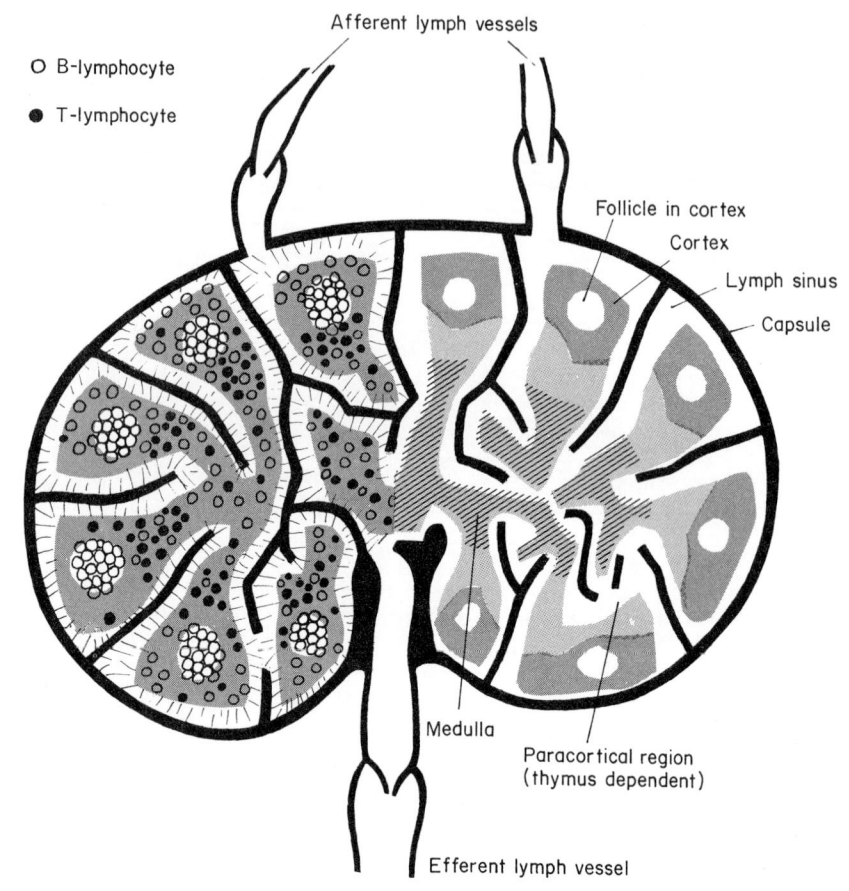

Fig. 50. Lymph node showing the areas with are dependent on the thymus and the bursa equivalent. ○ = B-lymphocytes, ● = T-lymphocytes. B-lymphocytes appear most numerous in the follicles, the regions where antibody formation takes place. T-lymphocytes are found mainly in the thymus-dependent paracortical region

lymphocytes. The nature of the corresponding receptors on the T-lymphocytes remains unclear. However, it seems that they may have certain principle similarities to those of the B-lymphocytes. The B-lymphocytes can be identified by the immunoglobulin receptors on their surface. In addition, they carry receptors for the complement factor C3 (Fig. 60C) and the Fc-portion of antibodies (Fig. 45). It is still difficult or impossible to distinguish between the many subpopulations of lymphocytes that seem to exist.

This division of the lymphoid system into T- and B-lymphocytes has obvious functional consequences for the two phenomena of tolerance and immune response which can follow the recognition of foreign material by lymphoid cells.

Although the mechanism responsible for the existence of immunological unresponsiveness is still unclear, it seems that T- as well as B-lymphocytes may be involved. For B-lymphocytes to respond it is necessary that they have the cooperation of 'helper' T-lymphocytes. This cooperation can obviously be prevented by 'suppressor' T-lymphocytes. Unresponsiveness may therefore mostly be the result of antigen inducing certain T-lymphocytes which actively prevent an immune response against the antigen. Earlier studies have suggested that even low doses of antigen can induce unresponsiveness in T-lymphocytes, low-zone tolerance. In contrast B-lymphocytes in the absence of T-cells require much higher doses for induction of unresponsiveness, high-zone tolerance.

Normally there is no response against self, so-called *natural tolerance*. This is presumably due to the fact that there are no T-lymphocytes responding against self which prevents the response of normally existing B-lymphocytes with receptors for self structures.

An immune response (Fig. 48) is the alternative outcome of the encounter between an antigen and the cells which possess the receptors for that antigen. Since the lymphoid system includes T- and B-cells and since both of these types of cells are stimulated by contact with the antigen, two effector mechanisms are produced.

When a receptor on a lymphoid cell fits with an antigen, the cell is stimulated to increased metabolism and cell division. This cell division leads to the production of an entire family or clone of daughter cells, each having the same genetic composition or genome as the original cell. Concurrent with this and as a result of the immune response, the cell line differentiates and the effector mechanism is developed depending on the type (T or B) of the original lymphocyte. The B-lymphocytes differentiate to plasma cells and form antibodies. Consequently, the circulating antibodies constitute one of the effector mechanisms of the immune response.

Instead of producing circulating antibodies, the antigen-stimulated T-lymphocytes synthesize other substances which are often called, lymphokines (see later). Together with a cytoxic activity which is present in the antigen-stimulated T-lymphocytes, these lymphokines give rise to the second effector mechanisn of the immune response, cell-mediated immunity (Fig. 49).

2. Characteristics of antigens

Before embarking on the topic of the immune response, it is necessary to give some particulars concerning the substances which act as antigens and which initiate the response. It has been mentioned already that the lymphocytes have a mechanism for the recognition of 'non-self' in contrast to self. With this in mind, we have to define antigens as material which is recognized by lymphocytes as 'non-self' and thereby stimulates specifically those cells to produce an immune response. However, not all foreign material is antigenic, i.e. capable of reacting with the receptors of lymphocytes in such a way that an immune response is developed. Antigens must have a certain molecular size and, more often than not, they must have a molecular weight which is greater than approximately 10 000. While material having molecular weight as low as 1 000–3 000 or even lower has been shown to be antigenic, this is the exception rather than the rule.

The portion of the structure of the antigen which fits and reacts with the receptors of the lymphocytes is called the *determinant* (Fig. 51). The classical work of Landsteiner demonstrated that the determinant is a chemically definable portion of the structure of the antigen molecule and that the characteristic specificity exhibited by the immunological reactions is due to the ability of the antibody to react with just that portion of the antigen, the determinant, to which it is directed. A single antigen molecule may have a large number of determinants; proteins are found often to have several determinants with a variety of structures. Antigens of the carbohydrate type may have a less complex structure, consisting of repeating units and often forming many similar determinants. A substance having a molecular weight which is too low to permit stimulation of the lymphocytes, but which can react with the corresponding antibody because it contains at least one antigenic determinant, is called a *hapten*. By reacting with antibodies, haptens can block the ability of the antibodies to react with complete antigen which contains the same determinant within the structure. Low molecular weight material, such as pharmaceuticals or a metabolite thereof (e.g. penicillin and penicilloyl), may be too small to be capable in themselves of inducing an immune response. However, they may become attached to various tissues e.g. blood cells, and so become capable of acting as *immunogens*, i.e. inducing an immune response. The antibodies which are thus produced can also react with the original pharmaceutical which in this case is a hapten. While the term immunogen implies the ability to induce an immune response, the term antigen implies the ability to react with the effector mechanism of the immune response. However, the term antigen is used often to cover both concepts.

For a substance to be capable of functioning as an immunogen (cause an immune response) and an antigen (capable of reacting with the completed antibody), it must have a rigid structure. Thus, gelatin is reported to be a poor antigen as its structure is unstable. Most proteins and carbohydrates of foreign origin which have a sufficiently high molecular weight can function antigenically. If these are derived from a different species, they are called *heteroantigens*. If they appear in different genetic forms within the same species, e.g. various plasma proteins and blood groups, they can also function antigenically. Such variants within the same species are termed alloantigens or *isoantigens* and account for the fact that blood for one individual can be antigenic for another individual. In special situations, the individual's own tissue can act antigenically in the same individual. This phenomenon is called *autoantigenity* and is discussed in greater detail on page 184.

3. Antibody formation

The formation of antibodies arises from the recognition of foreign substance by B-lymphocytes. This mechanism of recognition makes use of only a small portion of the structure of the antigen molecule, the determinant. Contact between the B-lymphocyte and the antigen is brought about most often by the intervention of antigen-carrying macrophages. Follicles containing collections of macrophages and B-lymphocytes can be found in the lymph glands. On exposure to an antigen, the B-cells containing the corresponding receptors become stimulated, begin to divide, produce antibodies, and differentiate into plasma cells (Fig. 51). For most antigens the B-cells require the cooperation of T-cells for antibody production to be included. The mechanism of this cooperation is not fully understood. However, it is obvious that T-cells do not only stimulate the B-cells but, in addition, control the B-cells and in certain cases can inhibit them and prevent their response completely as was mentioned in the above discussion of tolerance or immunological unresponsiveness. Furthermore, certain antigens, especially polysaccharides, can initiate antibody synthesis without the help of T-lymphocytes—such antigens are said to be 'T-cell independent' antigens.

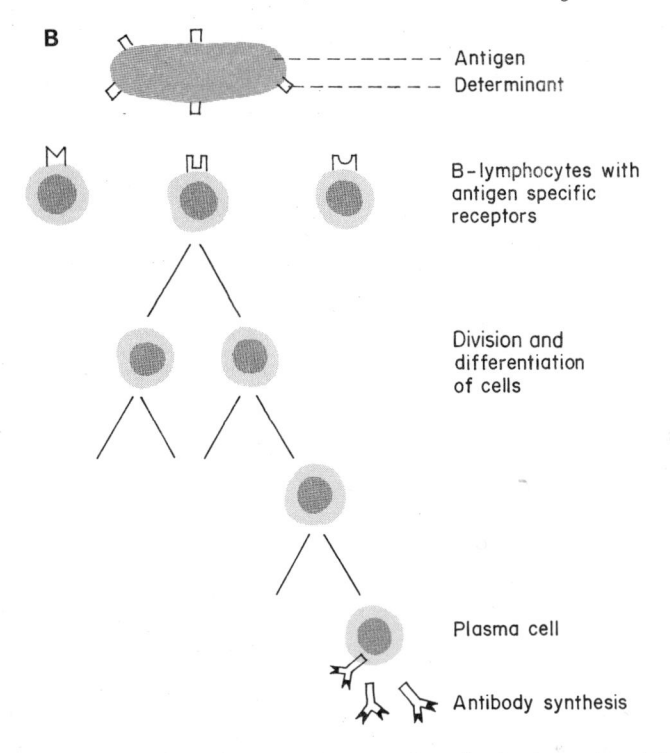

Fig. 51. Schematic representation of the mechanism of antibody formation. The antigen has structures on its surface, determinants, which fit with the receptors on the second of the three lymphocytes depicted in the upper row. The B-lymphocyte having the complementary suitable receptors is selected by the antigen and becomes stimulated. This results in division and differentiation of the cells. These cells begin to produce antibodies which have the same specificity as the receptors of the original B-lymphocyte. The final stage of the differentiation gives rise to antibody-producing plasma cells. The role of the macrophages in the antibody response, where they take up antigen and mediate its contact with the B-lymphocytes, is not shown in the figure; neither is the joint action of the B- and T-cells which is required for B-lymphocytes to become able to produce antibodies against most antigens

A B-lymphocyte possessing receptors which match the determinants of the antigen contains genetic information for the synthesis of antibodies which have the same specificity in their binding sites as do the receptors. This implies that the original cell and those cells which are derived from it, i.e. the entire cell clone, produce antibodies which display the same specificity towards the antigen as do the receptors of the original cell (Fig. 51). Furthermore, this means that all antibodies produced by the same clone of cells are identical with respect to immunoglobulin class, subgroup, and the various genetic markers (Km, Gm, or Am depending on the class of immunoglobulin, see Table 23). In addition, structures can be found which are unique for a particular clone of cells which give rise to a given antibody. These structures are to be found in the antigen-specific binding sites of the antibodies. Thus, the unique structural and functional heterogeneity has its cellular background in the various cell clones which produce them. Consequently, the immunoglobin fraction of blood is composed of the sum of a very large number of groups of antibodies, where all antibodies of a

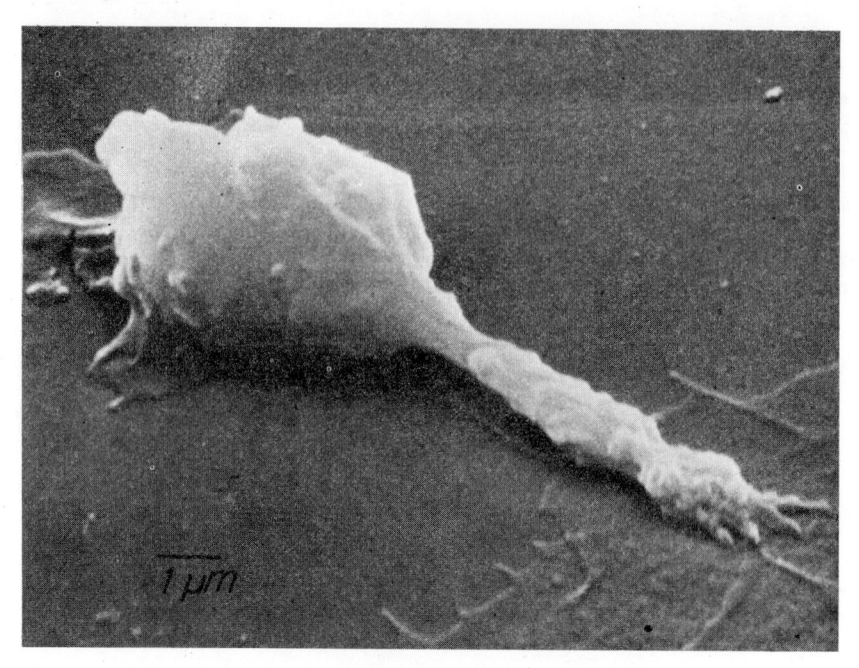

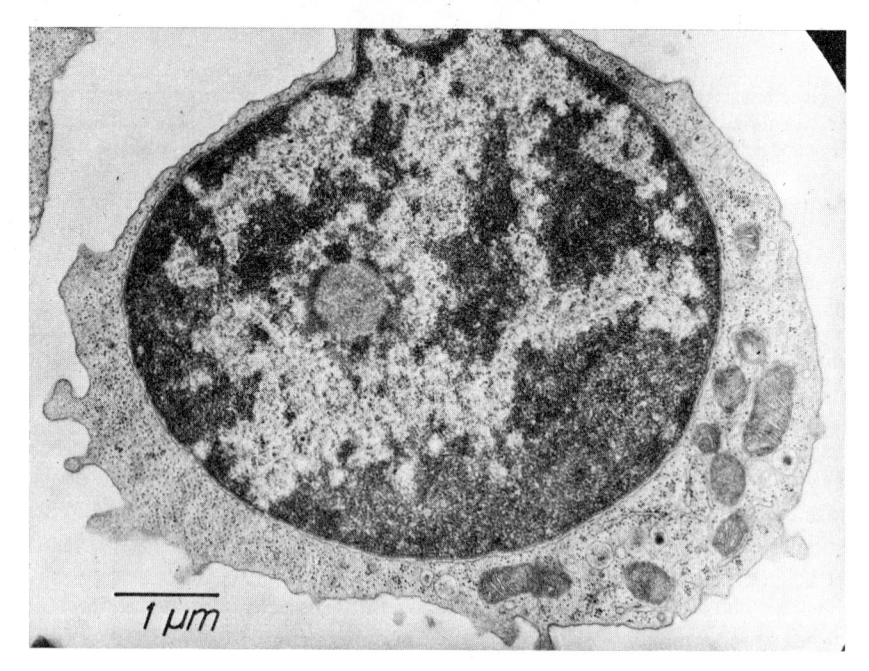

Fig. 52A. Photograph of a lymphocyte taken with scanning electron microscopy (photo, P Biberfeld)

B. Section through a small lymphocyte (electron microscopic photograph by L Lindholm, who is also responsible for C and D)

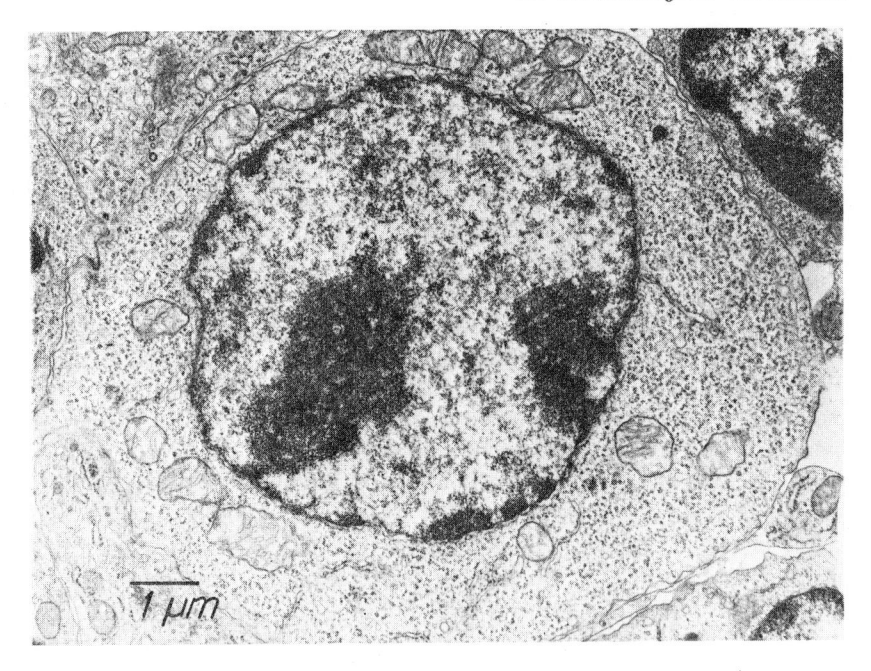

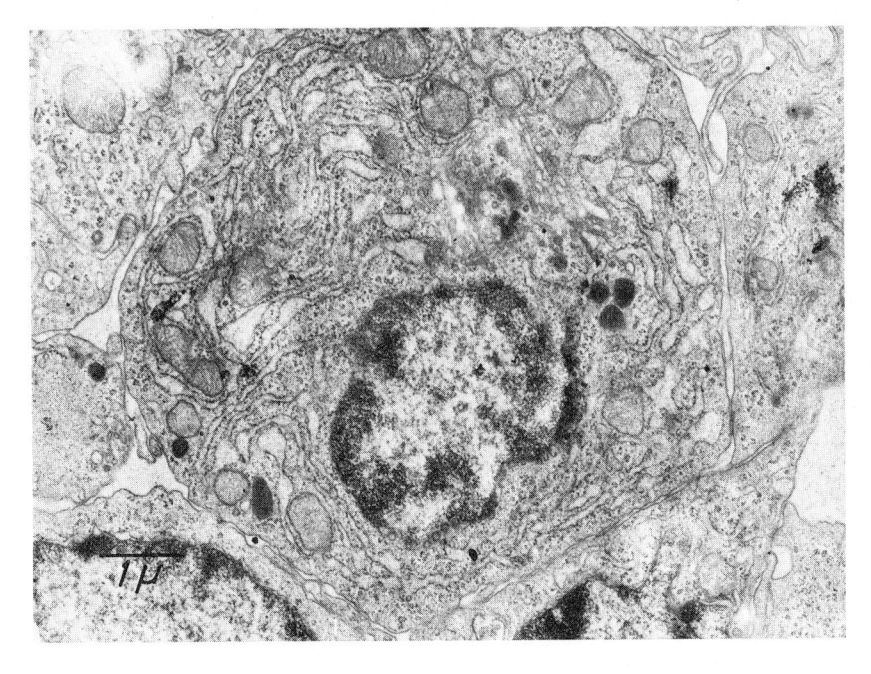

C. An antigen-stimulated lymphocyte which has differentiated into a lymphoblast. Note the large area of cytoplasm
D. Section through a plasma cell

given group are structurally completely identical and are produced by cells which belong to the same clone, i.e. they are derived from the same genome.

Not only the structural characteristics of a given antibody, such as its immunoglobulin class, but also its functional properties can be traced back to the cell which produced the antibody. One such functional property is the *association constant*, i.e. the strength of its binding to the antigen. This strength is a reflection of the degree of fit which exists between the binding site of the antibody and the structure of the antigen, i.e. determinant to which the binding site is matched. The greater degree of fit, the higher is the binding coefficient (*affinity*). The sum of the bindings which exist between the several different determinants of an antigen molecule and the binding sites on the antibody is called *avidity* (Siskind and Benacerraf, 1969). This avidity is a measure of the firmness of the binding which exists between the antigen and the corresponding antibody. The strength of the binding has a variety of different biological consequences, e.g. the efficiency of the neutralization of a toxin by toxin antibodies. In the case of an individual who is administered large amounts of antigen, one can picture a situation where the cells having receptors which show a somewhat low degree of fit, as well as those cells having the ideally fitting receptors, bind antigen and thereby become stimulated to produce antibodies. Thus, a spectrum of antibodies is present in the immune response which develops. At the one end the antibodies display a high *specficity*, i.e. *high degree of fit* and high avidity, and at the other end of the spectrum they have a poor specificity, a low degree of fit and a low avidity. On the other hand, if the individual is exposed to very low doses of antigen, only the cells which have a high avidity are capable of competing for the antigen. This is due to the fact that these cells bind most efficiently to the antigen. The outcome is the formation of antibodies which show high avidity and high specificity.

By thus viewing the relationship which exists between the avidity and the specificity of antibodies and their dependence on the specificity of the cell receptors which are stimulated by antigen, it becomes apparent that the specificity is a relative characteristic of immunological reactions. Antibodies having a high specificity for a particular antigen may show some degree of specificity for other structurally related antigens. In the case of the latter antigens, the degree of fit may be sufficient to produce a reaction, all be it weaker. If the strength of the reaction is greater than a certain threshold value, it can be of consequence in a biological system and thereby become apparent.

The antibodies which are produced by an antibody response can vary in their class of immunoglobulin as well as in their avidity. In the presence of small amounts of antigen, antibodies of the type IgM are most often the major product. On the other hand, in the presence of sufficient antigen this production of IgM antibodies is soon replaced by the formation of antibodies of the IgG type. These inhibit the continuation of the synthesis of IgM and are formed eventually in greater quantity than the IgM antibodies (Fig. 53).

When exposed to the same antigen for the second time, an individual produces a greater amount of antibody than was synthesized on the first exposure. Furthermore, the lag phase after the second contact is shorter. The antibodies produced in this case are mainly of the IgG type. The faster response of antibody which results from a second or higher successive stimulation by the same antigen and which gives rise to antibodies having a higher titre is called the *secondary response* or *anamnestic response*. This phenomenon has its basis in the *immunological memory*. After the first contact

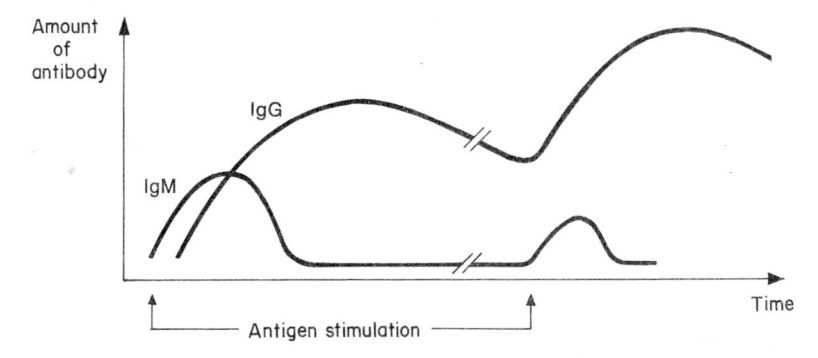

Fig. 53. The kinetics of the antibody response. An initial stimulation results in a primary immune response with the formation initially of antibodies of the IgM type. This is followed by the formation of antibodies of the IgG type, which inhibit the continuation of the synthesis of IgM. The second exposure to antigen results in the appearance of a secondary response. Here, the production of IgM is negligible, while that of IgG is fast and pronounced

with a particular antigen the resulting cell division produces a greater number of lymphocytes having receptors for this antigen than were present prior to the exposure (Fig. 54). Some of these cells are long lived memory cells (Fig. 49) and the next time the individual is exposed to the same antigen, there are present more cells which are capable of reacting, recognizing the antigen, and thereby stimulated to differentiate into antibody-producing cells. This results in the faster production of a greater number of antibodies which are directed against the antigen in question.

A secondary antibody response may be present even several years after the primary contact with the antigen. This is one of the explanations for the existence of a life-long immunity as a result of some infectious illnesses. Obviously the memory is continually involved and can be present for many years or even decades.

Some antigens give rise to an intense immune response while others are poor immunogens. For this reason, the terms 'strong' and 'weak' antigens are often used. It is probable that a greater number of cells recognize and become stimulated by the 'strong' antigens. Consequently, the strong antigens induce a more intense immune response.

4. Cell-mediated immunity

When the specific receptors of T-lymphocytes recognize and react with an antigen, the cells become stimulated and differentiate. Instead of leading to the formation of antibodies, this process gives rise to effector mechanisms of the cell-mediated immunity (Fig. 55). These stimulated T-lymphocytes are transformed into *lymphoblasts* and produce factors which are often given the collective name, *lymphokines*. These factors have not been examined in closer detail. Lymphoblasts specifically directed against certain tumour cells become cytotoxic against these tumour cells. Such T-cells are therefore called 'killer cells'. It is believed that a close contact between cells is required before this function can become operative. The extent of the function of diffusible cytotoxic factors in this reaction is unclear.

If certain lymphocytes attach via their special Fc-receptors to the Fc-portion of cell-bound antibodies, they can exert a cytotoxic effect on the cell. This reaction is distinct

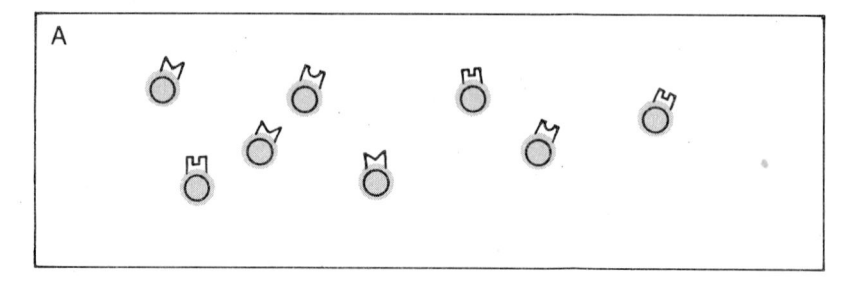

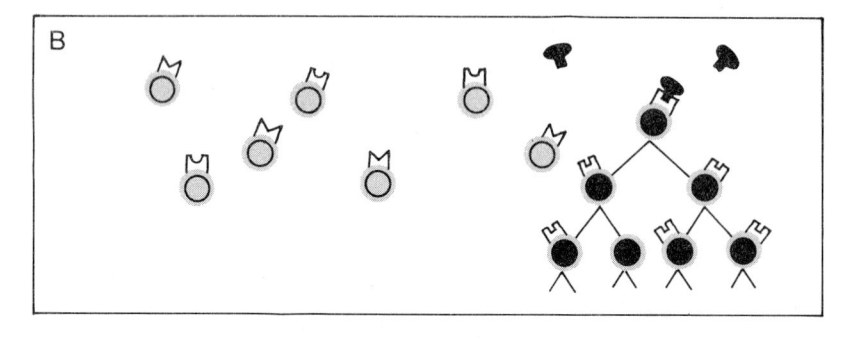

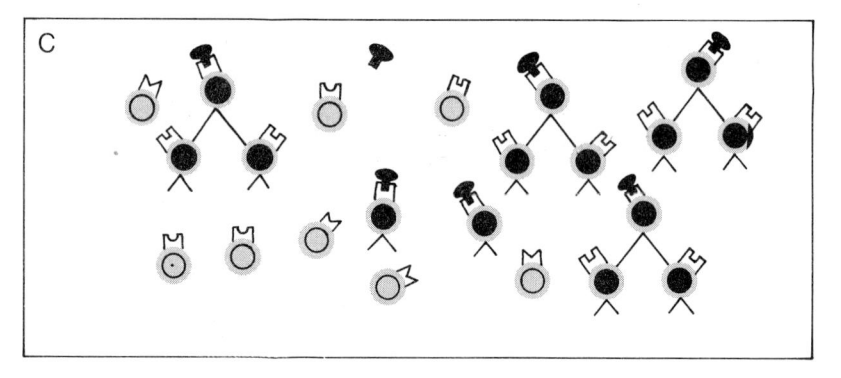

Fig. 54. A. Prior to stimulation an individual has a limited number of lymphocytes which possess receptors which fit a certain antigen
B. As a result of the primary antibody response, the cells undergo division. This results in an increased number of lymphocytes having receptors which fit the antigen
C. Following a primary antibody response, the individual has an increased number of cells which are capable of reacting with the antigen. These are long-lived memory cells and a later, second exposure to antigen causes a more pronounced response

from that involving cell-mediated immunity and its possible biological function is little known. The lymphocytes involved are not T-lymphocytes and are often called K-cells.

One type of lymphokine, *migration inhibitory factor* (MIF), can be measured by its ability to influence the movement of macrophages. Furthermore, the existence of lymphokines which have other effects on macrophages has been demonstrated. Of particular interest are the chemotactic effects which have been observed for granulocytes and especially for macrophages, as well as a macrophage-stimulating factor which causes these cells to become more efficient macrophages. The specific stimulation

II. Immunological mechanisms

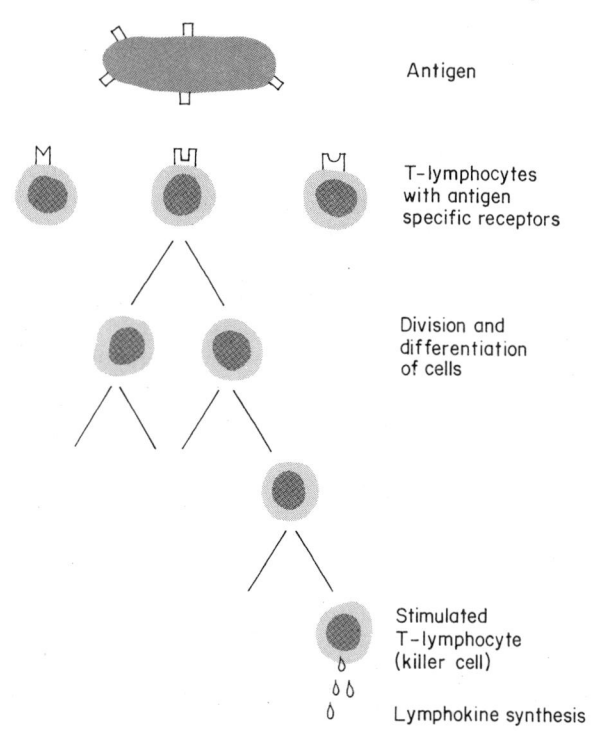

Fig. 55. Schematic representation of the development of cell-mediated immunity which arises during an immune response. The antigen reacts with a T-lymphocyte the receptors of which fit the determinants of the antigen. The T-lymphocyte becomes stimulated and undergoes division and differentiation. The resulting T-lymphocytes are cytotoxic killer cells and produce lymphokines and are responsible for the cell-mediated immune reaction

of T-cells with tumour antigen gives rise to the production of 'macrophage arming factor' which, in its turn, causes the macrophage to become cytotoxic against those tumour cells which present the antigen. In addition to their capacity to influence phagocytic cells, it would appear that lymphykines can exert mitogenic effects on lymphocytes other than those which are stimulated specifically. This causes the production of lymphokines in those cells which have not been stimulated specifically and functions probably as a reinforcing mechanism in cell-mediated immune reactions.

By injecting a suitable antigen, e.g. tuberculin, a cell-mediated immune reaction can be made to develop in skin. This produces a typical picture: a *delayed hypersensitivity reaction* where redness and induration develop after some 12 hours and reach a maximum after 2–3 days. This reaction is caused by the tuberculin-stimulated T-lymphocytes which release a skin reactive factor. It is also probable that other T-lymphokines, particularly those which influence phagocytic cells, contribute to the development of this reaction. Finally, it should be mentioned that the stimulation of lymphocytes by antigen can result in the formation of interferon. As will be seen later, this substance is of importance in the defence against some viral infections.

In addition to its role in the defence against infection, cell-mediated immunity is important in the mechanism for the rejection of transplants and possibly tumours. Consequently, the demonstration of cell-mediated immune reactions is of clinical

140 Immunoglobulins

significance. This can be carried out *in vivo* by causing the development of a delayed hypersensitivity reaction in skin or by various *in vitro* methods. These procedures are based on the knowledge that T-lymphocytes, on exposure to specific antigens or certain mitogens become stimulated and differentiate into lymphoblasts. The effect can be assayed by counting the number of blast cells or more accurately by measuring the increase in the metabolism in the form of ^{3}H-thymidine incorporation in the synthesized DNA. The production of lymphokines, especially MIF, can also be demonstrated.

To describe the immune response as the sum of two distinctly different mechanisms, antibody-mediated immunity and cell-mediated immunity, is to oversimplify the matter. It is probable that the cooperation which exists between the two systems is more pronounced than we have shown it to be. This is true of the functions of the regulation mechanism of the immune response in, among other things, the defence against infection. While the definite role of the macrophages remains unclear, it appears that these cells are of importance for the reactivity of B- as well as T-lymphocytes.

5. Antigen–antibody reactions

The reaction of antibody with antigen takes place between the binding sites of the antibody and those structures (determinants) of the antigen against which the antibody is directed. As was mentioned previously, the better the degree of fit between complementary loci (e.g. charged groups) of the two interlocking surfaces, the greater will be the binding energy and the more specific the reaction. It is essential that the degree of fit is extremely good if the forces which hold the antigen and the antibody together are weak and are very dependent on the distance between the two reactants. The lower degree of fit, the weaker the binding. On the other hand, a low degree of fit can be compensated by the participation of a large number of different antigenic structures in the reaction. Thus, an antibody can have a perfect fit and a high binding capacity for a certain structure but it can also bind, all be it less effectively, to other structures which are similar to but not identical with that which is structurally complementary to the binding site of the antibody. These less specific reactions of antibodies with antigens which are somewhat dissimilar in character, e.g. different kinds of related bacteria, are called *cross-reactions*. Such a cross-reaction of an antibody with two different bacteria

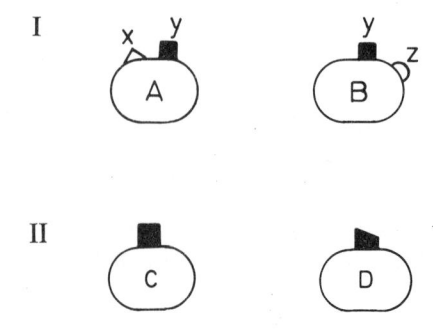

Fig. 56. I. Schematic representation of two different micro-organisms which cross-react because both have an identical structure on their surfaces, determinant *y*

II. Two different micro-organisms which cross-react because they each have on their surface a structure which is similar to that of the other micro-organism

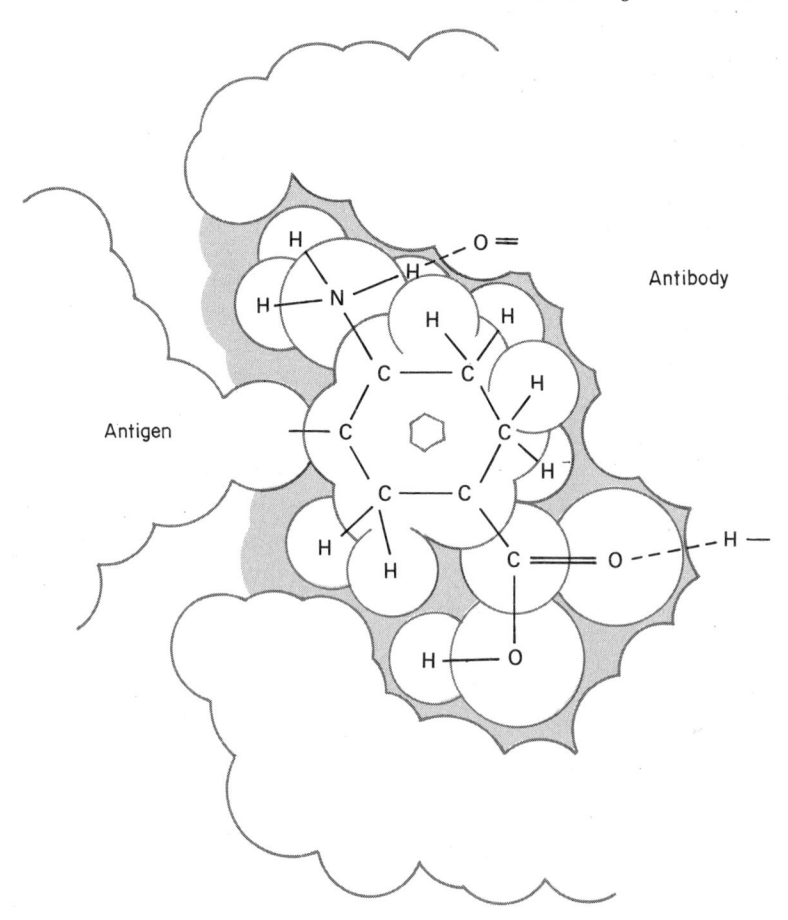

Fig. 57. Schematic representation of the binding of the determinant of the antigen with the binding site of the antibody. Two of the bonds which are responsible for holding the molecules together are indicated

can be caused also by the presence of identical structures or closely similar determinants (Fig. 56) on the two different bacteria.

The forces which hold the antibody and the antigen together are mainly van der Waals's forces with some contribution from hydrogen bonds and electrostatic bonds (Fig. 57).

The initial binding of antibody to antigen is called the *primary reaction*. This takes place very quickly and without producing any visible effects. This initial phase is followed by the *secondary manifestations*, which can be observed. When a soluble antigen comes into contact with a suitable antibody, it may be *precipitated*. For the precipitation reaction to take place, the antibody and the antigen must be present in a certain concentration ratio. This ratio is characteristic of each antigen-antibody system. If the reaction is carried out in a test tube, the observed precipitation is the sum of the individual precipitates arising from each of the antigen-antibody systems which are present Fig. 58A. If the antigen and the antibody are allowed to diffuse towards one another through an agar gel, they build concentration gradients. In this case, the

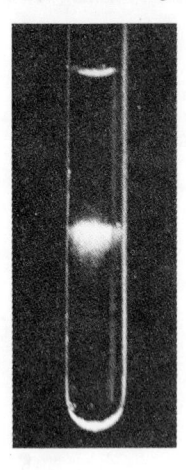

Fig. 58A. Precipitation performed in a test tube. The solution of antigen has been poured on top of the antiserum. A precipitate of antigen–antibody is formed where the two solutions meet

antigen–antibody systems which are present produce precipitates at various positions within the gel, depending on where their concentration relationships reach an optimum Fig. 58B. Analyses performed in this way permit (among other things) comparative studies of antigen preparations. The technique is usually called double *immunodiffusion* (Ouchterlony and Nilsson, 1973).

This provides a means whereby the presence can be demonstrated of many different components in a mixture, e.g. the various components of a bacterium or the different proteins of blood serum. The resolution of the analysis can be increased by first separating the antigens (e.g. by electrophoresis) and subsequently precipitating these with the corresponding antibodies. This is the underlying principle of the technique of *immunoelectrophoresis* (Fig. 58C). The immunodiffusion methods can also be adapted to quantitative determination of antigenic components. If an antigen is allowed to diffuse from a well into an agar gel containing antibodies against that antigen, ring-formed precipitates occur. The diameters of these precipitates are related to the concentrations of the antigen. This procedure is called, *simple radial immunodiffusion* (Fig. 58D) or the Mancini technique (Mancini et al., 1965). The amount of antibody in a sample can be determined by including a reference in the system. Alternatively, the antigen can be made to migrate more quickly into the antibody-containing agar by using electrophoresis. This procedure gives rise to rocket-like precipitation patterns, the heights of which are related to the concentrations of the antigens present (Fig. 58E). This method, 'rocket electrophoresis' or electroimmunoassay (Laurell, 1966) is used in the quantitative determination of antigenic components.

If the antigen is present as a particle, e.g. on the surface of a cell, the antigen induces the particles to clump together, *agglutinate* (Fig. 58F). The antibodies on an antigen which is present on a particular cell, e.g. red blood cells, can be demonstrated by so-called *direct agglutination* of the red blood cells. An estimation can be made of the concentration of the antigen by using a series of dilutions of the antibody solution or serum (titration). By attaching an antigen, e.g. a bacterial antigen, to particles such as red blood cells, one can test by *indirect agglutination* for antibodies against the antigen which is attached to the surface of the particles. In addition, the analysis can be made quantitative by employing a series of dilutions. If the antigen is present in the form of an active substance such as an enzyme, hormone, or toxin, its effect can be neutralized by

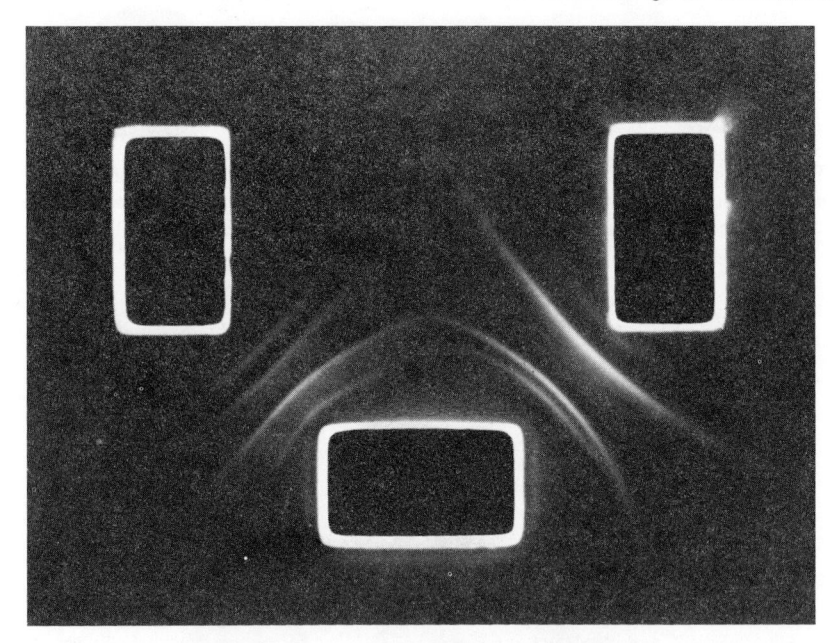

Fig. 58B. A so-called double diffusion analysis performed in agar gel. Two different preparations of streptococcal antigen, one in each of the two upper wells, can be compared by using an antiserum to streptococci in the lower well. Concentration gradients arise as the antigens and the antibodies diffuse from their respective wells into the gel and towards one another. A precipitate is formed at a position within the gel where a certain antigen and the corresponding antibody are present in such concentrations that the resulting antigen–antibody complex becomes insoluble. Since this concentration relationship is unique for each antigen–antibody system, the various precipitates will be formed at different positions within the gel and each precipitate will be indicative of a particular antigen. If both antigen preparations contain the same antigen, the corresponding precipitate for this antigen will have the form of a continuous arc, an interference reaction

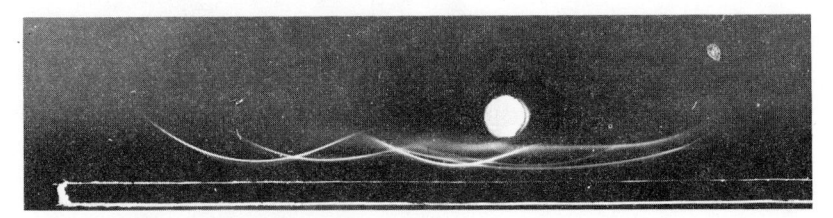

Fig. 58C. Immunoelectrophoresis. Human milk was placed in the round well and subject to electrophoresis (anode to the left). Following the electrophoresis, antiserum against milk was placed in the oblong well and allowed to diffuse into the gel. A precipitate was formed at the various positions of electrophoretic migration of the different milk proteins

using antibodies which are directed against that portion of the structure of the antigen which is responsible for its activity. Antibodies against the haemolysing toxin from streptococci, streptolysin, can thus be measured quantitatively by determining the degree of neutralization of the haemolytic activity by the antibodies.

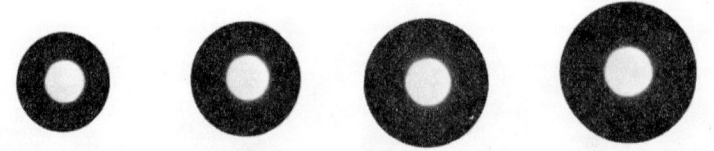

Fig. 58D. Simple radial diffusion. The agar gel has been mixed with antiserum against IgA and solutions of various concentrations of IgA have been placed in the round wells. The surface area of the 'ringformed' precipitates is related to the concentration of IgA

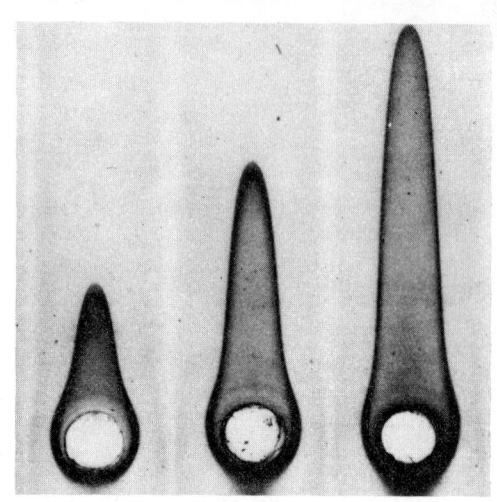

Fig. 58E. Electroimmunoassay (rocket electrophoresis) for the quantitative determination of antigen. The medium is an agar gel containing antibody. The antigen solutions are applied to the round wells and are subjected to electrophoresis. The height of the rocket-shaped precipitate is related to the concentration of antigen in the well

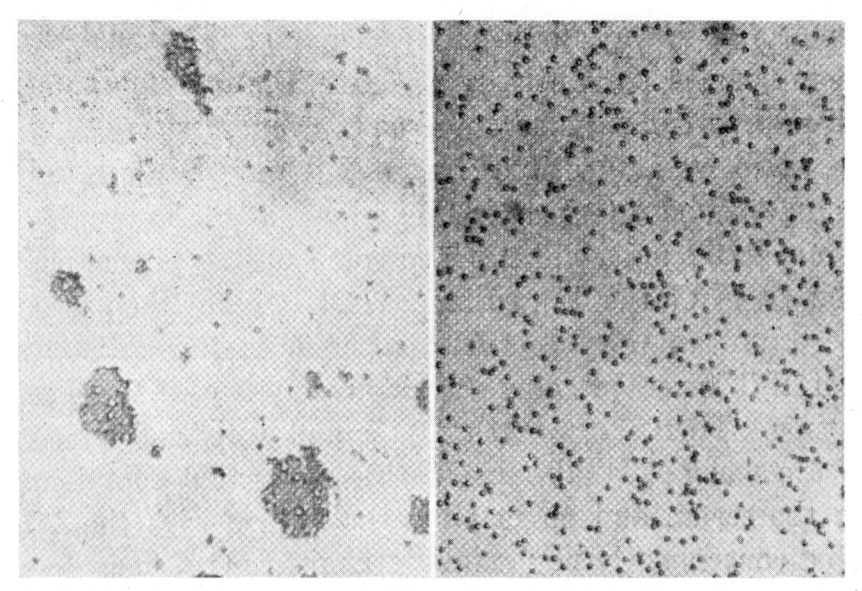

Fig. 58F. Red blood cells from sheep which have been agglutinated by using antibodies against these cells. The antibodies were obtained by immunizing rabbits with sheep blood cells. Non-agglutinated blood cells are shown for comparison in the picture on the right

Certain antigen–antibody systems activate a sequence of components of serum which is known as the complement system. This system, which is described in the next section, can be used in the so-called *complement binding reactions* in order to demonstrate that a complement-binding antigen–antibody reaction has taken place. This is one of the principles of the Wassermann reaction which is used to detect the presence of the autoantibodies against cardiolipin which appear in syphilis.

The secondary manifestations of antigen–antibody reactions such as precipitation, agglutination, neutralization, and complement activation are of great importance since they form the basis of the many different immunological methods which are used in microbiology and biochemistry. They provide a means of identifying and characterizing the fractions obtained during fractionation. They can also be used for the qualitative and quantitative analysis of hormones, pharmaceuticals, etc. They are useful for the identification of proteins, carbohydrates, and micro-organisms as well as for the detection and identification of the antibody response which appears in connection with infection or on exposure to foreign material, i.e. on vaccination or blood transfusion. Thus, they form the basis of diagnosis in bacteriology, virology, and blood group serology. Furthermore, they are used for diagnosis in connection with hypersensitivity, autoimmune phenomena, and transplant and tumour immunity. The usefulness of the reactions depends on their sensitivity and their specificity. As was mentioned previously, specificity is a relative term. However, the less specific reactions can be eliminated or can be controlled since the reactions in general can be manipulated so that only the most specific antigen–antibody reactions are visualized.

It should be mentioned here that techniques which are based on the use of antibodies have a limited applicability in those immunological reactions where cell-mediated immunity plays a crucial role. Such reactions are involved in transplant immunity, tumour immunity, and often defence against infection. In such cases, for a technique to be applicable it must be capable of demonstrating the involvement of T-lymphocytes in the activity. This can be accomplished by using the procedures which were outlined in Section 4, 'Cell-mediated immunity'. Techniques which are based on antigen–antibody reactions have been more readily available and have been developed more than those which involve T-lymphocyte reactions. However, the use of assays which involve the latter reactions are becoming more common.

Recent years have seen the development of techniques which are based on the primary reactions of antigen and antibody. In these cases, the binding of antigen to antibody can be demonstrated by marking the antigen with an enzyme, isotope, or a fluorescent substance. Examples of such methods are given in Figs. 59 and 71. These methods are often much more sensitive than those which are based on the secondary manifestations of the antigen–antibody reaction. Nanogram quantities of the antigen or antibody can often be detected. By using the technique of *radioimmunoassay*, which incorporates the use of isotope-labelled material, a variety of different substances can be measured quantitatively. These techniques have been made use of already in the form of the commercially available kits for the assay of various hormones. It is becoming common practice in these techniques to make the antibody insoluble by attaching it to the wall of a plastic tube, a particle, or a strip of paper, i.e. immunosorbent (Figs. 59 and 71). In this way, the antigen or antibody which reacts with the insoluble phase can be distinguished easily from the non-reactive material. The assay is simplified considerably and the sensitivity is enhanced. As will be seen

146 *Immunoglobulins*

Plastic tube

▶ Antigen

⊥ Antibody in patient's serum

(✳) Antihuman immunoglobulin
conjugated to alkaline phosphatase

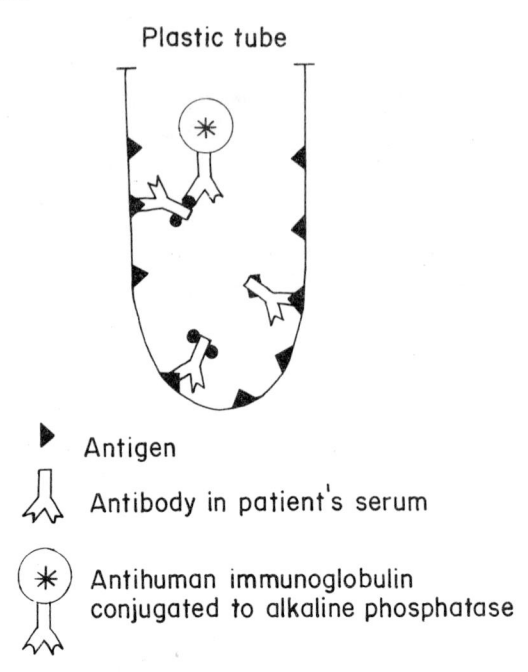

Fig. 59. Enzyme-linked immunosorbent assay (ELISA) where the antigen is bound to the walls of a plastic tube. If, for example, IgG antibodies are present in an added sample of a patient's serum, its presence can be demonstrated by using an anti-IgG serum which has been coupled to the enzyme, alkaline phosphatase. The greater the concentration of IgG in the patient's serum, the greater the amount of anti-IgG with enzyme which becomes bound to the walls of the plastic tube. Thus, the enzyme activity which remains after washing the tube is a reflection of the level of IgG antibodies to the used antigen in the patient. By coupling the enzyme to anti-IgM or anti-IgA serum, the patient's level of IgM or IgA antibodies against this antigen can be determined

later, diagnostic techniques which are based on the principles of immunosorbents are used in a variety of cases such as in allergy. The presence of different components in tissue can be demonstrated by using fluorescent-labelled antibodies. This technique can be applied in the diagnosis of immunological illnesses. In certain forms of glomerulonephritis, *immunofluorescence techniques* have been used to show the deposits of antigens, antibodies, and complement components in the glomeruli of the kidney.

The reaction of antigen with antibody has biological consequences. The above mentioned secondary manifestations of antigen–antibody reactions appear *in vitro*. There are also corresponding *in vivo* reactions which serve to eliminate material which is foreign to the body. Antibodies are an integral part of the body's apparatus for the defence against foreign antigenic material, such as micro-organisms, as well as against other antigenic material such as cells, tumour cells or even transfused blood, tissue transplants, and in some cases, pharmaceuticals. The mechanism of antibody action in these examples is described in detail in Sections III–VII which follow. They deal with infection, immunological illnesses, tumour immunology, transplant immunology, and blood group serology.

6. Complement

In the presence of fresh serum, antibodies which are directed against certain bacteria can cause injury to the cell membrane. This results in lysis of the cell. In the case of the red blood cells, this reaction results in the passage of haemoglobin through the cell membrane, haemolysis, and the eventual death of the red blood cells. This cytotoxic effect is mediated by what has been called serum complement and the phenomenon has long been used in the complement-binding reactions mentioned above.

It has long been known that complement is composed of several components. The research of the last 15 years, particularly that of Müller-Eberhard and co-workers, has contributed much to our understanding of the subject. Complement is composed of at least nine different components which include eleven distinct serum proteins. The designation and biological characteristics of these proteins are given in Table 25. Much attention has been devoted to the complement factors because of their biological implications and because of the fact that the functions of several serum proteins have been defined in this system. It has been shown that this system has many biological effects in addition to the lysis of some cells with which antibodies react. Before entering a more detailed description of these effects, it is helpful to comment on the sequence of reactions which make up the complement system.

A prerequisite for the activation of the complement sequence is the interaction of at least one molecule of IgM with an antigen or the interaction of two molecules of IgG with determinants which are sufficiently close together. Thus, the presence of only one molecule of IgM or many molecules of IgG per cell is required before the activation of complement on the surface of the cell can be accomplished. The first step in the sequence is the binding of the first component of the complement system, C1q, to the antibody or antibodies. In the presence of calcium, C1r and C1s bind to the first component (Figs. 60A and 61) thereby activating the C1s component of this complex to an esterase. This enzyme affects the C4 component in such a way that it becomes capable of binding to the surface of the cell. Following this, C1s affects C2 in such a way that in the presence of magnesium it forms a complex with C4 which becomes bound to the surface of the cell (Fig. 60B). This complex, C42, possesses enzymic activity and causes the proteolytic degradation of C3 into several fragments (Fig. 60C). One of these fragments, C3b, becomes attached to the surface of the cell and causes C5, C6, and C7 to bind successively to the surface of the cell to form a complex which subsequently binds C8 and C9. The activation of the sequence of C5–C9 results in injury to the cell membrane (Fig. 60D–E). The cell membrane is changed in such a way that when viewed through the electron microscope, small holes having a diameter of about 10 nm can be seen. These alterations to the cell membrane cause the leakage of material from the cell. This results in a breakdown to the osmotic balance, the cells undergo lysis, and die.

As was mentioned previously, this function of complement to produce cell lysis is only one of the many consequences of the activation of the complement system. Several fragments of the various complement factors, as well as the complexes of these factors which arise during the activation, have significant biological activity. As can be seen in Fig. 61, the fragmentation of C3 and C5 causes the appearance of so-called *anaphylatoxins* (C3a and C5a). These bring about the release of histamine by inducing degranulation of mast cells. Via its vascular effect, histamine adds to an in-

148 *Immunoglobulins*

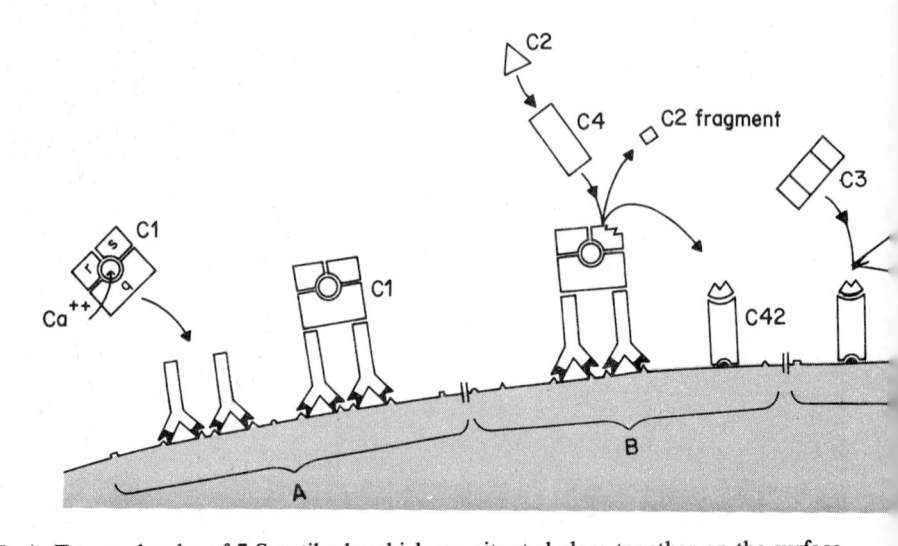

Fig. 60A–E. A. Two molecules of 7 S antibody which are situated close together on the surface of the cell activate the C1 complex which consists of C1q, C1r, C1s, and calcium
B. In its turn, C1 activates C4 and C2 which form a complex capable of activating C3
C. The activation of C3 results in the fragments C3a and C3b
D. The active fragment of C3, C3b, causes the binding to the surface of the cell of factors C5, C6, and C7
E. An aggregate of several molecules of C8 and C9 follows which causes the cell membrane to puncture. This causes a release of the contents of the cell and results in the death of the cell (lysis)

flammatory reaction. The fragments C3a and C5a, as well as the C567 complex, have chemotactic effects on neutrophil granulocytes. The granules of the accumulated phagocytic cells are easily released into the tissue phagocytosis and this is the major cause of the inflammation and injury to the tissue that results from complement activation. If this takes place locally in skin, a typical swelling arises (Arthus' reaction) which is always infiltrated by neutrophil granulocytes.

Furthermore, C3 can increase the efficiency of phagocytosis. This can be accomplished in several ways, one of which is the so-called immunoadherence. This implies that these structures which react with the antibody adhere to nearby cells and thereby increase the ease with which the antigen can be phagocytosed. In addition, C2b (a fragment of C2), possesses kinin activity adding to the inflammatory reaction. Further it seems that C1, C2, and C4 can take part in the neutralization of viruses, e.g. herpes virus.

The complement sequence and the various effects which are produced by its activation are represented in Fig. 61. The anaphylatoxins, chemotaxis, and enhanced phagocytosis contribute to the alterations of tissue which result in an inflammatory reaction. This arises also from the cytolytic reaction since it releases tissue-toxic cell constituents. Since inflammation and phagocytosis are important components of the defence against infection, the complement system has become of great biological interest. This is also due to the observations that the inflammatory reactions induced via complement can cause injury to tissue which sometimes can give rise to disease. Such tissue injuries are discussed in the chapter concerning immunological illnesses.

During the past few years, considerable interest has been shown in the alternative pathway for complement activation. This is thought to take place directly via C3 without prior activation of C1, C2, and C4 (Osler and Sandberg, 1973). A recently discovered serum protein, C3-proactivator (C3PA), is involved in this pathway. It is thought that activation via this route can be caused by lipopolysaccharides (endotoxins) and other substances which mostly are carbohydrates. It is possible that this type of complement activation can have importance in certain biological connections but this remains to be proven. An interesting serum protein, properdin, also takes part in this alternative pathway. This protein, in conjunction with C3b and C3PA, plays a role in the activation of C3. The mechanism of this activation is not yet completely clarified.

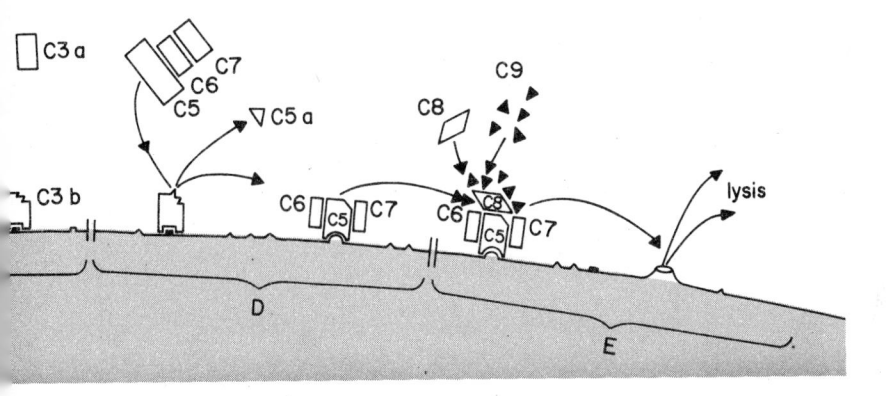

Evidence has been produced recently to suggest that the complement system and the coagulation system are interrelated. It is thought that the Hageman factor, via plasmin and kallikrein, can activate the complement sequence and that the complement factor, C6, is essential for the coagulation mechanism. The possible biological significance of the connection between the complement sequence and the coagulation mechanism, including fibrinolysis and the kinin system or inflammatory reactions, is unclear.

It is obvious that there should exist mechanisms whereby control can be exercised over the potentially dangerous complement system. Inhibitors of some of the complement factors are known to exist. By forming a complex with activated C1, *C1-esterase inhibitor* can block the enzymic activity of this component. This inhibitor is of particular interest since it is absent in cases of hereditary angio-oedema, where C2 and C4 become activated. This gives rise to the formation of the kinin active fragment, C2b, which is held to be responsible for the local oedema. Furthermore, C1-esterase inhibitor can inhibit kallikrein.

An important role of *C3b-inhibitor* is its prevention of the activation of C3 which normally takes place via C3b and C3-proactivator. If this were not the case, the complement system would be self-activating in the presence of sufficient active C3b. Furthermore, there exists an *anaphylatoxin inhibitor* which destroys the anaphylatoxin activity of C3a and C5a.

Complement plays a part in protection reactions as well as in those reactions which

Table 25. Components of complement

	C1q	C1r	C1s	C4	C2	C3	C5	C6	C7	C8	C9
Probable location of synthesis	Intestine Macrophages? Lymphocytes?	Intestine	Intestine	Macrophages? Bone marrow? Spleen?	Macrophages?	Macrophages?	Macrophages?	Macrophages?			
Concentration in serum (mg/l)	180		110	640	25	1600	80	75	55	80	230
Molecular weight	400 000	180 000	86 000	206 000	117 000	180 000	180 000	95 000	110 000	163 000	79 000
Sedimentation coefficient ($s^o_{20, w}$)	11.1	7.5	4.5	10.0	4.5	9.5	8.7	5.5	6.0	8.0	4.5
Electrophoretic mobility	γ_2	β	α	β_{1E}	β	β_{1C}	β_{1F}	β_2	β_2	γ_1	α_1
Sensitivity to heat	+				+					+	

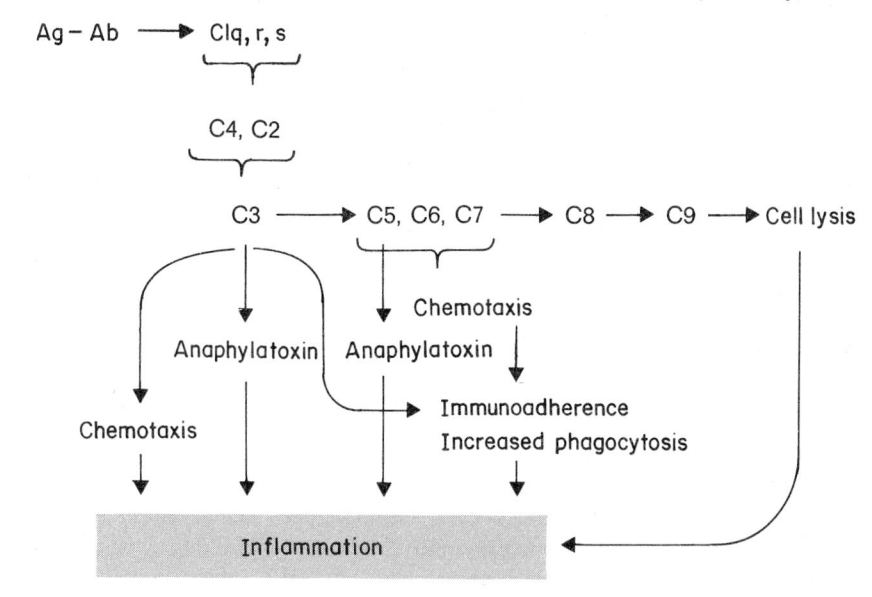

Fig. 61. Schematic representation of the complement sequence. Also shown are the various functions which arise from the activation of this sequence to produce an inflammation reaction

cause injury to tissue. Thus, the assay of the various complement factors is of practical interest. The total amount of complement activity in serum can be determined by its ability to induce haemolysis and the individual components such as C3 and C4 can be assayed quantitatively. Immunological techniques, particularly immunodiffusion techniques, are of help in these latter determinations, and can be of clinical importance since a lowered level of consumption of these components indicates an increased or occasionally decreased synthesis of complement components. This appears in certain conditions, such as glomerulonephritis and can be used as a measure of disease activity.

III. Defence against infection
LARS Å. HANSON

It is clear that the development of the lymphoid cells into a system of highly evolved and specialized cells is due to the valuable role which their mechanism of recognition of foreign material plays for survival. The specific immune response, with its two effector mechanisms, is often directed against foreign material such as invading microorganisms, bacteria, viruses, fungi, protozoa, and parasites. In many cases, the two effector mechanisms provide an effective means of protection which, however, is complemented by or is sometimes taken over by a series of other components. These components are listed in Table 26 under the heading: 'non-specific defence mechanisms'.

Table 26. Defence against infection

A. Non-specific defence mechanisms	B. Specific defence mechanisms
1. Genetic, constitutional components	1. Antibody-mediated immunity
2. Mechanical and chemical factors	2. Cell-mediated immunity
3. Interferon	
4. Properdin, complement	
5. Phagocytosis	
6. Inflammatory reactions	

1. Non-specific defence mechanisms

Non-specific mechanisms can be brought about by genetic and constitutional components. There are well-known examples of races showing increased sensitivity to certain infectious diseases, e.g. the high incidence of tuberculosis among North American Indians. A liability to attract tuberculosis can be seen even in certain families. The difference in susceptibility to various infectious diseases is even more pronounced when different species are compared. In this connection, it is interesting to note that many of the micro-organisms which are highly pathogenic for man are completely non-pathogenic for most other species. This is due to the specificity for certain hosts which has been developed by these pathogens. Their virulence factors have developed during evolution in such a way that they try to overcome the defence offered by the host. Thus, the host is forced to present defence mechanisms against these micro-organisms which attempt to invade the host, establish themselves via various infection pathways, and give rise to an infection (Fig. 62A). In healthy individuals, the attack by these micro-organisms is balanced by the defence against infection so that infection usually does not take place (Fig. 62B). On the other hand, if the number of micro-organisms is high or if they are unusually virulent, they can take over and cause infection. The outcome is the same if the individual's defence is lowered by poor health or defective immune mechanisms.

The foetus and the infant, which do not have fully developed defence mechanisms, can less easily combat the attempted invasion of micro-organisms. The same is true of old people whose various tissues have lower levels of function. Undernourishment and hormonal disorders, e.g. *diabetes mellitus*, Mb Cushing, and Mb Addison, cause partially defective defence mechanisms and consequently give rise to an increased susceptibility to infection.

Several mechanical and chemical factors are of considerable importance for the defence against the invasion of various micro-organisms. Skin and the mucous membranes constitute mechanical barriers. Similarly, the mucociliary apparatus of the respiratory tract and the coughing reflex constitute additional mechanical defence. Several components in sweat and secretions are capable of preventing the invasion of microbes. Such is the case with the fatty acids and the low pH of sweat, the low pH of gastric juice, and the relatively high levels of lysozyme and lactoferrin in exocrine secretions from various parts of the body. Lysozyme is an enzyme which can attack the mucopeptide layer which is present in the cell wall of many bacteria. Lactoferrin is an iron-binding protein which, because of its ability to compete with bacteria for iron, is known to have a bacteriostatic effect.

Viral infection of different types gives rise to the formation of a substance known as

III. Defence against infection

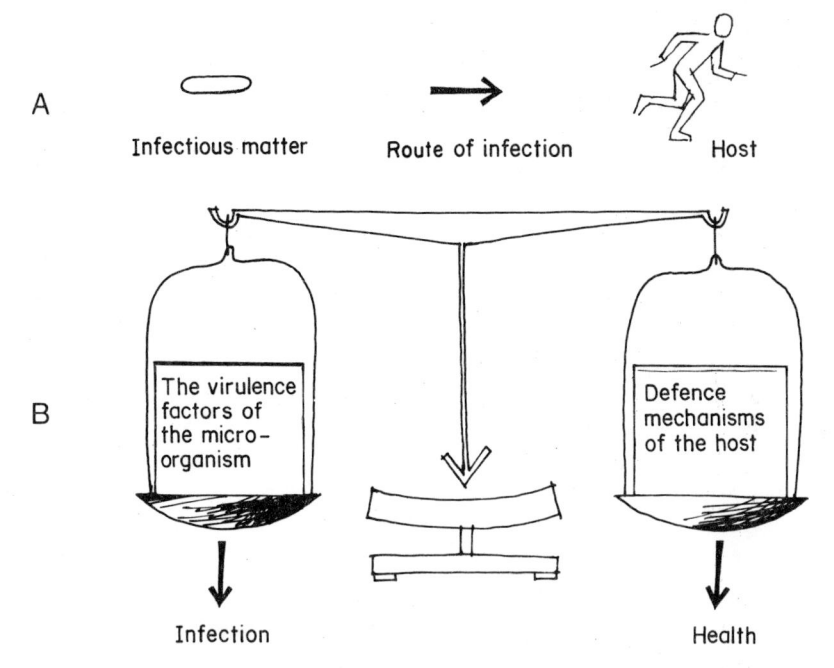

Fig. 62A. Micro-organisms follow various pathways to reach the host—man
B. The delicate balance between infection and health, with dose and virulence of invading microorganisms on one side and the host's defence mechanisms on the other

interferon. This substance has the ability to prevent the multiplication of various microorganisms, especially viruses. In a viral infection, interferon is produced much more quickly than the immune response and thus this substance plays an important role in the defence against viral illnesses. As was mentioned previously, cell-mediated immunity gives rise to the production of interferon. It was demonstrated recently that interferon can affect the lymphatic cells in such a way that the immune response becomes inhibited or stimulated. The biological significance of this is not known.

A substance, *properdin*, has been isolated recently from serum and has been shown to take part in the alternative pathway for the activation of complement, i.e. activation initiated directly via C3. While the full extent of the role of properdin in the defence against infection is unknown, it is clear that this substance takes part in virus inactivation and bactericidal reactions and that this is effected by the complement sequence C3–C9. The stimulation of phagocytosis is another result.

Phagocytosis, an important defence mechanism is mediated by the circulating blood granulocytes (Fig. 63A and B) and by the cells of the reticuloendothelial system. The latter is composed of monocytes in blood and the macrophages in different tissues e.g. histiocytes, Kupffer cells in liver, microglia in the central nervous system, and the so-called lateral cells of the spleen and bone marrow. The importance of these cells was demonstrated at the turn of the century by Metchnikoff who showed that they took up foreign material such as micro-organisms and enveloped it in small cysts, *phagosomes*, where the material was exposed to a variety of active substances including enzymes which are emptied into the phagosomes from the granules of the phagocyte. The substances kill and degrade the micro-organisms. During the process of phagocytosis

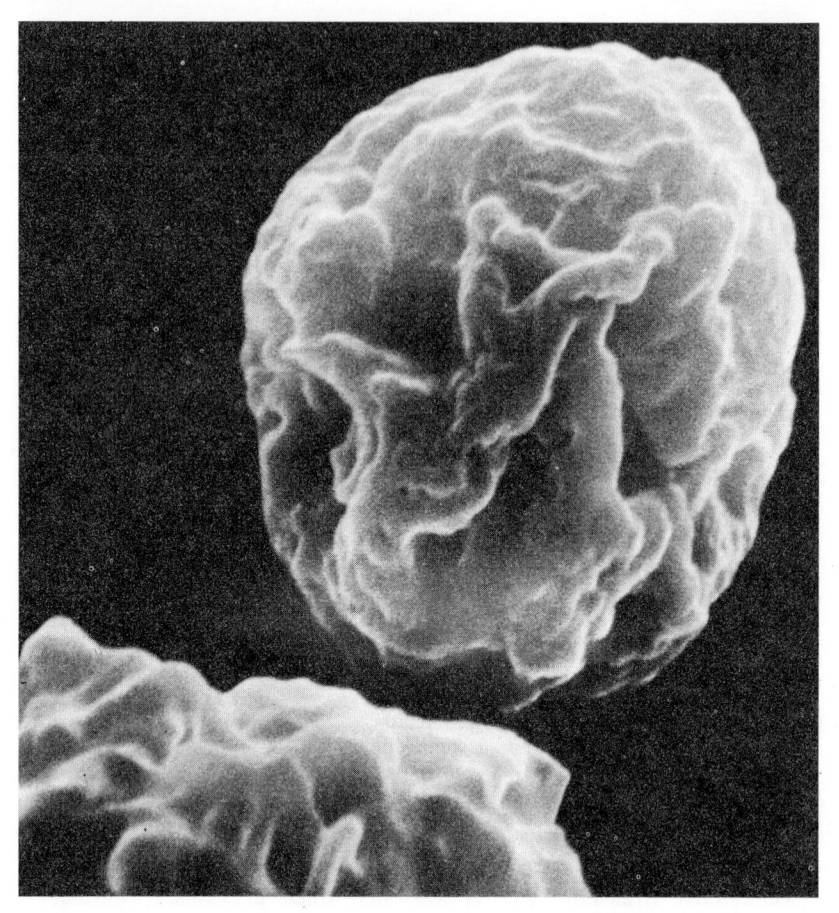

Fig. 63A. Pictures taken through a scanning electron microscope of blood leukocytes, most probably granulocytes (× 20 000)

some of the active substances in the granules are released from the cell giving rise to inflammation in the surrounding tissue. The phagocytic cells occupy a key position in the mechanisms which precipitate inflammatory reactions. This is evident from the finding that an inflammatory reaction cannot easily be developed in a laboratory animal from which phagocytic cells have been eliminated. Furthermore, only slight inflammatory changes are observed when patients suffering from agranulocytosis (a deficiency of white blood cells of the granulocyte type) become infected.

The circulating phagocytic white blood cells, granulocytes, often constitute a first line of defence against an invasion of micro-organisms (Fig. 64).

Several micro-organisms e.g. *Staphylococcus albus*, are easily taken up and killed by these cells (Fig. 65a). Thus, such bacteria have a very low capacity to induce illness; they are of low virulence and phagocytic cells provide a defence against such micro-organisms. There exist other micro-organisms which have virulence factors making them resistant to phagocytosis. Pneumococcus, which has polysaccharide capsule, is one such micro-organism (Fig. 65b). This polysaccharide capsule is a significant

III. Defence against infection 155

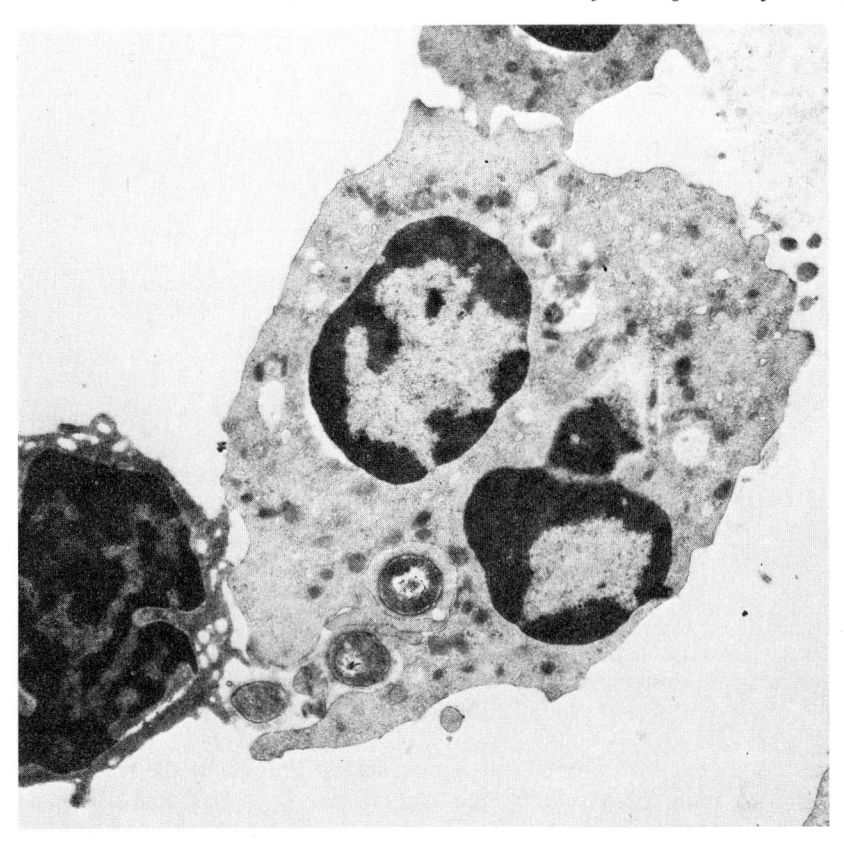

Fig. 63.B. Electron microscope picture of a granulocyte. The dark cell in the bottom left portion of the picture is a lymphocyte. Close to the lymphocyte and inside the granulocyte are seen three bacteria which have undergone phagocytosis. The bacterium which is located most deeply within the granulocyte is enveloped within a phagosome. It is here that the granules deposit their bacteria-destroying contents ($\times$ 20 300). Photographs A and B by S. Olling and C. Svalander

virulence factor of the pneumococcus and is said to be the only component of these bacteria which can help them give rise to infection in the face of the body's defence mechanisms.

There are other micro-organisms which can be taken up by the phagocytic cells but which have virulence factors making it possible for them to survive and sometimes multiply within these cells. Thus, *Staphylococcus aureus* and streptococci can produce toxins which inactivate or kill the host phagocytes (Fig. 65d). Mycobacteria are taken up by phagocytic cells but survive in these cells where they are protected against the defence mechanisms of secretions and serum (Fig. 65e). Thus, it is clear that the phagocytes by themselves do not provide an effective protection against the more virulent micro-organisms and additional means of defence are required to combat such micro-organisms. It is in this connection that antibodies have what is probably their most important function. Antibodies are capable of reacting with the surface of the micro-organisms e.g. pneumococci. Microbial uptake is facilitated via Fc- and C3-receptors on the granulocytes (Fig. 65c). The complement activation further improves the phagocytosis by release of chemotactic components. This process is outlined in Fig.

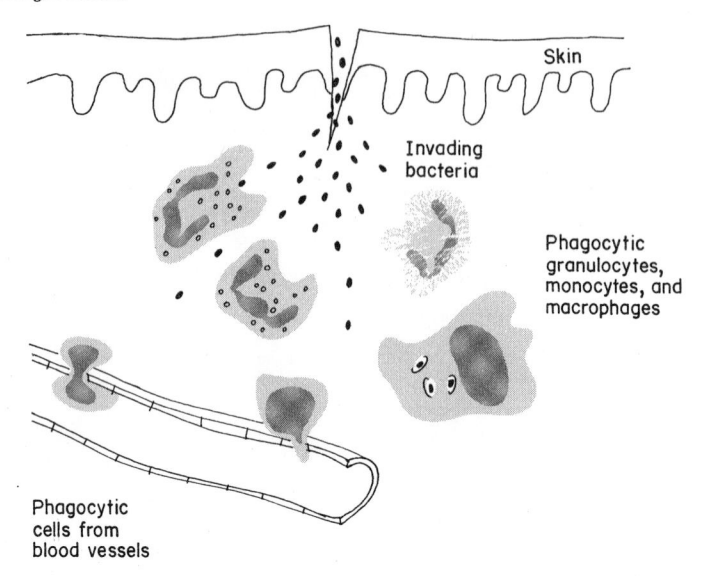

Fig. 64. Phagocytosis of bacteria which are invading a cut in the skin of an individual who has not previously been in contact with this micro-organism. Phagocytes, neutrophilic granulocytes in particular, make up the first line of defence against these micro-organisms. Monocytes also take part. However, this phagocytosis in non-immune individuals may be insufficient with the risk that the micro-organisms can multiply and spread via the lymphatics and blood vessels

66. When compared with Fig. 64, this figure demonstrates how the invading bacteria are dealt with more effectively by the phagocytes of an individual who possesses antibodies against the micro-organism in question. It should be mentioned here that in addition T-lymphocytes, which are responsible for cell-mediated immunity, can contribute to chemotaxis and to the activation of phagocytic macrophages.

It was shown recently that an acute phase protein, C-reactive protein, has a stimulating effect on phagocytic cells. This protein is formed rapidly on bacterial infections and may be of significance in defence.

2. Role of antibodies

The defence against infection often implies an intricate cooperation of a large number of different specific and non-specific mechanisms (Table 26). The specific mechanisms, i.e. the two effector mechanisms of the immune response, play an important part in this. However, the role played by these two mechanisms is dependent on the type of the invading micro-organism. The contribution of antibodies to the defence against infection is primarily the promotion of phagocytosis. This effect can be direct as in the case of antibodies to pneumococci (Fig. 65c) or it can be exercised indirectly via the complement system as shown in Fig. 61 and 66. The facilitation of phagocytosis is called opsonization and is primarily due to the phagocyte receptors for the Fc-portion of the antibodies. It is likely that the receptors which phagocytic cells have for C3b stabilize the Fc-binding, explaining the increased phagocytosis which is observed on activation of the complement system. Furthermore, antibodies are capable of providing protection by causing lysis of certain bacteria. This takes place via the complement

a Phagocytosis of *Staphylococcus albus*

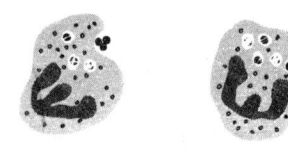

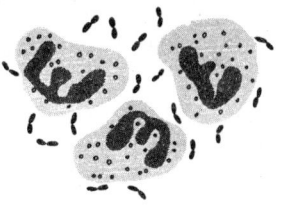

b Encapsulated pneumococci do not undergo phagocytosis in the absence of antibodies

Fig. 65(*a*). *Staphylococcus albus* which has undergone phagocytosis in granulocytes. These bacteria of low virulence are characterized by their vulnerability to uptake and subsequent killing by phagocytic cells. The picture shows how the bacteria are engulfed in the cavities (phagosomes) of the phagocytic cells where they are broken down
(*b*). The polysaccharide capsule of pneumococci acts as a virulence factor by preventing phagocytosis. Thus the pneumococci are present outside the granulocytes where they can multiply and continue to invade the neighbouring tissue

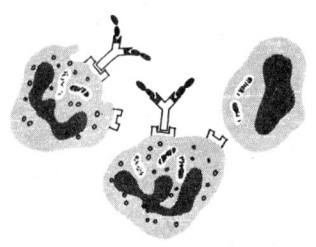

c Encapsulated pneumococci undergoing phagocytosis in the presence of antibodies

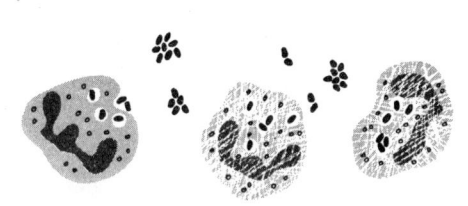

d *Staphylococcus aureus* undergoing phagocytosis

Fig. 65(*c*). Pneumococci in an individual who has antibodies against the capsule of the pneumococci can undergo phagocytosis by the granulocytes. This is due to these cells having special receptors which can attach to the Fc-portion of those antibodies which have reacted with the polysaccharide capsule as well as to C3b appearing on activation of complement. Thus the individual is immune to the pneumococci since the specific antibodies against the pneumococci enable phagocytosis to take place
(*d*). *Staphylococcus aureus* undergoing phagocytosis by granulocytes. These bacteria are more virulent than *Staphylococcus albus* and can clearly be taken up by the phagocytic cells. However, one of their virulence factors is a toxin which kills the granulocytes and permits survival of the staphylococci

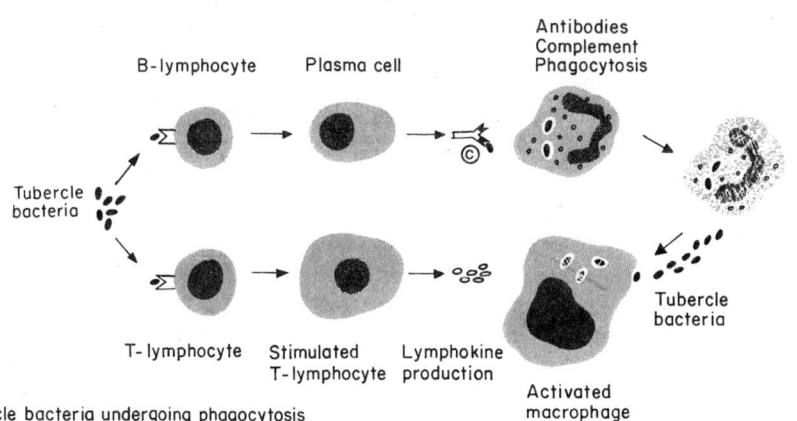

e Tubercle bacteria undergoing phagocytosis

Fig. 65(*e*). Infection with tubercle bacteria causes an immune response consisting of antibodies as well as stimulated T-lymphocytes. The phagocytosis of the bacteria by the granulocytes with help from the antibodies and complement does not result in the death of the bacteria, however, and immunity does not ensue. On the other hand, the cell-mediated immunity, which functions via the lymphokine-activated macrophages entails an effective phagocytosis and provides protection against tubercle bacteria

158 *Immunoglobulins*

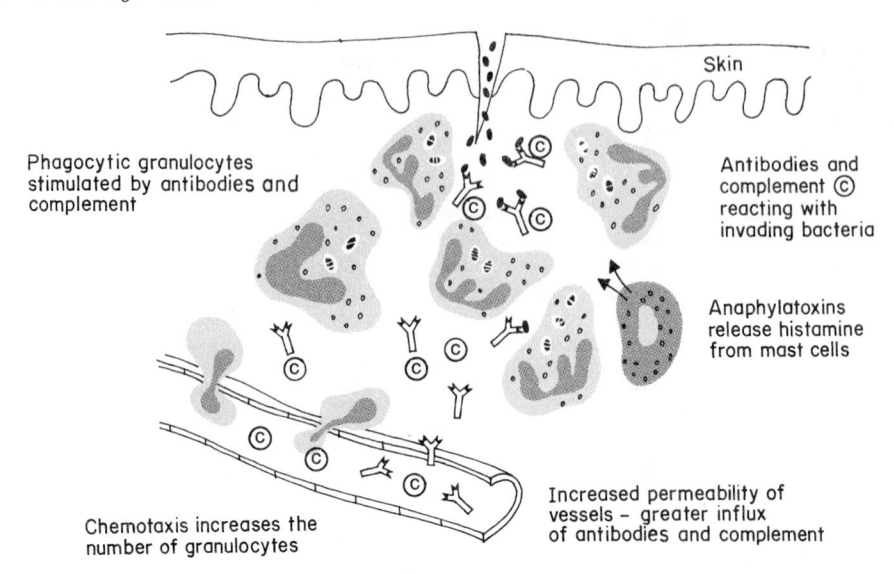

Fig. 66. Bacterial infection via a cut in the skin of an individual who has previously been in contact with the invading micro-organisms and has antibodies against them. Together with the complement ⓒ the antibodies activate phagocytosis by chemotaxis, immune adherence, agglutination, and the development of an inflammatory reaction. Thus the initial defence against the bacteria is comprised of granulocytes from the circulation. This is backed up by a specific defence in the form of antibodies and complement which activate the phagocytosis. The content of the granules of the neutrophil granulocytes is the most important contributor to the inflammatory reaction

system and is believed to occur with relatively few micro-organisms and, in particular, with certain gram-negative bacteria. Antibodies can also neutralize toxins. This property is of paramount importance in the protection against those bacteria, the pathogenicity of which is due to their production of toxins. Tetanus (lockjaw), diphtheria, and botulinus bacteria are examples of such bacteria. The presence of sufficiently high levels of neutralizing antibodies is enough to render the bacteria harmless and to give rise to complete immunity. The greater the avidity of the antibody, the greater is the neutralizing effect. Thus, IgG antibodies provide the most effective protection since they have generally the greatest avidity in an antibody response. Consequently, commercial preparations of gamma globulin which contain mostly IgG provide effective protection against infections which are caused by toxin-producing bacteria (Table 27). For several other bacteria such as streptococci, staphylococci and anthrax bacteria, where the production of toxin is only one of the virulent factors, the problem is more complex. In such cases, the protection is not mediated entirely by antitoxins, but instead other defence mechanisms such as phagocytosis are brought into play. In many infections, cell-mediated immunity also plays a role.

The ability of antibodies to neutralize viruses has a place of importance in the defence against infection. This effect blocks the virus and prevents it from entering those cells in which it can survive and eventually propagate in number. In the case of several viral infections, e.g. measles, chicken-pox, polio, epidemic hepatitis (hepatitis A), German measles, and complications of smallpox vaccination, it is known that antibodies play a decisive role in the development of immunity (Table 27). Effective

Table 27. Effects and doses of passive immunization with immunoglobulin

	Protection	Dose for prophylactic protection
Viral infection		
Measles	+	0.04 or 0.2 ml/kg ≥ 50 IE/ml (WHO)[c]
Vaccinia/variola[a]	+	2 ml ≥ 500 IE/ml (WHO)[d]
Varicellae[b]	+	5 ml ≥ 1/2 560 (complement binding)
Rubella[a]	+?	20 ml ≥ 1/1 024 (neutralization)[e]
Rabies[a]	+	15–40 IE/kg + vaccine (WHO)
Epidemic hepatitis[f]	+	0.02–0.04 ml/kg (WHO)[f]
Serum hepatitis	+	1/500 000 (indirect agglutination)
Adeno	+?	
Polio[g]	+?	
Parotitis[a]	+?	
Bacterial infection		
Tetanus[a]	+	250–500 IE (WHO)
Diphtheria[a]	+	500–1 000 IE (WHO)
Botulism[a]	+	
Pneumococcal infection	+	
Pertussis[a]	+?	
Staphylococcus aureus[a]	+?	
Pseudomonas aeruginosa etc.	+?	
Antibody deficiency syndromes		
(hypo- and dysgammaglobulinaemias)		
Primary	+	0.45–0.9 ml/kg every third week
Secondary—burns etc.	+	large amounts

[a] Immunoglobulin from convalescent serum and postvaccination serum.
[b] Immunoglobulin from convalescent serum following herpes zoster.
[c] The lower dose gives a modified, the higher dose a complete protection.
[d] Therapeutic effects have also been demonstrated in complications to smallpox vaccination. To prevent such (in for example eczema) a dose of 0.3 ml/kg is used.
[e] The accuracy of this titre has been questioned.
[f] For a continued protection during 4–6 months in massive exposure a dose of 0.06–0.12 ml/kg is recommended.
[g] The effectiveness of polio vaccination has eliminated the need for immunoglobulin as a prophylactic against polio.

protection against such diseases can be achieved by vaccination to establish a high antibody titre in blood—*active immunization*, or by injection with immunoglobulin to provide a good supply of antibodies—*passive immunization*. To achieve the desired result by using the latter method is not always easy. For example, it appears that the preparations of immunoglobulin which are available for the treatment of rubella (German measles) often do not contain sufficient antibody to give rise to an effective protection. It is essential that the preparation is given before the virus has become established intracellularly, where it is inaccessible to antibodies. Thus, the preparation of immunoglobulin should be given while the virus is still in the blood (viraemic phase) and preferably early in this phase.

Regular preparations of immunoglobulin have not proved to be helpful in cases of inoculation hepatitis, or serum hepatitis (hepatitis B). Recent investigations indicate, however, that high titred immunoglobulin preparations isolated from convalescent sera can provide protection.

While the mechanism of virus neutralization is not so well understood as that of toxin neutralization, it is likely that IgG antibodies produce a better effect than those of the IgM type and that complement compounds take part. In other cases of antibody-mediated protection, the reverse is true and antibodies of the IgM type are more effective than those of the IgG type in complement activation. This is also the case in the agglutination of microorganisms, a reaction which facilitates phagocytosis.

Commercially available preparations of immunoglobulin generally contain IgG to more than 90–95 per cent. Results obtained with immunoglobulin prophylaxis and therapy are summarized in Table 27. In this table, the doses which are based on the international standardization of WHO have a considerably higher degree of certainty than the others. In the case of the antibody-deficiency syndromes, the lower value corresponds to the lowest dose which, according to a study by the British Medical Research Council (1971), has proved to be effective. The higher dose (0.9 ml/kg per three-week period) should be tried if the lower one does not produce the desired effect.

It is thought that circulating antibodies do not always give rise to a particularly effective protection against infections which enter the body through the mucous membranes. It has been shown that the level of antibody in blood is not related to the protection against certain virus infections, e.g. caused by viruses of the myxo-, rhino-, or para-influenzae group. The protection against this virus is related to the level of antibody in the secretions of the respiratory tract. The antibodies which are found in exocrine secretions are mainly IgA antibodies of the secretory type. As has been mentioned in the chapter dealing with the structure of the immunoglobulins, these antibodies are dimeric molecules of IgA containing two extra polypeptide chains, the secretory component (SC), and the J(join)-chain. These stable molecules are resistant to proteolytic degradation and are more resistant to denaturation at low pH than are the serum antibodies. Thus, they are able to withstand the variety of environments offered by the different secretions of the body. Such IgA antibodies which are found in the secretion of the respiratory tract have been shown to provide protection against various rhino- and myxoviruses. Furthermore, secretory antibodies can prevent the attachment of bacteria to mucous membranes. This has been demonstrated for streptococci on the epithelium of the oral cavity and for cholera bacteria on the intestinal epithelium.

Most evidence indicates that the ability of secretory IgA antibodies to protect against viral and bacterial infections is dependent on their capacity to just bind microorganisms, which prevents contact with mucous membranes of the microbes, supposedly hindering the initial step in tissue invasion and infection. In contrast, there is no definite evidence to suggest that secretory IgA antibodies can activate complement or contribute to phagocytosis.

It is believed that secretory IgA antibodies which are formed locally in the respiratory tract, the gastrointestinal tract, the eyes, and urogenital tract can play an important part in the protection against many viral and bacterial infections. Consequently, much time has been devoted in recent years to the development of vaccines which can be administered via the mucous membranes to stimulate the local formation of the secretory IgA antibodies. Such antibodies are produced by plasma cells which are found close to the glandular structures under various mucous membranes (Fig. 67). These plasma cells are directly responsible for the production of the dimers of IgA which are found in secretory IgA. The dimers, together with the J-chains,

III. Defence against infection

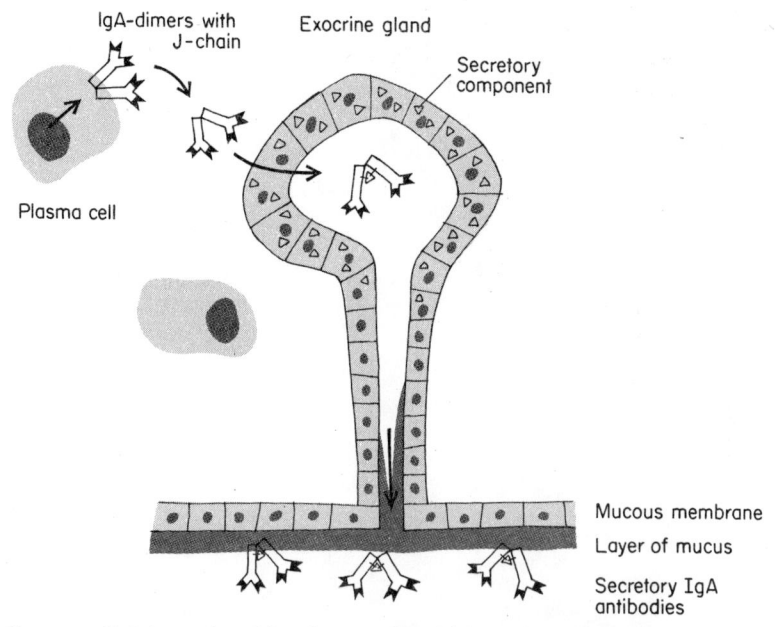

Fig. 67A. Secretory IgA is produced by plasma cells which are found in the vicinity of submucosal glandular structures. These plasma cells produce dimeric IgA held together by the J chain. Subsequently this molecule is coupled to a secretory component when the dimers pass through the epithelium of the glands where the secretory component is manufactured. The stable molecule of secretory IgA passes out into the layer of mucus on the mucous membrane and the secretion. Here, these locally produced antibodies take part in the defence of the mucous membranes

pass through or between the epithelial cells of the gland. In these cells, the secretory component is produced and coupled to the IgA dimers so that completed molecules of secretory IgA are released by the gland. These antibodies are subsequently found in the mucus and in the lumen (Hanson and Brandtzaeg, 1973).

It is believed that a special transport mechanism is required for the passage of these IgA antibodies from tissue to secretion. It is probable that the secretory component, which has a particular affinity for dimers of IgA, contributes to this selective transport. Thus, there is no significant passage of serum IgA from blood to secretion.

Evidence is accumulating that the large quantities of secretory IgA which are supplied to the infant by the mother's milk, can protect the gastrointestinal tract by preventing the invasion of bacteria through the mucous membrane. The antibodies are not resorbed, but function locally in the intestine by binding bacteria and viruses. A requirement for such a function is that the milk contains antibodies against microorganisms which are potentially pathogenic for the infant's intestinal tract. It has been difficult to explain the presence of secretory IgA antibodies against a large number of enterobacterial antigens in milk since these are not known to come into contact with the mammary gland where the local production of secretory IgA takes place. Recent data show that antigens exposing the Peyer's patches in the gut trigger IgA-producing cells. They leave via the lymph and blood and are carried to sites such as the mammary and salivary glands where local synthesis of secretory IgA takes place. Consequently, the maternal milk contains secretory IgA antibodies against those antigens exposing the intestinal lymphatic tissue of the mother. The breastfed infant is thereby elegantly

162 *Immunoglobulins*

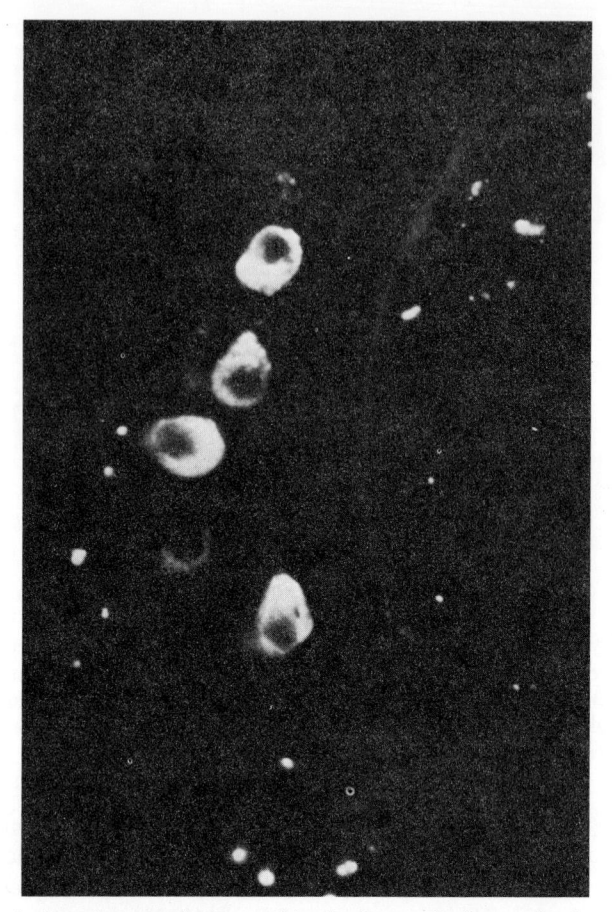

Fig. 67B. IgA-producing plasma cells detected in the tissue of salivary glands using the technique of immunofluorescence. Since the anti-serum has been labelled with a fluorescent marker and is specific for IgA, only cells containing IgA are seen ($\times 300$). Photograph by P Brandtzaeg

provided with antibodies against the pathogens present in its surroundings. At the same time the mother's intestinal mucosa will be seeded with these IgA-producing cells boosting her own local immunity.

Antibodies are formed in infections which are caused by fungi, protozoa, and worms. While it is not clear if all of these antibodies are of importance for the protection against such organisms, it is probable that they are significant in some cases e.g. in malaria. The same uncertainty applies to the IgE antibodies which are formed in large numbers in worm infections. The function of the eosinophils which is observed concurrently is unknown, but it is probably caused in part by eosinophilic chemotaxis brought on by IgE antibodies. Recent information suggests that the eosinophils may help in controlling the inflammatory reactions released by the IgE antibodies. They may also kill certain parasites.

It appears that antibodies play a more or less important role in the protection against various infections. The finding that they can cause damage to tissue has aroused much interest in recent years. This is caused by inflammatory reactions and is usually brought about by antigen–antibody complexes which activate complement (cf.

immune complex diseases). The normal defence mechanism can contribute to the symptoms of infection by causing inflammatory injuries, e.g. vasculitis, arthritis, nephritis, and encephalitis. It is possible that postinfectious arthritis, such as that appearing after vaccination with live rubella virus, can have such an origin. It is thought that the unbalanced immune response which can follow a defective cell-mediated immunity can result in the production of deficient immune elimination, increasing the risk of formation of immune complexes which are formed when attempting to eliminate the invader. This is believed to be the underlying mechanism for the tissue damage observed in the lepromatous form of leprosy. The combination of a reduced T-lymphocyte activity and a production of immune complexes is thought to be responsible for the late and lethal complication of measles and rubella, subacute sclerosing panencephalitis (SSPE), and may also be connected with multiple sclerosis (MS).

3. Cell-mediated immunity

For a long time, interest was focused mainly on the function of antibodies as a protection against infection. The cell-mediated immunity was seen primarily as a phenomenon which appeared in conjunction with the antibody response after exposure to various antigens. The interest was focused on the delayed hypersensitivity reaction which can be easily demonstrated by injecting tubercle bacteria, or a component from them called tuberculin, into the skin of individuals who have been vaccinated against or who are infected with such bacteria. It has become apparent that the cell-mediated immunity plays a role of great importance in the defence against many infections and that this role is in many cases more important than that played by the antibodies. Evidence to support this has come from studies which were carried out on patients who had defects in their cell-mediated immunity. These studies are described in a later section.

The function of cell-mediated immunity as a defence mechanism against infection is not quite understood. It is probable that the chemotactic activity for macrophages by the antigen-stimulated T-lymphocytes involved and the ability of lymphokines from these lymphocytes to increase phagocytosis can play an important part in the process. It has long been known that the macrophages of an immune individual are more effective in combating certain microorganisms than are those of a non-immune individual. This macrophagocytic activity does not have the specificity of immunological reactions, and macrophages which are stimulated by mycobacteria-specific T-lymphocytes are also more active towards *Listeria*. Obviously the non-specific increase in the activity of the macrophages is caused by the release of lymphokines from the specifically antigen-stimulated T-lymphocytes. Thus, in similarity to antibody-mediated immunity, cell-mediated immunity also functions via the stimulation of phagocytic cells. The lymphokine-activated macrophages are capable of killing highly virulent bacteria which are resistant to humoral antibodies, complement, and granulocytes.

A positive tuberculin test indicates that an individual has T-lymphocytes which, on specific stimulation with tuberculin, release lymphokines to give rise to the delayed hypersensitivity reaction in the skin. The occurrence of this reactivity against the tuberculin does not necessarily imply the presence of immunity against this illness. The individual who shows such a reaction usually has T-lymphocytes specific for other mycobacterial antigens which in contrast to tuberculin are virulence antigens. Reactivity towards these results in protection. Therefore, the observed reactivity of the T-cells to tuberculin can be used as an indicator but is not a specific measure of the immunity (Fig. 65e).

Cell-mediated immunity has been shown to be of particular importance in infections caused by micro-organisms which can act as intracellular parasites. Such microorganisms can undergo phagocytosis, but are not killed. Surviving intracellularly, they are protected from antibodies. This is the case in infections which are caused by *Brucella*, *Salmonella*, *Mycobacterium*, *Listeria*, intracellular viruses, and various fungi.

Cell-mediated immunity can provide protection against virus infections in two ways: via the viricidal effect of those macrophages which are activated by T-lymphocytes and via T-lymphocytes which are directed against viral antigen on the surface of infected cells and can act cytotoxically against these cells. When the cells are destroyed, the virus becomes exposed to neutralizing humoral antibodies. Furthermore, it is thought that antigen-stimulated T-lymphocytes release a substance which gives rise to the production of interferon, which plays an important role in the defence against virus infections by preventing the intracellular multiplication of the virus.

Ogra, Waldmann and others, who demonstrated the importance of the local production of antibodies for immunity against viral and bacterial infections, noticed recently (1974) that the locally induced cell-mediated immunity is also of importance for the protection against these infections. An understanding of this is essential for the preparation of effective vaccines against certain bacterial and virus infections.

It was mentioned earlier that the antibody-mediated defence against infection can give rise to tissue damage. It appears that the same is true of the cell-mediated reactions. This is evident in an intense tuberculin reaction which can lead to local necrosis and even to general symptoms, such as fever and malaise. The symptoms are caused by the cytotoxic T-lymphocytes, the activated macrophages, and the resulting inflammation. The damage can be serious if the reaction is extensive or if it involves tissues which include cells which are devoid of or have a limited capacity for regeneration, e.g. cells of the central nervous system. It is possible that cell damage of this type can be part of the pathogenesis of certain postinfectious encephalitis or central nervous system complications which can arise following infections such as measles.

4. Defects in the defence mechanisms

Man lives in a world of microorganisms, some of which are potentially pathogenic and can cause illness. Under normal conditions, the various defence mechanisms against infection balance the attempts of the microorganisms to colonize and invade the human body (Fig. 62). Infections can take place even under normal conditions if some part of the individual's defence becomes damaged. Such is the case in a skin lesion where bacteria can bypass the mechanical barrier which is normally created by the skin. In other cases, the dose of microbes may be so high that the micro-organisms can overcome even the normal defence mechanisms.

Certain individuals are more prone to infection than others. Today, we are much better equipped to pin-point the defects in the various defence mechanisms which can cause such illnesses. Studies which have been carried out during the last 20 years on patients who displayed such defects have provided new diagnostic and therapeutic possibilities. Furthermore, these studies have provided us with much useful information concerning the normal mechanisms of defence, their mode of action, and their significance.

The first case of recognised antibody deficiency syndrome was described by Bruton in 1952. The patient was a young boy who suffered from repeated infections which are caused primarily by pneumococci. Electrophoretic analysis of the boy's serum showed that it was practically devoid of the gamma globulin fraction. The patient was cured of his infections by being injected with gamma globulin and could thereafter lead an almost normal life. Following this report, several additional cases were discovered.

It soon became clear that there are many different kinds of defects in the mechanisms of defence against infections. These can be suitably classified on the basis of the development of the lymphoid cells and the phagocytic cells from the stem cells of bone marrow (Fig. 68).

Defects which arise in the development of stem cells via the myelocyte series into phagocytic cells result in the formation of different types of defective phagocytes. These defects can be quantitative as in granulocytopenia or qualitative as in chronic granulomatosis. Defects can arise also during the development of stem cells into the T- and B-lymphocytes of the lymphoid system. The type of defect is dependent on the stage during the development at which the defect arises. Abnormalities which affect the development of B-lymphocytes give rise to various forms of hypogammaglobulinaemia, i.e. antibody deficiency syndromes. Corresponding disorders in the development of T-lymphocytes give rise to a variety of defects in the cell-mediated immunity. Finally, defects can arise during the development of both systems. This causes the formation of combined defects which affect the functions of the T- and B-lymphocytes (Fig. 68).

Defects in non-specific defence mechanisms

Granulocytopenia

Acquired forms of granulocytopenia can appear after exposure to ionized radiation or as a result of drug reactions. They can also arise during the course of autoimmune diseases such as *lupus erythematosis disseminatus* or rheumatoid arthritis. Granulocytopenia is often the first symptom in acute leukaemia.

Granulocytopenia can be inherited in many forms which can be cyclic or non-cyclic. It can appear as an isolated condition or in combination with various diseases such as malabsorption, pancreas insufficiency, and different types of antibody deficiency syndromes.

In such patients, the dominating symptom is infections caused by staphylococci, streptococci, and pneumococci. This in itself indicates that the phagocytic cells are of particular importance in the defence mechanisms against such microorganisms. A recurring feature is stomatitis with necrotic changes in the oral cavity. The inflammatory reaction can be limited if the granulocytopenia is serious. This can be accounted for by the importance which is played by the contents of the granules of these phagocytes in precipitating an inflammatory reaction. Similarly, the fever need

166 *Immunoglobulins*

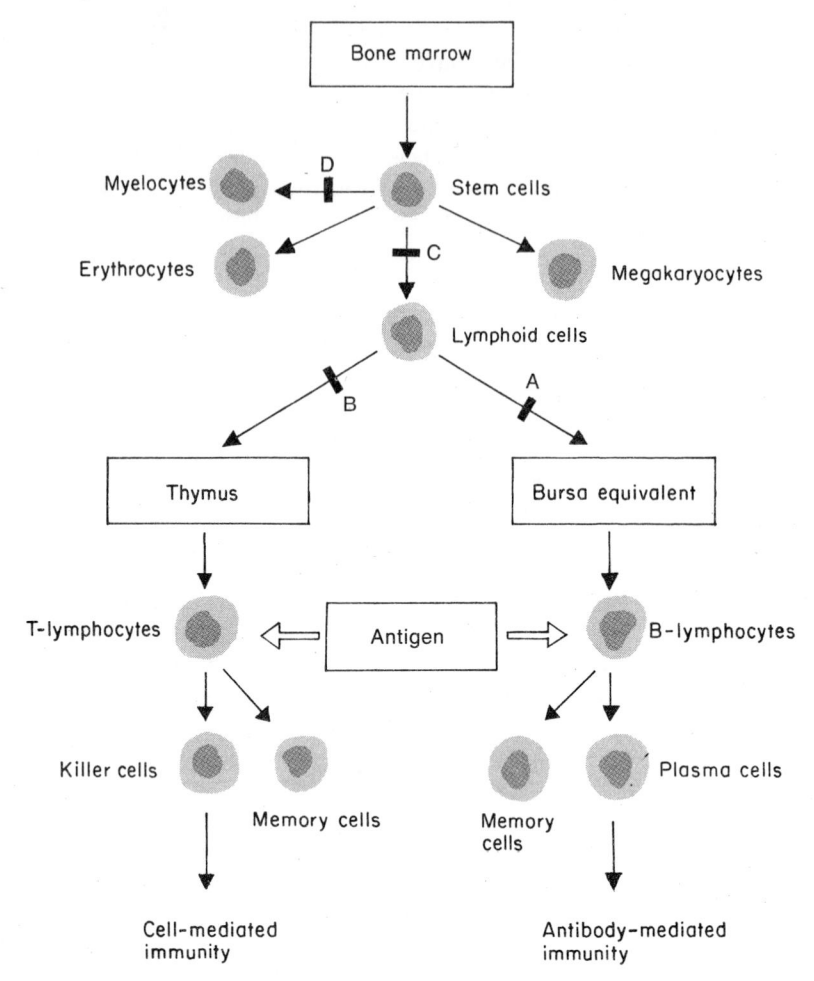

Fig. 68. A schematic representation of the lymphoid system showing possible localities of defects in the defence against infection
A. Defects in the development of immunocompetent B-lymphocytes giving rise to antibody deficiency syndromes
B. Defects in the development of immunocompetent T-lymphocytes giving rise to defects in the cell-mediated immunity
C. Possible locality of defects which affect the cell-mediated immunity as well as the antibody-mediated immunity
D. Defects in the development of myelocytes, i.e. phagocytic cells resulting in granulocytopenia or agranulocytosis

not necessarily be high in severe infections if the level of granulocytes is very low. This can probably be explained by the fact that pyrogenic substances which give rise to fever are derived primarily from granulocytes. However, pyrogenic bacterial components which cause the onset of fever are present in certain infections.

In the agranulocytosis patients, the stomatitis constitutes a breach from which generalized fatal infections can start. Such infections do not always respond to treatment with antibiotics or immunoglobulin. It is not unlikely that bone-marrow transplantation may prove in the future to be an effective therapy in many forms of agranulocytosis. In addition to the circulating phagocytic cells, the granulocytes, the macrophages constitute important phagocytic cells of the reticuloendothelial system. Quantitative and qualitative defects of the macrophages are not well known. However, it is not unlikely that the appearance of life-threatening infection in individuals who have been born without a spleen or who have their spleen removed, is due to an extensive loss of macrophage function. This may also explain the increased proneness to infection which is observed in patients who have dysfunction of the spleen during the course of sickle-cell anaemia.

Chronic granulomatosis

Chronic granulomatosis appears as an inherited, often sex-linked recessive illness. The clinical picture is dominated by repeated infections, being caused by staphylococci and gram-negative bacteria in particular. These infections are localized to the skin and to inner organs and result in the formation of granulomas.

The defect in the defence against infection in this illness has been localized to the phagocytic function of the granulocytes. These cells take up bacteria in the normal manner but are unable to kill them. The required increase in metabolic activity of the cells to kill the bacteria which have undergone phagocytosis is normally observed as an increase in the activity of the hexose monophosphate shunt in the phagocytic cells. This increase is not noted in patients suffering from chronic granulomatosis, probably because of an enzyme defect which, as yet, remains unidentified. The presence of the disorder can be detected by using a simple test, nitro-blue tetrazolium reduction test, NBT. The only form of therapy which is available at present is that involving the use of antibiotics. Therapy with immunoglobulins does not help and most of the patients die in their childhood or early adolescence.

Additional defects of phagocytosis

Isolated cases of various other types of phagocytosis disorders are known. In this connection, a patient suffering from widespread *Candida* infection was shown to have a deficiency of myeloperoxidase in his neutrophilic granulocytes and monocytes. It is thought that other defects occurring in the phagocytic cells also can be responsible for increased frequency of infections.

The *Chediak–Higashi* syndrome consists of a widespread defect in the structure of the lysosomes, resulting possibly from a microtubular defect. Patients suffering from this disease show pigment disorders and an increased frequency of infection. Similar syndromes can appear in cows, dogs, and mink.

These lysosomal disorders have also been shown to occur in the neutrophilic granulocytes, leading to the suggestion that deficient function of these cells is responsible for the increased susceptibility to infection. Recent observations suggest that these patients may respond to treatment with vitamin A. An increased incidence of malignant tumours in lymphoid tissue arises in conjunction with this disease. In these patients, as in other conditions where defects occur in the immune system, the increased susceptibility to infection can perhaps result in viral infections which give rise to the lymphoid tumours.

Complement defects

Since the complement system is known to intervene in a number of important functions such as phagocytosis and inflammation, it is to be expected that errors in this system can give rise to illness.

Hereditary angio-oedema is caused by an inborn defect in the activity of an α_2-globulin, the C1-esterase inhibitor, which under normal conditions inhibits the active esterase form of the C1-complex. Patients suffering from this disorder show repeated incidence of oedema in the gastrointestinal and the respiratory tract or the skin. Oedema in the respiratory tract can cause asphyxiation while that in the gastrointestinal tract can give rise to abdominal pain, often resulting in the patient being operated upon for suspected acute disease. It is most likely that the symptoms are caused primarily by the quinine active fragment, C2b, which is produced when C4 and subsequently C2 are activated by the C1 complex. Many of these patients respond excellently to treatment with tranexamic acid (AMCA) which obviously inhibits the enzymes which activate the C1-complex.

While *deficiencies of C1q and C2* have also been observed, it would appear that these do not give rise to any detectable defects, probably because the small amounts of these substances which do exist in the blood of such individuals are sufficient to permit normal function of complement. However, other disorders are often observed in these patients, including a condition which resembles *lupus erythematosus*.

A report has appeared of a man showing a deficiency of C3. Since childhood the patient suffered from repeated infections caused by a long series of different micro-organisms. The deficiency of C3 was caused by consumption of this factor through activation via the alternate pathway. This in turn arose from a deficiency of a C3b-inactivator which normally controls the activation of C3. As would be expected, his deficiency of C3 resulted in defective chemotaxis and phagocytosis as well as deficient bactericidal effect on gram-negative micro-organisms. An isolated deficiency of C3 has also been demonstrated.

The presence of a C5 deficiency has been detected in infants suffering from repeated infections by gram-negative bacteria. In these cases, uptake by phagocytic cells was shown to be defective. This could be normalized by the administration of normal plasma.

In some strains of rabbits, a deficiency of C6 has resulted in severe infections. As yet, few cases have been seen in man of deficiencies of Ch. C7, and C8.

Defects in specific defence mechanisms

Antibody deficiency syndromes appear in various forms (Table 28). In *congenital hypogammaglobulinaemia*) infantile sex-linked hypogammaglobulinaemia, Bruton) which occurs in boys, only very small amounts of IgA and IgM appear in the blood. A few months after birth, when IgG antibodies which have been supplied by the mother via the placenta begin to disappear, only low levels of IgG are found. Severe infections start to appear during the latter part of the first year of life. These are manifested as repeated attacks of pneumonia, gastroenteritis, meningitis, and septicaemia which are caused primarily by gram-positive bacteria such as pneumococci and streptococci, but can also be caused by staphylococci, *Haemophilus influenzae* as well as some other gram-negative bacteria. This shows the importance of antibodies in the defence against such bacterial infections. Viral infections, on the other hand, often run a normal course and induce immunity in these children. The reason for this is not immediately obvious but it may be that the very small amounts of antibody which the patients really have against various viruses are sufficient to give protection. Another possible explanation is that their normally functioning cell-mediated immunity and production of interferon can provide them with defence against viral infections.

The lymphoid tissue is practically devoid of lymphocytes in the reaction centres of the bursa-equivalent portion of the spleen and lymph glands (c.f. Fig. 50). There are no plasma cells in the lymph glands, spleen, bone marrow, or the mucous membrane of the intestine. The tonsils are poorly developed while the thymus is normal and almost normal amounts of circulating lymphocytes are found in the blood. The latter is due to the fact that the circulating lymphocytes are in about 80 per cent T-lymphocytes. The cell-mediated immunity of these patients is functionally normal. This can be demonstrated by skin tests which induce a delayed hypersensitivity reaction in the skin or by *in vitro* tests which demonstrate that the T-lymphocytes are stimulated normally by antigens or mitogens such as phythaemagglutinin (PHA).

It is striking that such patients show an increased incidence of various autoimmune disorders such as rheumatoid arthritis, autoimmune haemolytic anaemia and *lupus erythematosus disseminatus*. These findings in individuals who have impaired ability to produce antibodies would appear somewhat contradictory. There are those who propose that such conditions should be caused mostly by infection and should, therefore, appear more often in individuals who have an impaired defence against infection. In these children, certain tumours also appear more often than is normal. This can be taken to be a consequence of a diminished defence against 'foreign' cells in the form of tumour cells or possibly that the increased disposition towards infection results in the appearance of virus-induced tumours. It is not uncommon that these patients develop allergic reactions, particularly against those antibiotics which are required for their treatment.

The diagnosis is based on the repeated infections and on the defective antibody response to these infections and to various vaccines. It should be noted that only killed vaccines should be administered to these patients, as otherwise there is an increased risk for vaccination complications as has been observed with live polio virus vaccine.

The crucial test is of course the quantitation of serum immunoglobulins. This usually results in the detection of only some mg/l of IgA and IgM while the level of IgG in this type of hypogammaglobulinaemia can be up to 1 g/l. In the blood, no or only a few B-lymphocytes having antigen-binding immunoglobulin receptors are found. The analysis of these cases of immune disorders should also include the assessment of other defence mechanisms such as the cell-mediated immunity, phagocytosis, complement, C-reactive protein and, preferably, interferon. This assessment is important since combination of various defects in the defence mechanisms is not uncommon.

Good results can be achieved by regular supply of adequate doses of immunoglobulin (Table 27) and, in the presence of bacterial infection, by administering antibiotics. However, it is remarkable that the symptoms observed in the respiratory and in the gastrointestinal tracts persist or recur quite often despite the immunoglobulin prophylaxis. This can probably be explained by the fact that secretory IgA in these patients cannot be replaced by injecting immunoglobulin preparations. The reason for this is twofold. First, the commercially available preparations of immunoglobulin consist primarily of IgG and contain only very small amounts of IgA and, second, it seems that this IgA is in any case not transported over to exocrine secretions where secretory IgA has an important function in providing protection.

Hypogammaglobulinaemia of late onset has been called acquired, but judging from genetic studies, it would appear that it is hereditary like the early starting congenital form. These cases make up a heterogeneous group which is provisionally called *variable hypogammaglobulinaemia*. The histological picture is similar to that of the congenital type. In these patients, the level of immunoglobulins is somewhat higher than seen in the congenital form, but also here the picture is dominated by repeated infections. Intestinal disorders in the form of malabsorption, diarrhoea, and steatorrhoea are often observed.

Antigen-binding B-lymphocytes are found in the blood, but are unable to mature into plasma cells and to release synthesized antibodies. In some cases this block may be due to the activity of suppressor T-lymphocytes. It is not unusual to find that these patients also display some abnormalities of the various functions of the T-lymphocytes. In addition, they show an increased incidence of tumours especially in lymphoid tissues and the incidence of autoimmune diseases within the families is greater than normal. The diagnosis, prophylaxis, and therapy is identical to that for patients with congenital hypogammaglobulinaemia.

While a good assessment of the incidence of hypogammaglobulinaemia is not abailable, it is probable that the frequency is higher than 1/20 000. The most common form of the disease is variable hypogammaglobulinaemia.

Physiological hypogammaglobulinaemia which normally appears during infancy should not be confused with a pathological hypogammaglobulinaemia. The former condition appears as a consequence of the child at birth being without or having very low levels of IgA and IgM. The production of these immunoglobulins begins after the exposure of the child to various antigens in the surroundings, and the level of IgM rises quickly. At birth, however, the child has a higher level of IgG in its blood than does the mother since the maternal IgG is actively transported across the placenta to the foetus. These IgG antibodies are subsequently catabolized and the level reaches a minimum around 2–3 months after birth. Thereafter, an increase is observed as the child's own production of IgG takes over. During this period, there is usually no increased susceptibility to infection and consequently no reason for using immunoglobulin prophylaxis. However, the low level of IgM which is observed during the first months of life has been considered in connection with the increased incidence of gram-negative infections such as neonatal meningitis and septicaemia. It has not been demonstrated convincingly that the use of IgM-enriched immunoglobulin during this period of life has any prophylactic or therapeutic effect on full term children.

In some cases, a delay is observed in the child's production of immunoglobulin, giving rise to a *transient hypogammaglobulinaemia* and symptoms during the first two years of life. Temporary prophylaxis with immunoglobulin is justified in these cases.

Acquired hypogammaglobulinaemia can appear *secondary* to other illnesses e.g. in patients who have extensive burns, nephrosis, or who suffer from severe undernutrition. The condition may also appear secondary to malignant conditions such as leukaemia and multiple myeloma. In these patients immunoglobin prophylaxis is of doubtful value.

Conditions characterized by defects in a single or two classes of immunoglobulin are known as *dysgammaglobulinaemia*. This term covers also those cases where the defect is limited to subgroups of a single class of immunoglobulin. Furthermore, the designation covers a few cases where it is reported that the presence of a selective defect in the antibody production against certain microorganisms can be demonstrated. In most cases, the symptoms are dominated by bacterial infections. An increase in the number of infections is seen in *selective deficiency of IgA* in blood and secretion. These infections are often localized to the respiratory and the gastrointestinal tracts. Furthermore, there is an increased frequency of malabsorption, autoimmune phenomena and allergic reactions, and probably also tumours. This is caused presumably by the increased antigen contact via the mucous membranes as the normal protective mechanism in the form of secretory IgA no longer exists. However, there are reports of several individuals who have a selective deficiency of IgA but who do not show any symptoms. It is probable that in these cases some other defence mechanisms compensate for the defect. This can be achieved by local production of IgM and by increasing the serum level of IgG. Individuals who have also a deficiency of IgM cannot compensate for the deficiency of IgA and thus they usually have pronounced infection problems.

When the antibody deficiency is localized to a smaller fraction of the immunoglobulins, e.g. a deficiency of IgG2, electrophoresis of the patient's serum shows the presence of almost normal levels of gamma globulin.

It is probable that additional cases of immunodeficiency, particularly the selective forms, will be detected with the advent of more refined diagnostics. The selective defiency of IgA occurs in approximately one case per 700, making it the most common of the known immune defects. Because of the various manifestations of the disorder, which are over-represented in the deficiency of IgA, this defect is given in hospital statistics to have higher frequency.

It can be seen from the above that there is good reason to test for a deficiency of IgA in patients who show increased susceptibility to infection, malabsorption, and/or autoimmune disorders. Furthermore, testing for IgA deficiency is carried out for another important reason: the individual who is without IgA or who has low levels of this immunoglobulin runs a risk of contracting complications following blood transfusion and after being injected with immunoglobulin preparations containing IgA.

Data concerning the frequency of other immunodeficiencies are not available but it would appear that such cases are more common than was thought. With the diagnostic methodology which is available today, cases showing repeated infections should be examined for immune defects since these are therapeutic and prophylactic possibilities. For similar reasons, relatives of the individuals suffering from antibody deficiency syndromes should also be examined.

Various forms of defects of the *cell-mediated immunity* have been described (Table 28). A selective disorder of the thymus called *thymus alymphoplasia* (Nezelof) causes a defect in the function of the thymus, i.e. a defective ability to develop cell-mediated immune reactions while the antibody response appears to be relatively normal.

The simultaneous appearance of *thymus hypoplasia* and *defective parathyroid glands* (Di George's syndrome) is caused by an error in the development of the third and fourth pharyngeal pouches, from which both the thymus and the parathyroid glands

Table 28. Major defects in the defence against infection

I. Defects in non-specific defence mechanisms	II. Defects in specific defence mechanisms

A. Defects in phagocytosis
  quantitative: granulo-
  cytopenia
  qualitative: chronic
  granulomatosis
  (dysphagocytosis)
  Chediac–Higashi syndrome
B. Defects in complement
	A. Defects in antibody-mediated immunity
	  1. Congenital hypogammaglobulinaemia
	  2. 'Variable' hypogammaglobulinaemia
	  3. Physiological hypogammaglobulinaemia
	  4. Transient hypogammaglobulinaemia
	  5. Acquired, secondary hypogammaglobulinaemia
	  6. Dysgammaglobulinaemia
	B. Defects in cell-mediated immunity
	  1. Thymus alymphoplasia (Nezelof)
	  2. Thymus hypoplasia with parathyroidplasia (Di George)
	  3. Acquired defects
	C. Defects in both antibody and cell-mediated immunity
	  1. Thymus dysplasia with hypogammaglobulinaemia ('Swiss type', severe combined immunodeficiency, SCID)
	  2. Ataxia – telangiectasia
	  3. Wiskott–Aldrichs syndrome

originate. Also these patients show symptoms of an inability to develop cell-mediated immune reactions, but in addition, the deficiency of parathyroid hormone is seen in the occurrence of hypocalcaemia and convulsions.

Extensive defects in the cell-mediated immunity are followed by severe infections which are caused primarily by fungi and viruses. Prophylaxis with immunoglobulin is without effect and the patients die.

Recent experimentation with thymus transplantation has proved successful, however, but this approach is still in the experimental stage. A few cases of Di Geroge's syndrome have improved spontaneously.

Defects in the cell-mediated immunity have appeared secondary to other conditions such as undernutrition which also can lead to deficiencies in other defence mechanisms. It is probable that the deficient cell-mediated immunity is the major cause of the increased sensitivity to infection which is observed in undernourished persons. Impaired T-lymphocyte reactivity is seen in cases of Mb Hodgkin, sarcoidosis, and during several viral infections such as measles and influenza. The significance of this is as yet unknown but it may be connected with the fact that patients having Mb Hodgkin contract a greater number of infections caused by fungi, viruses (particularly *herpes zoster*), and certain bacteria.

Defects in both the antibody-mediated immunity and the cell-mediated immunity appear in various hereditary forms and are among the most severe immune defects, showing defective function of the T- and B-lymphocytes. The *severe combined immunodeficiency* (SCID), which was reported first in Switzerland and which is often called 'Swiss type', is particularly well documented. As is the case in other syndromes in which cell-mediated immunity plays a part, the first symptoms to appear often take the form of protracted *Candida* infection in the oral cavity and skin. The infection becomes more widespread and affects the lungs. There is a subsequent appearance of additional infections caused by viruses and other agents, e.g. *Pneumocystis carinii* which can also appear in congenital hypogammaglobulinaemia. The defective cell-mediated immunity of the children with severe combined immunodeficiency implies that injecting live vaccine such as the BCG-vaccine or the smallpox vaccine often results in severe, frequently fatal, complications due to growth of the vaccine strains.

The lymphoid tissue of these children is found to be devoid of T- and B-lymphocytes and a reduced number of circulating lymphocytes is noted in their blood. The thymus is rudimentary and shows a deficiency of lymphoid cells and Hassall's bodies. In some patients with SCID, defects in erythrocyte enzymes are causing lymphocyte destruction.

Functionally, stimulation with antigen fails to give rise to an antibody response and the ability to develop cell-mediated immune reactions is lost. The children die of severe infection during the first or second year of life. Therapy and prophylaxis with immunoglobulin or antibiotics cannot prevent this course of events. Recent experiments using transplantation of bone marrow cells have proved successful. This form of therapy has many unsolved problems, however, especially since these individuals who are without cell-mediated immune reactions are not capable of rejecting tissue containing foreign non-matching tissue antigens in the transplant. In many cases, the transferred immunocompetent tissue from the donor gives rise instead to severe reactions against the recipient (graft-versus-host reaction) which may result in the death of the patient. It is thought that a very high degree of match between donor and recipient is required in bone-marrow transplant. Recently, a new antigen system was discovered which may account for failures of many earlier bone-marrow transplants.

Several cases with variable forms of combinations of defective antibody and cell-mediated immunity have been encountered. As yet, these appear sporadic and are not included in the simplified patterns provided in Fig. 68 and Table 28.

Ataxia-telangiectasia is a syndrome which is dominated by progressive changes in the cerebellum giving rise to disturbance of the gait, telangiectasia of the skin and conjunctivae, and increased susceptibility to infection. The syndrome has not yet been allocated to a definite category of the immune defects but findings show defective function in the cell-mediated immunity as well as changes in the immunoglobulin patterns, and in particular, a deficiency of IgA. These patients often show repeated infection in the respiratory tract which is believed to be connected with the deficiency of IgA. Ataxia telangiectasia patients usually have an increased serum level of α-feto proteins. Its significance is unknown. While the therapeutic possibilities are few, it is possible that transplantation of immunocompetent tissues may prove useful even in these cases.

Wiskott–Aldrich syndrome consists of thrombocytopenia with ensuing bleeding tendency, eczema, and repeated infections. This disorder is hereditary and is sex-linked recessive but its more detailed nature has not been defined. It would appear that patients suffering from this disorder have difficulty in dealing with and responding to polysaccharide antigens. This is possibly due to deficient maturation of B-lymphocytes as judged from a similar disease appearing in a certain mouse strain. These patients often die in their early years of infection and, in some cases, of bleeding complications. Manifestations of allergy are common and very high levels of IgE have been found in many of these individuals. In addition to eczema, the patients often show allergy to drugs, making the problem of therapy a difficult one. Support for the diagnosis is to be found in the eventual detection of the hereditary nature of the disease and the occasional appearance of low levels of IgM and abnormally low isohaemagglutinin titres. Various defects of the cell-mediated immunity are often present in these patients causing an inability to develop cell-mediated reactions in skin against common antigens such as tuberculin from mycobacteria and antigens from *Candida*, streptococci, and mumps virus. Furthermore, it is usually found that their T-lymphocytes cannot be stimulated by mitogens such as phythaemagglutinin (PHA).

In this immunologic deficiency syndrome, as in most of the others (hypogammaglobulinaemia, ataxia telangiectasia, etc.), there is an increased incidence of malignant tumours which are most often localized to the lymphoreticular tissue. The prognosis is poor and attempted therapy using antibiotics and immunoglobulin have seldom proved successful. However, some positive results have been obtained recently in some cases by administering so-called *transfer factor*, a subcellular, low molecular weight component of lymphocytes. While this factor has not been characterized in greater detail, it is clear that it transfers some kind of stimulant of cell-mediated reactions e.g. tuberculin hypersensitivity. Recently, more promising results have been seen in patients with the Wiskott–Aldrich syndrome using a thymus extract called thymosin.

IV. Immunological diseases: allergies, immune complex diseases, and autoimmune diseases

LARS Å. HANSON

The mechanism of recognition which has developed in the form of the lymphoid system reacts with material which is foreign to the body and thereby protects its integrity. This mechanism, having obvious advantages for survival, has evolved into a system of major importance for the body's defence against microbes and other foreign components. It is clear, however, that damage to the body's own tissue can arise if these defence mechanisms which on stimulation always lead to some extent of inflammation, are precipitated in an unbalanced manner and become too extensive. In an attempt to simplify the description of the many possible types of immunological tissue damage, the conditions they may cause, and the mechanisms which give rise to them, the classification of the mechanisms into four types of reaction is summarized below in accordance with Coombs and Gell.

1. Mechanisms of immunological diseases

The *type 1 reaction*, the *immediate hypersensitivity reaction*, is characterized by antigen, in this case called the *allergen* (Fig. 69), reacting with the special antibodies (IgE) which cause these reactions. The IgE antibodies, which are also known as *reagins*, have a characteristic tendency to become bound by receptors on the histamine-rich basophilic

IV. Immunological diseases   175

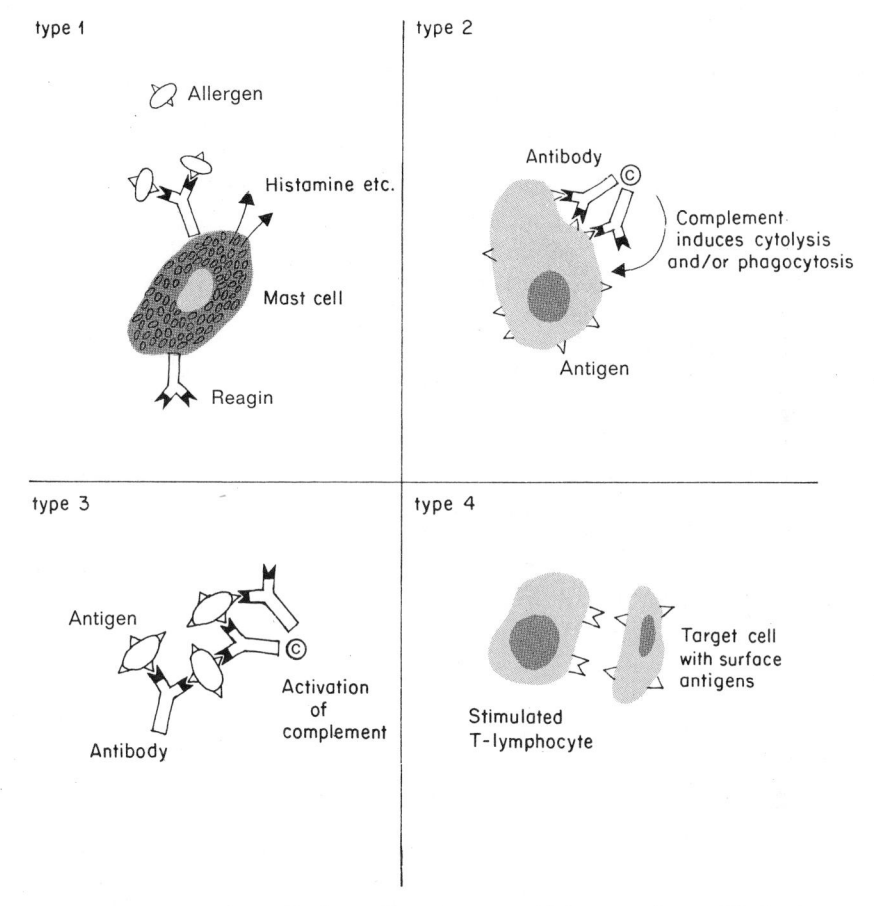

Fig. 69. The type 1 reaction, the immediate hypersensitivity reaction, following an allergen reacting with its specific reagins (IgE antibodies) which are attached to a mast cell or a basophil. This interaction between allergen and reagins causes the cell to release its granule content of histamine and other substances which give a specific form of inflammation with eosinophilic granulocytes. This is the mechanism which is responsible for atopic allergies, with symptoms of hay-fever, asthma, urticaria, anaphylactic shock, etc.

The type 2 reaction—the cytotoxic or cytolytic reaction. IgG or IgM antibodies react with surface structures on the cell and bring about activation of complement. As a result the cell undergoes lysis and/or phagocytosis

The type 3 reaction—the immune complex reaction. Complexes are formed between IgG antibodies and antigen. They activate complement which in its turn causes inflammation and tissue damage where the reaction takes place, especially due to the activity of neutrophilic granulocytes assembled via chemotaxis. The granule content of these cells are the major contributors to the inflammatory reaction

The type 4 reaction—the delayed hypersensitivity reaction. T-lymphocytes react with antigen on the surface of a cell. The T-lymphocytes are stimulated to become lymphoblasts and kill the antigen-carrying cell. An inflammatory reaction follows where macrophages are important cells, apparently the activated T-lymphocytes form lymphokines which are chemotactic for them

granulocytes in the blood and the mast cells which are found particularly adjacent to blood vessels in skin and mucous membranes. Due to the reaction between allergen and reagin, the cell is induced to release its granule contents of histamine and other active substances, giving rise to those symptoms which are characteristic for the immediate hypersensitivity reaction. Among the active components released is also a chemotactic factor specific for eosinophilic granulocytes. The release gives rise to a rapidly appearing inflammatory (weal and flare) reaction with many eosinophils.

The *type 2 reaction* consists of the *cytolytic or cytotoxic reaction* and is caused by antibodies which are directed against antigens on the surface of the cell (Fig. 69). This activates the complement system and the cell undergoes lysis or is taken up, with the help of antibody and complement on its surface, by phagocytic cells and is destroyed. Antibodies taking part in such a reaction belong to the IgM or IgG type and are directed against an antigen which is either part of the cell itself or a structure, e.g. a drug or a virus which antigen present on the cell surface.

The *type 3 reaction* is caused by the formation of *immune complexes* by antigen and IgG antibodies which bring about the activation of the complement system (Fig. 69). The inflammatory alterations which are induced by such an activation of complement can give rise to various degrees of tissue damage depending on the localization of the immune complexes. The neutrophilic granulocytes which assemble due to the chemotactic activity of activated complement, are primarily responsible for this type of inflammation.

The *type 4 reaction* consists of the *delayed hypersensitivity reaction* where stimulated T-lymphocytes having receptors for antigenic structures on the surface of a cell come into contact with such a cell. The antigenic stimulus turns the lymphocyte into a lymphoblast which kills the antigen carrying cells and releases lymphokines. The delayed tissue reaction is precipitated. It includes the inflammatory reactions induced via cell-mediated immune mechanisms, where macrophages play a key role.

Finally, a further mechanism exists where leucocytes become cytotoxic towards target cells via antibodies against these cells. Such leucocytes, often called K-cells, may be lymphocytes or macrophages and bind to the antibodies in cases of virus-infected cells as well as tumour cells, but its biological importance is still unknown.

2. Atopic allergies

The most common type of hypersensitivity reactions are the *atopic* allergies, which are caused by type 1—the immediate hypersensitivity reaction. These conditions include asthma, hay-fever, nettle-rash (urticaria), Quincke's oedema, atopic eczema and the generalized form anaphylactic shock. It is characteristic of these hypersensitivity reactions that they appear in individuals who have an inherited tendency to react to material which is completely harmless for normal individuals. The exact nature of the factors in patients who show these hypersensitivity reactions is not known.

The *allergens*, the substances which bring about the symptoms, are often pollen from various plants such as grass, or even trees. In Sweden, the birch tree is a particular offender in this connection. In the USA ragweed is the most common allergen. Food products, and skin epithelium of domestic animals such as dogs, cats, and horses are further examples of common allergens. While the properties which cause a substance to be a potent allergen are not fully understood, certain common features, such as a moderately high molecular weight, have been demonstrated in a few allergen groups. The component of birch pollen which acts as an allergen is characterized by its fast diffusion from the grain of the pollen (Fig. 70). This may be one explanation why just

IV. *Immunological diseases* 177

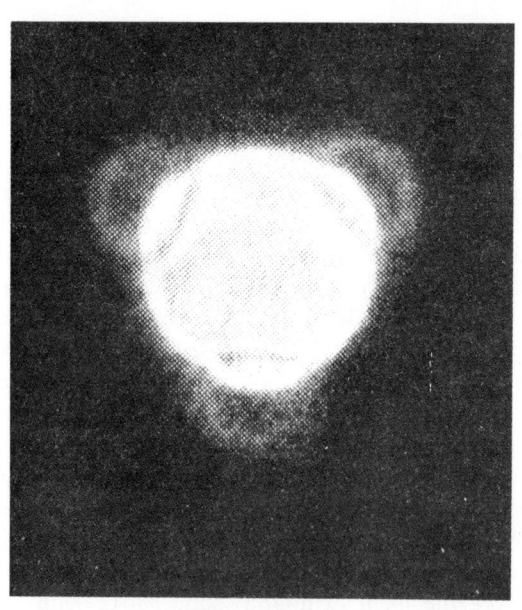

Fig. 70. Pollen from a birch tree has been placed on a layer of agar which contains antibodies against the allargen of this pollen. The allergen quickly diffuses into the agar from the three openings in the pollen grains and thereby comes into contact with the antibodies. They precipitate the allergen, forming semicircular lines outside the three openings in the pollen grain. Photograph by I. Belin

this substance, of all the components of the pollen, can trigger allergy. Furthermore, it has been observed that pollen of such a size that it can travel deep into the respiratory tract gives rise to symptoms more often than do particles of pollen which are larger, e.g. pollen from coniferous trees.

Reagins, the special antibodies which belong to class E of the immunoglobulins, and which have the capacity to become attached to receptors on mast cells and basophilic granulocytes, occupy a key position in atopic patients. In normal individuals the serum level of IgE is very small having a maximum of approximately 100–200 μg/l. A much higher value, sometimes as high as several thousand μg/l, is found in the serum of atopic patients. However, it is unclear whether or not this production of higher levels of IgE antibodies is sufficient in itself to explain the greater disposition of these patients to hypersensitivity reactions. The production of IgE antibodies against various antigens can be induced in non-atopic individuals without the appearance of symptoms.

Plasma cells which are often localized to mucous membranes are responsible for the production of IgE antibodies, suggesting local synthesis. The IgE formation is obviously dependent on T-lymphocyte helper function. The control of IgE production by suppressor T-cells seems deficient in atopic patients.

Structural studies performed on isolated myeloma proteins of the IgE class have demonstrated the presence of a longer heavy chain than is seen in immunoglobulins such as IgG. Investigations are under way to attempt to define the structure of this chain which furnishes these IgE antibodies with their cell-attaching ability. The allergen–reagin reaction on the surface of a mast cell causes release of those substances which precipitate the symptoms of allergy. A drop in the intracellular level of cyclic

AMP induces the release of histamine from these cells, the granules of which are rich in histamine and other substances. Histamine causes contraction of smooth muscles, increased permeability of small blood vessels, and increased secretion from the various glands in the gastrointestinal and respiratory tracts. Furthermore, a substance known as Slow Reacting Substance-A (SRS-A) is formed and released and is of considerable importance for the initiation of allergic symptoms. As with histamine, the secretion of SRS-A is brought about by a drop in the level of cyclic AMP which is induced by the allergen-reagin reaction. SRS-A causes a prolonged tightening of the bronchi. Kinins, which can cause a drop in blood pressure, as possibly certain prostaglandins are further examples of substances which may be of importance. The eosinophilia accompanying immediate hypersensitivity reactions is due to a specific chemostatic factor also produced and secreted by the mast cells. The eosinophils form and secrete histaminase which may modulate the effect of the histamine release, as well as a factor which blocks SRS-A.

The *symptom picture* depends on the location of the allergen–reagin reaction with the subsequent of the release of the various active substances. If the *shock organ* is the skin, the result can be nettle-rash; the patient will suffer from hay-fever if the reaction occurs in the nose, and asthma if it occurs in the lungs. If the reaction is more general, e.g. following injection of a substance to which the individual is hypersensitive, the manifestations are more dramatic and take the form of anaphylactic shock with the sudden onset of breathing difficulties and a drop in blood pressure. This can cause death within a few minutes of receiving the injection.

Diagnosis. While the diagnosis is simple in typical forms of allergy such as hay-fever and allergic conjunctivitis, the picture can be more complicated in other cases. Furthermore, difficulties are often encountered when attempts are made to identify the substance or substances which have caused the patient's complaint. In such cases, knowledge of an exact background to the illness can provide valuable information. The patient who complains after horse-riding or after picking daisies can be quickly treated for hypersensitivity to horse dandruff in the first case and pollen from daisies in the latter. However, the background history may require complementary information from various diagnostic tests. It is here that *skin tests* are of particular value.

In skin testing, the substance which is suspected of being responsible for the hypersensitivity is injected in a very small dose into the skin. The various active components, histamine etc., are released in the region of the injection, if the patient has mast cell-fixed reagins against the injected substance. A few minutes later, a weal and flare reaction appear, i.e. an immediate hypersensitivity reaction.

As patients who do not show any signs of suffering from the substance in question can also display some positive skin tests, the diagnosis may require confirmation by *provocation tests*. Here, the substances which have evoked an intensely positive skin test and which are suspected from the history are tested on the individual by either applying them dropwise in the nose or eyes or by allowing the individual to inhale them in very small quantities. If this gives rise to characteristic symptoms in the form of nasal catarrh, conjunctivitis, or asthma there are good grounds to propose that the individual really has symptoms of clinical relevance on exposure to these substances. However, these analyses are relatively time-consuming and are sometimes troublesome for the patient. In isolated cases, there is even a risk for continued allergic symptoms or anaphylactic shock.

On the basis of the discovery that the reagins belong to the immunoglobulin class E

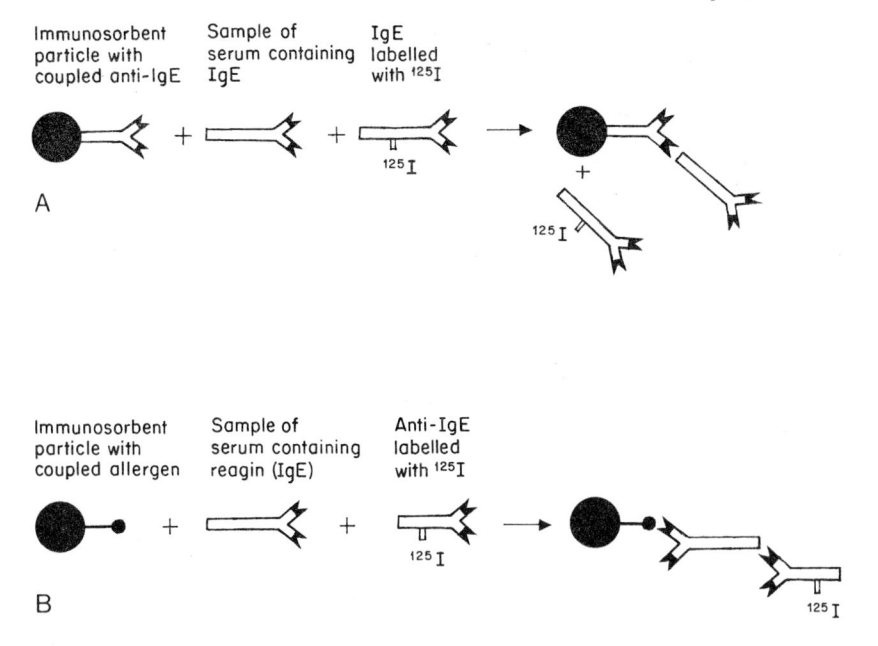

Fig. 71. A. The principle of RIST (Radio ImmunoSorbent Test). The method, which is used for the quantitative determination of IgE, employs anti-IgE which has been rendered insoluble by coupling to an insoluble phase. This anti-IgE is allowed to react with the IgE in the sample of serum to be tested, to which has been added a known amount of IgE, labelled with radioactive iodine. The IgE of the serum sample competes with the labelled IgE for the anti-IgE and the amount of iodine-labelled IgE which is not bound to the anti-IgE gives a measure of the IgE in the original sample of serum

B. The principle of RAST (Radio AllergoSorbent Test). The method is used for the determination of the amount of specific reagin against a certain allergen. The allergen is rendered insoluble by coupling it to an immunosorbent. The sample of serum which is to be tested is added to the allergen. A complex is formed between the reagin of the sample and the allergen. The amount of reagin having IgE character is determined by allowing radioactively labelled anti-IgE react with this complex. Thus, the amount of radioactivity which is recovered bound to the complex is a measure of the amount of reagin which is present in the original sample of serum

(Ishizaka in the USA, Johansson and Bennich in Sweden), techniques were developed for the quantitative determination of IgE in blood. The method, *Radio ImmunoSorbent Test* (Fig. 71A), usually abbreviated RIST, can be employed to demonstrate the high levels of IgE which are present in approximately 60 per cent of atopic individuals. The overlap between normal values and those which are pathologically increased is relatively extensive and hence, the assay of IgE is of limited value except in some cases where the diagnosis of atopic allergy requires further support.

At the same time, a method for the determination of reagins against various allergens was developed. This is generally called RAST (Radio AllergoSorbent Test, Fig. 71B). This method enables a survey of the patient's serum content of reagins which are suspected of being responsible for his or her symptoms. Good agreement, for most allergens more than 75 per cent, has been demonstrated between the results of RAST and those of provocation tests. The RAST method is as useful as the skin test but the number of allergens which are sufficiently well characterized to permit their use in the assay is still somewhat limited, although rapidly increasing.

It may prove practically difficult and expensive to introduce *in vitro* methods such as RAST to cover all possible allergens. Furthermore, allergy-like symptoms appear in cases such as endogenic asthma and certain types of urticaria where to date the participation of IgE antibodies has not been demonstrated. The diagnosis of allergic diseases can therefore not be done in the laboratory but requires the skill of a clinical allergist.

Specific therapy must be based on the painstaking evaluation of those substances which are responsible for the patient's ailment. When this is known, the first line of attack should be to attempt to remove them from the patient's surroundings. This can usually be done easily in the case of hypersensitivity to dogs or cats, but can be quite another matter when the ailment is caused by dust or pollen which cannot be eliminated so easily.

Instead, attempts should be made to decrease the individual's hypersensitivity to such substances. This can be done by repeated injections of small, increasing amounts of the substance in question, so-called *hyposensitization*. Using this technique, considerable improvement can be obtained in approximately 70 per cent of those patients who suffer from hay-fever. While the underlying mechanism of this is not clear, the results of several studies suggest that the injections initiate the production of IgG antibodies against the allergen. It is supposed that these antibodies, by virtue of their higher avidity, are more efficient than the IgE antibodies in the binding and hence can block the allergen and prevent it from reacting with the IgE antibodies. In addition, it has been demonstrated that IgG antibodies against the same allergen are capable of inhibiting the synthesis of IgE. Since the reactions involved are immunologically specific, the success of a hyposensitization treatment depends on the correct choice of allergen for use in the injections. This requires a correct diagnosis on the basis of history, skin tests or RAST and, in some cases, provocation tests.

Unspecific therapy. Much time and effort have been devoted to the search for preparations which are capable of blocking the release of symptom-evoking substances such as histamine. The only preparation which is presently available is di-sodium chromoglycate (Lomudal®) but this is not soluble and therefore comes to a halt at the mucous membranes. In spite of this, promising results have been obtained in cases of hay-fever and extrinsic asthma.

Adrenergic substances which stimulate β-receptors give rise to increased levels of intracellular cyclic AMP. This blocks the release of histamine and SRS-A from the allergen-exposed mast cells. Furthermore, it is known that prostaglandins type E1 and E2 can produce a similar effect via different receptors, but this has not as yet been applied in therapy.

Theophyllamine can block the enzyme, phospho-di-esterase, which is responsible for the breakdown of cyclic AMP. This produces an increased level of cyclic AMP and inhibits the release of histamine besides its effects on the target cells in the lungs. Expectorants are important compounds for therapeutic use and in difficult cases cortisone is required. The mechanism of action of cortisone remains essentially unresolved. However, its anti-inflammatory effect via influence on lymphocytes and phagocytes and its effect on the production of histamine are probably of consequence in atopic allergy.

3. Drug allergies

Atopic individuals, i.e. patients who show an inherited tendency to develop allergies of the immediate hypersensitivity type, can also show allergic manifestations to various drugs. Such allergies are often manifested as type 1 reactions. All four types of reaction can be expected, however, especially in patients who are not obviously atopic.

Hypersensitivity to penicillin is a good example of this. Detailed studies have shown that the hypersensitivity reaction to penicillin is not precipitated directly by the drug itself, but is brought about by metabolites of this drug, especially a group called penicilloyl. This metabolite seems to function as an allergen primarily by becoming coupled to protein impurities in the penicillin. Via type 1 reaction, penicillin can cause symptoms such as skin changes (nettle-rash), asthma, and even the generalized reaction

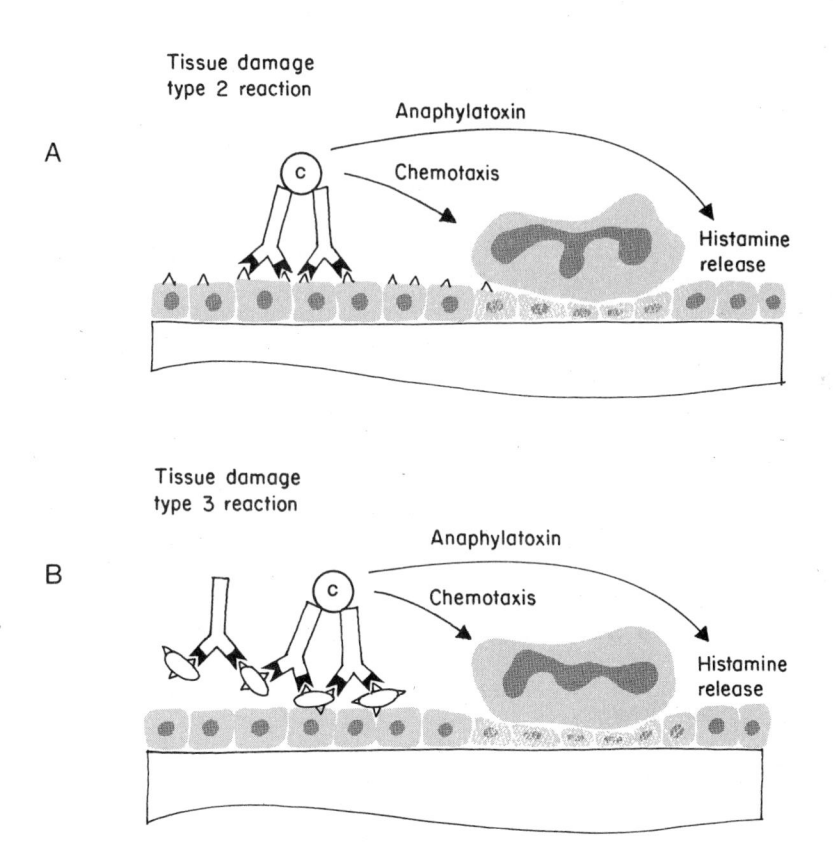

Fig. 72. A. Type 2—cytolytic or cytotoxic reactions where antibodies against cell-bound antigen activate the complement system Ⓒ to give rise to anaphylatoxin production, chemotaxis, and infiltration by neutrophilic granulocytes. These granulocytes may cause inflammation and tissue damage, besides engulfing the antibody-coated cells
B. Type 3—immune complex reaction where antigen–antibody complexes activate the complement system Ⓒ giving rise to production of anaphylatoxin, chemotaxis, and infiltration by neutrophilic granulocytes. These granulocytes can damage neighbouring tissue by the inflammation caused by release of their granulae content on phagocytosis

of anaphylactic shock. Via the type 2 reaction, the cytotoxic or cytolytic reaction, penicillin can give rise to haemolytic anaemia. Here, metabolites of the drug become fixed to the surface of cells and antibodies against these products react subsequently with the cells and destroy them. Consequently the patients suffer from Coombs-positive haemolytic anaemia. The same condition can be evoked by other drugs such as alpha-methyldopa and the identical mechanism can be responsible for thrombocytopenia or leukopenia. Damage to other tissue can also arise (Fig. 72A).

Less commonly, drugs can induce tissue damage via the type 3 reaction. These changes are caused by the formation of immune complexes and can occur in the kidneys. In addition, contact allergies can be induced by drugs via the type 4 reaction.

The above account demonstrates that the use of one method for the diagnosis of drug allergies, for example aiming at type 1 reactions, is inadequate. Instead, techniques which cover all four possible mechanisms must be employed.

4. Contact allergies

Contact allergies appear most often in individuals who have a hereditary predisposition for such allergies. This heredity is different from that of atopic individuals. Contact allergies, like professional eczema, are frequent and can be caused by allergy to chemicals, including drugs as has been mentioned previously. They are delayed type hypersensitivity reactions, i.e. type 4 reactions, which implies that they are precipitated via antigen-stimulated T-lymphocytes.

Dinitrochlorbenzene (DNCB) can sensitize and evoke a delayed hypersensitivity reaction in about 95 per cent of healthy adults. Consequently, this chemical is used to determine whether or not an individual has a normal ability to develop this reaction and hence possesses functioning T-lymphocytes. A positive reaction in a sensitized individual reaches a maximum after two to three days.

Besides an accurate history, the diagnosis of contact allergy is based on skin tests where the suspected material is brought into prolonged contact with the patient's skin in so-called contact or patch tests.

If the offending substance cannot be eliminated, symptomatic therapy must be applied. Here, cortisone preparations are used to check the inflammatory changes. Occasionally, hyposensitization of contact allergy can be carried out.

5. Immune complex diseases

If an individual is vaccinated with material to which he or she has become immune because of previous vaccination with the same material, a widespread swelling can sometimes appear in the injected area. This reaction usually appears a few hours following the injection and disappears gradually within one to two days. The reaction appears between the time required for an immediate (type 1) reaction developing in minutes and that required for a delayed (type 4) hypersensitivity reaction, taking 24–48 hours. This intermediate reaction is due to formation of complexes between the injected antigen and the antibodies which had arisen from the previous vaccination. In accordance with the type 3 reaction, these complexes activate complement and precipitate an inflammatory reaction. On the activation of the complement sequence, this reaction is characterized by the formation of chemotactic factors. These factors induce the accumulation of neutrophilic granulocytes where the complexes have deposited (Fig. 61). The complexes undergo phagocytosis but at the same time the granules content of the phagocytic cells is partly released to leak out of the granulocytes. The granules contain various enzymes and other active substances which damage surrounding tissue. Furthermore, anaphylatoxins are produced during the complement activation causing the release of histamine which in turn increases the permeability of the blood vessels, setting free fluid and adds to the inflammatory reaction. This phenomenon is called *Arthurs' reaction* and constitutes the localized form of the immune complex reaction (Fig. 72B).

The classical form of the generalized immune complex reaction is *serum sickness*. This is manifested when serum from a different species is injected intravenously in an individual who subsequently produces antibodies against proteins of the foreign serum. On the appearance of these antibodies, antigen–antibody complexes are formed which accumulate in vessel walls, particularly those of cardiac muscle and in the kidneys and joints. Here, the complement system is activated by the complexes and the chemotactically-active components trigger off an invasion of neutrophilic granulocytes. These cells cause inflammatory changes and hence tissue damage. Since cases requiring prophylactic or therapeutic treatment with protein from a different species are nowadays very few, this form of serum illness is now rarely seen. Such treatment is usually carried out using human material such as human antitetanus immunoglobulin.

The clinical picture of immune complex-induced inflammation is not without interest since several conditions have been shown to be subject to similar deposition of antigen–antibody complexes with the appearance of tissue damage. Thus, it has been demonstrated that changes appear in the lungs of individuals who have antibodies against certain kind of inhaled organic dust and that these changes are precipitated via a type 3 reaction. In pigeon-breeders' disease, the patient has antibodies against the pigeon's serum protein. These proteins are present in the pigeon's dried faeces and are inhaled in the form of dust by the breeder. In so-called farmer's lung the induced antibodies are directed against *Micropolyspora faeni* and *Termoactinomyces vulgaris* which are present in mouldy hay. Recent data indicate that such material may also activate complement directly via the alternate pathway. This results again in complement-mediated inflammation. Patients suffering from *diabetes insipidus* who inhale pitressin through the nose can produce antibodies against the hormone. If the hormone reaches the lungs on inhaling, the patients may develop lung symptoms because of the formation there of complement-activating immune complexes. Considerable interest has been devoted to the fact that immune complexes are deposited very often in the kidneys where they can give rise to various forms of nephritis. The prognosis for patients with *lupus erythematosus* is seriously aggravated by glomerulonephritis which is caused by the deposition of complexes of DNA and anti-DNA in the glomeruli. These complexes activate complement which again induces inflammation via neutrophilic granulocytes accumulating in the glomeruli where they produce the characteristic picture of nephritis. Similarly, the form of nephritis which arises in patients suffering from malaria is obviously caused by the formation of complexes between malaria antigens and antibodies which are deposited in the glomeruli of the kidneys where they activate complement and give rise to tissue damage. Additional forms of nephritis are caused by different antigens from microorganisms, viruses, and tumours via similar type 3 reactions.

It is believed that certain forms of vasculitis (periarteritis nodosa), arthritis (rheumatoid arthritis) and carditis can also be caused, or aggravated, by immune complexes. Recent findings show that the deposition of immune complexes in the skin may be an important pathogenic factor in the lepromatous form of leprosy. Furthermore, many of the symptoms which are seen in the second stage of syphilis may be evoked by immune complexes.

The formation of antigen–antibody complexes is a common and normal occurrence serving to eliminate the antigen, but under certain circumstances they give rise to tissue damage. Very little is known of the nature of these circumstances. Experiments using animals have demonstrated that vasodilatation is required before the immune complexes can be deposited in the vessel walls and cause damage. Histamine and various vasoactive amines may be capable of inducing such changes in the blood vessels. In rabbits, this may be caused by an immediate hypersensitivity reaction (type 1 reaction) with the subsequent formation of a platelet-aggregating factor, PAF. The aggregated thrombocytes release vasoactive substances, serotonin in the case of rabbits (Henson and Benveniste, 1971).

6. Autoimmune diseases

The so-called autoimmune diseases are precipitated by immunologic mechanisms. These diseases include conditions where the immunologic reactions are, or are assumed to be, directed against self-tissue, i.e. 'autoantigens'.

The phenomena of immunology were defined in the introduction as being caused by the ability of the lymphoid cells to react with material which is recognized as 'non-self' as opposed to that which is recognized as 'self'. According to this definition, the existence of autoimmune reactions would appear to be impossible. Naturally, some form of disorder in the recognition mechanisms of the lymphoid cells could be responsible for the development of a reactivity against 'self'. This could take place if the lymphoid cells were not tolerant towards 'self' tissue. Until recently, it was thought that lymphoid cells having receptors directed against 'self' tissue could not exist. Investigations have demonstrated, however, that B-lymphocytes which can react with human thyroglobulin are present in the circulation. It was believed previously that this globulin was present only in the follicles of the thyroid gland and had no contact with lymphoid tissues. Thus, the appearance of autoantibodies against thyroglobulin may have resulted from a damaged thyroid gland which released thyroglobulin. This globulin would then come into contact with lymphoid cells which would recognize it as 'non-self' and give rise to the production of autoantibodies. Recent results have shown, however, that small amounts of thyroglobulin normally exist in the blood circulation. Consequently, there must be other explanations for the appearance of autoantibodies against thyroglobulin.

T-lymphocytes having reactivity against 'self' tissue are not as common as such B-lymphocytes. This observation and the fact that T-lymphocytes are required for the production by B-lymphocytes of antibodies against most antigens is probably of prime importance for our understanding of the problem of autoimmunity. That T-lymphocytes do not usually react against 'self' tissue may be explained by the fact that they are easily made tolerant. Thus, on exposure of the cells to small quantities of the antigen to which the receptors of the T-lymphocytes are best fitted, the cells are made specifically non-reactive. This is known as 'low zone' tolerance. The B-lymphocytes, however, are more difficult to make tolerant. They require higher concentrations of antigen before they become tolerant—'high zone' tolerance. It is thought that this is the reason for the non-existence of T-lymphocytes having reactivity against autoantigens which appear in high concentrations e.g. serum albumin, or very low concentrations e.g. thyroglobulin.

B-lymphocytes, on the other hand, are reactive towards autoantigens which are present in low concentrations only. The presence of B-lymphocytes which are reactive towards substances to which they are exposed in high concentrations, e.g. serum albumin, has not been demonstrated (Allison, 1973).

It is generally believed that T-lymphocytes exercise a control over the B-lymphocytes. Even if B-lymphocytes have receptors which are specific for autoantigens, the production of autoantibodies does not begin until helper T-lymphocytes are stimulated. Thus the production of autoantibodies is not a normal event as the T-lymphocytes are tolerant to 'self' tissue. Specific suppressor T-lymphocytes are presumably of major importance in this control of potential autoantibody-producing B-cells.

However, T-lymphocytes can be stimulated in various different ways so that they can cooperate with B-lymphocytes in the production of autoantibodies. In viral infections, virus-specific antigens can appear on the surface of the infected cell. These antigens can activate T-lymphocytes which in turn stimulate the B-lymphocytes to produce antibodies against the autoantigens on the surface of the cell (Table 29). This explains the fact that autoantibodies are present in a variety of viral infections such as mononucleosis, influenza, measles, *herpes simplex*, and coxsackie. An alternative possibility is the infection of the lymphocytes by the virus.

Similarly, autoantibodies can appear if a drug becomes coupled to the surface of cells and if this drug acting as a hapten specifically stimulates T-lymphocytes. Here again, B-lymphocytes can produce antibodies against the autoantigens on the surface of the cells. This may possibly be the course of events in the syndrome, very similar to *lupus erythematosus*, which can appear after exposure to certain drugs such as hydralazine and procainamide. Those antibodies against red blood cells which appear after exposure to α-methyldopa may have a similar genesis.

Autoantibodies can even appear in conjunction with some bacterial infections such as leprosy and syphilis. In syphilis, the antibodies against cardiolipin which are demonstrated by the Wassermann reaction are autoantibodies. The mechanism behind the production of these antibodies may be similar to that described above since it is known that several chronic bacterial infections may act as an adjuvant stimulating the T-lymphocyte system. Once again this unspecific stimulation of T-cells may help B-lymphocytes having receptors for autoantigens to produce antibodies against these (Table 29). Furthermore, certain bacterial antigens are mitogenic and can give rise to direct stimulation of B-cells with autoantibody formation ensuing.

The frequency of occurrence of autoantibodies increases with age. Furthermore, the function of T-lymphocytes is reduced in the aged. Experimental evidence supports the proposal that this deficiency in the T-lymphocyte function can give rise to a deterioration in the control over these B-lymphocytes which are potential producers of autoantibodies. Thus, the appearance of autoantibodies in ageing experimental animals can be prevented by transferring T-lymphocytes from younger animals. In an animal

Table 29. Possible mechanisms of autoimmunity

Normally, T-lymphocytes tolerate 'self' tissue because of the presence of low zone tolerance against autoantigens.
On the other hand, B-lymphocytes are tolerant only towards autoantigens which are present in high concentration (high zone tolerance).
However, the function of B-cells generally requires the cooperation of T-helper lymphocytes and is controlled by T-suppressor lymphocytes.

Autoimmunity can appear if

1. T-lymphocytes are stimulated specifically by viral antigens on the surface of the virus-infected cell. Through cooperation of the T-cells, B-lymphocytes may produce autoantibodies against the cell.

2. T-lymphocytes are stimulated specifically by a drug which is coupled to the surface of a cell. Through cooperation of the T-cells, B-lymphocytes can produce autoantibodies against the antigens on the cell.

3. T-lymphocytes are stimulated unspecifically by the adjuvant effect of chronic infections such as leprosy, tuberculosis, or syphilis. The production of autoantibodies is induced by the cooperation of the T-cells with B-lymphocytes.

4. Deteriorated function of T-lymphocytes with increasing age can give rise to a defective control by T-cells of the B-cells which have receptors for 'self' tissue. Thus B-cells may produce autoantibodies.

5. Extrinsic antigens which cross-react with 'self' tissue may be capable of inducing an immune response which may also be directed against autoantigens.

6. Mitogenic effects on B-lymphocytes of certain microbial antigens may induce autoantibody formation without the help of T-lymphocytes.

---

strain spontaneously attracting autoimmune disease, it has been shown that the symptoms appear after suppressor T-lymphocytes have diminished.

Another explanation of the existence of autoantibodies is that they arise as a result of an immune response against antigens which cross-react with autoantigens. Such cross-reactions are not unusual and have been observed between streptococci and cardiac tissue, streptococci and kidney tissue, coli bacteria and kidney tissue, and between coli bacteria and the mucous membrane of the large intestine. The latter type of cross-reaction may possibly be a pathogenic factor in ulcerative colitis.

Autoantibodies appear more often than autoimmune diseases. The presence of autoantibodies does not imply the presence of tissue damage which is based on autoimmune reactions. However, it is clear that in certain connections autoantibodies can precipitate tissue damage via the cytolytic or cytotoxic type 2 reaction. Goodpasture's syndrome and autoimmune haemolytic anaemia are examples of this. Goodpasture's syndrome, which consists of glomerulonephritis and pulmonary bleeding, is due to autoantibodies against the basal membranes of the lungs and kidney glomeruli.

Autoantibodies can cause tissue damage via a type 3 reaction by forming complexes with their autoantigens. In this way, the form of nephritis which often appears in systemic *lupus erythematosus* is caused by the formation of immune complexes between DNA and anti-DNA. These complexes are deposited in the glomeruli to give rise to glomerulonephritis via a type 3 reaction.

It is believed that the pathogenic mechanisms of some autoimmune conditions may be cell-mediated immune reactions (type 4) which can cause tissue damage. This implies the existence of T-lymphocytes which have receptors against 'self' tissue. Such cells have been detected in animal experiments (Cohen and Wekerle, 1973). However, under normal conditions the interaction of these cells with autoantigens is prevented, probably by specific factors in serum. It has been suggested that these controlling factors may be antibodies, antigen-antibody complexes, or the autoantigen in a soluble non-immunogenic form.

It is remarkable that infection and autoimmunity are related in many cases. It would appear that the phenomenon of autoimmunity is often induced by infection, agreeing with the observation that autoimmune conditions are more common in patients with immune defects which increase the frequency of infection. Continued research in this field and the investigation of those factors which normally control the tolerance of autoantigens and thereby prevent autoimmunity, may provide further insight into this problem.

A presentation of tissue damage which is caused by immunologic mechanisms would be incomplete without the mention of isoimmunization e.g. Rh immunization, transfusion complications, and the rejection of transplants. These will be dealt with in the following sections.

V. Transplantation immunology

GÖRAN MÖLLER

Immunology has become of particular practical use in the field of transplantation surgery. Because of the presence of antigens which are foreign to the host, a transplant which is transferred from one individual to another is normally always rejected. Thus, the host becomes immunized against these antigens and by an immunological reaction rejects the transplant. The antigens which are responsible for the immunization are called transplantation or histocompatibility antigens. The immune response initiated against such antigens is characterized by the development of humoral antibodies and cell-mediated immunity. It is generally accepted that the rejection of the transplant is caused primarily by the cell-mediated immunity and that humoral antibodies can directly or indirectly take part in the reaction.

1. Histocompatibility antigens

The cells of all individuals contain histocompatibility (or transplantation) antigens. These antigens are genetically determined by genes in several loci in different chromosomes. However, within each species there is one major dominating system of transplantation antigen, MHS (major histocompatibility system). In man it is called HLA, in mouse H-2. In addition to this major system there are several weaker (minor) antigenic systems. Histocompatibility antigens are characterized by being:

1. genetically determined,
2. dominantly inherited,

3. highly polymorphic,
4. present on nucleated cells,
5. cell surface structures,
6. capable of inducing an allograft reaction.

The HLA system in man is well characterized and is the major histocompatibility system in man. Each individual carries four distinct loci on each chromosome in pair No. 6. There are three loci, HLA-A, -B, and -C, which house genes that determine serologically detectable structures present on all nucleated cells. This means that each individual is characterized by the antigens determined by these genes, 1–2 antigens of the A locus, 1–2 of the B locus, and 1–2 of the C locus. Thus, each individual has maximally 6 such antigens on its cell surface. Since the number of alleles (alternative genes) is high within each locus, the probability that two unrelated individuals are HLA identical is small.

Another HLA locus is termed -D (earlier nomenclature MLC locus). Products of this locus are not present on all nucleated cells, but are represented on B-lymphocytes, endothelial cells, monocytes, and spermatocytes. HLA-D antigens are known to induce a reaction in mixed lymphocyte cultures, and it has been established recently that HLA-D antigenic compatibility is of prime importance in kidney transplantation to avoid transplant rejection and in bone marrow transplantation to avoid a fatal graft-versus-host reaction. HLA-D antigens have been defined until recently mainly by cellular *in vitro* techniques.

In addition to these genes, the HLA region contains genes for complement factors C′2, C′4, and possibly also one of the chains in the C′8 structure, as well as genes for blood groups Chido and Rodgers, and Factor B (Bf) of the properdin system.

Furthermore, there is reason to believe that the human major histocompatibility gene region contains genes that determine immune reactivity (IR genes) since all counterparts of the HLA region in other animal species contain such genes. Second, indirect evidence for this assumption is accumulating since many different diseases in humans are associated with particular HLA haplotypes in families or with specific HLA antigens in random patient materials.

2. Immune reactions against transplanted tissue

As with all other antigens, the transfer of allogenic tissues to a host induces an immune response. This results in the production of antibodies by B-cells and the development

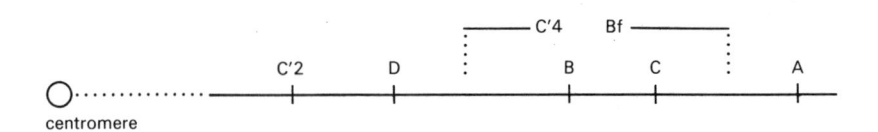

Fig. 73. Schematic representation of the HLA region and its loci. The HLA chromosomal region comprises four distinct HLA loci, which are closely linked. One allele for each locus is present on each chromosome. Three loci, HLA-A, -B, and -C contain genes for antigens expressed on all nucleated cells. HLA-D antigens are present only on some nucleated cells. For further details see text

Table 30. Properties of mouse T- and B-cells

Properties	T	B
Large amounts of immunoglobulin on the surface	−	+
Release antibodies after stimulation by antigen	−	+
High rate of recirculation	+	−
Antigens	T-dependent	T-independent
Activated by mitogens	PHA[a], ConA[a]	LPS[a] and other polyclonal B-cells' activators
Receptor for the Fc part of immunoglobulins	+	+
Receptor for complement factor 3	−	+
Receptor for sheep blood cells	+	−
Receptor for certain viruses (e.g. EB virus)	−	+

[a] PHA = Phytohaemagglutinin.
[a] ConA = Concanavalin A.
[a] LPS = Lipopolysaccharide from gram-negative bacteria.
[b] Immunologically activated T-cells can have receptors.

of cell-mediated immunity by activated T-cells. Various properties of T- and B-cells are summarized in Table 30. T-cells can react with antigen and bind it to their surface. While the binding of antigen to B-cells is known to occur via immunoglobulin. This is not the case with T-cells. The reaction of T- and B-cells with histocompatibility antigens is basically the same as with other antigens. There is, however, one notable difference namely, the frequency of antigen-sensitive cells (the proportion of cells in the body which can react with histocompatibility antigens) is very high (1–4 per cent), when compared with the frequency of antibodies which are reactive towards all other known antigens (1 in 10^4–10^5 cells). This unusually large fraction of immunocompetent cells which is directed against the transplantation antigens or other individuals has attracted a great deal of theoretical interest. Recent work has shown that the specificity of the antigen-binding receptors on the T-cells is not the same as that of the immunoglobulin receptors on the B-cells. The T-cells have a high ability to react with transformed histocompatibility antigens (altered self).

This has been demonstrated experimentally by employing various systems where the histocompatibility antigens were changed by the interaction with haptens or viruses. The finding that T-cells effectively recognize transplantation antigens and virus-infected cells and kill these cells by reacting with the virus-transplantation antigen complex suggests that the normal function of the T-cells is to defend the individual against virus infections by removing the virus-infected cells from the organism.

3. The effector function

The development of an immune response to transplantation antigens results in the rejection of the transplant usually 10–12 days after the transplantation. *In vivo* experiments have shown that the mechanism of rejection is caused by cell-mediated

190   Immunoglobulins

immunity. It is generally believed that the T-cells are responsible for the rejection since removal of T-cells by neonatal thymectomy or by treatment with antilymphocyte serum completely abolishes rejection. Actually, certain transplants can be rejected by humoral antibodies alone. The mechanism of rejection has been studied in detail using *in vitro* experiments. These experiments are based primarily on tissue culture methods where various types of target cells are mixed with lymphocytes from immunized individuals. These *in vitro* systems have demonstrated the existence of three different types of rejections (Fig. 74):

1. Humoral antibodies can react with target cells and bind complement. The target cells die as a consequence of cell membrane lysis caused by complement. The target cells must contain a high concentration of transplantation antigens for this mechanism to be efficient.

2. It has been shown that T-cells are capable of killing target cells in tissue culture. Killing requires very close contact between the T-cell and the target cell and it has been shown that humoral cytotoxic factors are not responsible for cytotoxicity. Furthermore, the cytotoxic effect of the T-cells is not due to the release of antibodies and there is no evidence to suggest that complement takes part in the reaction. In order that the T-cells can exhibit a cytotoxic effect, it is necessary that they bind to the target cells with the help of their receptors. As a result of this close contact, the T-cell is transformed into a killer cell. Although the exact mechanism of the cytotoxic effect is not known, it is likely that it is non-specific and mediated by some enzymic reaction.

3. Finally, there is clear evidence for cooperation between antibodies and lymphocytes in a certain cytotoxic reaction. Humoral antibodies can bind to target cells without causing injury to these cells because of the lack of complement participation. However, when lymphocytes are added to antibody-coated target cell, they bind to the Fc part of the antibodies since certain lymphocytes possess receptors for the Fc portion of immunoglobulin. When this reaction has taken place, the lymphocytes are transformed into cytotoxic cells and are competent to kill the targets. As yet defined K (killer)-cells can carry out this cytotoxic reaction. These three mechanisms have been demonstrated *in vitro* and probably exist *in vivo*. Through a so-called hyperacute reaction antibodies can also reject transplanted tissue, e.g. a transplanted kidney. Furthermore, T-cells alone can reject the transplant. Finally, there is reason to believe that the antibody induced cell-mediated immune reaction can be of importance in certain cases of transplant rejection although the evidence is not very sound.

4. Clinical aspects

Since the cause of transplant rejection is an immune reaction against transplantation antigens, primarily the dominant HLA antigens, it is clear that clinical work aims at transplanting between individuals who are identical with respect to their HLA systems. This is accomplished by determining the individual HLA antigens of the donor and thereafter selecting the most compatible recipient. Even in cases of complete HLA identity, immune reactions against non-HLA antigens can arise. For this reason, the recipient is treated with immunosuppressive drugs.

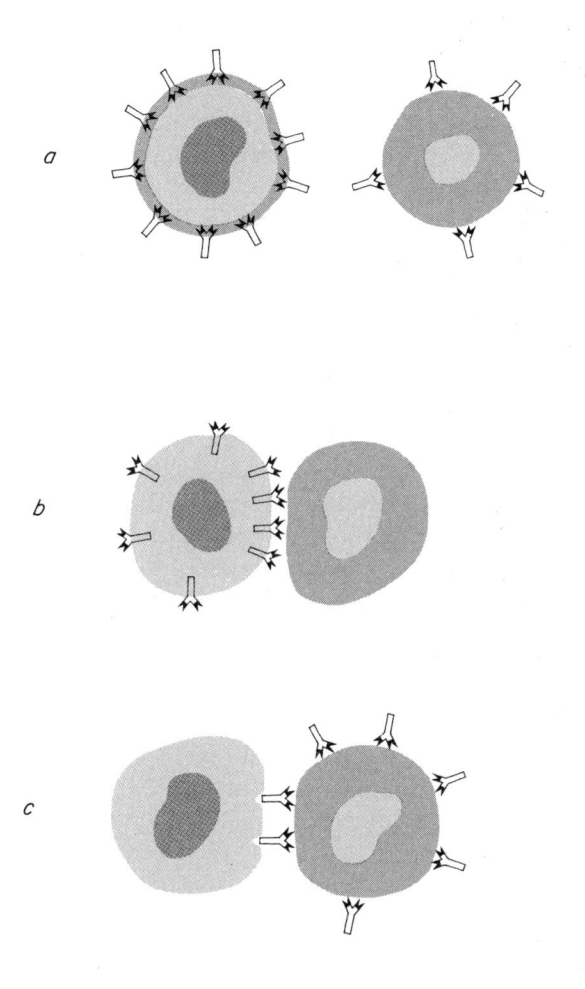

Fig. 74.
(a) Humoral antibodies plus complement
Humoral antibodies which are directed against the target cells can react with the antigens on these cells and thereby bind complement (greying in the left figure). If the antigen concentration on the target cell is high (left cell) the cell membrane is lysed and results in the death of the cell. If the antigen concentration is low as in the right cell, complement is not bound and the cell survives
(b) Cell-mediated immunity.
T-lymphocytes (the cell on the left) bind to the target cell via their antigen-specific receptors. The T-cell is thereby transformed into a killer cell which can kill other cells which are in close contact with it. Complement, antibodies or other soluble factors are not responsible for the death of the target cell
(c) Antibody-induced cell-mediated immunity.
Antibodies are present on the target cell (cell on the right) but this does not result in the death of the cell since complement is not present. Lymphocytes which have receptors for the Fc-fragment of antibodies (left cell) can bind to the antibody-coated target cell and kill it. While the mechanism of the cell death is not known, close contact is a necessity and it would appear that soluble substances are not involved. The nature of the killer cell is obscure as yet

HLA typing

To help in the choice of donor and recipient, the lymphatic cells from these individuals are typed using antibodies, which are directed against different HLA antigens. A cytotoxic reaction is used for this purpose. Antibodies against a certain HLA antigen are added to lymphocytes in the presence of complement. If the cells have the corresponding antigen, they are killed. Thus by using all the known HLA antigens, the individual's HLA composition can be determined. Each individual has a maximum of eight HLA antigens. Twins from the same egg have, of course, identical antigens. The genetics of the HLA system imply that 25 per cent of the members of a family are identical. It is unlikely that unrelated individuals can be HLA identical, but such a situation can exist. In clinical connections, the difference in the HLA systems of two individuals is described in terms of degrees of identity: A1, identity between members of the same family; A2, identity between parents and children; A3, identity between non-related persons; B, compatibility, i.e. the transplant does not contain antigens which are not present in the recipient, but the recipient has antigens which are not present in the transplant; C, the transplant contains a foreign HLA antigen; D, the transplant contains two foreign HLA antigens; E, the transplant contains three foreign HLA antigens; F, the recipient has preformed antibodies against the transplant. Such antibodies can be due to blood transfusion, pregnancy, or an earlier transplantion.

In general, clinical results show that the survival of kidney is best (80 per cent) in A-transplants and worst in F-transplants. The exact difference between C-, D-, and E-transplants is still not well characterized. In recent years it has been shown that HLA-D locus compatibility is of fundamental importance for the survival of the transplant. It is probable that the rejection reaction is activated by the interaction of T-cells with HLA-D products. The activated T-cells can then bind to target cells which have HLA-A, -B, or -C antigens which distinguish the donor from the recipient. Thus, HLA-D incompatibility is required for the activation of cytotoxic effector cells, but it is not necessary for the ability of the activated cells to kill foreign cells.

Mixed lymphocyte culture

The most important factor in the rejection reaction is the cellular immune reaction. A test, the so-called *mixed lymphocyte culture* reaction (MLC), assays the cellular immunity *in vitro*. This involves the mixing in a test tube of lymphocytes from two individuals whereby the lymphocytes react immunologically against each others' foreign antigens. The reaction is manifested by cell division, morphologic transformation, and the development of so-called killer cells. The reaction can be made unidirectional by, e.g., treating one population of lymphocytes with compounds which inhibit the DNA synthesis, thereby permitting the assay of the DNA synthesis in the other population. Thus, a study can be made of the immunological reaction of one lymphocyte population against the other. Since the reaction requires 6–7 days for completion, it can not be used in cases of acute transplantation, but since it measures a relevant immunological reaction it is probable that it will find use in transplantations where live donors are employed. Since we are beginning to be able to assay HLA-D incompatibility serologically, new possibilities for the selection of donor and recipient have become available. The results which have been obtained from transplantations which have been carried out between individuals who are HLA-D compatible (but are incompatible with respect to HLA-A, -B, or -C antigens) are also promising. It is not improbable that the rejection reaction can be practically completely controlled by ensuring that the donor and the recipient are both HLA-D compatible.

5. Immunosuppression

Even in cases of donor and recipient where there is HLA identity, there is an immunological reaction against non-HLA antigens. Thus, it is important to minimize this reaction which can be achieved either specifically or unspecifically.

Unspecific methods

Physiocochemical methods are based on the knowledge that certain compounds or treatments suppress the immunological defence. X-ray radiation kills lymphocytes these cells and is therefore immunosuppressive. Various chemicals such as cortisone have an analogous effect and are therefore immunosuppressive. Substances which inhibit the synthesis of DNA (azathioprin) have been shown to be very active in human transplants and compounds such as actinomycin which affect the synthesis of RNA are used clinically. Since the effect of these compounds is not limited to the chemical processes of lymphocytes but affects all other cells, the substances are unspecific and produce toxic effects on the hematopoietic system and the gastrointestinal tract. However, because of the rapid cell division which takes place in the immune system they have a relatively selective effect on this system. On the other hand, T- and B-cells are both affected explaining the finding that the production of antibodies and the cell-mediated immunity against all antigens are equally impaired. The success of immunosuppression using these methods demands a delicate balance between the survival of the transplant and that of the patient. There are also biological compounds which are immunosuppressive. The most widely used is antilymphocyte globulin (ALG) which is an antiserum directed against human lymphocytes and is raised in a different species of animal, usually horse. Immunosuppression is obtained when patients are injected with this serum. The mechanism of action of ALG is well documented. Following injection, ALG reacts with lymphocytes circulating in blood and these are removed by phagocytosis in the liver and spleen. As most of the circulating lymphocytes and T-cells, a rather selective removal of these cells is achieved. This diminishes the strength of the rejection reaction while the immune response to the so-called T-independent antigens remains intact. Since the majority of T-independent antigens are of bacterial origin, a selective effect is produced on the cell-mediated immunity while the production of antibodies against many pathogenic bacteria remains intact.

Specific methods

It is expected that immunological tolerance and enhancement will be introduced in the future. Human experiments have not yet been carried out to any great extent. In tolerance, the aim is to inject soluble HLA antigens either by themselves to induce tolerance or labelled with radioactive isotopes to bring about *antigen suicide*, i.e. the antigen binds to the receptors on the lymphocytes and because of the radioactive radiation kills the lymphocytes. Immunologic enhancement is based on the principle that antibodies are capable of inhibiting immunologically competent lymphocytes by competing in the reaction for the antigen. The principle has been of practical use in the prophylaxis of Rh immunization. Furthermore, experiments have demonstrated that many transplanted tissues can easily be made to survive by injecting the recipient with blocking antibodies which are directed against the transplant. As yet, enhancement has not become widespread in clinical usage.

VI. Tumour immunology

GÖRAN MÖLLER

Tumour immunology has been a topical subject for the past 15 years, but unlike transplantation immunology only a few practical results have been obtained. Since patients, doctors, and scientists are motivated by the same wish, the topic is surrounded by emotional factors. This common motive is one side of tumour immunology which has not been particularly positive, since wishful thinking has to a large extent dominated the subject. Tumour immunology can be suitably divided into three parts: tumour antigens, immune reactions, and the concept of immunological surveillance.

1. Tumour antigens

There are at present two types of tumour antigens: (a) tumour-specific and (b) tumour-associated embryonic antigens.

(a) Due to experiments which made use of transplantation of tumours in identical individuals (inbred mice) tumour-specific antigens were discovered early. It was demonstrated that an individual could be immunized against his/her own tumour so that a later transplantation of the tumour did not lead to the growth of a tumour. The antigen was specific for the tumour and was not present in the individual's normal cells. Using this transplantation system the following has been shown (Table 31). Tumours which are induced by chemical or physical agents each have different antigens, even if two tumours have been induced by the same agent on two different sides of the same mouse. Irrespective of the histological type of tumour, those which

Table 31. Tumour-specific antigens in mouse

Tumours induced by	TSTA[a]	Cross-reactivity within each aetiologic group
Chemical agents	+	−
Radiation	+	−
Virus:		
polyoma (DNA virus)	+	+
Moloney (RNA virus)	+	+

[a] TSTA = tumour-specific transplantation antigens.

are induced by viruses have identical antigens if they are caused by the same virus. These results, which have been obtained using laboratory animals, are not in complete agreement with those obtained in human experiments where there is evidence to suggest that tumours of the same histological type have the same antigen in different individuals. Thus, lung cancer cells in various individuals have the same antigen despite the fact that there is a large amount of evidence in favour of the idea that lung cancer in man is a chemically induced tumour.

(b) Tumour-associated antigens appear in connection with certain tumours but can appear also in normal cells. Tumour-associated antigens are normally present in embryonic cells of the same organ, but these disappear in the normal cells of the adult to become evident again when the cells become tumorous. One example of such antigens is the so-called carcinoembryonic antigen (CEA) which is present in tumour cells in the gastrointestinal tract (and is released into serum) and which is present even in the embryonic cells in these regions. The antigen appears in various other pathologic conditions and because of its production by the foetus is present also in pregnant women. Another analogous antigen is α-fetoprotein which is present in liver cancer and in the embryonic liver cells. In may be that these antigens will be of diagnostic importance but this remains unclear. Nevertheless, they can be put to prognostic use by assaying the antigen and thereby permitting early detection of any growth of the tumour.

2. Immune reactions

As was the case in the rejection of organ transplants, it has been demonstrated in mice that transplantation of tumours can give rise to antibodies and cell-mediated immunity. There is evidence for the existence of immune reactions against self-tumours in humans and it has been shown that kill lymphocytes and humoral antibodies both appear. In recent years much interest has centred around the finding that certain humoral antibodies which are directed against the patient's own tumour can inhibit the cell-mediated immunity (blocking antibodies). This is a classical example of immunological enhancement and is thought to be one factor contributing to the growth of a tumour in the presence of the cell-mediated immunity. Thus there should exist a balance between killer lymphocytes and the blocking antibodies which contribute to the growth of the tumour. However, this has not been demonstrated in any system. Furthermore, there are examples of 'unblocking' antibodies which impair the effect of the blocking antibodies. It is not clear how these antibodies take part in *in vivo* reactions against tumour. It is possible that they are merely an *in vitro* artefact.

3. Immunological surveillance

Immunological surveillance is held as a fundamental concept in tumour immunology. They thought behind this idea is that the tumour cells which arise as a result of genetic alterations such as mutations often appear in the body but that these neoplastic cells are normally eliminated by the cell-mediated immune reaction which is directed against the tumour-specific antigens. It has also been proposed that the normal function of the

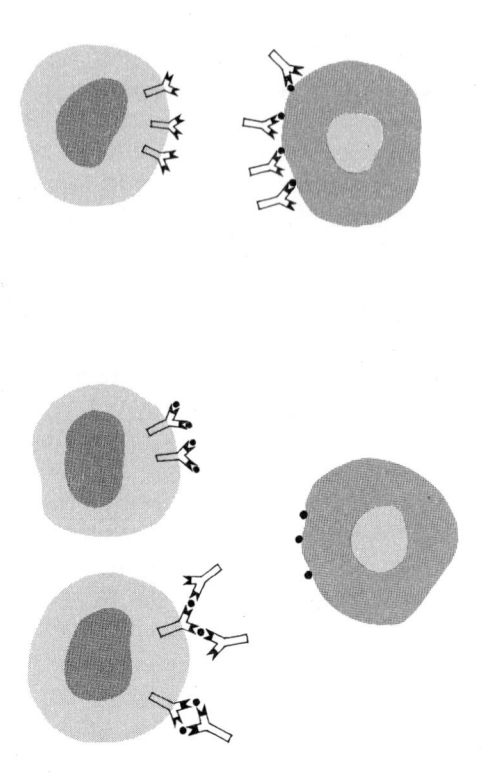

Fig. 75. Two examples of the mechanism of blocking antibodies. In the first case, top figure, humoral antibodies react with a target cell (on the right). Thus the killer lymphocytes (left cell) which have receptors for the target cell can not react with this cell and consequently a cytotoxic effect does not occur. In the second case, lower figure, the killer cells have been blocked because their receptors have interacted with an antigen–antibody complex or with soluble antigens which are released by the target cell. Since the receptors of the killer lymphocytes are blocked, they can not bind to the target cell and a cytotoxic effect does not arise

cell-mediated immunity (T-cells) is to reject tumours and that this type of immunity serves to prevent the appearance of neoplastic cells. This hypothesis is supported by the finding that patients who lack a cell-mediated immunity as a result of, for example, certain congenital immune defects, show an increased frequency of tumours. Furthermore, patients who have undergone transplantation and who have therefore been treated with immunosuppressive drugs have also a higher frequency of tumours. On the other hand, this hypothesis does not fit with the fact that a complete lack of the cell-mediated immunity, occurring for example after treatment with antilymphocyte serum, does not result in a higher tumour frequency. Furthermore, there is one type of mouse strain which is totally devoid of T-cells and which consequently can not reject any transplants, but which does not develop tumours. Finally, it can be mentioned that those tumours which appear in patients who have immune defects or in immunosuppression normally represent a relatively rare form of tumours which are predominantly limited to the lymphatic system. Therefore, it has been supposed that the cell-mediated immunity makes the patients more susceptible to infections by viruses which may induce tumours. This increased susceptibility to viral infections should not be confused with the concept of immunological surveillance which is based on the postulate that the system of T-cells normally prevents the appearance of neoplastic cells. In other words, there is at present no concrete evidence for the existence of immunological surveillance.

4. Practical applications of tumour immunology

As yet, tumour immunology has not reached the stage of practical application. However, there are several theoretical ways which can be followed. It is most likely that tumour immunology will be developed for diagnostic and eventual prognostic use in tumour illnesses. Tumour-associated antigens such as CEA may be used to diagnose cancer in the gastrointestinal tract. If this method turns out to be capable of detecting cancer at an earlier stage than other methods, if the specificity of the reaction is such that other illnesses do not give misleading positive results, and if it results in better prognosis for the patients, the method can have practical applications. At present there is no evidence to suggest that these stipulations can be met.

In certain tumour illnesses, the cell-mediated immune reactions have been shown to be related to the patient's prognosis following the removal of a tumour by the customary methods. Thus, the strength of the cell-mediated immunity when measured *in vitro* has been high in cases where the tumour failed to return but was low when the tumour did return. If this is the case, then a way is open for the assessment of the patient's prognosis following traditional treatments. However, since the immune reactions are particularly complex it is unlikely that such a strong connection should exist in many cases. It would appear that the advent of therapy and prophylaxis for tumour illnesses will not take place in the immediate future. The hypothetical therapy is based on the idea that the immune system could be activated to kill the tumour. Comprehensive experiments have been carried out using unspecific activation of the immune system by, for example, BCG-vaccination and other so-called adjuvants but the effects have been either weak or have resulted in an increased growth of the tumour. The possibility of making use of the specificity of the immunological system, e.g. the ability of antibodies to react with tumour-specific antigens, would appear to be a realistic alternative. By binding radioactive isotopes or compounds which are toxic for the cells to the antibodies, use can be made of the specificity of the antibodies to localize the toxic factors to the tumour and to destroy these cells without damaging the normal cells. Such methods have not as yet been used in the human system.

The possibility of vaccinating against cancer, i.e. prophylaxis against tumour illnesses, is for the time being merely speculation. However, if it can be shown that certain forms of tumour are caused by virus, that these viruses can be purified and the antigenic extract obtained and if the individual can be immunized, the possibility remains that the appearance of certain types of tumours can be prevented. However, the problem is that tumour viruses are often transmitted from parents to children (vertical transmission) while direct horizontal contagion is thought to be rare. However, by manipulating the immunological system (so-called immunological engineering) there are certain possibilities of controlling virus-induced tumours to some extent.

VII. Blood group serology
BENGT GULLBRING

A. Introduction

1. Definitions

Blood group serology is of special importance because of its practical applications, such as transfusion treatment and the prophylaxis and treatment of haemolytic diseases in new-born babies. Blood group serology has contributed much to our understanding of the laws of human genetics. The blood group systems have been of use in forensic medicine, they have also been of great importance in anthropology where valuable information has been obtained concerning man's migration. These wanderings of man have been reflected in the frequency of variation of the blood group genes geographically and within peoples. Our knowledge in the latter area has increased to such an extent that it surpasses what we know of other genes within the plant and animal world.

In this section, the term 'blood group' is used to describe the occurrence of inherited antigens on the surface of red blood cells. This term is also used to describe differences in these antigens. Furthermore, differences in the blood of various individuals which are designated by heredity could also be included under the term 'blood group', but such is not the case. Similarly, 'belonging to a certain blood group system' signifies that a system of antigens is inherited independently of another system.

2. Cell membrane

The antigens of the erythrocytes are localized to the cell membrane. A clearer picture of the topographic and chemical location of the antigens in the structure of the membrane has come as a consequence of our increased insight into the structure of the cell membrane. A double layer of lipids, mostly phospholipids, forms the basic structure of the cell membrane (Fig. 76).

This structure contains a hydrophilic and a hydrophobic portion which are thought to be orientated so that the hydrophobic lipid portion, which is composed of fatty acid chains, faces in towards the centre of the membrane and the hydrophilic non-lipid portion

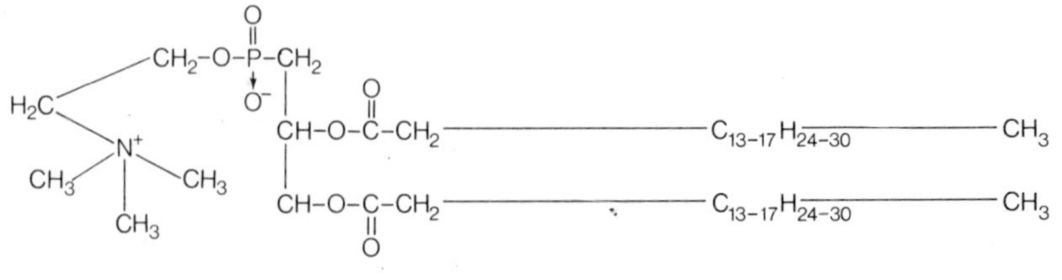

Fig. 76. The structure of a typical phospholipid, lecithin (phosphatidyl-choline). Coupled to the molecule of glycerine are two long fatty acid chains and the phosphate ester of choline. The fatty acids make up the hydrophobic lipid portion of the molecule and the hydrophilic non-lipid portion is composed of ionized choline and phosphate. Other phospholipids vary in the fatty acid composition and in the composition of the hydrophilic portion of the molecule

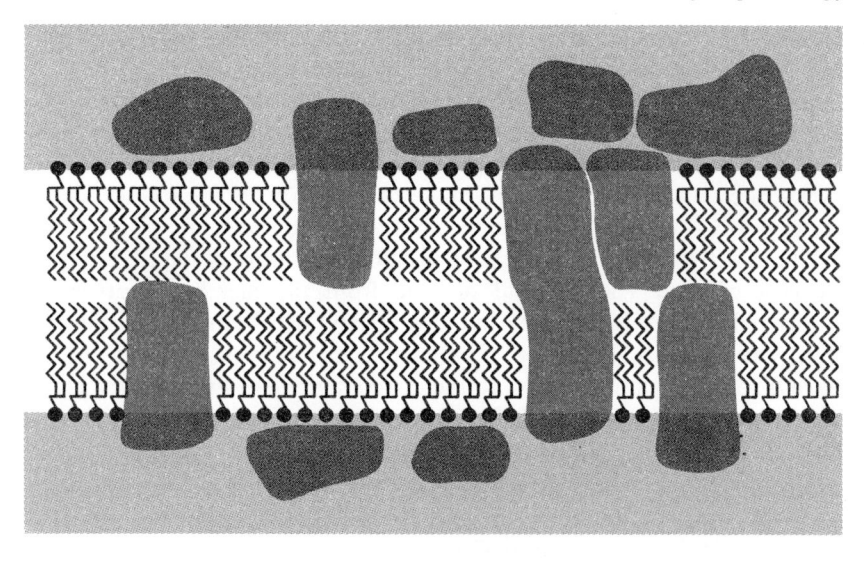

Fig. 77. A schematic representation of the structure of the biological membrane. The basic structure is composed of phospholipid molecules which are situated side-by-side in two opposed layers. The shaded areas represent protein molecules. These molecules can have variable positions in relation to the double layer of phospholipid, e.g. on the surface, partial or complete penetration of the membrane. According to F. Fox, *Scient. Amer.*, **226** (1972) p. 36. Published with the permission of the copywright holders—Scientific American Inc

faces outwards. The membrane even contains proteins which give it its mosaic-like structure (Fig. 77). This palisade-like construction provides the membrane with its plasticity which is of great importance for the structural changes which the red blood cells undergo during, for example, passage through the capillary network. This structure provides also a relatively high degree of 'self healing' in the case of membrane damage.

The membrane contains a variety of different proteins. Immunological experiments have shown that there are at least 200 antigens on the erythrocytes and that many of these antigens are proteins.

3. Erythrocyte antigens

The erythrocyte antigens are protein or lipid in nature. Glycoproteins which are localized to the surface of the red blood cells and which have antigenic activity are known to exist. To this group of antigens belong M-, N-, S-, and Fy^a-antigens which are labile to proteolytic enzymes.

Treatment with the enzyme sialidase (neuraminidase) results in the removal of sialic acid from the surface of the erythrocytes and destroys the sites of M and N but does not affect the majority of other antigens on the red cells. Among the best known of the receptors on the surfaces of blood cells are those which react with phytohaemagglutinin (PHA). A red blood cell contains between 3.4×10^5 and 5.0×10^5 such receptors on its surface. The total number of receptors on the surface of the cell can be more than this since this figure represents the number of receptors which are available to PHA. Thus, it is possible that other receptors exist but these are so close together that they are not available for determining with PHA. The topographic form of the surface of the cell can even manifest itself as crypt formations.

Treatment of the erythrocytes with proteolytic enzymes may increase the uptake of blood cell antibodies. This has been interpreted to mean that for example sialomucopeptide which normally makes up a part of the cell surface and which is cleaved off by the enzyme, normally prevents some uptake of antibody. The enzymic treatment of erythrocytes is of great importance in the routine serological laboratory.

Interesting experiments have been carried out on the nature of the Rh antigen, which probably is a protein. The removal of lipid from the membrane of erythrocytes considerably reduces the Rh activity but this activity can be restored also by adding lipid which has been obtained from Rh-negative membranes. Morgan and Watkins (1969) have made great contributions to the understanding of the chemical compounds which carry the blood group specificity of the ABO system.

4. Blood group antibodies

Blood group antibodies have been demonstrated in the immunoglobulin classes IgG, IgM, and IgA. Details of the various antibodies can be found in the text which deals with the respective blood group system. The most common property is that they belong to immunoglobulin class IgG or IgM.

Certain properties of the antibodies are summarized in Table 32. Most of the routine methods which are used to demonstrate that antibodies have reacted with an erythrocyte antigen are based on a simple observable agglutination reaction. The ability of IgM antibodies to agglutinate red blood cells suspended in physiological saline is of great practical importance. Antibodies which display this ability are often called 'complete'. Antibodies which are devoid of this ability are called 'incomplete' and are generally IgG antibodies. However, it has been shown that these IgG antibodies react with red blood cells suspended in physiological saline just as efficiently as complete antibodies, but an observable agglutination is not produced. Blood cells which have bound antibodies as a result of such a reaction are usually called sensitized or coated. Differences in the ability to agglutinate blood cells in physiological saline is believed to be due to:

1. The length of the antibody molecule.
2. The repulsive effect of the electrical charge on the blood cell.

Table 32. Some properties of the antibodies belonging to various classes of immunoglobulins[a]

Property	IgG	IgM	IgA
Agglutination of red blood cells suspended in saline	No	Yes	(Yes)
Cause haemolysis *in vitro*	Yes	Yes	No
Temperature optimum	37°C	4–20°C	4–20°C
Complement binding	Yes	Yes	No
Transferred across placenta	Yes	No	No
'Natural' occurrence	No	Yes	?
Appear after immunization	Yes	No	Yes

[a] Given properties are the rule, exceptions occur.

3. The density of antigen sites on the surface of the blood cell.

Various methods have been used to obtain observable agglutination reactions, even with incomplete antibodies. The most common are:

1. Enzymic treatment.
2. Using a macromolecular environment, e.g. albumin.
3. Reduced ionic strength.

All of the above methods have an effect on the electrical potential at the surface of the blood cell.

The electrical charge on the surface of the cell is negative and is greatly determined by sialic acid. When the blood cells are suspended in an electrolyte, an ionic cloud is built around the cell. A potential, *zeta potential*, is created which is dependent on the charge on the surface of the cell and which determines the size of the ionic cloud and the distance between the individual cells. In physiological saline, this distance is greater than 25 nm.

The molecules of IgM and IgG are believed to have a length of 100 nm and 25 nm respectively. Thus, since the IgM molecules can bridge a wider gap between blood cells than can IgG these antibodies give rise to agglutination. The distance between blood cells in a saline suspension is such that this difference is decisive (Fig. 78).

The surface of the erythrocyte is probably not smooth but is provided with crypts and protrusions. This structure and a great number of antigen sites on the surface may explain why certain IgG antibodies such as IgG anti-A and anti-B can agglutinate of red blood cells suspended in saline.

On treating with various proteolytic enzymes such as papain, the sialomucopeptides are cleaved and sialic acid is thereby released from the surface of the cell. This results in a drop in the zeta potential and provides an opportunity for the IgG antibodies to bridge the gap and give rise to agglutination. It is also possible that the enzymic treatment exposes more antigen sites.

Incomplete antibodies can agglutinate red blood cells in a suspension which contains macromolecules such as albumin. This is due to the increase in the dielectric constant of the suspension medium which subsequently decreases the zeta potential.

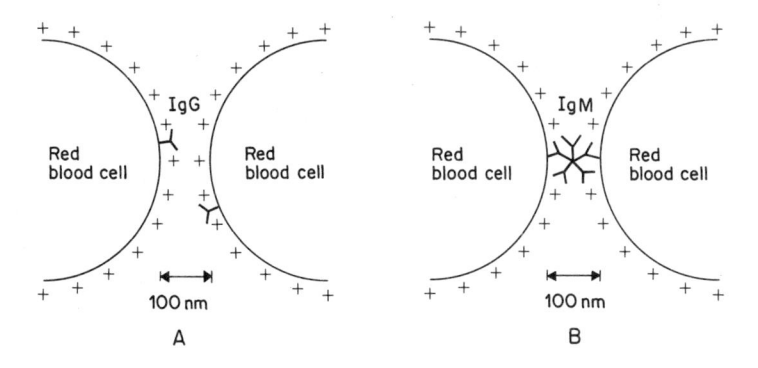

Fig. 78. A schematic representation of how the ion cloud which appears around the negatively charged red blood cells in saline suspension prevents the molecules of IgG from causing agglutination (A). Because of their greater length, the molecules of IgM can bridge the gap between the blood cells and can thereby give rise to agglutination (B)

The reaction between antibody and antigen can be increased markedly by using a suspension medium which has a low ionic strength. This is thought to be due to a reduction in the ion cloud which surrounds the blood cells. The method is best applied in conjunction with antiglobulin sera (see below) or in automated blood grouping techniques such as the Autoanalyser.

The reaction between the antigen on the erythrocyte and the antibody is affected also by pH but this is of no practical consequence in routine work. It has been reported that a pH of 5–6 is required for the demonstration of certain antibodies within the MN blood group system. The temperature optimum is not the same for each antibody. The difference is probably a reflection of the different kinds of binding which are involved.

In Table 32 the term 'naturally' occurring antibodies is used. This term appears often in the literature and should be interpreted to mean 'occurring without prior immunization with blood cell antigens'. On the other hand, there is a substantial amount of evidence which suggests that immunization during the first year of life against certain intestinal bacteria antigens which cross-react with the antigens of the ABO system gives rise to these so-called naturally occurring antibodies within the ABO system and even in the MNS, Lewis, and P systems. They have temperature optima which are lower than 37°C and some of them do not react over 25°C. Some of these, e.g. most of the Lewis antibodies, bind complement.

5. Antiglobulin sera for the demonstration of antibodies (Coombs's test)

Coombs's test makes use of antiserum against human globulin (which is the substance of incomplete antibodies) to demonstrate the presence of incomplete antibodies. Antiglobulin serum is obtained by immunizing a suitable animal, usually a rabbit, with human serum or the globulin which has been isolated from human serum. The test was described as early as 1908 but fell into oblivion to be revived by Coombs et al. (1945).

The test has been of great importance in blood group serology. While IgG antibodies such as anti-Rh do not agglutinate Rh-positive blood cells which are suspended in saline, they bind to the cells. These so-called sensitized blood cells can then be agglutinated by antiglobulin serum. In this reaction where anti-Rh is used as example, the incomplete antibodies constitute the antigens for the antiglobulin serum (Fig. 79). A reaction of this type which involves first an interaction between the erythrocyte antigen and the antibody and then the antiglobulin serum is usually called indirect (indirect Coombs's test). The term 'direct' is usually applied when the sensitizing (i.e. the binding of incomplete antibody to the blood cells) takes place *in vivo*, e.g. in haemolytic diseases of the newborn.

Antiglobulin serum has had its varied usage in the demonstration of antibodies in serum (e.g. in the serological compatibility testing), in the grouping of the different erythrocyte antigens with known IgG antisera and in the diagnosis of haemolytic diseases.

The antiglobulin serum which is used contains mostly anti-IgG but also anticomplement. The presence of anticomplement in the sera is important and necessitates special techniques for the preparation of antiglobulin sera. Red blood cells which have reacted with complement-binding antibodies are subsequently agglutinated by anticomplement serum which is directed against the complement factors C3b and C4.

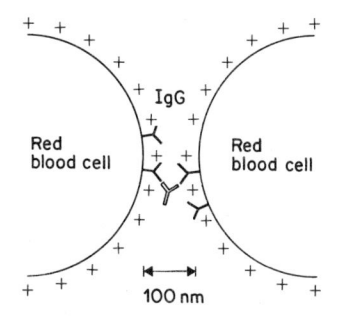

Fig. 79. A schematic representation which shows how molecules of antiglobulin (unfilled symbol) can cause agglutination of red blood cells suspended in saline and to which IgG molecules (filled symbols) have been bound (compare Fig. 78)

6. Frequency of blood group antibodies

The frequency of occurrence of various blood group antibodies in a population is of interest. Many factors are involved, e.g. the frequency of individuals with or without a stimulating antigen, the frequency of individuals who can be stimulated, and the ability of the antigen to act as an immunogen.

In connection with the frequency of antigens it will be merely mentioned here that some antigens are found in almost all individuals in a population, so-called public antigens, while others are found only rarely, so-called private antigens.

By carrying out voluntary immunization of Rh-negative men throughout the world to obtain anti-Rh(D), our knowledge of the effect of such an immunization has increased. The results have shown that approximately 70 per cent can be immunized, so-called responders, and that the remaining 30 per cent do not produce anti-Rh(D).

By studying the immunization which has arisen during pregnancy, it has been found that antibodies of the Rh-system are dominant. An English survey of 2 024 cases of incomplete antibodies which was carried out in 1964 demonstrated that 94.7 per cent belonged to anti-D or anti-CD. In only 36 cases (1.8 per cent) did the antibody belong to a blood group system other than Rh. Probably the dominance of the Rh system will remain, even if reduced, because of the regular administration of Rh antibodies to the Rh-negative mother who gives birth to a Rh-positive baby, so called Rh prophylaxis. A Swedish survey (Nilsson, 1967) which was carried out in the days prior to the introduction of Rh prophylaxis and which covered 11 094 sera obtained during antenatal care showed the presence of a single antibody in 366 cases and the presence of more than one antibody in 79 cases. The type and frequency of these antibodies are provided in Tables 33 and 34. Even in this material the dominance of antibodies of the Rh system is evident.

There is very little information available concerning the frequency of antibodies having different specificities within a sample of patients who are in need of transfusion. Information obtained from such an analysis is not so reliable since several factors are involved, e.g. the composition of the patient sample, the frequency of earlier transfusions and pregnancies, the methods used in the blood grouping laboratory, and the choice of blood for the transfusion.

Table 33. The incidence of the appearance of a single antibody in the sera of pregnant woman (antenatal care) or at the time of delivery (Nilsson, 1967)

Antibody	Number
Rh system	
Anti-D	244
Anti-C	1
Anti-c	15
Anti-E	19
Anti-e	1
Anti-C^w	2
Kell system	
Anti-K	21
Anti-k	1
Lewis system:	
Anti-Le^a	49
Anti-Le^b	3
Duffy system	
Anti-Fy^a	9
Vel system	
Anti-Ve	1
Total	366

Table 34. The appearance of more than one antibody in the sera of pregnant woman (antenatal) or at the time of delivery (Nilsson, 1967)

Antibody	Number
Anti-D+C	52
Anti-D+E	5
Anti-D+Jk^a	1
Anti-D+Le^a	7
Anti-D+C+E	1
Anti-E+Fy^a	1
Anti-E+c	4
Anti-C^w+K	1
Anti-C^w+Jk^b	1
Anti-K+Le^a	1
Anti-K+Fy^a	1
Anti-Le^a+Le^b	3
Anti-Fy^a+Jk^b	1
Total	79

B. Genetics of blood groups

The genetics of blood groups is more or less complicated according to the level of ambition which is to be satisfied. The belonging to a certain blood group is determined by the antigens on the surface of the red blood cells and is genetically designed.

Table 35. Fundamental features of the ABO system

Genotype	Phenotype	Reaction with anti-A	Reaction with anti-B
AA AO	A	+	−
BB BO	B	−	+
OO	O	−	−
AB	AB	+	+

Complicating factors such as the interference of other genes do not generally take place. The blood group antigens of the known systems are regulated by autosomal chromosomes. Only one exception is known namely, the Xg system. The demonstration of the presence of an erythrocyte antigen usually implies the existence of the corresponding gene. Interaction of other genes is uncommon and, even in these cases, the effect of the individual gene manifests itself. Possible complicatons which could arise as a result of different genes having indistinguishable effects do not occur.

It is usual that neither dominance nor recessivity arise. A pair of allelic genes determines the presence of two separate antigens recognizable with antisera against each of the antigens.

The blood cells of the heterozygote react with both antisera. These relatively simple relationships are the basis of our knowledge of this subject which has become rather complicated. The occurrence of blood group antigens is probably an early result of gene activity. Furthermore, various antigens can be carried by the same molecule, e.g. AB individuals do not possess two different molecules, one for each antigen, but instead they have one molecule which carries both antigens. A detailed account of the human system of blood groups can be found in Race and Sanger: *Blood Groups in Man* (1975).

C. ABO and Lewis systems

1. ABO system

Because of its practical importance, the ABO system is one of the most important blood group systems. The discovery of this by Landsteiner at the turn of the century opened the way for transfusion treatment.

The ABO system is determined by three alleles, *A*, *B*, and *O*. The phenotypes (antigens) which are determined by these genes can be demonstrated by making use of their reactions with anti-A and anti-B sera.

It is characteristic that antibodies against antigens A and B normally appear in accordance with Table 36. Furthermore, the A antigen can be subdivided into subgroups of which A_1 and A_2 are the most common. Approximately 80 per cent of individuals having A antigens have the A_1 form, the remainder have the A_2 form. Antisera having the specificity of anti-A_1 is available and provides the possibility of subdividing individuals with A antigens. Since there is no antibody with anti-A_2 specificity, those individuals whose blood contains A antigens but which does not react with anti-A_1 sera are described as being A_2. Anti-A_1 sera can appear as an irregular

Table 36. Antigens and antibodies in the ABO system

Group	Subgroup	Antigens on red cells	Antibodies in serum
A	A_1 A_2	$A_1 + A$ A	anti-B (anti-A_1 in ~1% of A_2 subjects)
B	—	B	anti-A anti-A_1
0	—	none	anti-A anti-A_1 anti-B
AB	A_1B A_2B	$A_1 + A + B$ $A + B$	none (anti-A_1 in 25% of A_2B subjects)

antibody in individuals who have the blood group A_2 or A_2B. Furthermore, it has been found that the normally occurring anti-A (present in individuals who have O- or B-group) can be subdivided into anti-A which reacts with A_1 as well as A_2 cells and an anti-A_1 which reacts only with A_1 cells. The subgroups, A_1 and A_2, are important in practical connections. The existence of further subgroups is known but these will not be discussed here.

The strength of the reaction between the A antigens and anti-A serum can be depicted by: $A_1 > A_1B > A_2 > A_2B$. Thus A_2B is the weakest A antigen combination. Consequently, in routine grouping it should be ensured that the test sera which are used for the demonstration of the A antigen react distinctly with the A_2B combination.

The B antigen can not be subgrouped in a way which is analogous to A_1–A_2. Variants which react weakly have been described but the incidence is low.

2. Antibodies within the ABO system

As can be seen in Table 36, anti-A and anti-B are present normally in serum when the corresponding antigen is missing from the red blood cells. These antibodies are usually described as *naturally occurring*. It is meant by this that they appear without any obvious immunization having taken place previously via for example transfusion or pregnancy. Antibodies generally belong to the IgM class of immunoglobulins but IgG anti-A or anti-B may at the same time be present. In certain cases they can even belong to the IgA class. Following immunization with A or B antigen in, for example, ABO-heterospecific pregnancy (where the ABO system of the mother and foetus are incompatible) an increase is seen in the level of IgG antibodies within the ABO system of the mother. Under optimal conditions, antibodies IgG and IgM can both produce haemolysis. While agglutination is the most important reaction in routine assays, a haemolytic reaction is occasionally seen. Inattention here can result in the reaction being classified as negative. Careful examination shows that most anti-A sera are potentially haemolytic. This is most easily brought about if the serum to blood cell ratio is held high or if the anti-A serum is completely fresh. The effect is more difficult to demonstrate if the serum is stored for a matter of a few hours. This is due to the presence in the serum of complement factors which are sensitive to storage. Furthermore, the haemolytic effect is more easily demonstrated if the A-blood cells have been stored. These facts should be kept in mind in the routine blood grouping and serological compatibility testing of suitable blood for patients. As has been mentioned above, the agglutination reaction rather than the haemolytic reaction is used for the routine serological demonstration of antigen–antibody reactions. Thus, one should be well aware of the fact that for example anti-A sera can very efficiently cause the haemolysis of A blood cells which have been stored in saline for a period of one to four days. Even blood cells which have been stored more than one week as clotted blood or more than three weeks as ACD blood increase the possibility of haemolysis in the *in vitro* testing of the type mentioned above. In practice, undesirable haemolytic effects which are believed to be caused by complement are usually avoided by treating the serum at 56°C for 30 minutes.

3. Reactions towards transfusion which are caused by incompatible ABO blood

The term 'incompatibility' refers to the situation where the recipient possesses antibodies which shorten the survival time of the transfused erythrocytes. The clinical effect of such an incompatibility is variable. Among the factors which are involved are the volume of the transfusion, the rate of breakdown of the transfused blood cells, the type of the erythrocyte antigens and the density of antigen sites on the red cells and the properties of the recipient's antibodies such as titre, class of immunoglobulin, and complement binding ability. In certain cases, the phagocytic properties of the reticuloendothelial cells are also a contributing factor.

A distinction is usually made between the breakdown of the blood in the recipient's bloodstream, so-called intravascular haemolysis and that which generally takes place in the spleen and liver, so-called extravascular haemolysis.

The important rule in blood transfusion that the recipient should not possess antibodies which are directed against the red cells of the donor is of special relevance in the case of the ABO system. This system has naturally occurring antibodies (Table 36) which in the case of transfusion in an incorrect grouping can lead to a serious haemolytic transfusion reaction. The transfusion of A-blood to an O-recipient generally gives rise to intravascular lysis of the red cells. The red blood cells in a unit of blood (450 ml) are broken down within the space of an hour or less. The extent of the breakdown is regulated primarily by the titre of the recipient's antibodies. There is normally sufficient complement in the recipient's blood to permit haemolysis of the donor cells. For further information on the haemolytic transfusion reactions, their treatment, and prevention the reader is referred to textbooks on transfusion therapy.

4. ABO incompatibility as a cause of haemolytic diseases in the newborn

Haemolytic diseases in the newborn which are caused by ABO incompatibility between mother and foetus do exist but are relatively uncommon when compared with the frequency of incompatible births. Depending on the parameter(s) which are used for the assessment of suspected haemolytic diseases, Mollison suggests a minimum incidence of 1 in 150 births having icterus and that in approximately 1 in 3 000 of all newborn the haemolytic disease is so serious that treatment is required. In a Swedish survey (Nilsson, 1967) of just over 10 000 births exchange transfusion was carried out in 63 new-born babies because of ABO haemolytic disease, i.e. a considerably higher frequency. Furthermore, it should be observed that these figures concern only A- or B-children of mothers who belong to blood group O. Rosenfield (1955), on examining blood samples taken from 1 480 umbilical cords, found that 39 of these gave positive direct antiglobulin tests (Coomb's test). Of these 39, 38 had mothers with blood group O. Even the children who underwent exchange transfusions in the above mentioned Swedish survey belonged to O-mothers. There are reports which suggest that O-mothers have a higher frequency of antibodies within the ABO system which can pass through the placenta, i.e. IgG antibodies. Similarly, it has been shown that group B children have a somewhat lower frequency of haemolytic diseases than children belonging to group A.

5. The Lewis system

The Lewis system is regulated by the gene *Le* and by the allele *le*. This system is hardly a blood group system in the usual meaning of the term but is more a system which affects the appearance of macromolecules in the fluids of the body. These macromolecules are absorbed by the red blood cells and their antigenic properties can consequently be detected by using the usual techniques of blood grouping. There are two antigens in the Lewis system namely, Le^a and Le^b. In secretions such as saliva and milk these antigens are glycoproteins, but in plasma they are glycolipids. They have antibodies which are denoted anti-Le^a and anti-Le^b. With the help of these the phenotypes listed in Table 37 can be demonstrated within the Lewis system. In the newborn the Lewis antigens are either not developed or only poorly developed.

The antibodies anti-Le^a and anti-Le^b are naturally occurring and are present primarily in Le(a− b−)-individuals, who are reported to have antibodies (generally anti-Le^a) in a frequency of 20 per cent. The antibodies are almost always IgM. Lewis antibodies do not give rise to haemolytic diseases in the new-born. This is because of their IgM character and the poorly developed antigens of the newborn. As a rule, Lewis antibodies do not give rise to transfusion reactions but the appearance of such reactions has been reported.

6. ABH and Lewis antigens in secretion

The antigens on the red blood cells in these systems are as a rule glycolipids. However, water soluble blood group substances have been identified in the secretions

Table 37. Lewis phenotypes in red blood cells

Phenotype	Frequency in adults
Le(a+b−)	23%
Le(a−b+)	74%
Le(a−b−)	3%

(saliva) of certain individuals. These substances are glycoproteins. A gene, *Se*, regulates the appearance of these substances. If an individual has inherited this gene in a single or double set, *Sese* or *SeSe*, then he/she has blood group substances belonging to the ABO system in the secretions and is usually called a secretor. If the individual has inherited only the allelic gene, *sese*, the term non-secretor is applied.

The production of ABH substance is represented schematically in Fig. 80. It is thought that a precursor substance is acted on by a gene, *H*, which virtually all individuals possess, and that this precursor substance is transformed to H substance. In the presence of an *A* and/or *B* gene most but not all of the H substance is transformed into A and/or B substance. The *O* gene does not affect the H substance. Furthermore, as can be seen in the figure, water soluble ABH substances appear in secretions such as saliva if the *Se* gene is present in a single or double set. If this gene is missing, i.e. genotype *sese*, there is no ABH substance present in saliva.

An extremely rare genotype, *hh*, is due to the lack of *H* gene and is responsible for the 'Bombay' type. Since there is no conversion of the precursor substance into H substance the presence of *A* and *B* or *Se* genes can not be manifested. Their blood cells do not react with anti-A or anti-B sera and their serum contains anti-A, anti-B, and anti-H. They are usually denoted 'O_h'. Even if the *Se* gene is present in these individuals, their saliva does not contain ABH substances. The discovery of the 'Bombay' type has even demonstrated that the genes *H* and *h* are inherited independent of the ABO genes. The union of an individual belonging to the 'Bombay' type with one who belongs to group O may give rise to offspring whose blood group is A or B. This is due to the fact that the 'Bombay' individual may have gene *A* or *B*, even if it does not give recognizable effect in the phenotype, and that this gene is inherited by the child who receives an *H* gene from the other parent. Judging by the uncommonness of the 'Bombay' type, this happening is a rarity but implies that parents who both seem to be group O can have children who are group A or B.

A schematic representation of the sequence of events in the production of Lewis substances is given in Fig. 81. It is believed that the *Le* gene converts a precursor

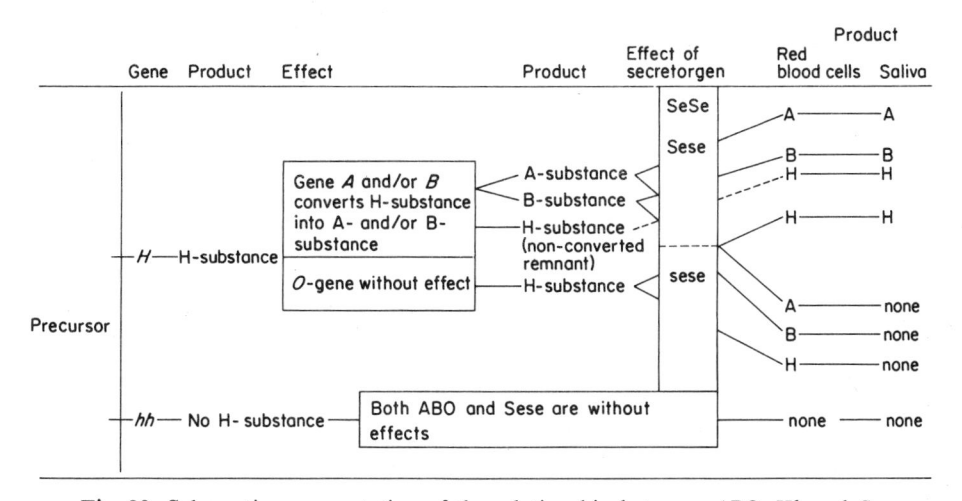

Fig. 80. Schematic representation of the relationship between *ABO*, *Hh* and *Sese*

Fig.81. Schematic representation of the Lewis system

Gene	Product	Effect	Product Red blood cells	Product Saliva	Red blood cells Lewis type
$LeLe$ / $Lele$	Le^a-substance	The genes H and Se convert Le^a-substance to Le^b-substance	Le^b	Le^b Le^a*	Le(a−b+)
		The genes H and se do not effect Le^a-substance	Le^a	Le^a	Le(a+b−)
$lele$	No Le-substance		No Le-substance	No Le-substance	Le(a−b−)

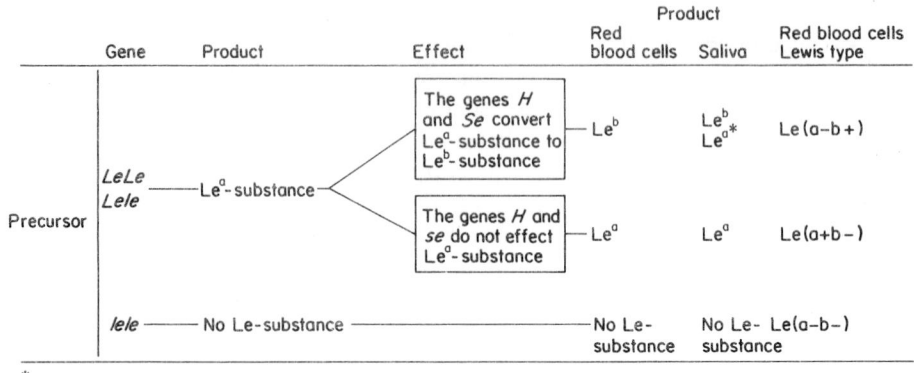

*Remaining unconverted Le^a-substance

substance to Le^a substance. There is much evidence to suggest that the precursor substance in this case is the same as that for the ABH substances. The allelic gene is without effect on the precursor substance. The Se and H gene, in a single or double set, convert Le^a substance to Le^b substance. An individual who has at least one Le, Se, and H gene is of the Le (a− b+) type. As is evident in the figure, the H and Se genes do not bring about a complete conversion of all formed Le^a substance into Le^b substance. Some remaining Le^a substance can be detected in saliva. Individuals who have the genotype $sese$ can not convert the formed Le^a substance. This implies that the presence of Le and H gene but lack of Se gene makes the individuals Le (a+ b−). Individuals having two le genes do not convert the precursor substance to Le^a substance and the possible presence of the Se and H gene are without effects and the type is Le (a− b−).

7. Chemical composition of blood group substances

The blood group substances which can be demonstrated in secretion are glycoproteins which have molecular weights in the region of 300 000. Approximately 15 per cent of the molecule consists of peptides. Carbohydrate chains are coupled to the peptides determine the A, B, H, or Lewis serological activity. The specificity is subject to the sequence and type of coupling of the individual sugar residues within the terminal and subterminal portions of these chains. In Table 38 can be seen the genes which determine the various transferases as well as how these affect the chains.

D. Rh system

The discovery of the Rh system has been of multiple importance. It has contributed much to our understanding of human genetics and made diagnosis and treatment possible in several types of haemolytic diseases of the newborn. Prophylactic treatment for the avoidance of Rh immunization can now be carried out. The importance of the system in the daily transfusion work is consolidated and is shared only by the ABO system. The discovery of the Rh system at the beginning of the 1940s signalled the beginning of a rapid development and expansion within the field of blood group serology. This was due above all else to the studies of Landsteiner and Wiener on the erythrocyte antigens of the *Rhesus* monkey and the clinical observations of Levine and Stetson.

The presence or lack of an antigen, denoted D or Rh_o, within the Rh system determines wheather a person should be denoted 'Rh-positive' or 'Rh-negative'. Approximately 85 per cent of all individuals are Rh-positive. Individuals who are devoid of the D antigen, i.e. are Rh-negative, can be immunized by the antigen either by transfusion of Rh-positive blood or during pregnancy if the foetus is Rh-positive.

1. Nomenclature

Two nomenclatures are used to describe the antigens and the genetic combinations of the Rh system. These two nomenclatures are based on two different understandings of the background to the system. Both nomenclatures are often used side by side in practical work.

According to A. S. Wiener, the system is built of multiple alleles. Thus there is a

Table 38. Gene products of *H*, *Le*, *A*, and *B* (Morgan and Watkins, 1969)

Gene	Gene product	Structures coupled by enzyme	Terminal structure of carbohydrate chain	Serological specificity
H	α-L-frucosyl-transferase (1)	α-Fuc	β-Gal(1–3)-GNAc ↑ α-Fuc	H
Le	α-L-frucosyl-transferase (2)	α-Fuc	β-Gal(1–3)-GNAc ↑ α-Fuc	Le[a]
H and *Le*	α-L-frucosyl-transferases (1 and 2)	α-Fuc	β-Gal(1–3)-GNAc ↑ ↑ α-Fuc α-Fuc	Le[b]
A	α-N-acetyl-galactosami-nyltransferase	α-GalNAc	α-GalNAc→β-Gal(1–3)-GNAc | α-Fuc	A
B	α-D-galacto-syltransferase	α-Gal	α-Gal→β-Gal(1–3)-GNAc | α-Fuc	B

Gal = galactose, GNAc = N-acetylglucosamine, Fuc = fucose.
GalNAc = N-acetylgalactosamine.
The arrows indicate the site of the effect.

212 *Immunoglobulins*

Table 39. The Rh system

RBC factors	RBC agglutinogen	Alleles	Alleles	RBC antigen
Rh_0, rh′, hr″ hr′ hr″	← Rh_1 ← rh	← R^1 ← r	$D \rightarrow$ or $d \rightarrow$	D or 'not-D'
Rh_0, rh″, hr′ Rh_0, hr′, hr″ rh′, hr″ rh″, hr′ Rh_0, rh′ rh′, rh″	← Rh_2 ← Rh_0 ← rh′ ← rh″ ← Rh_z ← rh_y	← R^2 ← R^0 ← r' ← r'' ← R^z ← r^y	$C \rightarrow$ or $c \rightarrow$ $E \rightarrow$ or $e \rightarrow$	C or c E or e
Multiple alleles			Linked genes	

series of eight alleles. Each allele determines an agglutinogen which has two or more antigenic factors on the erythrocytes. However, R. A. Fisher, R. Race, and Ruth Sanger claim that the system consists of three adjacent loci where each locus has two alternative genes (*linked gene theory*) which are responsible for the erythrocyte antigens. This implies that a complex of three genes in the latter case corresponds to one gene in the first theory. It is essential to realize that the existence of an antigen which is determined by the allele *d* has not been demonstrated. This should be taken to mean that blood cells not agglutinated by anti-D sera are 'non-D'. Apart from this the system of 'linked genes' is based on antithetic antigens so that when for example the C antigen is determined by the *C* gene, the c antigen can not be determined simultaneously by the same locus on the same chromosome. As the antigens C and c are inherited on their individual chromosomes, the C and c antigens can both be found on the red blood cells. In connection with the clinical importance of the D antigen, it is worth mentioning here that in the alternative nomenclature the presence of this antigen is signified by an 'R' at the beginning of the notation for such complexes.

Concerning the sequence of the genes, Race and Sanger claim that a lot of evidence suggests that *C* (or *c*) and *E* (or *e*) but not *D* and *E* are related. Strictly speaking, this should produce a linear sequence of *D C E*.

The alleles and the gene combinations according to the two theories, together with their frequency of occurrence in the Swedish population are given in Table 40.

2. Frequencies of Rh types

The Rh types vary with population. From the frequency table (Table 40) it can be seen that the most common combination is *CDe/cde* which has a frequency of $2 \times (0.4037 \times 0.3821) = 0.309$ or 31 per cent. Next comes the combination *CDe/CDe* with 0.163 or 16 per cent and for *cde/cde*, which is routinely denoted 'Rh-negative', the frequency is 0.145 or 15 per cent. Table 40, which is by no means complete, shows nine haplotypes which provide 45 different combinations.

3. Rh antibodies

Several different antibodies have been identified within the Rh system. Only a few of these will be mentioned here, and the nomenclature which is most often used is that of Fisher. From studies performed on individuals who were immunized either as a result of transfusion or pregnancy, the existence of antibodies against the antigens C, c, D, E, and e have been demonstrated. These antibodies are called anti-C, -c, -D, -E, and -e respectively. The existence of an antibody having the specificity anti-d has not been demonstrated. Table 41 shows the reaction pattern of various combinations of Rh antigens with the above mentioned antisera.

Apart from the agglutinogens used in the nomenclature of Wiener, the table includes also the customary Swedish notation, namely Rh-positive (84 per cent), Rh-partial (1 per cent) and Rh-negative (15 per cent). In Sweden, this nomenclature has long been in use and includes the notation 'Rh-partial'. Such an individual is devoid of the D antigen and can therefore be immunized against this antigen. This implies that such an individual when pregnant or when receiving a blood transfusion should be equated with a Rh-negative individual. Thus such an individual should be given Rh-negative blood and Rh prophylaxis according to the principles for Rh-negative individuals. On the other hand, Rh-partial blood donors should be designated Rh-positive.

4. The D antigen

The strength of the D antigen is variable. A weak D antigen, denoted D^u, was described early. The D^u antigen could often be demonstrated only by using an antiglobulin serum (indirect Coombs's test) and is determined by an allele of the D gene which is denoted D^u. On closer examination, the group of individuals who are designated as D^u has been shown to be heterogeneous. It is thought nowadays that the Rh (D) antigen consists of an antigen which has at least four parts. The various parts are generally present in full extent but they can sometimes be poorly developed or can be missing completely.

In Sweden the D^u type of Rh-positive individuals are judged to be Rh-positive. They

Table 40. The frequency of Rh gene combinations in the Swedish population (Heiken and Rasmuson, 1966). The symbol 'R' implies that the D antigen is determined and 'r' implies that this is not the case

According to Wiener	According to Fisher	Frequency
R^1	CDe	0.4037
r	cde	0.3821
R^2	cDE	0.1670
R^0	cDe	0.0186
R^{1w}	C^wDe	0.0198
r''	cdE	0.0030
r'	Cde	0.0049
R^z	CDE	0.0008
r^y	CdE	rare

Table 41. The reaction of Rh antisera with various Rh antigen combinations

Serum	Rh-positive							Rh-partial		Rh-negative
	Rh_1Rh_1 CDe/CDe	Rh_1rh CDe/cde	Rh_2Rh_2 cDE/cDE	Rh_2rh cDE/cde	Rh_0rh cDe/cde	Rh_1Rh_2 CDe/cDE	rh'rh Cde/cde	rh''rh cdE/cde	rh rh cde/cde
anti-D	+	+	+	+	+	+	−	−	−
anti-C	+	+	−	−	−	+	+	−	−
anti-E	−	−	+	+	−	+	−	+	−
anti-c	−	+	+	+	+	+	+	+	+
anti-e	+	+	−	+	+	+	+	+	+

may be given Rh-positive blood in transfusion but should not be given so-called Rh prophylaxis. The evidence suggests that it is extremely rare for a D^u individual to produce anti-D following a transfusion with D-positive blood. The classification of D^u individuals varies from country to country.

5. Special antigens within the Rh system

Several antigenic variants have been detected within the Rh system. Only a few which are of special interest will be mentioned here.

The *G antigen* was discovered by Allen and Tippett (1958). These workers showed that the G antigen exists in all gene complexes except *cde* and *cdE*. This provided an explanation for the finding that pregnant woman of the genotype *cde/cde* could produce a supposed 'anti-CD' despite the fact that the child's father was lacking the C antigen. It was now shown that it was a question of anti-D+G. Similarly, a *cde/cde* woman who produced a supposed 'anti-CD' by being immunized by a *Cde/cde* foetus was shown to be anti-C+G. Furthermore, it has been found in the intentional immunization of Rh-negative individuals by $Rh_0(cDe/cde)$ blood cells that these produce antibodies which react with cells which have the C but not the D antigen. This is due to the fact that the Rh_0 cells have the G antigen and that the serum contained anti-D+G.

Furthermore, an explanation is provided for the finding that anti-C is seldom produced by Rh-positive individuals while on the other hand, an antibody which reacts with C+ cells and which is anti-G is often produced by Rh-negative individuals.

Most 'anti-CD' sera are believed to contain anti-D+G or anti-D+C+G.

The C^w antigen

This antigen has been taken to be an alternative gene to C. For example, the gene combination C^wDe can appear instead of CDe. If C^w blood is transfused into a person who has the C antigen an immunization can take place and antibodies which have the specificity of anti-C^w can be demonstrated. A similar immunization can take place also during pregnancy. Most anti-C sera react with blood cells which possess the C^w antigen. The C^w antigen is relatively rare, occurring in less than 2 per cent of the population.

Rh_{null}

There have appeared reports of just over ten individuals who had blood cells which did not react with any of the known Rh antibodies. This blood type has been denoted Rh_{null} and is extremely rare.

	Normal	Bombay	Rh$_{null}$
ABO	+	−	+
Rh	+	+	−
Anaemia	−	−	+

$\dagger$ = ABO - antigen

▨ = Rh - antigen

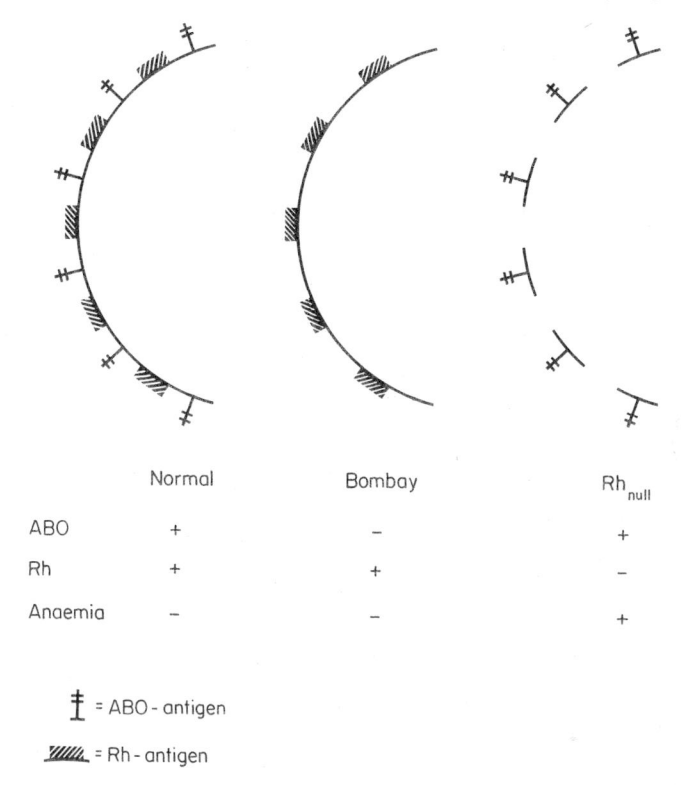

Fig. 82. The appearance of antigens and signs of anaemia in individuals of the Bombay and Rh$_{null}$ type. According to Levine et al. (1973)

The changes which are undergone in Rh$_{null}$ are probably more extensive than those which affect the Rh system. In this respect, an association has been found in most cases of Rh$_{null}$ with a mild haemolytic process with spherocytosis. This points to the presence of damage to the membrane and the notation 'Rh$_{null}$ disease' has been used in such cases.

Figure 82 provides a representation of the relationships which exist between Rh$_{null}$ and 'Bombay' (see the ABO system) blood, and normal blood from individuals who have normally developed antigens. While these two blood groups are very rare, they are of great interest and have contributed to our understanding of various genetic products and sequence effects.

6. Rh immunization

Interest in the immunizing capabilities of the Rh antigens continues to be high. This is due partly to the fact that inadequate blood grouping and compatibility testing can result in transfusion reactions due to the Rh antigens. The relatively high frequency of Rh antibodies has been mentioned previously (page 204). The appearance of anti-D following blood transfusion is rare since particular attention is paid to this antigen in the routine choice of blood. Antigens other than D within the Rh system can occasionally give rise to antibodies. The possibility of detecting such antibodies in routine work is good and can be carried out by using adequate methods in the compatibility test. However, the presence of such antibodies may greatly limits the choice of compatible blood.

216 *Immunoglobulins*

```
           Homozygote                    |          Heterozygote
   Father              Mother            |   Father              Mother
   CDe/CDe      x      cde/cde           |   CDe/cde      x      cde/cde

 CDe/cde  CDe/cde  CDe/cde  CDe/cde      | CDe/cde  CDe/cde  cde/cde  cde/cde
 _____/         | _____/  _____/
          All Rh-positive                |    Rh-positive         Rh-negative
```

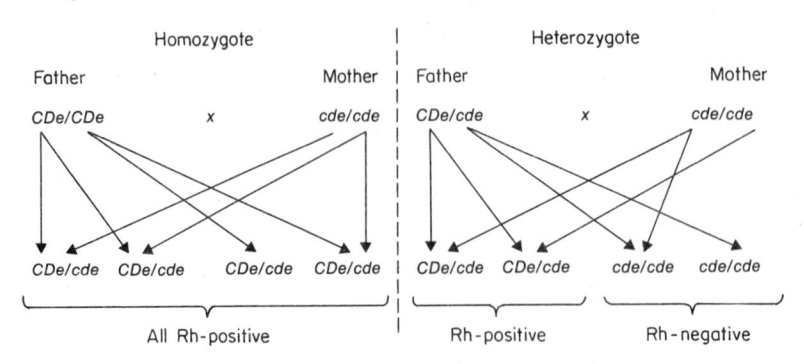

Fig. 83. The possible Rh types of a child who has a Rh-negative mother and a father who is either homozygous or heterozygous Rh-positive

The major cause of the interest in Rh immunization is of course the importance of the Rh antibodies in the haemolytic diseases of the newborn. In approximately every tenth pregnancy the woman is Rh-negative while the foetus is Rh-positive. There are roughly three *DD* homozygotes for every four *Dd* heterozygotes. The consequence of this is evident in the example provided in Fig. 83. As a result of these relationships the chance that a Rh-negative woman can have two successive pregnancies where the foetus is Rh-positive is somewhat less than 50 per cent. When this fact is taken into account with the knowledge that the second pregnancy with a Rh-positive foetus contributes to a great extent to haemolytic diseases in the newborn, the disease could theoretically occur in such a high per cent. However, this disease is seen only in approximately 6 per cent of women who are pregnant for the second time with a Rh-positive foetus and who have not been subjected to Rh prophylaxis.

Mollison reports that approximately 0.8 per cent of Rh-negative woman have anti-Rh *present by the end of their first pregnancy* with a Rh-positive foetus and that the figure became almost 1 per cent if only woman who gave births to ABO compatible, Rh-positive children were considered. A survey of 909 Rh-negative women, whose first child was Rh-positive and ABO compatible showed that there were 21 cases (2.3 per cent) of immunization by the third day after delivery. This higher figure is probably due to a greater sensitivity of the method which was used for the detection of the antibody, e.g. enzyme-treated cells. Mollison reports further that approximately 7 per cent of Rh-negative mothers who did not receive Rh prophylaxis and whose first children were Rh-positive and ABO compatible, showed the presence of antibody *within a period of six months following parturition* In a Finnish survey (Eklund and Nevanlinna, 1973) which followed 1 012 Rh-negative women over a period of nine months following parturition, the frequency of immunization was 3.5 per cent (4.3 per cent for ABO compatible). These women were not given Rh prophylaxis during this period. This frequency is considerably lower than that which is normally given.

The significance of the amount of bleeding from foetus to mother (TPH, transplacental haemorrhage) can be seen in the results of a survey which was carried out on Rh-negative mothers whose first children were Rh-positive and ABO compatible. In those cases where foetal blood cells could not be detected in the blood circulation of the mothers at the end of the pregnancy, antibodies could be detected in 3 per cent of these cases over a period of six months following parturition. On the other hand, approximately 20 per cent of those mothers who showed the presence of 0.1 ml of foetal blood cells in their circulation had detectable antibodies over the same period of time. The presence of 0.1 ml or more foetal blood cells was detected in approximately one-fifth of women at the time of birth.

It is interesting to note that if a Rh-negative woman who has given birth of a Rh-positive, ABO-compatible, child gives birth to yet another such child, the frequency of those who have Rh antibodies at the end of the second pregnancy is roughly 17 per cent. This implies that for every woman who has detectable Rh antibodies after the first pregnancy, there is one woman who becomes primarily immunized but who requires further stimulation through a second pregnancy in order to produce detectable antibodies.

The *influence of the ABO system* on Rh immunization has been known since the 1940s. ABO incompatibility gives partial protection against this immunization but how this takes place is not fully understood. In a study where 24 Rh-negative individuals were injected with ABO-compatible, Rh-positive, blood cells, 17 individuals produced anti-Rh while only 4 of 32 who were injected with ABO-incompatible blood cells produced anti-Rh. The partial protective effect of ABO incompatibility in Rh immunization can be seen in pregnancy. Some observations made by Nevanlinna and co-workers in Finland are of particular interest. These investigators have found, in cases where the mother became immunized, that it was 4 times more common for the child who preceded the first child with haemolytic disease to be ABO compatible than incompatible. The ill children were just as often ABO compatible as not. This implies that ABO incompatibility does not give protection in cases where the mother is Rh immunized. It has also been pointed out that the protective effect of ABO incompatibility is greater in cases where the mother belongs to the O-group. Thus the protection in B-man with O-woman is twice that in B-man with A-woman. In the case of mother and child, the protection offered by incompatibility is greater in cases of A-incompatibility (about 90 per cent) than in B-incompatibility (about 50 per cent).

Several theories have been suggested for the explanation of the partial protective effect of ABO incompatibility. Among these is the theory of *clonal competition* which proposes that there exists more cells producing antibodies within the ABO system available to take up the incompatible ABO antigen than those which produce anti-Rh. Mollison concludes that ABO incompatibility provides its partial protection through a breakdown of the red blood cells in the liver. This localization would then be an unfavourable site for the induction of immune responses. The possibility that the anti-A and anti-B induced lysis of red blood cells can alter the immunogenicity of the Rh antigen has not been excluded. On the other hand, in the Rh prophylaxis some specific mechanism prevents the Rh antigen from reaching the antibody forming cells.

7. Rh prophylaxis

Freda and co-workers (1966) presented a clinical study which showed that Rh immunization of Rh-negative woman could be prevented by the passive administration of anti-D gamma globulin at the time of delivery. The significance of this so-called Rh prophylaxis was obvious and national preventive programmes were introduced in several countries. It is worthwhile noting that there is a relatively good protection implied by ABO incompatibility between mother and foetus and that only a relatively small dose of passively administered anti-D is necessary. In the previously mentioned Finnish report on 1 012 mothers who were not given prophylaxis, 35 (3.5 per cent) became immunized and only one of these had given birth to a ABO incompatible child. It is obvious that the size of the protective dose is considerably lower than that which is required to react with all of the Rh sites on the foetal red blood cells in the mother's circulation. In Sweden it is customary to give a protective dose of 250 μg of anti-D gamma globulin intramuscularly within 72 hours following parturition. In the Finnish material, which appears representative of Scandinavia, there were 17 (0.13 per cent) immunized mothers among the 12 720 mothers who received Rh prophylaxis and who were followed up during four to six months following parturition. The failure rate of the protective effect can also be studied by determining the frequency of mothers who become immunized by a Rh-positive foetus during a second pregnancy. In the Finnish material consisting of 1 027 mothers, this frequency was found to be 1 per cent (10 cases). Rh prophylaxis is not given to mothers who are already immunized. In the Finnish survey there were 7 467 first-time mothers and of these, 26 (0.35 per cent) became immunized before parturition and as such were not given Rh prophylaxis.

It is obvious that Rh prophylaxis provides a considerable amount of protection against Rh immunization. The failure rate is low (0.13 per cent) and is lower than the risk for immunization (0.35 per cent) *during pregnancy*. A reduction of this immunization is an important goal on the way to a more effective prophylaxis. Clinical experiments are being undertaken to study the possibility of giving Rh prophylaxis during pregnancy. Encouraging results have been obtained in some countries such as Canada. This prophylaxis does not cause any damage to the foetus.

A second situation where the passive administration of anti-D can be important for the prevention of Rh immunization is the incorrect transfusion of Rh-positive blood into a Rh-negative patient. In such instances, the dose of anti-D which is used is considerably higher than that which is used in the normal prophylaxis. In one such case at the Karolinska Hospital, Stockholm, a 14-year-old Rh-negative girl was given 300 ml of Rh-positive blood. During a period of nine days following the transfusion, the girl was given a total dose of anti-D which was 27 times greater than the normal dose used in prophylaxis. After the period of nine days the transfused red cells had disappeared from the patient's circulation and an examination six months later showed no signs of Rh immunization. There is a Swedish recommendation that 4 000 μg of anti-D should be given to prevent the onset of Rh immunization following the incorrect transfusion of 500 ml of Rh-positive blood.

E. Certain blood group systems of clinical interest

The ABO and Rh systems have been described in detail here because of their importance in clinical medicine. Some additional systems will be presently described in less detail.

The introduction of the antiglobulin technique for the detection of antibodies resulted in the discovery of several different blood group systems. Three such systems are discussed below. The reader who requires a more detailed account of these is referred to the excellent monograph of Race and Sanger.

1. The Kell system

The Kell system was discovered in 1946 shortly after the introduction of the antiglobulin technique for clinical usage. Two antigens were detected within this system and these were denoted K (Kell) and k (Cellano). The former antigen is present in approximately 9 per cent of the population. Individuals are either homozygous (KK) or heterozygous (Kk) with respect to the gene, K, which determines the K antigen. Only 1 in approximately 500 individuals is lacking the k antigen, i.e. genotype KK. This together with the fact that the k antigen has a relatively weak immunizing ability, makes the incidence of individuals who have developed the anti-k antibody rare. However, apart from the ABO and Rh systems anti-K is the most common immune antibody but it too is relatively uncommon.

Anti-K can be produced by immunization during pregnancy. According to Mollison, the calculated risk for haemolytic disease appearing in a case where the mother is K-negative and pregnant for the second time with a K-positive foetus, is 1 in 4 000. In this case Mollison assumes that the K-antigen is 10 times less antigenic than D in the Rh system.

Both antibodies can cause haemolytic transfusion reactions. The detection of the antibody (anti-K) in the compatibility testing of blood will as a rule not give great practical difficulties – 91 per cent of the donors are lacking in the antigen. On the other hand the detection of anti-k seriously limits the choice of available blood donors – 0.2 per cent of the donors are devoid of this antigen. Fortunately, the latter situation is uncommon.

2. The Duffy system

The Duffy system is regulated by two alleles Fy^a and Fy^b. The most common antibody in this system is anti-Fy^a, which can cause haemolytic transfusion reactions. Anti-Fy^a may cause haemolytic diseases in the new-born, although this is uncommon.

3. The Kidd system

The Kidd system has two alleles, Jk^a and Jk^b. Approximately 25 per cent of the population are homozygotes for Jk^a i.e. phenotype Jk(a+b−), 50 per cent are heterozygotes having the phenotype Jk(a+b+), and the remaining 25 per cent are homozygotes for Jk^b and have the phenotype Jk(a−b+). The antibodies anti-Jk^a and anti-Jk^b are uncommon. The former antibody was discovered in a woman who had given birth to a child which had haemolytic disease. Both of these antibodies can cause haemolytic transfusion reactions.

Table 42. The Duffy system (Mollison, 1972)

Genotype	Phenotype	Reaction with anti-Fy^a	anti-Fy^b	Frequency %
$Fy^a Fy^a$	Fy(a+b−)	+	−	17
$Fy^a Fy^b$	Fy(a+b+)	+	+	49
$Fy^b Fy^b$	Fy(a−b+)	−	+	34

Proteins taking part in coagulation and fibrinolysis

I. Factors and mechanisms involved in blood coagulation
LARS-OLOV ANDERSSON and RAGNAR LUNDÉN

The fundamental principles of the mechanism of blood coagulation were formulated over 100 years ago by Alexander Smith at the Virchows Institute in Berlin. In 1905, Morawitz, Fuld, and Spiro presented a coagulation theory which is now called the classical theory (Fig. 84).

Several additional factors of significance in coagulation were later discovered. These of course influenced the classical theory but it still remains the nucleus of the new coagulation scheme. The designation of the various coagulation factors soon became an important question and a committee on the nomeclature was formed in 1954. This body recommended that the coagulation factors should be allocated roman numerals. Stipulated information about the properties of a potential factor is required before the substance becomes recognized as a coagulation factor and is given a number. Furthermore, there must be strong evidence to show that a deficiency of the factor gives rise to haemorrhagic diathesis. Various properties of the factor must be experimentally established, e.g. the temperature stability, adsorption to barium sulphate, kaolin and Celite, the ability to be dialysed, occurrence in various plasma fractions, and the electrophoretic characteristics. The method for isolation of the factor should also be supplied as well as reproducible methods for measuring the activity of the factor. The lifetime of the factor in human blood must also be established. While the chemical identification of the factor is not required, the role in the coagulation mechanism must be established.

At present there are 13 factors which have been approved by the committee. These are as follows:

  I   Fibrinogen
 II   Prothrombin
III   Thromboplastin (thrombokinase)

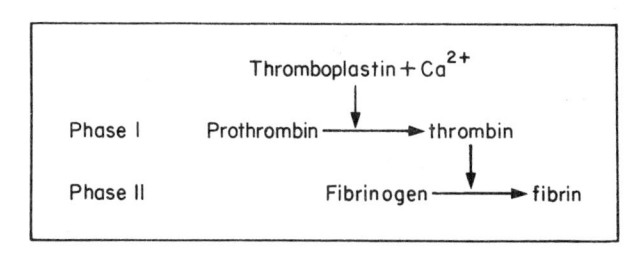

Fig. 84. The classical theory of coagulation.

IV Ca^{2+}
V   Factor V (proaccelerin, Ac-globulin)
VI   Accelerin (activated Factor V)
VII Proconvertin
VIII Haemophilia A-factor (AHF)
IX   Haemophilia B-factor ('Christmas factor')
X   Stuart factor
XI   Haemophilia C-factor
XII Hageman factor
XIII Fibrin stabilizing factor

Several different coagulation schemes have been presented. Total agreement concerning the course of events in the coagulation process does not exist. A summary of the various coagulation schemes is provided in Inga Marie Nilsson's book *Haemorrhagic and Thrombotic Diseases* (1973). An example of a mechanism is that presented hypothetically by Birger Blombäck in 1966 (Fig. 85), according to which, the process can be divided into three phases: the production of thromboplastin, the conversion of prothrombin into thrombin, and finally, the formation and stabilization of fibrin.

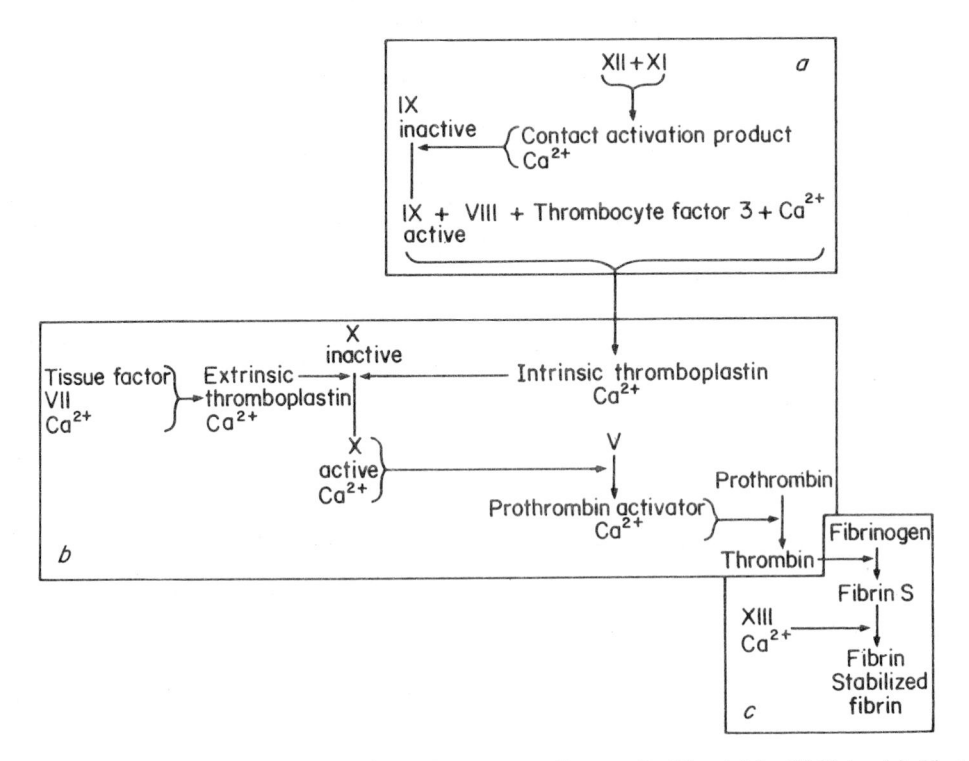

Fig. 85. The hypothetical coagulation scheme according to B. Blombäck (1966a). (a) First phase = the production of plasma thromboplastin. (b) Second phase = the conversion of prothrombin into thrombin. (c) Third phase = the conversion of fibrinogen into fibrin

II. Fibrinogen and fibrin formation
BIRGER BLOMBÄCK

1. Occurrence and role

Fibrinogen is defined as that protein in blood and tissue extract which in the presence of thrombin is transformed into an insoluble product which is called fibrin. Fibrinogen exists in the blood plasma of all vertebrates and a protein similar in character to fibrinogen is found in many invertebrates. Accordingly, lobster lymph contains a protein which aggregates in the presence of tissue extract from the same species and thereby becomes insoluble.

It is generally accepted that the most important biological role of fibrinogen is that of a precursor to the thread-like material, fibrin, and that its most important function is that as the structural element in haemostatic blood clots formed at injured endothelium surfaces in the circulating system. This does not mean that the importance of fibrinogen is limited entirely to the haemostatic mechanisms of the organism. Evidence that fibrinogen/fibrin should have other functions is suggested by the fact that only a small proportion of the circulating fibrinogen is necessary for an adequate haemostasis. Furthermore, there is evidence suggesting that fibrinogen/fibrin could be of great importance in wound healing.

Fibrinogen belongs to a group of proteins whose concentration in blood increases markedly following infection. The latter situation has given rise to the suggestion that fibrinogen may play some role in the organism's defence against infection. The occurrence of a clotting protein in the haemocytes of the horseshoe crab (*Limulus polyphemus*) is interesting in this connection (Solum, 1973). This protein aggregates when in contact with bacteria endotoxin. Nakamura et al. (1976) have isolated the coagulation protein in a *Limulus* species. The protein has a molecular weight of 17 000 and has sequence homologies with the Bβ-chain of human fibrinogen. It was shown that an enzyme in the haemocytes in the presence of endotoxin split two bonds in the protein. Following this limited proteolysis, aggregation of the remaining protein occurred. Interesting enough, the enzyme was shown to possess a Factor Xa like specificity for synthetic substrates and vertebrate Factor Xa in the presence of endotoxin converted the coagulogen to its active form (Iwanaga pers. comm.). The *Limulus* enzyme had, however, no effect on vertebrate fibrinogen even in the presence of endotoxin. These findings provide a basis for the speculation that the fibrinogen in mammals has developed possibly from an ancestral protein, which is still preserved in the invertebrates where it is in readiness to prevent infection. Is the agglutination of staphylococci in the presence of mammalian fibrinogen a function reminiscent of such an ancestral protein?

More than a hundred years have passed since Denis de Commercy and Olof Hammarsten carried out their pioneering studies of isolating fibrinogen from plasma and its conversion into fibrin in the presence of thrombin. We have gained a considerable knowledge of the physicochemical and molecular properties of fibrinogen over the past hundred years. However, in spite of all the information at hand today, we can merely speculate as to how the fibrin fibre is built up of individual, activated fibrinogen units.

Hopefully studies on fibrinogen structure and of fibrin formation will give us insight into the processes which govern clot formation in the blood vessels and will therefore aid our understanding of this most crucial event in normal haemostasis and in thrombosis, be it localized or generalized as in intravascular coagulation. In a broader perspective, fibrin formation may also serve as a model of the dynamics involved in the formation of biological fibres.

In what follows, I shall give a summary of the most important physicochemical and chemical properties of fibrinogen, the molecular basis of its transformation to fibrin, and finally its physiological importance in health and disease. The reader who requires a more detailed understanding of this subject is referred to the review work of Scheraga and Laskowski (1957); Blombäck (1967); Laki (1968); Doolittle (1973); Murano (1974); Mosesson and Finlayson (1976); and Gaffney (1977a,b).

2. Physicochemical properties

Various physicochemical properties of fibrinogen are presented in Table 43. Fibrinogen is a plasma protein of which more than 90 per cent consists of amino acids. The amino acid composition is similar in different animal species (Cartwright and Kekwick, 1971). Approximately 4–5 per cent of the weight is made up of covalently bound carbohydrate which in its turn is composed of neutral sugar, glucosamine, and sialic acid. The molecule contains also small amounts of ester-linked phosphoric acid and sulphuric acid.

On the basis of its diffusion and sedimentation properties, fibrinogen is estimated to have a molecular weight of 340 000 (Table 43). Light scattering measurements have suggested a molecular weight of approximately the same value.

By quantitative determination of the NH_2-terminal amino acids of fibrinogen, it has been concluded that the molecule is a dimer (cf. Blombäck, 1967). The two identical halves each consist of three polypeptide chains, Aα, Bβ, and γ, which are connected by disulphide bridges. The two half molecules are also joined to each other via disulphide bridges (Blombäck and Blombäck, 1972). The molecule can be represented by the formula (Aα, Bβ, γ)$_2$. There is evidence suggesting that fibrinogen in circulation blood consists of a population of somewhat different molecules. By studying the solubility of fibrinogen in ethanol-water mixtures we can distinguish between three types of fibrinogen: one with

Table 43. Physicochemical and chemical parameters of bovine fibrinogen

Molecular weight	340 000	
Sedimentation coefficient ($s^0_{20,w}$)	7.7–7.9 · 10^{-13} S	
Diffusion coefficient ($D^0_{20,w}$)	2.0 · 10^{-7} cm^2/s	Cf. Scheraga and Laskowski (1957)
Specific viscosity [η]	0.25 dl/g	
Partial specific volume (V)	0.71–0.72 cm^3/g	
		Cf. Doolittle (1973)
Frictional ratio (f/f^0)	2.34	
Molecular volume	3.7 × 10^3 nm^3	Marguerie and Stuhrmann (1976)
Degree of hydration (g/g protein)	6	
Extinction coefficient ($E^{1\%}_{280}$)	16.25	
Isoelectric point (IP)	5.5	Cf. Scheraga and Laskowski (1957)
α-Helix content (%)	33	Mihalyi (1965)

high, one with low, and one with intermediate solubility (Mosesson and Alkjaersig, 1967). The fibrinogen having low solubility in ethanol–water has been shown to be associated with the cold-insoluble globulin of plasma (for reference see Mosesson and Finlayson, 1976). Whether the fibrinogen in this complex has properties different from those of the remaining plasma fibrinogen, has not as yet been investigated. The fibrinogen most used in investigations is that form which has intermediate solubility. Unless otherwise stated, this is the type of fibrinogen which is referred to here.

Fibrinogen having high solubility in ethanol–water has somewhat lower molecular weight. It probably arises as a consequence of plasmic degradation of fibrinogen as this process has been shown to give rise to products having high solubility (Mosesson et al. 1974).

One cause of the heterogeneity of fibrinogen with regard to solubility may therefore be the occurrence of proteolytic degradation of the molecule during its circulation in blood. NH_2-terminal analysis of fibrinogen suggests that the heterogeneity may be explained, in part, by the occurrence of degradation at the NH_2-terminal portion of the peptide chains (cf. Blombäck, 1967).

The susceptibility to plasmin, in early stages of fibrinolysis, of terminal segments of the chains of intact fibrinogen has been demonstrated in several studies (Mills and Karpatkin, 1970; Gaffney and Dobos, 1971; Lahiri and Shainoff, 1973; Ly et al., 1974).

The carboxy-terminal of the Aα-chain of fibrinogen is the first site of attack when the protein is degraded by plasmin. Degradation of the Bβ-chain from the NH_2-terminal also occurs at fast rate and the γ-chain is the most resistant to plasmic attack.

Another cause of heterogeneity is the existence of charge heterogeneity in the oligosaccharide and phosphate residues which are bound to the peptide chains (Gaffney, 1971). Charge heterogeneity has been demonstrated by chromatography of fibrinogen in DEAE–cellulose (Finlayson and Mosesson, 1963; Mosher and Blount, 1973). According to Mosher and Blout, fibrinogen is separated into three distinct fractions (Fig. 86). The separation in fractions is due to the occurrence of two different

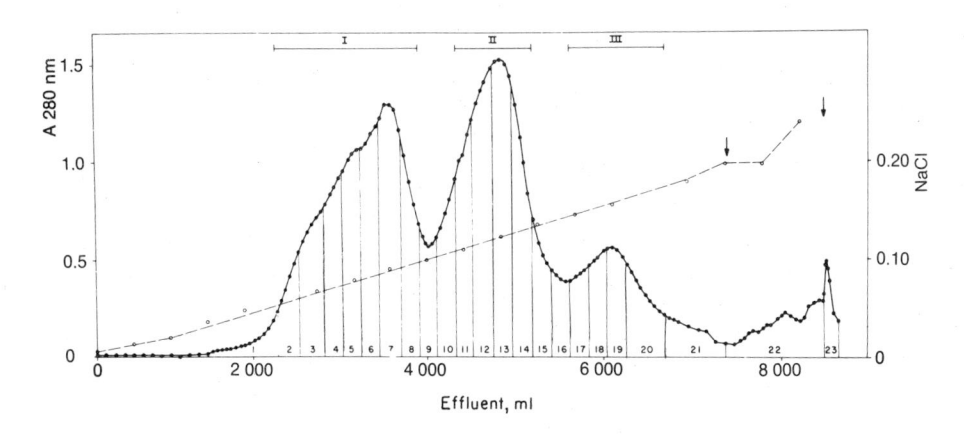

Fig. 86. Chromatogram of bovine fibrinogen on DEAE–Sephadex A 50. ●-●: UV-extinction; ○-○: NaCl concentration. The three fractions are indicated with roman numerals. From Mosher and Blout, 1973

γ-chains in fibrinogen. The fibrinogen in the first fraction contains γ-chains of one type while the fibrinogen in the third fraction has γ-chains of another type. The intermediate fraction contains fibrinogen having γ-chains of both types. Nevertheless, Mosher and Blout found that even fibrinogen in these chromatographically pure fractions was heterogeneous. This superimposed heterogeneity appeared to be a consequence of differences in protein-bound phosphate. As a result of their experiments, Mosher and Blout suggested that as many as 36 slightly different fibrinogen molecules could exist in the blood of any one individual.

What does in reality an average fibrinogen molecule look like? Hydrodynamic measurements indicate that the fibrinogen molecule is a rod- or ellipsoid-shaped particle having a length of 40–50 nm and a length/width ratio of 5 to 10 (Scheraga and Laskowski, 1957). However, the interpretation of the hydrodynamic data is dependent on the degree of hydration of the molecule. Data presented in recent years indicate that the molecule may contain as much as 6 g of water per gram of protein (Marguerie and Stuhrmann, 1976). This extremely high degree of hydration suggests that the molecule has a swollen lattice-like structure. Marguerie and Stuhrmann suggested on the basis of their data that the most likely shape of fibrinogen in solution was an oblate disk although a rodlike structure was also compatible with the data.

As with the hydrodynamic measurements, electron microscopic investigations have failed to yield unambiguous results. Hall and Slayter (1959) found that the molecule was a structure made up of three spherical particles, bound together by a thread-like structure. Köppel (1970) was unable to verify this structure but obtained instead pictures showing spherical particles which appeared to have the form of a pentagondodecahedron. Köppel assumed that the chains of the protein were surface orientated while the inside was filled with water. Using the freeze-etching technique Bachmann et al. (1975) have produced electron microscopic pictures of a structure which is believed to represent the hydrated fibrinogen molecule (Fig. 87). The idealized molecule takes the form of a cylinder with rounded ends. It has a length of 45 nm and a width of 9 nm. Irregular forms of the molecule were also observed. The form observed by Bachmann et al. requires a high degree of hydration. Consequently, the molecular volume of the hydrated molecule will be 7 times greater than the 'dry volume' calculated solely from data of molecular weight and partial specific volume. By applying electron microscopy to a dry preparation of fibrinogen, a different picture of the molecule was produced, which was fairly consistent with the results of Hall and Slayter. Therefore, the model of Hall and Slayter may represent an artefact produced by dehydration of the native fibrinogen molecule.

Tooney and Cohen (1972) have crystallized a derivative of fibrinogen lacking a small portion of the carboxy-terminal region of the Aα-chain of the molecule. The crystals were shown by electron microscopy to have an ordered structure where the unit cell had the dimensions 9 nm × 45 nm, i.e. the same dimensions as Bachmann et al. (1975) found for non-crystalline but hydrated rod-shaped fibrinogen molecules. Stryer et al. (1963) found in low-angle X-ray diffraction studies that the axial repeats in the hydrated fibrinogen molecules were 22.6 nm. This number may represent the length of each half-molecule in a dimer of about 45 nm. This would then indicate that the half-molecules of fibrinogen are joined in the centre of a rod-shaped particle.

I have chosen this model of fibrinogen in my deliberations on symmetry and functional properties of the molecule. It should be pointed out, however, that the actual

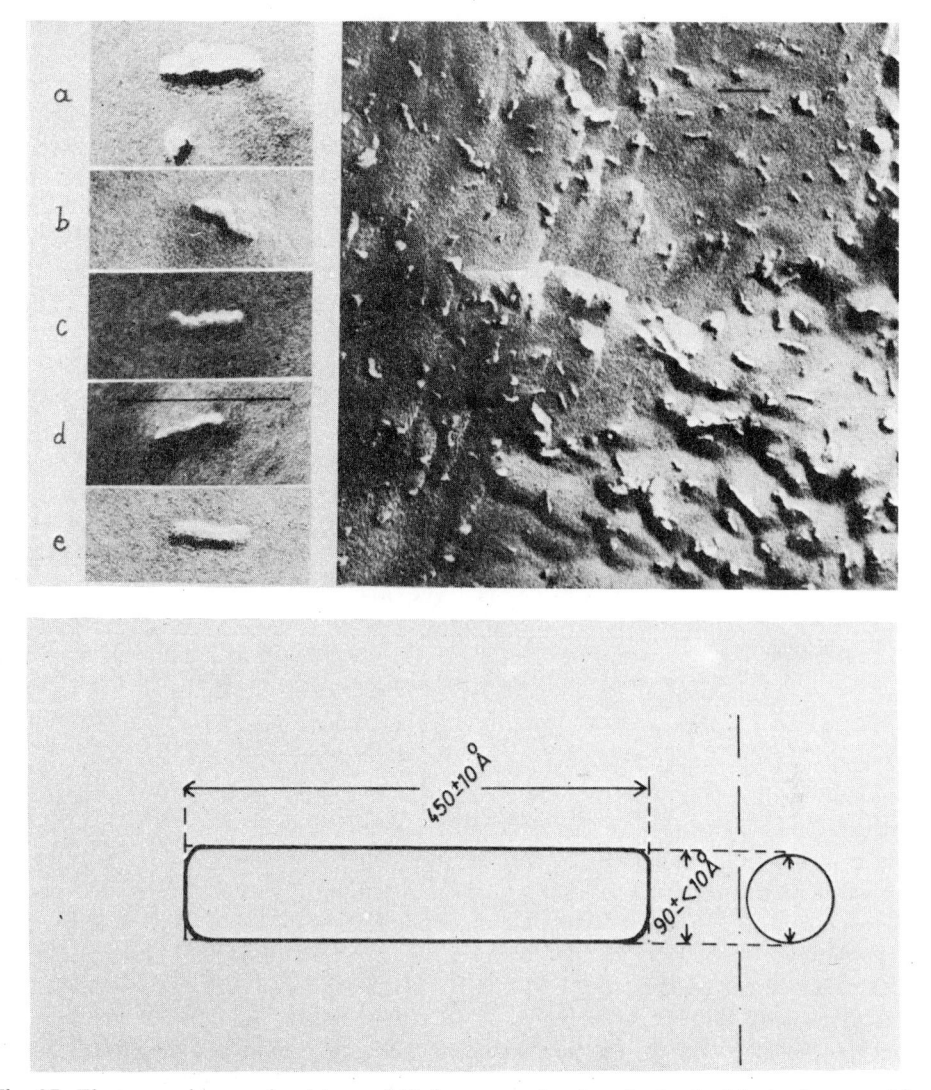

Fig. 87. Electron microscopic picture of fibrinogen molecules obtained with the freeze-etching technique. The right upper part of the picture shows a typical population of molecules. The left upper part of the picture shows various atypical forms present in the population of molecules. The lower part of the picture shows the most likely shape and dimensions of the molecule. By courtesy of Dr K. Lederer, 1973

shape of the molecule is of minor importance in this respect. Most of the models proposed for fibrinogen are candidates for such deliberations as long as they have a twofold symmetry.

3. The subunits and prosthetic groups of fibrinogen

Following sulphitolysis of the disulphide bridges, Henschen (1964) was able to isolate the composite polypeptide chains (Aα, Bβ, and γ) of fibrinogen. Similar results have

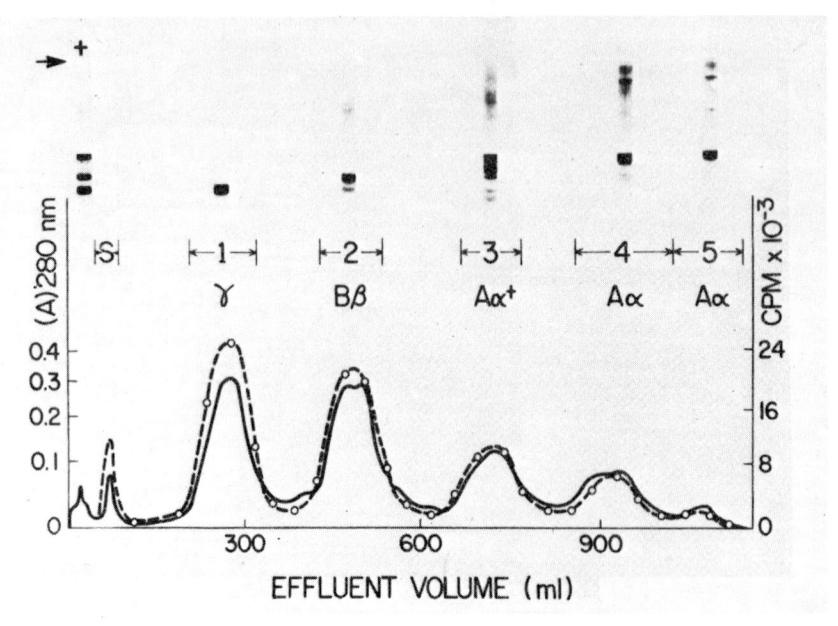

Fig. 88. Chromatogram of S-carboxymethylated (^{3}H) fibrinogen on carboxymethylcellulose.—: extinction at 280 nm. ○-○: radioactivity. In the upper part of the diagram are inserted the polyacrylamide gel patterns of the fractions. From Murano, 1974

been achieved by other workers following carboxymethylation or oxidation of the disulphide bridges (Fig. 88). As only three types of chains could be demonstrated in these experiments and as the intact molecule has been shown by NH$_2$-terminal analysis to have six chains, it would appear that the molecule is composed of three polypeptide chains in a paired dimer. The amino acid composition of carboxymethylated human fibrinogen and its isolated polypeptide chains is shown in Table 44. Polyacrylamide electrophoresis of the polypeptide chains in the presence of sodium dodecylsulphate indicates molecular weights of: Aα 64 000, Bβ 57 000, and γ 48 000. These values are in good agreement with those obtained from sedimentation equilibrium studies. The molecular weight values for the chains suggest a minimum molecular weight of 170 000 for a fibrinogen unit. Consequently the molecular weight of 340 000 attributed to the intact fibrinogen is satisfied by the formula (Aα, Bβ, γ)$_2$.

As one would expect from the observations carried out on intact fibrinogen, heterogeneity has been demonstrated to exist also in the isolated polypeptide chains of the molecule. Murano (1974) mentions at least four variants of the Aα-chain having different chromatographic and/or electrophoretic mobility.

The prosthetic groups of fibrinogen consist of ester-bound phosphate and sulphate as well as carbohydrate. In the case of protein-bound phosphate in human fibrinogen, this is bound partially as serine phosphate in the NH$_2$-terminal portion of the Aα-chain (Aα3 Ser) (cf. Blombäck, 1967. As Aα3 Ser is only phosphorylated to 30 per cent one could conclude that a significant amount of the heterogeneity between different molecules exists because of the extent of phosphorylation. Phosphate is also bound to other parts of the molecule but these are, as yet, not localized. Sulphate is bound as tyrosine-O-sulphate in the Bβ-chain in several animal species (Krajewski and

Table 44. Amino acid analysis of human fibrinogen and its isolated polypeptide chains. (From Cartwright and Kekwick, 1971)

Amino acid	Mole per 10^5 g protein or peptide			
	γ-chain	β (B)-chain	α (A)-chain	Native fibrinogen
Lysine	66.9	67.0	58.9	65.1 ± 1.0
Histidine	18.4	20.2	17.6	18.0 ± 0.2
Arginine	35.5	36.8	59.0	47.1 ± 0.4
Aspartic acid	108.1	119.1	106.3	106.5 ± 3.3
Threonine	51.9	45.5	60.5	53.2 ± 1.7
Serine	51,2	60.3	85.3	71.2 ± 5.0
Glutamic acid	104.7	113.8	99.2	99.4 ± 0.7
Proline	27.6	42.1	54.9	42.1 ± 1.4
Glycine	74.9	85.2	99.0	84.7 ± 3.6
Alanine	52.4	51.8	36.8	41.5 ± 0.9
Half-cystine	17.7	28.0	16.0	21.0 ± 0.4
Valine	38.2	44.9	44.8	40.0 ± 2.5
Methionine	16.9	27.9	16.7	18.9 ± 1.2
Isoleucine	37.7	35.6	39.2	36.0 ± 0.4
Leucine	55.2	54.3	50.4	54.2 ± 0.5
Tyrosine	40.4	38.2	17.8	29.6 ± 1.1

Blombäck, 1968) but this is not the case in human fibrinogen, where a sulphated tyrosine residue is located in some other not yet characterized region of the molecule.

The carbohydrate portion of human fibrinogen is bound to both the γ- and Bβ-chains (Gaffney, 1972). It is uncertain whether the Aα-chain contains carbohydrate residues. The saccharide chains are heterogeneous. They are in general composed of approximately ten monosaccharide residues; the chains are branched and built up of mannose, galactose, glucosamine, and sialic acid. Sialic acid and galactose are situated in the terminal position. The polysaccharide chain is, according to Mester, linked to the polypeptide chain via an asparagine residue (cf. Blombäck, 1972). The compound constituting the link between carbohydrate and protein has been isolated in the form of 2-acetamide-1-N-(4-L-aspartyl)-2-deoxy-β-D-glucosylamine (Mester, 1969). In the γ-chain of human fibrinogen a heterogeneous carbohydrate moeity is most likely bound in this fashion to γ 52 Asn (cf. Blombäck et al., 1976). Further information on the occurrence of carbohydrate in fibrinogen assay may be found in a review on the topic by Blombäck (1972).

The heterogeneity of fibrinogen is adequately explained by the heterogeneity which exists in its isolated chains. As I briefly mentioned earlier, the heterogeneity may result from limited proteolytic degradation caused by exo- and endopeptidases, amidases, and phosphatases. One can also imagine a situation where various amounts of carbohydrate and phosphorous have been incorporated into different molecules during biosynthesis or the production of genetically different molecules. In fact it has been demonstrated that differences exist in the amino acid compositions of different γ-chains suggesting that possibly several types of genes are involved in the synthesis (Henschen and Edman, 1972). We also know that in one fibrinogen, fibrinogen Detroit, an amino acid substitution exists in the Aα-chain (Blombäck et al., 1968b).

4. The primary structure of fibrinogen

The amino acid sequence of fibrinogen is presently under investigation in several laboratories. When we have obtained sufficient insight into the primary structure of fibrinogen, we can understand better the function of the molecule and of diseases where an abnormal function exists. However, a full understanding of the function will probably not be provided by even an elucidation of the primary structure of the molecule. To arrive at this, we probably require an elucidation of the tertiary structure by X-ray crystallography. In any event, the unravelling of the primary structure is a prerequisite to solve the puzzle of the tertiary structure in a meaningful way.

Two types of fragmentation have been of fundamental use in solving the primary structure of fibrinogen. The first type of fragment has been produced using *cyanogen bromide*, a chemical which reacts with methionine residues in a protein. Methionine is converted into homoserine in the process and the amino acid residue which follows is cleaved. In order to place the CNBr-fragments in the intact structure use is made of fragments produced by cleaving with *plasmin* or other proteolytic enzymes. The structures of these will form overlaps between different CNBr-fragments and thereby facilitate the deduction of a unique amino acid sequence for the intact chains.

CNBr-fragments. Cleavage of human fibrinogen with CNBr results in some 30 fragments with molecular weight ranging from less than 2 000 to up to 60 000 (Blombäck et al., 1968a; Gårdlund et al., 1977). Several of these fragments have been isolated in pure form. Interest has been directed primarily towards those fragments which contain disulphide bridges (Table 45). The reason for this is that these bridges often play a decisive role in maintaining the conformation of the protein, and it can be supposed that the primary structure in the proximity of the disulphide bridges is also of importance in determining the function of the protein. Fibrinogen contains 28–

Table 45. Fragments of fibrinogen obtained with cyanogen bromide and plasmin, K denotes the K value for the counter-current system: 2-butanol: 2% CF_3COOH: 0.1% CH_3COOH (2:1:1). (From Gårdlund et al., 1977)

	Moles per mole Fbg	Mol. wt.	Number of chains	Chain identity	S–S per mole Fbg	K
Cyanogen bromide fragments						
N-DSK (Hil-DSK)	1	58 000	2×3	Aα, Bβ, γ	11	0.1
Hi2-DSK	2	28 000	1	α	2	0.1
Ho1-DSK	2	42 500	5	α, β, γ	12	6.2
Ho2-DSK	2	7 000	1	β	2	3.0
Ho3-DSK	2	7 000	2	γ	2	3.0
CNBr-1	2	6 000	1	α	0	—
CNBr-2	2	10 000	1	β	0	—
CNBr-3	—	14 000	1	α	0	—
Plasma fragments						
D	2	85 000–100 000	3	α, β, γ	15–16	—
E	1	50 000	2×3	Aα, Bβ, γ	11	—
PL-1	2	50 000	1	α	2	—
PL-2	2	20 000	1	α	0	—

29 disulphide bridges. The largest CNBr-fragment, having a molecular weight of 58 000, is composed of NH$_2$-terminal fragments of the three chains of fibrinogen (Aα, Bβ, and γ). This fragment, which represents approximately 16 per cent of the entire molecule, contains approximately one-half of the disulphide bridges of the molecule and is given the name 'NH$_2$-terminal disulphide knot' or N-DSK.

Following reduction and alkylation, the chain fragments of N-DSK have been isolated by gel filtration and chromatography. The Aα-chain fragment exists in three molecular forms. Apart from the common form, there is also a phosphorylated variant and a variant which is one amino acid shorter at the NH$_2$-terminal end of the chain. The latter has probably arisen as a result of cleavage of fibrinogen in blood by exopeptidases. The phosphorylated variant may very well be the primary product of biosynthesis, which after secretion from the cell is dephosphorylated in the presence of phosphatases. The γ-chain of N-DSK also displays microheterogeneity which, as is the case for the γ-chain of intact fibrinogen, is dependent on the heterogeneity of the polysaccharide bound to the peptide chain. The amino acid sequence of the chains has been determined by stepwise degradation using the phenylisothiocyanate method of Edman.

The structure of the Aα-chain of N-DSK is shown in Fig. 89 (cf. Blombäck et al., 1976). In the phosphorylated variant (AαP) the phosphoric acid is bound to serine in position 3 and in the variant (AαY), alanine is missing in position 1. Thrombin rapidly cleaves the bond between 16 Arg and 17 Gly in both N-DSK and the isolated Aα-chain fragments, releasing fibrinopeptide A (Aα 1–16). The bond between 19 Arg and 20 Val is cleaved at a much slower rate.

Besides the Aα-chain of N-DSK additional portions of the Aα-chain have recently been sequenced by Hessel (1975); Doolittle et al, (1977a); Gårdlund (1977). In all 198 residues are now known from the NH$_2$-terminal end of the chain. Partial sequences of the CNBr-fragments of the chain including the COOH-terminal portion have also been determined (Doolittle et al., 1977b).

The primary structure of the Bβ-chain of N-DSK is seen in Fig. 89 (cf. Blombäck et al., 1976). In the Bβ-chain thrombin cleaves slowly the 14 Arg–15 Gly bond with release of fibrinopeptide B. The chain consists of 118 amino acid residues. One structural detail of interest is the presence of pyroglutamic acid in the NH$_2$-terminal position. This probably arises after the biosynthesis of the chain by ring closure which takes place between the γ-carboxy and α-amino groups of glutamine. Furthermore, repeating sequences occur frequently in the Bβ-chain. It is possible that these repeated units are an indication of some special regularity in the secondary or tertiary structure of the chain.

The complete primary structure of the entire Bβ-chain will certainly be elucidated in the near future since the primary structure of all its CNBr-fragments has recently been reported by Lottspeich and Henschen (1977a,b).

The γ-chain fragment of N-DSK contains 78 amino acid residues (cf. Blombäck et al., 1976). The structure is represented in Fig. 89. This fragment contains carbohydrate, which is bound to the β-amide group of asparagine in position 52. This is the only position of attachment of carbohydrate in the entire γ-chain. The carbohydrate portion consists of mannose, galactose, glucosamine, and sialic acid. Galactose and/or sialic acid are the terminal residues in the carbohydrate chain which is branched. Because the carbohydrate chains in certain fibrinogen molecules have two sialic acid residues while others have one (or none), there exists a charge heterogeneity in the γ-chain fragment

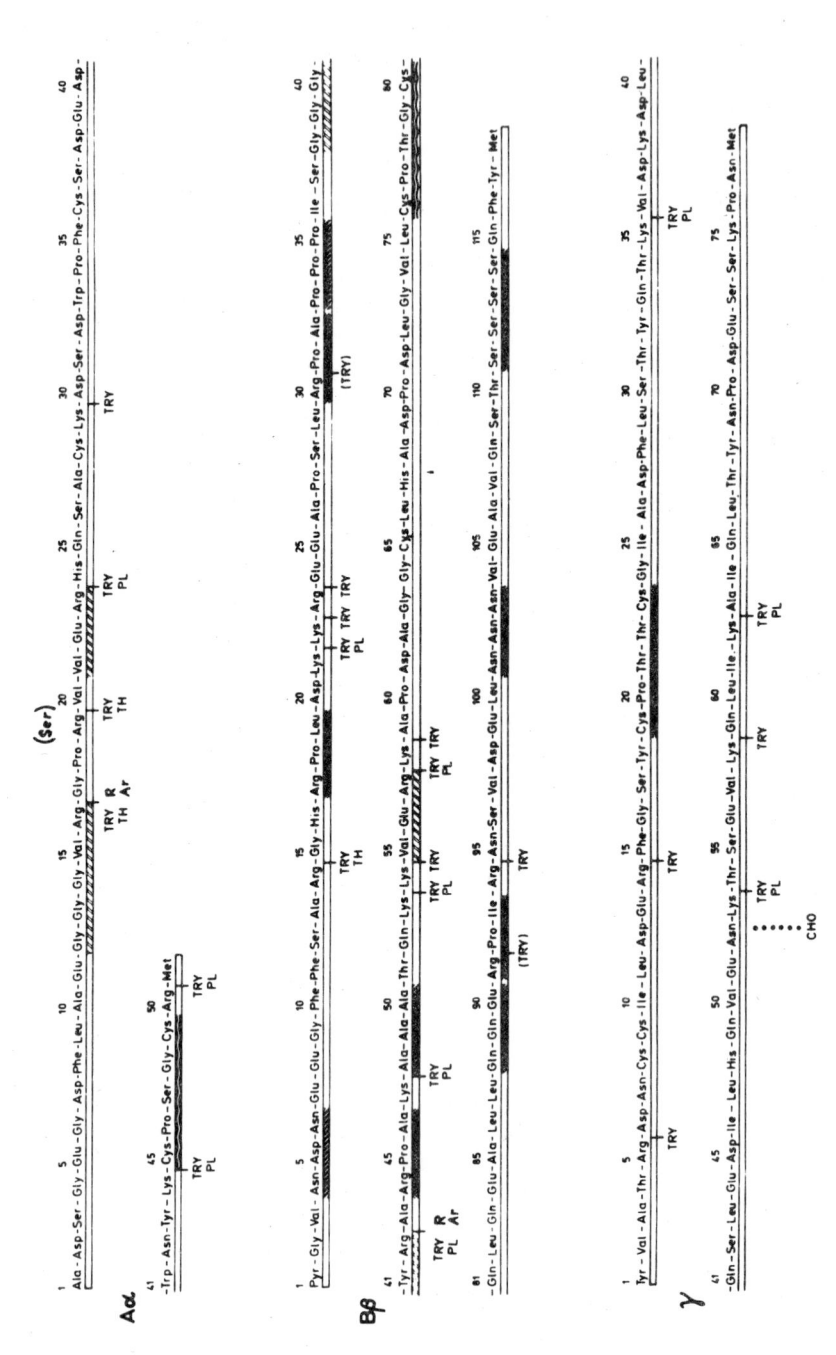

Fig. 89. The amino acid sequences of the Aα-, Bβ- and γ-chains of N-DSK. TH, R, Ar, TRY and PL: positions of cleavage by thrombin, Botroxobin, Arvin, trypsin and plasmin. CHO carbohydrate chain. From B. Hessel, Primary structure of human fibrinogen and fibrin. Thesis 1975. Chemistry Dept., Karolinska Institutet, Stockholm, Sweden

which can be seen in electrophoresis of not only the γ-chain of N-DSK but also in electrophoresis of the intact γ-chain.

In a recent communication by Lottspeich and Henschen (1977b) the essentially complete sequence of the γ-chain was described. It consists of about 410 residues.

Disulphide bridges in N-DSK. The combined molecular weight of the three chain fragments of N-DSK was calculated to be 29 900. As the molecular weight of N-DSK is 58 000 it follows that this probably represents a dimeric structure of three pairs of chains. The conclusion that N-DSK is a dimer implies also that the fibrinogen molecule itself has the same overall structure.

The arrangement of disulphides is depicted in Fig. 90 (cf. Blombäck et al., 1977). As can be seen in this diagram, the two halves of the molecule are connected by symmetrical disulphide bridges in the Aα- and γ-chains. These disulphides have twofold, symmetry axis. In Fig. 90 it can also be seen that the three chains in each half-molecule are linked by disulphide bridges. In this way a particularly compact knot is formed in the molecule (encircled in the diagram). Disulphide exchange appears to take place in this area of the molecule. Evidence for this is the fact that certain disulphide-containing peptides have been isolated which are not compatible with the structure shown in Fig. 90. Instead, they suggest a different arrangement of some disulphide bridges (see inset in Fig. 90). The exchange probably takes place during the isolation of the various disulphide-containing peptides.

Other CNBr-fragments. The disulphide-containing peptides of the remaining CNBr-fragments have all been isolated but their sequences have been only partially determined (Gårdlund et al., 1977). The general properties of the fragments are given in Table 45. The number of disulphides in the various CNBr-fragments of fibrinogen match the 28–29 found in the molecule by Henschen (1964). Besides N-DSK, no disulphide fragments from other parts of the molecule have been shown to contain symmetrical disulphides indicating that the half-molecules in fibrinogen are covalently linked only in the NH_2-terminal portion of the molecule.

Besides the above mentioned disulphide-containing fragments, a number of CNBr-fragments have been isolated (Table 45) which have been shown to be of special importance since they provide overlaps with the fragments produced on degradation of the molecule with plasmin. Figure 91 shows how various CNBr-fragments are arranged in the structure of fibrinogen.

Plasmin fragments. Plasmin has a more narrow specificity than trypsin when digesting fibrinogen. Plasmin rapidly cleaves bonds in the carboxy-terminal portion of the Aα-chain. On the other hand, bonds are also cleaved in both the NH_2- and carboxy-terminal portions of the Bβ-chain. Even the γ-chain is hydrolysed by plasmin, but at a rate which is considerably slower than that for the other two chains (for review see Doolittle 1973; Murano 1974; Gaffney 1977a,b). The cleavage by plasmin follows a typical pattern as shown by Marder et al. (1969). The cleavage produces first a group of fragments which is called X. If digestion is continued a population of degradation products arises which is called Y. The final products of the digestion are the so-called 'core' fragments, D and E, together with a number of smaller fragments (Table 45). Fragment Y is of interest since it is produced from fragment X by release of 1 mol of fragment D per mole. Hence, fragment Y appears to be composed of 1 mol of fragment E and 1 mol of fragment D. Consequently, it is an intermediate arising from an

234 *Proteins taking part in coagulation and fibrinolysis*

Symmetry/axis

Aα - Cys-Lys-Asp-Ser-Asp-
     28

Aα - Cys-Lys-Asp-Ser-Asp-Trp-Pro-Phe-Cys-Ser-Asp-Glu-Asp-Trp-Asn-Tyr-Lys-Cys-
     28   36   45

Bβ - Cys-Leu-His-Ala-Asp-Pro-Asp-Leu-Gly-Val-Leu-Cys-Pro-Thr-
     65   76

γ - Cys-Cys-Ile-Leu-
    8 9

γ - Cys-Cys-Ile-Leu-Asp-Glu-Arg-Phe-Gly-Ser-Tyr-Cys-Pro-Thr-Cys
    8 9   21

Pro-Ser-Gly-
    23

Cys-Arg-
    44

Cys-Pro-Thr-Cys
    61

Cys-Gln-Leu-
    80

Alternative arrangement of disulphides:

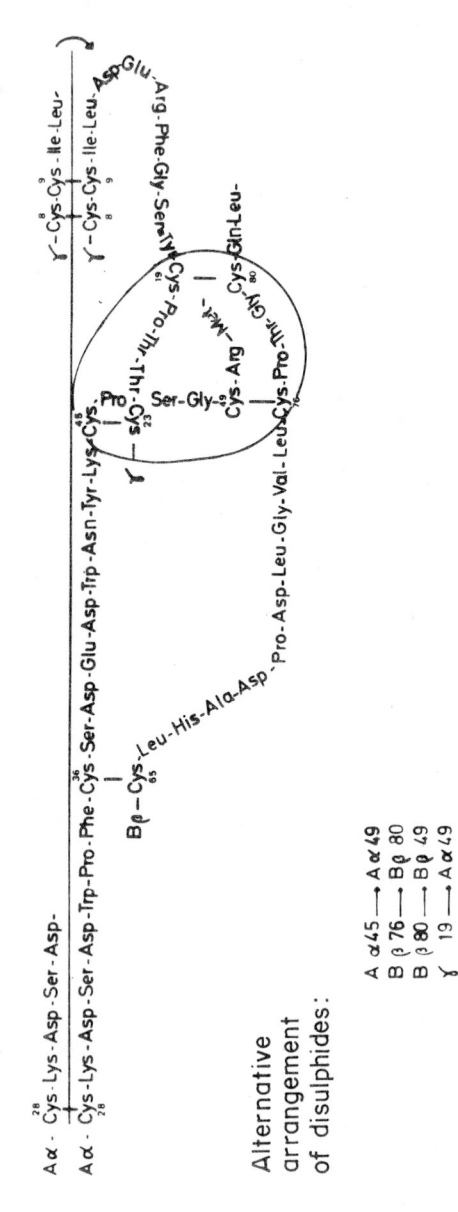

A α45 ⟶ A α49
B β76 ⟶ B β80
B β80 ⟶ B β49
γ 19 ⟶ A α49

Fig. 90. The arrangement of the disulphide bridges in N-DSK. The disulphides in the circled region are the so-called labile disulphides, i.e. those found to take part in disulphide exchange. Alternative arrangements in this area are known to exist, see Blombäck, Hessel, and Hogg, 1976

II. Fibrinogen and fibrin formation   235

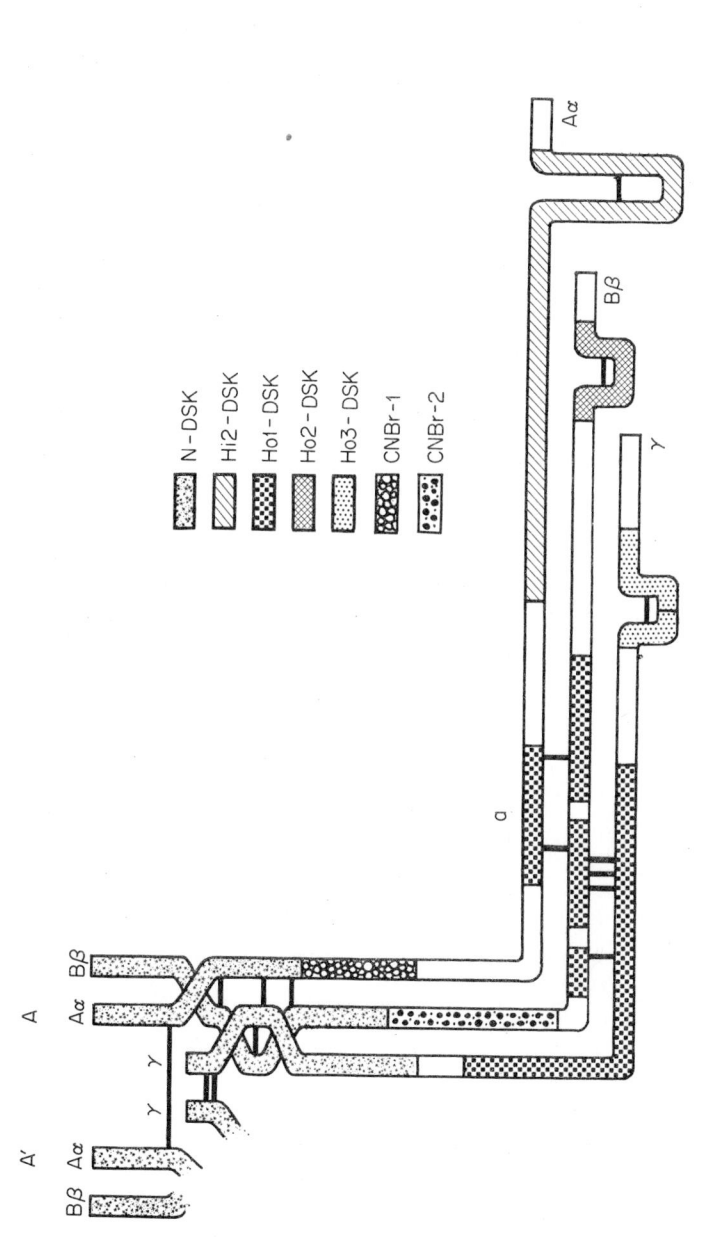

Fig. 91. Schematic representation of the fibrinogen half-molecule with the remaining half-molecule partially indicated. Cyanogen bromide fragments are inserted in the structure. Black bars indicate disulphide bridges, A and a indicate the localization of polymerization domains. Of the corresponding domains (A', a') on the contralateral side only the localization of the A' domains is indicated

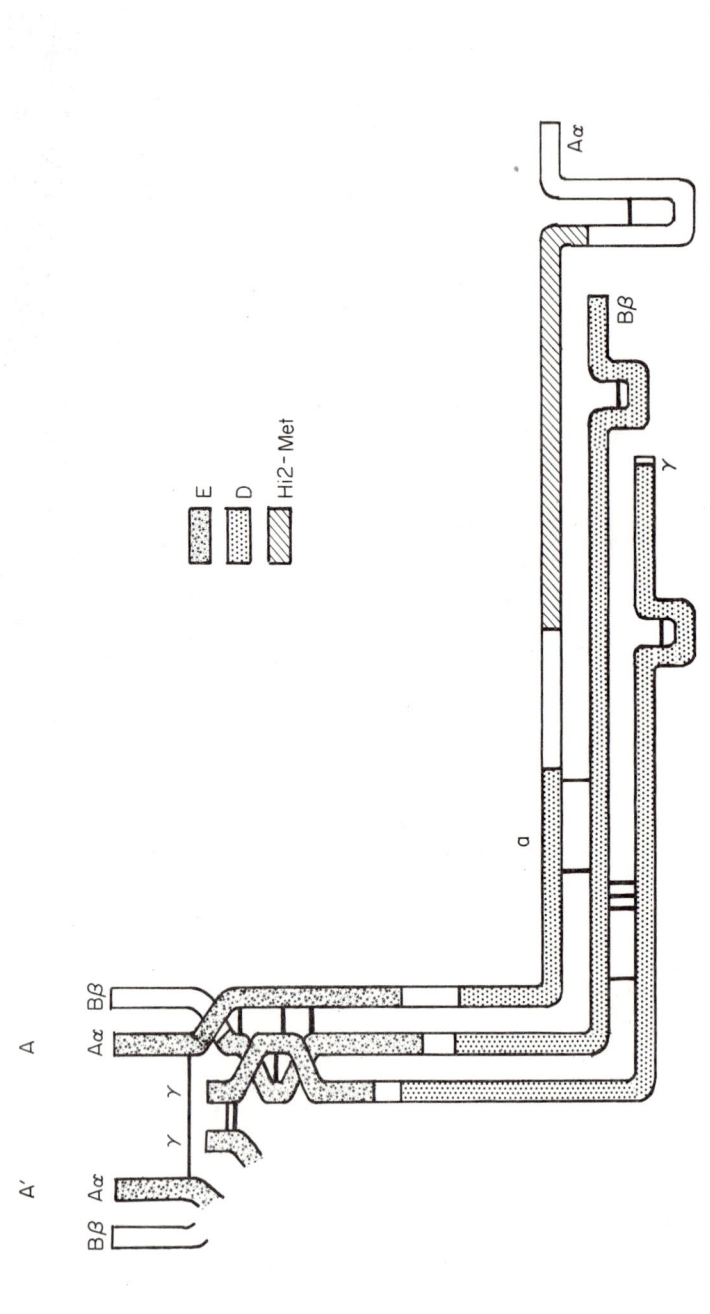

236 *Proteins taking part in coagulation and fibrinolysis*

Fig. 92. Schematic representation of the fibrinogen half-molecule with the remaining half-molecule partially indicated. Plasmin fragments are inserted in the structure. E and D indicate classical plasmic fragments. Hi2-Met stands for one of the remaining major fragments isolated from a plasmic digest of fibrinogen. Regarding explanation for A, A', and a see Fig. 91

unsymmetrical cleavage of fragment X. The positions of some plasmin fragments within the fibrinogen molecule are depicted in Fig. 92. By comparing Figs. 91 and 92 it can be seen that fragment E has a considerable portion of its structure in common with N-DSK (cf. Blombäck et al., 1976). In contrast to N-DSK, fragment E is devoid of the first 53 amino acid residues of the Bβ-chain and the carboxy-terminal portion of the γ-chain in N-DSK. Furthermore, fragment E has a somewhat longer Aα- and Bβ-chain than N-DSK. Based on the structure of the latter extensions it became possible to isolate CNBr-fragments providing overlaps in the Aα- and Bβ-chains in fragment D (schematically represented in Fig. 93).

Most investigators have isolated fragment D as a monomeric structure. Since fibrinogen is a dimer, it follows that there must exist two D fragments per molecule of fibrinogen. It should be mentioned that dimeric types of fragment D have also been proclaimed by Mosesson et al. (see Mosesson and Finlayson, 1976). However, a dimeric rather than a monomeric fragment D would not necessarily change the general conclusions arrived at in this report with regard to the overall structure of fibrinogen. In my further deliberations I will only consider the case when fragment D is monomeric. Fragment D consists of three chains which have their respective origins in the Aα-, Bβ-, and γ-chains of fibrinogen (cf. Blombäck et al., 1976). It has been found that the γ-chain of fragment D has structures in common with the carboxy-terminal portion of the γ-chain of N-DSK (Fig. 93). Furthermore a CNBr-fragment has been isolated from the Bβ-chain, providing an overlap between this chain in fragment E and fragment D (Gårdlund, 1977). Another CNBr-fragment from the Aα-chain forms an overlap between fragment E and the α-chain in fragment D*. No CNBr-fragment has been found up until now which provides overlap between carboxy-terminal plasmic fragments and the α-chain of fragment D.

5. Fibrin—the ordered structure of fibrinogen

The fibrinogen–fibrin transformation takes place after removal of two acidic peptides from the NH$_2$-terminal portion of the Aα- and Bβ-chains. The molecular weight of the

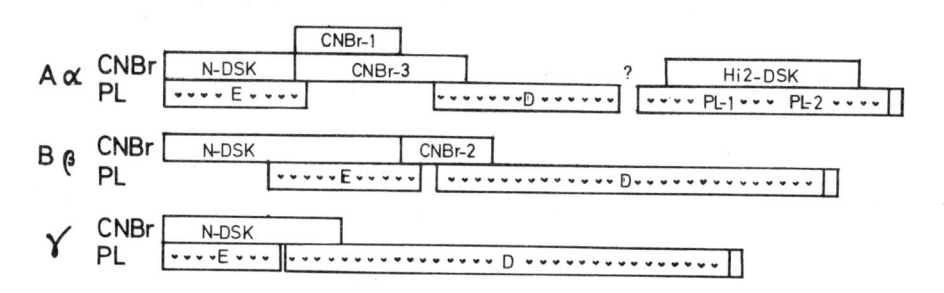

Fig. 93. Schematic representation showing the overlaps between CNBr and plasmic fragments in the three chains of fibrinogen. The principal fragment to which the chain fragments belong are indicated in the diagram

*This fragment was obtained by limited treatment of fibrinogen with CNBr (Gårdlund, personal communication 1974).

fibrinopeptides varies between 1 500 and 3 000 depending on the species from which they have been isolated (for review see Blombäck, 1967; Doolittle, 1973). Depending on their origin in the chains of fibrinogen the peptides are denoted as either fibrinopeptide A or fibrinopeptide B. The release of these peptides is effected by hydrolytic cleavage, catalysed by thrombin. Thrombin is a trypsin-like enzyme which in protein substrates has a narrow specificity. Of the few hundred trypsin-sensitive bonds in fibrinogen, only four are cleaved by thrombin, resulting in release from the fibrinogen molecule of two molecules each of fibrinopeptides A and B.

Fibrinopeptide A is always released first (Fig. 94). After a lag-phase, the release of fibrinopeptide B is greatly accelerated. Polymerization of the thrombin-activated fibrinogen molecules begins even before measurable amounts of fibrinopeptide B have been released. Fibrinopeptide A from various species shows a marked homology in amino acid sequence. This is especially true for the structure in close proximity to the thrombin-sensitive arginyl–glycyl bond (16 Arg-17 Gly in human fibrinogen) (Fig. 95). The preservation during evolution of structures in fibrinopeptide B is not as evident as is the case with fibrinopeptide A (Fig. 96). Thrombin has primarily affinity for structures in the Aα-chain, explaining the release of fibrinopeptide A without a lag-phase. The specificity with regard to the Aα-chain is dependent on a short amino acid sequence around the thrombin-susceptible bond. Thus it would appear that all of the elements required for recognition by thrombin are present in the first 51 amino acid residues of the Aα-chain. Studies of kinetic parameters in thrombin-susceptible substrates have suggested that the sequence Aα 8–23 in human fibrinogen is of prime importance for the fibrinogen–thrombin interaction. The sequence Aα 33–51 is also of some importance in guiding the interaction (Blombäck et al., 1977; Scheraga, 1977). The importance

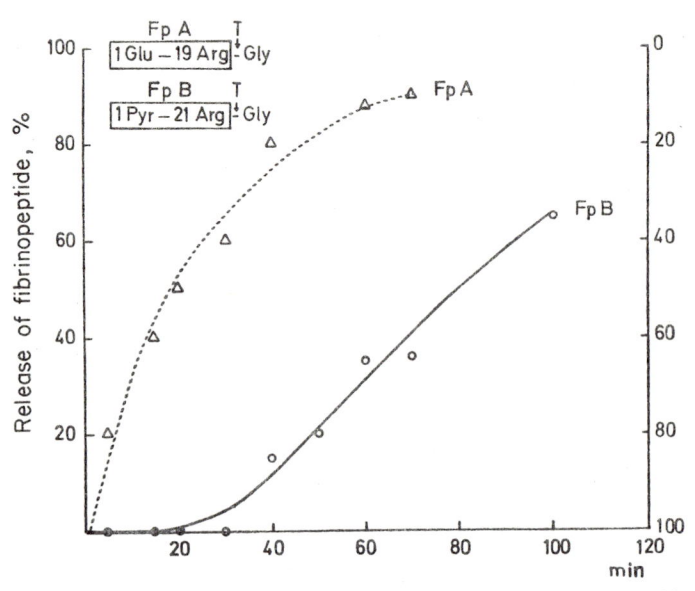

Fig. 94. Release of fibrinopeptides A and B from bovine fibrinogen after addition of thrombin. ---- fibrinopeptide A; —— fibrinopeptide B. The susceptible bonds are shown in the upper part of the figure

of structures residing in fibrinopeptide A for thrombin–fibrinogen recognition was already postulated on the basis of comparative structural studies of fibrinopeptide A in different animal species (cf. Blombäck et al., 1977).

In fibrinogen Detroit (Blombäck et al., 1968b) a mutation has taken place at position 19 in the Aα-chain where an arginine in normal fibrinogen has been replaced by serine. This mutation has taken place in the constant (or invariable) portion of the chain. In fibrinogen Detroit thrombin releases fibrinopeptide A at almost the same rate as from normal fibrinogen. This suggests that the arginine residue at position 19 in normal fibrinogen does not play a major role in the binding of thrombin to its substrate.

The polymerization of fibrinogen can be explained by intermolecular interaction of functional domains within the molecule after activation by thrombin (Blombäck and Blombäck, 1972). It appears that the fibrinogen molecule has two sets of functional domains (Fig. 91). One set of domains became active on release of fibrinopeptide A. This set consists of the domains A and A' which are located in N-DSK in the NH_2-terminal part of the molecule and the domains a and a' which are located in fragment D in the COOH-terminal part of the molecule. The domains A and A' are indeed structurally identical but because the half-molecules in fibrinogen have one twofold axis of symmetry these halves will not appear identical. On viewing from any one direction, we see the polypeptide chains of one side of the molecule, while the corresponding chains of the other half of the molecule present their reverse sides (Fig. 97). The same reasoning applies for the steric arrangement of a and a' which also are structurally identical. This mode of symmetry in the molecule is supported by the chemical investigations which show that the half-molecules of N-DSK (AA' domains) are joined by three symmetrical disulphide bridges, one in the Aα-chain and two, juxtapositioned, in the γ-chain (Blombäck et al., 1976; cf. Blombäck et al., 1977). This leaves us, for steric reasons, with the conclusion that there exists only one twofold axis of symmetry, i.e. by turning the molecule 180° the new reflection can not be distinguished from the original one. Since the symmetry displayed by the smallest parts of a unit must also apply to the whole we conclude that the complementary domain aa' in fragment D must have the same symmetry. These conclusions regarding symmetry obviously apply to any shape the fibrinogen molecule eventually may turn out to have.

In our model of the molecule the release of fibrinopeptide A takes place in the domains A and A'. Through the release of fibrinopeptide A a rearrangement or conformational change takes place in these domains, thereby exposing a structure which is active in polymerization. The activated domains have the ability to interact with the domains a and a', respectively, in another fibrinogen—or thrombin-activated fibrinogen molecule (i.e. fibrinmonomer). The domains a and a' are functional in fibrinogen as it circulates in blood, but as long as activation of the domains A and A' has not taken place, polymerization and clot formation do not occur. As each fibrinogen molecule consists of two half-molecules, each having two active domains, we can easily visualize how a fibrin thread can arise via 'end-to-end' joining of an activated A or A' site in the NH_2-terminal portion of one molecule to an a or a' site in another molecule (Fig. 98). In this model each molecule in the fibre covers half of the preceding one.

The other set of functional domains is very likely activated on release of fibrinopeptide B. We assume that this set of domains also consists of two complementary structures which we denote BB' and bb', respectively (Fig. 91). The location of these domains in the molecule is not yet known.

Proteins taking part in coagulation and fibrinolysis

	19	18	17	16	15	14	13	12	11	10	9	8	7	6	5	4	3	2	1	
			N-ALA	ASP	SER	GLY	THR	GLU	GLY	ASP	PHE	LEU	ALA	GLU	GLY	GLY	GLY	VAL	ARG-OH	MAN
			N-ALA	ASP	SER	VAL	THR	GLU	GLY	ASP(GLU)	PHE(LEU	ALA	GLU	GLY	GLY	GLY	VAL	ARG-OH	GIBBON
			N-ALA	ASP	THR	GLY	THR	GLU	GLY	ASP	PHE	LEU	ALA	GLU	GLY	GLY	GLY	VAL	ARG-OH	RHESUS MONKEY
			N-ALA.	ASP.	THR.	GLY.	ASP.	GLY.	ASP.	PHE)ILE	(THR.	GLU.	GLY.	GLY)	VAL	ARG-OH	DRILL			
			N-VAL	ASP	PRO	GLY	LYS	GLY	THR	GLU	PHE	ILE	ASP	GLU	GLY	ALA	GLY	VAL	ARG-OH	RABBIT
		N-ALA	ASP	THR	GLY	THR	SER	GLU	PHE	ILE	(ASP	GLY	ALA	GLY	ILE)	ARG-OH	RAT			
							N-THR	ASP	THR	GLU	PHE	ILE	ALA	ALA	GLY	ALA(ALA	GLY)	ARG-OH	GUINEA PIG
			N-THR	ASN	VAL	LYS	GLU	SER	GLU	PHE	ILE	ALA	GLU	GLY	GLY	VAL	ARG-OH	MINK		
			N-THR	ASP	VAL	LYS	GLU	SER	GLU	PHE	ILE	ALA	ALA	GLY	ALA	GLY	VAL	ARG-OH	BADGER	
			N-THR	ASN	SER	GLY	GLU	GLY	GLU	PHE	ILE	ALA	GLU	GLY	VAL	GLY	VAL	ARG-OH	DOG, FOX	
			N-THR	ASP	GLY	LYS	GLY	GLY	GLU	PHE	ILE	ALA	GLU	GLY	GLY	GLY	VAL	ARG-OH	BROWN BEAR	
			N-GLY	ASP	VAL	GLN	GLY	GLU	GLU	PHE	ILE	ALA	GLU	GLY	GLY	GLY	VAL	ARG-OH	CAT, LION	
			N-THR	ASP	THR	LYS	GLU(SER.	ASP.	GLU	PHE	LEU	ALA	GLU	GLY	GLY.	GLY.	VAL)	ARG-OH	GRAY SEAL	
					N-THR	GLU	GLY	GLY	GLU	PHE	LEU	HIS	GLU	GLY	GLY	GLY	VAL	ARG-OH	HORSE, MULE 1	
			N-THR	LYS	THR	GLU	GLY	GLY	GLU	PHE	ILE	SER	GLU	GLY	GLY	GLY	VAL	ARG-OH	DONKEY, MULE 2	
			N-THR	LYS	THR	GLU	GLY	GLY	GLU	PHE	ILE	GLY	GLU	GLY	GLY(GLY.	VAL)	ARG-OH	ZEBRA 1		
			N-THR	LYS	THR	GLU	GLY	GLY	GLU	PHE	ILE	SER	GLU	GLY	GLY(ALA.	GLY.	VAL)	ARG-OH	ZEBRA 2	
			N-THR	THR	VAL	GLU	GLN(SER.	GLY.	GLX)	PHE(LEU.	ALA.	GLU.	GLY.	GLY.	GLY)	ARG-OH	COLLARED PECCARY			
			N-ALA	GLU	VAL	GLN	ASP	LYS	GLY	GLU	PHE	LEU	ALA	GLU	GLY	GLY	GLY	VAL	ARG-OH	PIG, BOAR
		N-THR.	ASP.	PRO.	ASP.	ALA.	ASP.	LYS.	GLY.	GLY.	(GLU)	PHE(LEU.	ALA.	GLU.	GLY.	GLY.	VAL)	ARG-OH	LLAMA		
		N-(THR.	ASP.	PRO.	ASP.	ALA.	ASP.	LYS.	GLY.	GLY.	GLU)	PHE(LEU.	ALA.	GLU.	GLY.	GLY.	VAL)	ARG-OH	VICUNA		
			N-THR	ASP	PRO	ALA	ASP	LYS	GLY	ASP	PHE	LEU	ALA	GLU	GLY	GLY	GLY	VAL	ARG-OH	CAMELS
			N-THR	ASP	PRO	ALA	ASP	PRO	GLY	ASP	PHE	LEU	THR	GLU	GLY	GLY	GLY	VAL	ARG-OH	OX
		N-GLU	ASP	GLY	SER	ASP	PRO	PRO	SER	GLY	ASP	PHE	LEU(ALA.	GLU.	GLY.	GLY.	GLY.	VAL)	ARG-OH	EUROPEAN BISON	
		N-GLU	ASP	GLY	SER	ASP	PRO	GLY	ALA	SER	GLY	ASP	PHE	LEU	ALA	GLU	GLY	GLY	VAL	ARG-OH	CAPE BUFFALO
					N-GLU	ASP	GLY	SER	ASP	PRO	PRO	GLU	PHE	LEU(ALA.	GLY.	GLY.	GLY.	VAL)	ARG-OH	WATER BUFFALO
	N-GLU	ASP	GLY.	SER.	ASP.	GLY.	VAL	ALA	SER	GLY.	GLU.	PHE.	LEU.	ALA.	GLU.	GLY.	GLY.	GLY.	VAL)	ARG-OH	SHEEP
	N-ALA	ASP	PRO	ASP	ALA	VAL	GLN	GLY	GLY	GLU	PHE	LEU	ALA	GLU	GLY	GLY	GLY	VAL	ARG-OH	PERSIAN GAZELLE
			N-ALA	ASP	SER	ASP(PRO.	ALA.	ASP.	LYS.	GLY.	GLY.)	PHE	LEU	ALA	GLU	GLY	GLY	GLY	VAL	ARG-OH	PRONGHORN
			N-THR	ASP	SER	ASP	PRO	VAL	GLY	GLY	GLU	PHE	LEU	ALA	ASP.	GLY.	ALA.	THR,	GLY)	ARG-OH	REINDEER
			N-THR	ASP	SER	ASP	PRO	ALA	GLY	GLY	SER	PHE(LEU.	PRO.	GLU.	GLY.	GLY.	GLY.	VAL)	ARG-OH	MULE DEER	
			N-SER	ASP	SER	ASP	PRO	ALA	GLY	GLY	GLU	PHE	LEU	ALA	GLU	GLY	GLY	GLY	VAL	ARG-OH	MUNT JAK
	N-(ALA.	ASP.	GLY.	SER.	ASP.	PRO.	ALA.	SER.	GLY.	GLU.	PHE(LEU.	THR.	GLU.	GLY.	GLY.	GLY.	VAL)	ARG-OH	SIKA DEER		
	N-ALA	ASP	GLY(SER.	ASP.	PRO.	ALA.	SER.	GLY.	GLU.	PHE)LEU.	ALA.	GLU.	GLY.	GLY.	GLY.	VAL)	ARG-OH	RED DEER			
	N-ALA	ASP	GLY	SER	ASP	PRO	ALA	SER	GLY	ASP	PHE	LEU	ALA	GLU	GLY	GLY	GLY	VAL	ARG-OH	AMERICAN ELK	
	N-(ALA.	ASP.	GLY.	SER.	ASP.	PRO.	ALA.	SER.	GLU.	GLU.	PHE)LEU.	ALA.	GLU.	GLY.	GLY.	GLY.	VAL)	ARG-OH	KANGAROO		
					N-THR	LYS	ASP	GLY	THR	ASP	PHE	ILE	ALA	GLU	GLY	GLY	GLY	VAL	ARG-OH	WOMBAT
				N-THR	LYS	THR	GLU	GLY	SER	SER	PHE	LEU	ALA	GLU	GLY	GLY	GLY	VAL	ARG-OH	LIZARD	
					N-GLU	ASP	THR	GLY	THR	PHE	GLU	GLU	GLY(GLY.	GLY.	GLY.	HIS,	VAL,	VAL)	ARG-OH	

Fig. 95. Fibrinopeptide A from different animal species. The amino acid sequences have been elucidated by Blombäck (1970) and by Doolittle and co-workers (1973). (Figs. 95 and 96 are from M.O. Dayhoff: *Atlas of Protein Sequence and Structure.* Washington, D.C.: National Biomedical Research Foundation, 1972, Vol. V, p. D. 87) Mule has equal amounts of horse and donkey fibrinopeptides. In zebra two types of fibrinopeptides have been found

21	20	19	18	17	16	15	14	13	12	11	10	9	8	7	6	5	4	3	2	1	
							⊏GLU	GLY	VAL	ASN	ASP	ASN	GLU	GLU	GLY	PHE	PHE	SER	ALA	ARG-OH	MAN
							⊏GLU	GLY	VAL	ASX	ASX	ASX	GLX	GLX	GLY	LEU(	PHE.	GLY)	ALA	ARG-OH	ORANGUTAN
								⊏GLU(	GLY.	VAL.	ASX.	ASX.	ASX.	GLX=	GLY.	LEU)	PHE(	GLY.	ALA)	ARG-OH	GIBBON
							⊏GLU(	GLY.	VAL.	ASX,	GLY)	ASN	GLU	GLU	GLY	LEU	PHE	GLY	GLY	ARG-OH	GREEN MONKEY
												N-ASN	GLU	GLU	SER	PRO	PHE	SER	GLY	ARG-OH	RHESUS MONKEY
							⊏GLU(	GLY.	VAL.	ASX,	GLY,	ASX.	GLU.	GLU.	GLY.	LEU)	PHE.	GLY	GLY	ARG-OH	DRILL
								N-ALA	ASP	ASP	TYR	ASP	ASP	GLU	VAL	LEU	PRO	ASP	ALA	ARG-OH	RABBIT
							N-ALA	THR	THR	ASP	SER	ASP	LYS	VAL	ASP(	ILE,	LEU,	SER.	ALA)	ARG-OH	RAT
		N-HIS	TYR	TYR	ASP	ASP	THR	ASP	GLU	GLU	GLU	ARG	ILE	VAL	SER	THR	VAL	ASP	ALA	ARG-OH	DOG
		(⊏GLU.	TYR.	TYR.	ASP.	ASP.	THR.	ASP.	GLU.	GLU.	GLU.	ARG.	ILE.	VAL.	SER.	THR.	VAL.	ASP.	ALA)	ARG-OH	FOX
	N-ILE	ILE	ASP	TYR	TYR	ASP	GLU	GLY	GLU	GLU	ASP	ARG	ASP	VAL	GLY	VAL	VAL	ASP.	ALA.	ARG-OH	CAT
		N-ILE	ASP	TYR	TYR	ASP(	GLU.	GLY.	GLU.	GLU.	ASP)	ARG(	ALA,	VAL,	GLY)	PHE(	VAL.	ASP.	ALA)	ARG-OH	LION
		N-LEU	ASP	TYR	ASP	HIS	GLU	GLU	GLU	ASP	GLY	ARG	THR	LYS	VAL	THR	PHE	ASP	ALA	ARG-OH	HORSE
		N-LEU	ASP	TYR	ASP	HIS	GLU	GLU	GLU	ASP	GLY	ARG	THR	LYS(	VAL.	THR.	PHE.	ASP.	ALA)	ARG-OH	DONKEY
		N-LEU	ASP	TYR	ASP	HIS	GLU	GLU	GLU	ASP	GLY(	ARG.	ALA.	LYS.	VAL.	THR.	PHE.	ASP.	ALA)	ARG-OH	ZEBRA
		N-ALA	ILE	ASP	TYR	ASP	GLU	ASP	GLU	ASP	GLY	ARG	PRO	LYS	VAL	HIS	VAL	ASP	ALA	ARG-OH	PIG
		N-ALA	THR	ASP	TYR	ASP	GLU	GLU	GLU	ASP	ASP	ARG	VAL(	LYS.	VAL.	ARG.	LEU.	ASP.	ALA)	ARG-OH	LLAMA
		N-(ALA.	THR.	ASP.	TYR.	ASP.	GLU.	GLU.	GLU.	ASP.	ASP)	ARG	VAL	LYS	VAL	ARG(	LEU.	ASP.	ALA)	ARG-OH	VICUNA
		N-ALA	THR	ASP	TYR	ASP	GLU	GLU	GLU	ASP	ASP	ARG	VAL	LYS	VAL	ARG	LEU	ASP	ALA	ARG-OH	CAMELS
⊏GLU	PHE	PRO	THR	ASP	TYR	ASP	GLU	GLY	GLN	ASP	ASP	ARG	PRO	LYS	VAL	GLY	LEU	GLY	ALA	ARG-OH	OX
(⊏GLU.	PHE.	PRO.	THR.	ASP.	TYR.	ASP.	GLU.	GLY.	GLU.	ASP.	ASP.	ARG.	PRO.	LYS)	VAL	GLY	LEU	GLY	ALA	ARG-OH	EUROPEAN BISON
⊏GLU(	PHE.	PRO.	THR.	ASP.	TYR.	ASP.	GLU.	GLY.	GLU.	ASP.	ASP.	ARG.	PRO.	LYS)	SER(	GLY.	LEU.	GLY.	ALA)	ARG-OH	CAPE BUFFALO
⊏GLU(	PHE.	PRO.	THR=	ASP.	TYR.	ASP.	GLU.	GLY.	GLN.	ASP.	ASP.	ARG.	PRO)	LYS(	LEU.	GLY.	LEU.	GLY.	ALA)	ARG-OH	WATER BUFFALO
	N-GLY	TYR	LEU	ASP	TYR	ASP	GLU	VAL	ASP	ASP	ASN	ARG	ALA	LYS	LEU	PRO	LEU	ASP	ALA	ARG-OH	SHEEP
	⊏GLU	TYR	SER	ASP(	TYR.	ASP.	GLU.	VAL.	GLU.	GLU.	ASP.	ARG.	PRO.	LYS)	SER	ARG(	VAL.	ASP.	ALA)	ARG-OH	PERS GAZELLE
⊏GLU(	PRO,	SER=	ASP.	TYR.	TYR.	ASP.	GLU.	GLU.	GLU.	ASP.	ASP)	ARG	ALA	LYS	LEU	ARG(	LEU.	ASP.	ALA)	ARG-OH	PRONGHORN
⊏GLU	HIS	LEU	ALA	ASP	TYR	ASP	GLU	VAL(	GLU.	ASP.	ASP)	ARG	ALA	LYS	LEU	HIS	LEU	ASP	ALA	ARG-OH	REINDEER
⊏GLU	HIS	LEU(	ALA.	ASP.	TYR.	ASP.	GLU.	VAL)	ASP	ASP	ASP	ARG	ALA	LYS(	LEU.	HIS.	LEU)	ASP	ALA	ARG-OH	MULE DEER
⊏GLU(	HIS.	SER.	THR=	ASP.	TYR.	ASP.	GLU.	VAL.	GLU.	ASP.	ASP)	ARG	ALA	LYS(	LEU.	HIS.	LEU.	ASP.	ALA)	ARG-OH	MÙNT JAK
(⊏GLU.	HIS.	SER.	THR.	ASP.	TYR.	ASP.	GLU.	GLU.	GLU.	GLU.	ASP.	ARG.	ALA.	LYS.	LEU.	HIS.	LEU.	ASP.	ALA)	ARG-OH	SIKA DEER
(⊏GLU.	HIS.	SER.	THR.	ASP.	TYR.	ASP.	GLU.	GLU.	GLU.	GLU.	ASP.	ARG=	ALA	LYS=	LEU.	HIS.	LEU.	ASP.	ALA)	ARG-OH	RED DEER
⊏GLU(	HIS.	SER.	THR=	ASP.	TYR.	ASP.	GLU.	GLU.	GLU.	GLU.	ASP)	ARG	ALA	LYS(	LEU.	HIS.	LEU.	ASP.	ALA)	ARG-OH	AMERICAN ELK
N-SER	PHE	ASP	TYR	ASP	ASP	ASP	THR	GLY(	GLU,	GLY,	GLY,	GLY,	VAL,	LYS,	SER,	SER,	VAL,	ASP,	ALA)	ARG-OH	KANGAROO

Fig. 96. Fibrinopeptide B from different animal species. The amino acid sequences have been elucidated by Blombäck and co-workers (see Blombäck, 1970) and by Doolittle and co-workers (see Doolittle, 1973). 1.

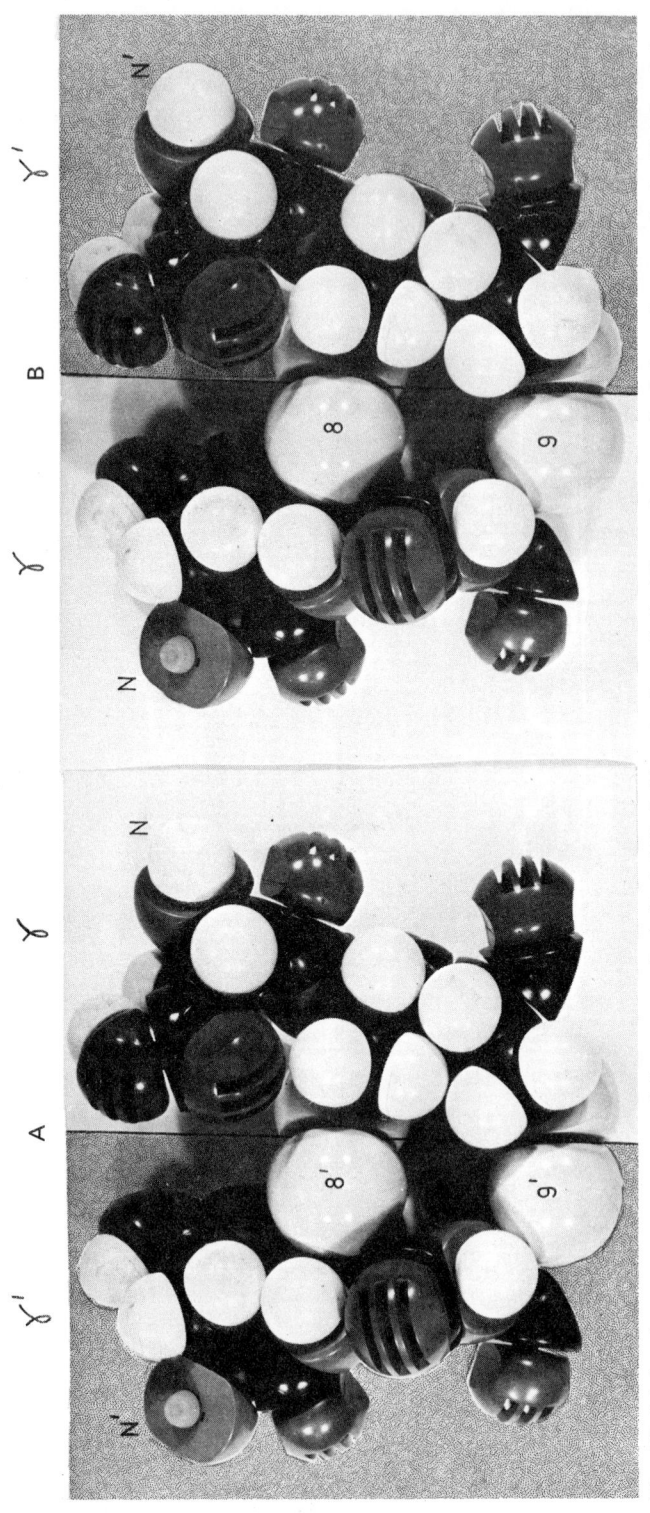

242 *Proteins taking part in coagulation and fibrinolysis*

Fig. 97. Molecular arrangement around the symmetrical disulphide bridges in the γ-chain. The amino terminals have been marked with N and the sulphur atoms with 8 and 9, respectively; (*a*) before and (*b*) after rotation of the molecule 180°. It is evident from these pictures that it is not possible to distinguish between the two γ chains (γ and γ') after rotation

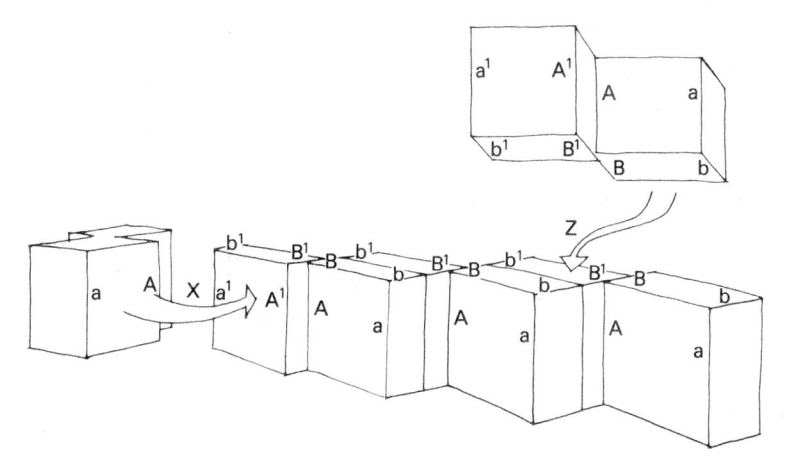

Fig. 98. Schematic representation of fibrin thread formation. In this model, rectangular boxes have been used as building units. These are joined in a double molecule having a twofold symmetry. The domains AA′–aa′ are thought to be situated at the opposite ends on the broad sides of the boxes while the domains BB′–bb′ are located at opposite ends of the narrow sides of the boxes. A polymer arises through 'end-to-end' polymerization by the domain a or a′ binding to the complementary domain A or A′(X). In a similar manner, 'side-to-side' polymerization takes place, causing branching of the initial polymer by combining of the narrow sides of the boxes (Z). The arrows indicate the binding position of the units

As previously mentioned the thrombin-induced release of fibrinopeptide B requires prior release of fibrinopeptide A. This is most likely the result of a conformational change which takes place in the molecule on release of fibrinopeptide A. In this way, fibrinopeptide B becomes accessible to thrombin and following its release the interaction BB′ and bb′ occurs. However, the release of fibrinopeptide B is slow until, after a lag-phase, the release is dramatically accelerated. This acceleration appears to be a result of the BB′ and bb′ interaction. The polymerization involving these sites appears to induce an additional conformational strain on the Bβ-chain thereby facilitating the release of fibrinopeptide B.

Evidence for the existence of two sets of complementary binding domains in fibrinogen–fibrin conversion is found in the fact that removal of fibrinopeptide A alone by the snake venom enzyme, Bothroxobin, gives rise to a polymer which is different from that which forms when both fibrinopeptide A and B are released in the presence of thrombin. In the latter case, the polymer is more compact than that obtained in the presence of Bothroxobin (cf. Blombäck et al., 1977). Further evidence for the existence of two sets of polymerization domains is obtained from investigations of fibrinogen Detroit. In this fibrinogen the AA′ and aa′ domains are inactive even after release of fibrinopeptide A. On release of fibrinopeptide B, however, polymerization occurs indicating that an independent polymerization site has been activated.

We believe that the course of events as shown in Fig. 99 takes place during fibrin formation in the presence of thrombin. These events occur invariably in an isolated fibrinogen–thrombin system and also when blood is allowed to clot, the fibrin formed seems to be predominantly type II fibrin. It is likely that proteins present in the blood are important in the control of the production of fibrin II. In the presence of antithrombin III (and especially together with heparin) the thrombin formed would

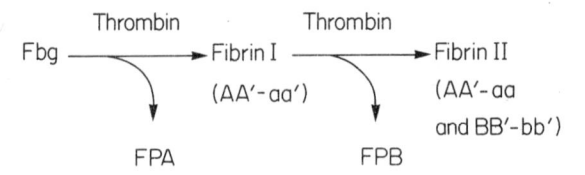

```
                Thrombin              Thrombin
        Fbg ─────────────▶ Fibrin I ─────────────▶ Fibrin II
             ╲              (AA'-aa')   ╲           (AA'-aa
              ▼                          ▼          and BB'-bb')
             FPA                        FPB
```

Fig. 99. Proteolytic events in the formation of fibrin in the presence of thrombin
FPA: fibrinopeptide A; FPB: fibrinopeptide B

rapidly be neutralized. This would favour formation of fibrin I rather than fibrin II. We believe that in fibrin II formation blood is restricted to the site of a lesion in the vessel wall. There the concentrations of procoagulant factors, including thrombin, are the highest, a situation which will favour more formation of fibrin II at this point than in the surrounding bloodstream.

It is obvious that when the BB' and bb' domains are active in polymer production, this would reinforce the fibre formed by AA' and aa' interaction alone. The involvement of the BB' and bb' domains also provides a simple means of branching the fibrin fibre to produce an intricate polymer network. Figure 98 depicts a model of how these domains operate in 'end-to-end' and 'side-to-side' polymerization. While I have chosen to use rectangular boxes in this model, the actual form is of no importance. We can extend the play with all these domains by allowing, as H. W. Thomas* in Cardiff has done, the succeeding activated dimer units to combine with the preceding ones at an angle of 120°. In such a way a protofibril is produced having a threefold screw symmetry. If we assume that the resulting 'protofibrils' are, through interaction of the BB' and bb' domains, aggregated in a sixfold screw symmetry, then a polymer would be produced which is in good agreement with the picture obtained through electron microscopic studies of a fibrin fibre. In the schematic model of the fibrin polymer which is shown in Fig. 98, it has been assumed that all the domains have the same binding energy. Of course, it is also possible that this is not the case. It is just as likely that both negative and positive cooperative effects play a part and thereby change considerably the geometry of polymerization.

The actual localization of one (AA' and aa') of the two sets of domains involved in polymerization of the domains rests primarily with studies concerning the affinity between fragments of the fibrinogen molecule and various insoluble fibrinogen and fibrin derivatives (Kudryk et al., 1974; cf. Blombäck et al., 1976). If fibrinogen is covalently coupled to Sepharose and then activated with thrombin or Bothroxobin, the conjugate displays specific adsorption properties. Regardless of mode of activation the activated conjugates adsorb specifically fibrinogen from plasma and fragment D from a plasmin digest of fibrinogen. Apparently, activation of the fibrinogen–Sepharose conjugate exposes structures (AA') which have the possibility of interacting with structures present in fragment D (aa'). Since intact fibrinogen also binds to the conjugate, we must assume that the latter structures are exposed in fibrinogen as it circulates in blood. We concluded from these studies that the domains A and A' are activated by release of fibrinopeptide A and that the complementary domains, a and a', are located in the fragment D portion of the molecule.

The next question concerns the localization of the domains A and A'. The fact that

---

*Personal communication, 1970.

these appeared to be activated by release of fibrinopeptide A suggested that the domains were located in the NH_2-terminal portion of the molecule. The NH_2-terminal fragment, N-DSK, was of special interest in this connection as it constitutes approximately 16 per cent of the intact fibrinogen molecule and carries the NH_2-terminal of both fibrinopeptide A and B. We conjugated this fragment with Sepharose and were able to show that this, like the fibrinogen–Sepharose conjugate, on activation with thrombin specifically adsorbed fibrinogen as well as fragment D from plasmin digested fibrinogen. As was expected N-DSK in solution, on activation with thrombin, was shown to bind to the fibrinogen–Sepharose conjugate (cf. Blombäck et al., 1976).

The structures in N-DSK which are activated or exposed after activation with thrombin or Bothroxobin and which are responsible for the interaction with fragment D may be present in the first 43 NH_2-terminal amino acid residues in the Bβ-chain and/or the carboxy-terminal portion of the γ-chain. This suggestion is derived from the fact that fragment E, which contains all of the structures of N-DSK except the above mentioned residues in the Bβ- and γ-fragments, binds to a much smaller extent to the fibrinogen–Sepharose conjugate after activation with thrombin. In fibrinogen Detroit, where 19 Arg has been replaced by serine, polymerization does not occur on release of fibrinopeptide A. It is therefore likely that this amino acid residue in normal fibrinogen is involved somehow in the interaction. As mentioned previously clotting does not occur in fibrinogen Detroit unless release of fibrinopeptide B takes place. We believe that the polymerization observed in fibrinogen Detroit represents interaction at independent polymerization sites, BB'–bb'. The BB' sites may also be located in N-DSK since N-DSK activated with Bothroxobin does not bind as efficiently to fibrinogen–Sepharose as does N-DSK activated with thrombin. There is so far no indication as to the location of the bb' sites in fibrinogen.

There are, no doubt, structures in or around the symmetrical disulphide bridges which also play, directly or indirectly, a fundamental role in the structural integrity and function of the polymerization domains. Thus, it has been shown that thioredoxin-catalysed reduction of the symmetrical disulphide bridges in the Aα- and γ-chains of fibrinogen, caused a total loss of the ability of fibrinogen to form fibrin. This phenomenon can not be ascribed to a change in the proteolytic activity of thrombin as the rate of release of fibrinopeptide A from the reduced fibrinogen is the same as that for the unreduced material (cf. Blombäck et al., 1976).

There may be a number of constituents in blood, including proteins and ions, which interact with fibrinogen and thereby stabilize it in a certain conformation. Calcium ions are known to bind to fibrinogen at three, high affinity, binding sites, one of which appears to be lost at pH values under 7 (Marguerie et al., 1977). This binding of calcium may explain why calcium ions protect fibrinogen against thermal denaturation (Ly and Godal 1973). Confirming earlier work (for references see Blombäck, 1967 and Marguerie et al., 1977) we have found in a recent study that calcium ions exert a pronounced effect on the polymerization step in the fibrinogen–fibrin transition and they do not influence the proteolytic stage that precedes polymerization (Blombäck et al., 1978). More interesting in our study, however, was the finding that in the presence of calcium ions the transition from coarse to transparent clot (Ferry and Morrisson, 1947) did not occur in the alkalium pH range. Therefore, calcium may bind to a group or groups in the protein having an apparent pK value in this range, thereby stabilizing the protein and allowing for the formation of a compact fibrin structure. It can only be a guess as to which groups are involved, but α- and ε-amino groups as well as tyrosine OH-groups are possible candidates. Two of the three high affinity binding groups demonstrated by Marguerie et al., 1977 would be expected to be involved in this binding.

We consider that the conclusions concerning the polymerization of fibrinogen, drawn from the investigations using the fibrinogen- and N-DSK–Sepharose conjugates also apply to physiological fibrin formation. Thus, it is known, that fibrinolytic degradation products of fibrinogen, in particular fragments X and Y and fragment D, inhibit the polymerization of fibrinogen (Budzynski et al., 1967). Furthermore, it is known that a pronounced bleeding tendency occurs in clinical states where the concentration of these degradation products is high. The presence in blood of fragment D or related fragments is expected to cause the inhibition of the formation of a normal fibrin polymer by interaction with the AA′ domain of fibrin monomers. Because the fragments are monovalent, no further elongation of the polymers can take place from the N-DSK end of the polymer. In fact, it was shown by Bang (1964) that the fibrin network formed in the presence of fibrinogen degradation products has an appearance which differs from the normal in that it is more fragile. Strong support for our notion is given by findings with fibrinogen Detroit using normal and abnormal fibrinogen coupled to Sepharose and subsequently activated by thrombin. The conclusion drawn from these experiments was that the N-DSK portion (AA′ domains) of the fibrinogen Detroit molecule, after activation, had no ability to bind to fragment D (aa′ domains) of normal fibrinogen. On the other hand, the fragment D portion of fibrinogen Detroit possesses normal binding properties. Under the conditions of these experiments no activation of the BB′ domains appeared to take place despite the fact that fibrinopeptide B was released. Nevertheless, the domain in fibrinogen Detroit carrying the mutation (Aα19 Arg→19 Ser) has anomalous binding properties while the fragment D domain with apparently normal structure has normal binding properties. The fact that patients with dysfibrinogenaemia Detroit have a haemorrhagic diathesis and that fibrinogen Detroit has a much delayed clotting time in the presence of thrombin strongly support the notion that there exists a relationship between the mutation in the AA′ domains (defective binding properties) and the impaired haemostasis seen in these patients.

In our discussion of the location of the domains in the fibrinogen molecule, we have made use of the picture of the molecule which our chemical investigations have provided. Such a representation is, by necessity, linear. We can now ask ourselves: where are the domains situated in the tertiary structure of the molecule? Assuming that the electron microscopic pictures of Bachmann et al., 1975 (Fig. 100) represent the native hydrated molecule we can suggest where in the molecule the domains AA′—aa′ are located (Blombäck et al., 1976). According to Bachmann et al., the average fibrinogen molecule has the shape of a cylinder with rounded ends. Careful examination of different pictures of the molecules, reveals that many of them differ appreciably from this idealized form (Fig. 100).

One sees forms which appear to be puckered in the middle or are bent at the ends. The authors suggest that this indicates that the molecule has an appreciable flexibility. However, one could also interpret the electron microscopic pictures from another standpoint. The different forms may possibly represent various projections of a rigid molecule. In Fig. 101, I have depicted our interpretation of how two half-molecules may be joined to produce the molecular form which is observed by electron micros-

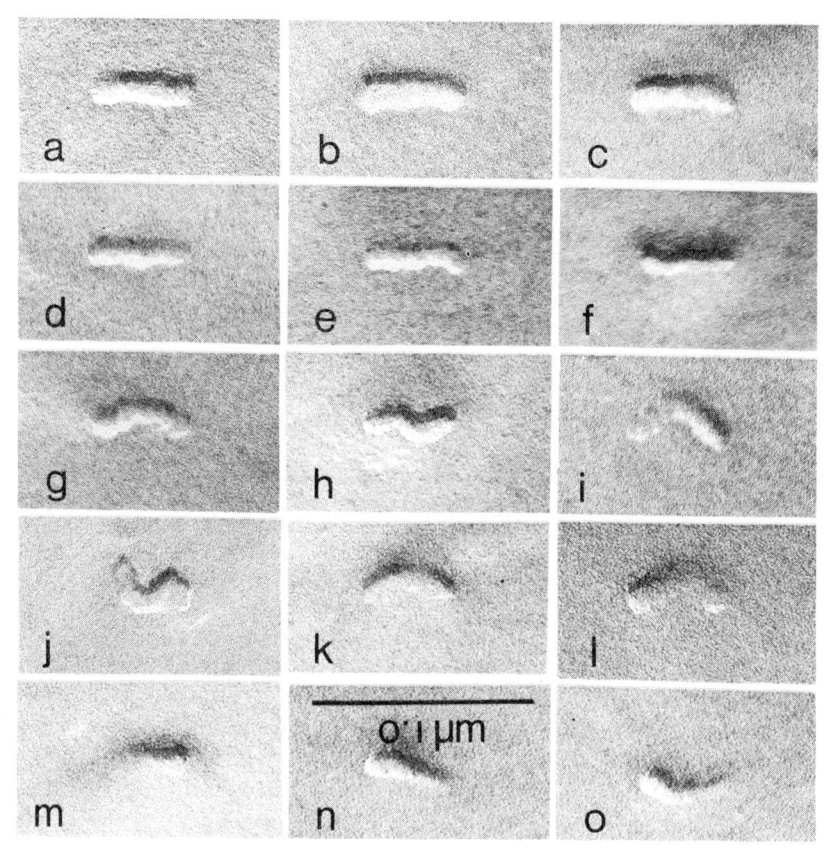

Fig. 100. Electron microscopic pictures of fibrinogen molecules taken by using the freeze-etching technique. From Bachmann et al., 1975. Photograph by courtesy of K. Lederer

copy. The puckered form (Fig. 100) may represent a picture of a double molecule in which two rod-shaped half-molecules are linked via their NH$_2$-terminal ends with a twofold axis of symmetry. Most of the pictures seen in Fig. 100 will then fit a representation of the molecule in a projection which is more or less perpendicular to the former. The remaining forms which are seen in Fig. 100 are either partially concealed or have forms (i and j) which are not consistent with our interpretation. In our interpretation of the electron microscopic pictures, which also takes into account hydrodynamic and X-ray diffraction measurement in fibrinogen, the domains, AA' must be located in the central joining portion of the molecule. It may be that the domains, BB' and bb', are located in the same part of the molecule. In Fig. 101 I have also attempted to show how two fibrinogen molecules are orientated when interaction takes place in the AA' and aa' binding domains.

6. Stabilizing the fibrin polymer

The fibrin polymer which is formed after activation with thrombin undergoes secondary transformation through the introduction of covalent cross-linking between glutamine residues in the γ-chain of one molecule and lysine residues in the γ-chain of

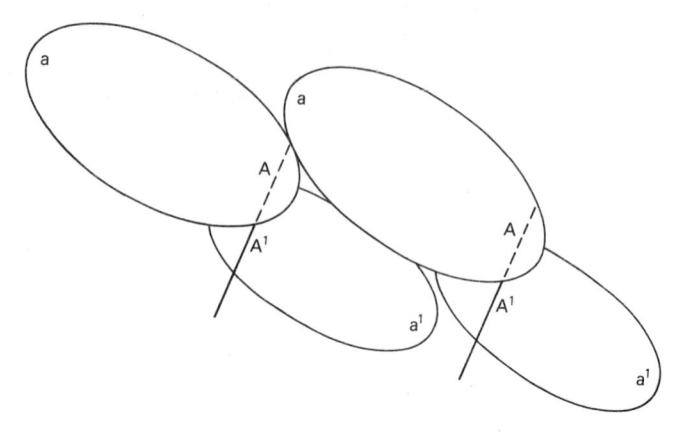

248 *Proteins taking part in coagulation and fibrinolysis*

Fig. 101. Interpretation of the electron microscopic pictures of the fibrinogen molecule. The drawing shows one projection of two molecules combined through the binding domains AA′ and aa′ when activated by thrombin. Each molecule consists of two half-molecules joined in a twofold symmetry by the symmetrical disulphides, creating clefts between the two half-molecules

another molecule (Doolittle, 1973; Lorand, 1972). In the initial phase of polymerization, these residues are brought into juxtaposition. In the presence of activated transglutaminase (Factor XIII) and calcium ions, condensation between the γ-chains takes place between the γ-carbonyl group of glutamine and the ε-group of lysine with concomitant release of ammonia (Fig. 102). Factor XIII is present in plasma and platelets, where it exists as an inactive precursor. It is activated by thrombin, probably by limited proteolysis. The α-chain of fibrin also undergoes intermolecular cross-linking but it is still unclear if the reaction mechanism is the same as that involving the γ-chains. The resulting stabilized fibrin is insoluble in urea solution and other solvents which dissolve non-stabilized fibrin.

On digestion of cross-linked fibrin with plasmin, fragment D appears, at least at some stage of the digestion, in a dimeric form (for review see Gaffney, 1977a,b). This

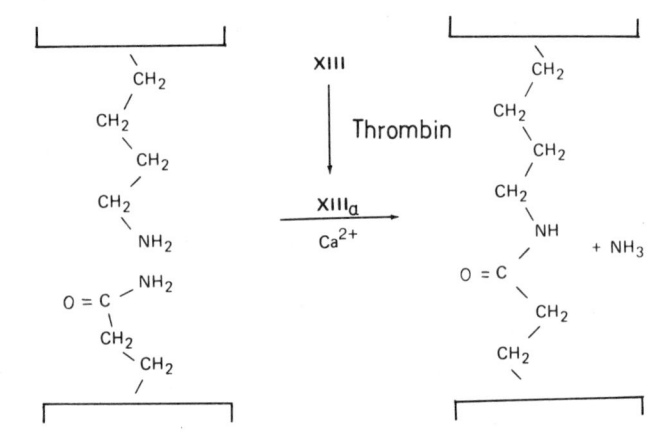

Fig. 102. Formation of ε(γ-glutamyl) lysine cross-links through condensation of glutamine and lysine side-chains. Adapted from Doolittle, 1973

dimer contains cross-linked γ-chains. This fragment may be useful in the differentiation between primary fibrinolysis of fibrinogen and fibrinolysis of fibrin already present in blood and other organs (see section on 'Fibrinogen in health and disease'). It appears that in cross-linked fibrin the α-chains are much more resistant to plasmin than in non-cross-linked fibrin.

7. The antigenic structure of fibrinogen and the location of epitopes and other structural elements

Marder et al. (1969) have with the use of antisera raised against fibrinogen demonstrated that the molecule has several antigenic determinants. Two of these determinants have their structural origin in fragment E and fragment D which arise from degradation of fibrinogen with plasmin. Fragments X and Y also have specific determinants and there also exist determinants which are unique for intact fibrinogen. By using antibodies which have been raised against fragments of fibrinogen, e.g. plasmin or CNBr-fragments, one can elucidate the antigenic structure of the molecule as well as obtain information concerning the location of these determinants (or epitopes) in the three-dimensional structure. Plow and Edgington (1973, 1975) have demonstrated that fragments D and E possess determinants (neo-epitopes) which are not expressed in the intact molecule. Kudryk et al. (cf. Blombäck et al., 1976) showed that the antigenic determinants in N-DSK were localized mainly in certain portions of this structure. Furthermore, it was shown that anti-N-DSK cross-reacted to only a small extent with intact fibrinogen and with fragment E, the latter having a considerable portion of its structure in common with N-DSK. However, after cleavage with CNBr, fragment E reacted to the same extent as N-DSK. This may suggest that the antigenic determinants are not only buried in fibrinogen but also in fragment E. Fragment E in comparison with N-DSK has chain extensions on its Aα-and Bβ-chains. These extensions are removed on treatment with CNBr. One possible explanation is that the extensions are folded in such a way as to hide the epitopes in fragment E. Other interpretations of these results are also feasible but I shall not venture upon these in this connection.

Results obtained from investigations using thioredoxin also indicate that certain structures of N-DSK are buried in the intact fibrinogen molecule. It has been shown that only 2 or 3 of the 11 disulphide bridges located in the N-DSK portion of fibrinogen are reduced by thioredoxin (Blombäck et al., 1976). In isolated N-DSK, all are reduced. It is interesting that the bonds which are reduced in intact fibrinogen constitute the symmetrical disulphides. We favour the idea that the disulphides which hold together the two half-molecules of fibrinogen are surface exposed whereas the interchain disulphide bridges are located in portions of the molecule which are hidden.

In general, antibodies which have been raised against the hydrophobic structures of fibrinogen do not react with the intact fibrinogen molecule. Furthermore, the disulphide bridges in these are not available for reduction by thioredoxin in intact fibrinogen. We suppose, therefore, that the hydrophobic fragments lie hidden in the molecule. On the other hand antibodies raised against hydrophilic structures in the molecule appear to be different. These antibodies react also with the intact fibrinogen molecule and the disulphide bridges in the structures are reduced by thioredoxin. Such a hydrophilic fragment (Hi2–DSK) is situated in the carboxy-terminal portion of the

Aα-chain and is released from the molecule in the early phase of a plasmic digestion (Blombäck et al., 1976). Most of the disulphide bridges in fibrinogen thus appear to be buried in 'core' structures in the interior of the molecule. They are without doubt of great importance for maintaining the stability of the molecule and as such are kept out of reach of the reducing systems of the organism.

8. Fibrinogen in health and disease

Fibrinogen is a *sine qua non* for normal haemostasis. Its primary role in this process is to form a fibrin network around the platelets which adhere and aggregate around small lesions in the vessel wall. A stable haemostatic plug of platelets is thereby created. If fibrin formation for some reason fails, the platelet plug will eventually be swept away and bleeding restarts. Cross-linking of the fibrin formed may also be important for consolidation of the haemostatic plug.

The normal fibrinogen concentration is 2–3 g/l plasma. Fibrinogen belongs to a group of 'reactive proteins' and increases in the level of fibrinogen in the blood are observed in many conditions. In infection the fibrinogen level in blood increases markedly, this being the major cause of the increased red cell sedimentation rate seen in these conditions. In neoplastic diseases one sees just as often, increased fibrinogen levels. In the postoperative states or after trauma, there is also generally an increase in the blood fibrinogen level. It is probable that the increased fibrinogen levels are caused by increased synthesis.

Increased synthesis can parallel increased catabolism. If the catabolism increases more than the synthetic capacity of the organism, the result will be a fall in the level of blood fibrinogen. Such an imbalance may arise in liver diseases. This phenomenon is most common in states of intravascular coagulation. This condition should be distinguished from thrombosis. The latter condition which is a local pathological phenomenon will be described later. In intravascular coagulation, fibrinogen catabolism increases because of disseminated deposition of fibrin in the blood vessel system. Uncontrolled activation of fibrinogen may take place following entrance into the blood of substances which promote conversion of prothrombin into thrombin. Intravascular coagulation is a serious condition which usually, paradoxically, one can say, manifests itself as a bleeding diathesis. It can arise as a complication in several diseases with different pathogenesis. It is found for example in abruptio placentae, after trauma, in shock, during haemolytic crisis, neoplastic diseases, etc. The diagnosis is difficult. The fibrinogen concentration in blood is often quite low but need not necessarily be so. The concentration of other clotting factors is also often reduced. A valuable tool for the diagnosis of intravascular coagulation was recently introduced (Nossel et al., 1974). This is a radioimmunological method for the measurement of fibrinopeptide A. As the release of fibrinopeptide A is a measure of the degree of activation of fibrinogen molecules, the level of this peptide reflects the pathological process and its intensity. In intravascular coagulation there is a substantial rise in the level of fibrinopeptide A (FPA). The fibrinopeptide A level is also elevated in thrombosis if the thrombosis is extensive.

In a rare congenital disease, afibrinogenaemia, there is an apparent lack of fibrinogen. These patients have a strong bleeding tendency. Coagulable protein can not be demonstrated in the blood and fibrinogen is absent when measured by immunological methods. This does not mean that these patients are devoid of a fibrinogen-like protein. It is possible that an abnormal fibrinogen molecule is present lacking the antigenic determinants which are typical for normal fibrinogen.

Congenital hypofibrinogenaemia is a more common condition than afibrinogenaemia. There exists hardly any increased bleeding tendency in these patients. It has been speculated that these patients may possibly be heterozygotes with regard to a afibrinogenaemia trait.

During recent years, reports have appeared of patients who have a functionally defective fibrinogen. The condition is usually described by the term: dysfibrinogenaemia. So far, some 20 families afflicted with functionally abnormal fibrinogen have been described. The most characteristic finding is a lengthening of the 'thrombin time' of plasma. In other words, the time taken for coagulation of the plasma on addition of thrombin is longer than normal. To distinguish the different types of abnormal fibrinogen from each other, they have been given the name of the town or district where the discovery was made. Most of the patients described were believed to be heterozygotes, and they usually present only a minor haemostatic defect. In the case of fibrinogen Detroit one member of the afflicted family was found to be homozygous with regard to the abnormality (Blombäck et al., 1968b). This fibrinogen, named fibrinogen Detroit, is inherited according to an autosomal dominant pattern (Mammen et al., 1969). The homozygotes have a severe bleeding diathesis and unlike the heterozygotes, their plasma does clot very slowly in the presence of thrombin.

Fibrinogen Detroit is an example of the dramatic functional consequences which a small change in amino acid sequence may have. The mutation (Aα 19 Arg → Ser) has occurred in the invariable part of the structure, i.e. that part which has been preserved in the course of mammalian evolution. Evidently, this portion of the Aα-chain is critical for polymerization. However, this does not necessarily mean that the affinity of thrombin for this chain is lower than in normal fibrinogen. In fact, it has been demonstrated that fibrinopeptide A is released from fibrinogen Detroit and that the rate of release appears to be almost normal. Hence, we suppose that the mutation brings about secondary changes in the conformation of fibrinogen in such a way that one of the domains which is normally active in polymerization remains dormant even after release of fibrinopeptide A. In Fig. 103 I have depicted how the functional disorder may be brought about. Through a conformational change, which takes place after the release of fibrinopeptide A, the polymerization domains in N-DSK (AA') in one molecule and fragment D (aa') in another combine in the normal situation. In fibrinogen Detroit, no conformational change takes place, or if it does, the change in conformation is not compatible with the combination of the two domains. Though activation of the BB' domains can take place in fibrinogen Detroit this is a slow process and, furthermore, if a polymer eventually forms by this route it would be expected to have a structure different from that of the normal fibrin strand.

Thrombosis is one of the major diseases in our society. This is appreciated when we understand that in patients undergoing surgery, 30–40 per cent develop postoperative thrombosis which give clinical symptoms in about 10 per cent. Much progress has been achieved in the fight against thrombosis during the past 10 years due mainly to the introduction of anticoagulants such as heparin and dicoumarol in the treatment and prophylaxis of thrombosis. However thrombosis is still a major problem in our communities.

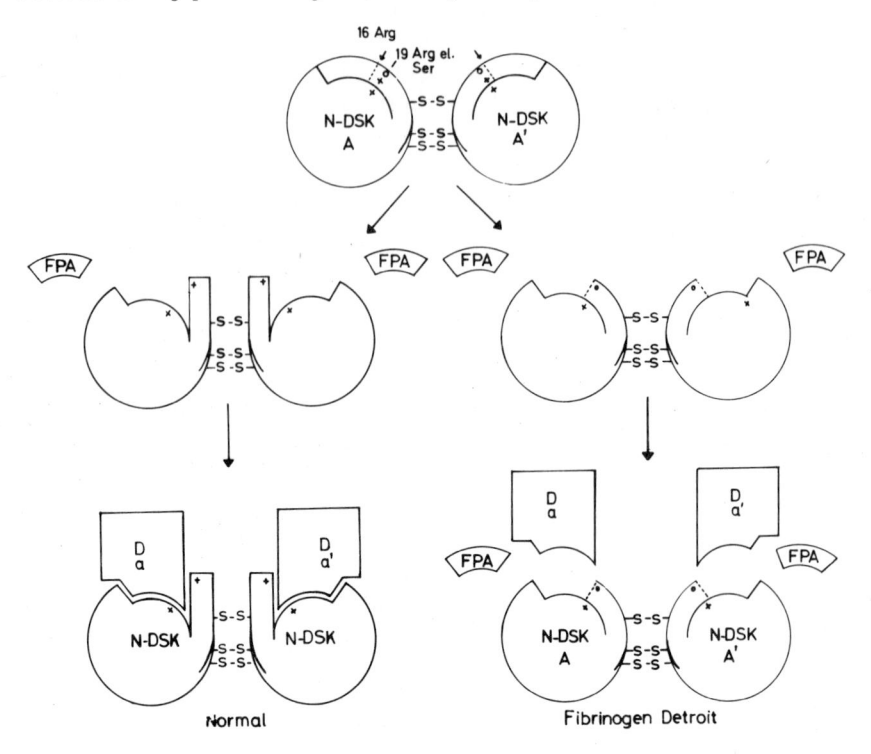

Fig. 103. Interaction between the polymerization sites in normal fibrinogen and fibrinogen Detroit. The figure shows a situation in which no conformational change occurs in the N–DSK domain of fibrinogen Detroit on release of fibrinopeptide A. FPA: fibrinopeptide A. o: denotes charge of neutral amino acid Aα19 Ser in fibrinogen Detroit

In the classical description of venous or arterial thrombosis the role of fibrinogen in formation of the obstructive structure is more or less crucial. In venous thrombi the fibrin network provides the structural framework of the clot in which red cells and other cellular components are trapped. This is what Virchow called the red thrombus. In arterial thrombi on the other hand the clot structure is much more compact. Here the clot structure is built up by a mass of platelets in which fibrin strands are laid down. This is the so-called white thrombus. The two types of thrombi reflect the physical conditions under which they are formed. On the venous side where the blood flow is slow an initial thrombus formed at a site of a lesion in the vessel wall has a chance of growing in the direction of the bloodstream. The explanation of this is that the slow flow favours a relatively high concentration of procoagulant factors at some distance from the lesion.

On the arterial side when the flow is rapid the clot will enlarge primarily by aggregation of platelets at the site of lesion. Fibrin formation is restricted to the mass of platelets but nevertheless it will stabilize this mass which under unfavourable conditions will grow step by step until the vessel is occluded.

There appears to be more a quantitative than a qualitative difference between a 'normal' haemostatic plug and a thrombus or one can say that the haemostatic plug of platelets is just a non-occluding thrombus (Copley, 1974). What then are the factors controlling the growth of the haemostatic plug? Virchow, in the middle of the last century, mentioned three factors of importance in the formation of a pathological thrombus. These were: blood flow, vessel wall, and constituents of the blood. Thus a predisposing factor for thrombus formation is a slow blood flow which may be caused by heart disease or diseases of the veins. Destruction of the endothelial lining of the blood vessels may also be a predisposing factor since it results in extensive platelet deposition which acts as a nucleus for fibrin formation, eventually leading to thrombosis. Last, but not least, constituents of the blood may play a decisive role in determining whether a haemostatic plug remains as such or grows to an obliterating clot structure known as a thrombus. Increased levels of coagulation factors may favour thrombus formation merely on an enzyme-kinetic basis. However, more important, the level of inhibitors of coagulation (e.g. antithrombin III) or of fibrinolysis may play a major role in controlling the growth of a haemostatic plug.

Let us also consider the consequences which formation of different types of fibrin may have on the thrombotic process (see preceding section). It appears to me that the control mechanisms for compartmentalization of type II fibrin to the very site of the endothelial lesion may play a major role in confining the haemostatic process. In this control all the parameters of the triad of Virchow are of importance. Extensive formation of type II fibrin rather than type I fibrin would be expected to have a better chance to lead to formation of an obstructive thrombus since this type of fibrin is more compact than type I fibrin and appears to be more resistant to degradation by fibrinolytic enzymes.

9. Epilogue

Further progress in thrombosis research is, I believe, intimately coupled with basic research on biochemical events in blood coagulation. Fibrinogen, the structural element of the blood-clot is always somehow involved, not only in physiological haemostasis but also in thrombus formation. In order to understand haemostasis and thrombosis it is indispensable to know more about the functional states of this molecule under different physiological and pathophysiological conditions. In order to reach this goal we must know more about its primary structure, its physicochemical characteristics, its shape, its interaction, etc. or to quote Goethe: 'Wer sie nicht kennte die Elemente, ihre Kraft und Eigenschaft, wäre kein Meister über die Geister'. The trail of research on fibrinogen which I have described on these pages has not come to an end—it is just in its beginning.

III. Thrombin and prothrombin

STAFFAN MAGNUSSON

A. Limited proteolysis as a means of regulation

The concept of proteolysis or cleavage of peptide bonds in proteins was originally associated with the nearly complete degradation of food protein to amino acids and dipeptides in the digestive tract. There is also another kind of strictly limited and highly specific proteolytic process, where only a single or very few peptide bonds are cleaved in large proteins that contain several hundred peptide bonds. Such selective limited proteolysis is an essential element in the regulation of many biological systems, not only blood coagulation and fibrinolysis, but also the complement system, the zymogen activation in the digestive tract, the release of peptide hormones from prohormones (proparathyroid hormone, proinsulin, proglucagon, and others), the release of vasoactive polypeptides (angiotensin, bradykinin), the control of virus assembly where key proteins that occur as elements of the virus structure will only fit the structure after specific proteolytic tailoring. Other examples are the penetration of the egg cell membrane by the sperm cell, the expression of growth characteristics in cultures of cells that have been malignantly transformed by virus infection. As a rule in the biosynthesis of extracellular proteins in eukaryotic organisms an N-terminal peptide fragment is cleaved off from the 'fresh' ribosomal product before the new protein molecule can pass through the cell membrane. The proteolytic enzymes that catalyse these specific reactions differ from the digestive enzymes mainly in two respects. In most cases the active enzyme has a higher and more exactly defined substrate specificity than for example trypsin. Furthermore, the structures of the their zymogens are considerably larger than those of the digestive enzymes. This 'extra' structure in the zymogens of the regulatory enzymes is engaged in specific interactions with other structures, such as proteins, phospholipids, metal ions, and membrane structures, facilitating selective steering of the activation of a particular zymogen, such that it can occur only under a set of well-defined conditions, apparently different for each specific zymogen.

At present prothrombin–thrombin is the best known of these regulatory zymogen-enzyme systems as far as structure and function relationships are concerned. Therefore, it is of some interest for the general understanding of such processes even outside the field of blood coagulation.

B. Historical outline

Thrombin was originally defined as the blood plasma (serum) enzyme that catalyses blood clotting. Its specific substrate protein, fibrinogen, was isolated in relatively pure form in the 1890s (O. Hammarsten). Through the work of Alexander Schmidt it became clear that in the circulating blood plasma thrombin occurs as an inactive zymogen, prothrombin. Arthus and Pagès showed that rapid activation of prothrombin to thrombin requires calcium ions. These facts as well as the function of thrombokinase (thromboplastin), then thought to be a phospholipid-containing tissue protein preparation, as an accelerator of the activation, were combined in 1905 to form the clotting theory of Morawitz. Bordet and Delange found that certain inorganic salts of low solubility could be used as rather specific adsorbents for prothrombin. Specifically barium sulphate, calcium phosphate, aluminum hydroxide, and magnesium hydroxide have been used in purification methods for prothrombin. In the middle of the 1930s Eagle concluded that prothrombin is activated to thrombin by limited proteolysis and that thrombin is a proteolytic enzyme. The development of two different test systems for measuring the prothrombin activity in blood plasma, namely the two-stage test (Warner, et al., 1936; later modified by Ware and Seegers, 1949) and the one-stage test by Quick were prerequisites not only for the purification of prothrombin and thrombin but also for the studies by Dam and his co-workers of the function of vitamin K and those of Link of the isolation, structure determination, and synthesis of dicoumarol, an 'antagonist' of vitamin K. These studies showed that vitamin K is required for the biosynthesis of active prothrombin and that this synthesis is inhibited by dicoumarol. Dicoumarol and other synthetic vitamin K antagonists have found widespread use since the 1940s; in controlled dosage for the prevention and treatment of thrombosis; in uncontrolled dosage as rat poison. Treatment of patients with dicoumarol and related derivatives is generally monitored by the one-stage test of Quick or methods evolved from it such as the P-P method of Owren and co-workers and later the thrombotest method.

C. Thrombin—structure and function

1. Function and specificity

Thrombin is a proteolytic enzyme of the same type as the endopeptidases of the pancreatic juice, trypsin, chymotrypsin, elastase, and kallikrein, namely a serine protease. Thus, it has an active site that can be inactivated with diisopropylfluorophosphate (DFP), which binds specifically to one of the 16 serine residues in the thrombin structure (Ser-195 in Fig. 105). Like trypsin thrombin catalyses the cleavage of small synthetic lysine or arginine substrates, for example tosyl-L-arginine methyl ester (TAMe) (Sherry and Troll, 1954) and tosyl-L-lysine methyl ester (TLMe) (Elmore and Curragh, 1963). While trypsin cleaves practically all arginyl and lysyl bonds in proteins, only very few proteins are substrates for thrombin. This is true even for denatured proteins which are usually better targets for proteolytic attack. In the late 1940s Bailey, Bettelheim, Lorand, and Middlebrook in Cambridge showed that the thrombin-catalysed conversion of soluble fibrinogen to fibrin monomer, that polymerizes spontaneously to form insoluble fibrin—the matrix of the blood clot—involves a limited proteolysis of the fibrinogen with release of fibrinopeptides (see Fibrinogen and fibrin formation page 223). In addition to this, the 'classical' substrate protein for thrombin, several other proteins and polypeptides are now known which are cleaved selectively by thrombin. In those cases where the amino acid sequence is known, it has been found that the thrombin-sensitive arginine or lysine residue is preceded by Pro or by Val, Leu or Ala. For many of the thrombin-sensitive proteins it appears that the thrombin-catalysed cleavage is probably essential for the activation and/or inactivation of the protein and that thrombin functions as a regulator. The best documented case is the activation by thrombin of Factor XIII to Factor XIII_a (plasma trans-glutaminase

256 *Proteins taking part in coagulation and fibrinolysis*

or 'cross-linking factor'). This coagulation factor catalyses the formation of amide bonds from γ-carboxyl groups in glutamine residues to ε-amino groups in lysine residues and makes the fibrin much less soluble. Thrombin also catalyses the cleavage of the arginyl bond in position 156 of bovine prothrombin. This cleavage probably functions as a regulator of prothrombin activation. Both coagulation Factors V and VIII can apparently be activated by thrombin.

Thrombin can also initiate the aggregation of platelets and may therefore play an important role in the development of arterial thrombosis. The exact mechanism for the function of thrombin in platelet aggregation is not clear.

Buchanan and co-workers have recently found that thrombin acts as a mitogen in fibroblast cultures and more efficiently than other serine proteases, such as trypsin, chymotrypsin, and plasmin. They interpreted this to mean that thrombin also plays a role in wound healing.

2. Primary structure

The primary structure of bovine thrombin has been known since 1974 (Magnusson *et al.*, in Hemker and Veltkamp, 1975). The molecule is composed of two polypeptide chains. The A-chain consists of 49 amino acid residues and has a molecular weight of 5 700 (Fig. 104). The B-chain consists of 259 amino acid residues (Fig. 105). It also contains approximately 5 per cent carbohydrate. The molecular weight of the protein part of the B-chain is 29 700. The molecular weight for the protein part of the entire thrombin is then 35 400. Including the contribution from the prosthetic carbohydrate part the total comes to 37 300. The active site of thrombin is located in the B-chain. The amino acid composition is given in Table 46. Of the four disulphide bridges in thrombin three are internal in the B-chain, the fourth connects the A- and the B-chains. Recently, the amino acid sequences of the two chains of human thrombin have been determined. The homology with bovine thrombin is very strong and except for the fact that residues 1–13 of the human thrombin A-chain have been cleaved off during activation all the conclusions drawn from our knowledge of bovine thrombin seem to apply to human thrombin.

```
           1                                              10
        Thr-Ser-Glu-Asp-His-Phe-Gln-Pro-Phe-Phe-

        -Asn-Glu-Lys-Thr-Phe-Gly-Ala-Gly-Glu-Ala-

        -Asp-Cys-Gly-Leu-Arg-Pro-Leu-Phe-Glu-Lys-

        -Lys-Gln-Val-Gln-Asp-Glu-Thr-Gln-Lys-Glu-

        -Leu-Phe-Glu-Ser-Tyr-Ile-Glu-Gly-Arg
```

Fig. 104. The A-chain of thrombin contains 49 amino acid residues. The molecular weight is 5 721. Before activation the A-chain constitutes the sequence 275–323 of prothrombin

```
 16  17  18  19  20  21  22  23  24  25  26  27  28  29  30  31
 Ile-Val-Glu-Gly-Gln-Asp-Ala-Glu-Val-Gly-Leu-Ser-Pro-Trp-Gln-Val-

 32  33  34  35  36 36A  37  38  39  40  41  42  43  44  45  46
-Met-Leu-Phe-Arg-Lys-Ser-Pro-Gln-Glu-Leu-Leu-Cys-Gly-Ala-Ser-Leu-

 47  48  49  50  51  52  53  54  55  56  57  58  59  60  61  62
-Ile-Ser-Asp-Arg-Trp-Val-Leu-Thr-Ala-Ala-His-Cys-Leu-Leu-Tyr-Pro-

 63  64  65 65A 65B 65C 65D 65E 65F 65G 65H 65I  66  67  68  69
-Pro-Trp-Asx-Lys-Asn-Phe-Thr-Val-Asp-Asp-Leu-Leu-Val-Arg-Ile-Gly-

 70  71  72  73  74  75  76  77  78  79  80  81  82  83  84 84A
-Lys-His-Ser-Arg-Thr-Arg-Tyr-Glu-Arg-Lys-Val-Glu-Lys-Ile-Ser-Met-

 85  86  87  88  89  90  91  92  93  94  95  96  97  98  99 99A
-Leu-Asp-Lys-Ile-Tyr-Ile-His-Pro-Arg-Tyr-Asn-Trp-Lys-Glu-Asn-Leu-

100 101 102 103 104 105 106 107 108 109 110 111 112 113 114 115
-Asp-Arg-Asp-Ile-Ala-Leu-Leu-Lys-Leu-Lys-Arg-Pro-Ile-Glu-Leu-Ser-

116 117 118 119 120 121 122 123 124 125 126 127 128 128A128B128C
-Asp-Tyr-Ile-His-Pro-Val-Cys-Leu-Pro-Asp-Lys-Gln-Thr-Ala-Ala-Lys-

129 130 131 132 133 134 135 136 137 138 139 140 141 142 143 144
-Leu-Leu-His-Ala-Gly-Phe-Lys-Gly-Arg-Val-Thr-Gly-Trp-Gly-Asn-Arg-

145 146 147 147A147B147C147D147E 148 149 150 151 152 153 154 155
-Arg-Glu-Thr-Trp-Thr-Thr-Ser-Val-Ala-Glu-Val-Gln-Pro-Ser-Val-Leu-

156 157 158 159 160 161 162 163 164 165 166 167 168 169 170 171
-Gln-Val-Val-Asn-Leu-Pro-Leu-Val-Glu-Arg-Pro-Val-Cys-Lys-Ala-Ser-

172 173 174 175 176 177 178 179 180 181 182 183 184 184A 185 186
-Thr-Arg-Ile-Arg-Ile-Thr-Asn-Asp-Met-Phe-Cys-Ala-Gly-Tyr-Lys-Pro-

187 188 188A188B188C188D 189 190 191 192 193 194 195 196 197 198
-Gly-Glu-Gly-Lys-Arg-Gly-Asp-Ala-Cys-Glu-Gly-Asp-Ser-Gly-Gly-Pro-

199 200 201 202 203 203A203B 204 205 206 207 208 209 210 211 212
-Phe-Val-Met-Lys-Ser-Pro-Tyr-Asn-Asn-Arg-Trp-Tyr-Gln-Met-Gly-Ile-

213 214 215 216 217 219 220 221 221A 222 223 224 225 226 227 228
-Val-Ser-Trp-Gly-Glu-Gly-Cys-Asp-Arg-Asn-Gly-Lys-Tyr-Gly-Phe-Tyr-

229 230 231 232 233 234 235 236 237 238 239 240 241 242 243 244
-Thr-His-Val-Phe-Arg-Leu-Lys-Lys-Trp-Ile-Gln-Lys-Val-Ile-Asp-Arg-

245 245A245B
-Leu-Gly-Ser
```

Fig. 105. The B-chain of thrombin contains 259 amino acid residues. The molecular weight is 29 683 for its protein part. Before activation it constitutes residues 324–582 of prothrombin. The numbering system for chymotrypsin is used to facilitate comparison of thrombin with other serine proteases, for example the pancreatic ones. The B-chain has one prosthetic carbohydrate group, consisting of glucosamine, mannose, galactose, and sialic acid. It is bound to Asn-65B. The oligosaccharide constitutes about 5 per cent of the weight of the B-chain, making the total molecular weight approximately 31 250

Table 46. Amino acid compositions calculated from the sequences of prothrombin and its different activation products. Molecular weights calculated from the sequence, with approximate additions for the carbohydrate substituents. Gla = γ-carboxyglutamic acid, CHO = carbohydrate

	Prothrombin	A-fragment	S-fragment A-chain	Thrombin	B-chain	Thrombin and neoprothrombin-T	Neoprothrombin-s	'Pro' fragment
Asp	34	4	13	3	14	17	30	17
Asn	25	10	5	1	9	10	15	15
Asx	1	—	—	—	1	1	1	—
Glu	43	11	11	8	13	21	32	22
Gln	18	2	4	4	8	12	16	6
Gla	10	10	—	—	—	—	—	10
Gly	48	11	12	4	21	25	37	23
Ala	34	10	10	2	12	14	24	20
Val	35	9	5	1	20	21	26	14
Met	6	1	—	—	5	5	5	1
Ile	20	4	1	1	14	15	16	5
Leu	46	10	9	3	24	27	36	19
Pro	35	10	9	2	14	16	25	19
1/2Cys	24	10	6	1	7	8	14	16
Trp	14	3	2	—	9	9	11	5
Lys	31	5	2	4	20	24	26	7
His	9	2	—	1	6	7	7	2
Arg	45	15	8	2	20	22	30	23
Ser	36	11	9	2	14	16	25	20
Thr	29	10	5	3	11	14	19	15
Phe	20	4	3	6	7	13	16	7
Tyr	19	4	4	1	10	11	15	8
Total	582	156	118	49	259	308	426	274
Molecular weight	66 098 +3 CHO c. 75 500	17 973 +2 CHO c. 25 500	12 775	5 721	29 683 + CHO c. 31 500	35 386 +CHO c. 37 200	48 143 +CHO c. 50 000	30 730 +2 CHO c. 38 300

3. Homology with serine proteases and haptoglobin

A comparison of the entire B-chain sequence with the amino-acid sequences of chymotrypsin, trypsin, and elastase shows a clear homology, which is especially pronounced in those parts of the structure that have turned out to be of central importance for enzyme function and for the zymogen activation mechanism in the case of the pancreatic enzymes. From 30 to 35 per cent of the amino acid residues in the B-chain are identical with their corresponding amino acids in chymotrypsin, trypsin, or elastase. This degree of homology means that the B-chain and the pancreatic serine proteases have an evolutionary relationship and have evolved through repeated duplication and consequent divergent evolution of the gene that provided the code for their common ancestral protein. During evolution all these serine proteases have retained their catalytic function, but their substrate specificity has developed in different directions. Haptoglobin which consists of two polypeptide chains, one α-chain and one β-chain, is also a member of the serine protease family from an evolutionary point of view because its β-chain is strongly homologous both with the pancreatic serine proteases and with the B-chain of thrombin. The ongoing sequence determination of the haptoglobin β-chain (Kurosky et al., 1974) shows that the latter can be regarded as a serine protease that has 'lost' its catalytic activity by an exchange of Ser-195 for an Ala-195.

4. Tentative tertiary structure

A highly probable consequence of the extensive sequence homology with the pancreatic serine proteases is that the tertiary structure of the thrombin B-chain, which is not yet known, will turn out to be principally the same as those of chymotrypsin, elastase, and trypsin, with the 'extra' amino acids that occur in thrombin (indicated with a figure + a letter in Fig. 105), so-called 'insertions', lying on the 'surface' of the molecule. The soundness of this argument is supported by the fact that the hypothetical tertiary structure models of elastase and trypsin, that were constructed by Hartley by substituting the sequences of these enzymes into the coordinates for the tertiary structure of chymotrypsin (determined by Blow and co-workers), turned out to have been amazingly good approximations of the real tertiary structures that were solved a year or two later (Shotton and Watson; Stroud and co-workers). Therefore, it seems reasonable to predict that the *catalytic activity of thrombin* is due to an active centre with Ser-195, His-57, and Asp-102 with the same 'charge relay' enzyme mechanism as chymotrypsin. The *specificity for Arg-* (or Lys-) residues in the substrate is probably due to the β-carboxyl group in Asp-189 which in that case constitutes the bottom of a 'side-chain pocket' that is 'lined' with Gly-216 and Gly-226. Such 'pockets' occur in both chymotrypsin and trypsin but in elastase Gly-216 and Gly-226 are replaced by Thr and Val whose side chains block the 'entrance' to the pocket. The sequence Ser-Trp-Gly-214-216 of the thrombin B-chain probably serves as a 'secondary binding site' for the amino acid residues in the three positions P2–P4 (in the substrate) immediately preceding the Arg (or Lys) (P-1) at which cleavage takes place. If this concept of substrate binding to thrombin is correct, it probably implies that the detailed structure in the area around position 99 determines the 'secondary' substrate specificity, i.e. which amino acid residues can be accepted for a thrombin substrate in the positions immediately preceding the Arg at which cleavage occurs. Precisely this area is one of those that are rather different in sequence between for example chymotrypsin, thrombin, and Factor X_a. A consequence of this fact is that we shall have to await the determination of the real tertiary structures of thrombin, Factor X_a, and the other clotting proteases by X-ray crystallography before we can hope to understand the 'secondary' substrate specificity of these enzymes in sufficient detail to permit intelligent tailoring of highly specific inhibitors and substrates for these enzymes.

The three internal disulphide bridges in the B-chain connect Cys-42 with Cys-58, Cys-168 with Cys-182, and Cys-191 with Cys-220, corresponding to three of the four disulphide bridges that are common to the pancreatic serine proteases. The fourth, Cys-136 to Cys-201, is missing in thrombin, and also in Factors X and X_a, but it does occur in plasmin. The disulphide bridge that connects the two thrombin chains involves Cys-22 in the A-chain and Cys-122 in the B-chain. Cys-122 also contributes to the inter-chain bridge of chymotrypsin, haptoglobin, and probably Factor X_a as well as one of the two inter-chain bridges in plasmin.

5. Partial homology/analogy with angiotensin and with luteinizing hormone (LH)

The sequence homology between the thrombin B-chain and the other serine proteases is not equally pronounced in all parts of the structure. In a couple of the less strongly conserved regions thrombin shows unexpected sequence similarities with angiotensin (Fig. 106) and in a third region with part of the β-component of luteinizing hormone (LH) (Fig. 107). The latter homology is especially interesting, because the two sequence

```
                                    Ace        Renin
            1              5         ↓      10  ↓
A:  Asp – Arg – Val – Tyr – Ile – His – Pro – Phe – His – Leu – Leu – Val – Tyr – Ser
B:  Asp – Arg – Val – Tyr – Val – His – Pro – Phe – His – Leu


C:  Asp – Lys – Ile – Tyr – Ile – His – Pro – Arg – Tyr – Asn – Trp – Lys – Glu – Asn
                                                ↑
                                            Thrombin

D:  Leu – Ser – Asp – Tyr – Ile – His – Pro – Val – Cys – Leu – Pro – Asp – Lys – Gln
```

Fig. 106. Sequence homology between angiotensin and two peptide sequences in the B-chain of thrombin
A: The sequence 1–14 is a part of angiotensinogen.
A and B: The sequence 1–10 is angiotensin I and the sequence 1–8 is angiotensin II from cow (B), horse (A), and human (A)
C and D: The two sequences 86–99 and 114–127 in the B-chain of thrombin that are homologous with angiotensin
Identical positions are underlined. Arrows indicate the peptide bonds that are cleaved by thrombin, renin, and ACE (angiotensin converting enzyme)

```
                                                                              168
IA:  – Val – Leu – Gln – Val – Val – Asn – Leu – Pro – Leu – Val – Glu – Arg – Pro – Val – Cys –

IB:  – Val – Leu – Pro – Val – Ile – – – – Leu – Pro – Pro – Met – Pro – Glu – Arg – Val – Cys –

IC:  – Met – Leu – Leu – Gln – Ala – Val – Leu – Pro – Pro – Val – Pro – Glx – Pro – Val – Cys –

              182
IIA: – Asn – Asp – Met – Phe – Cys – Ala – Gly – Tyr – Lys – Pro –
             CHO
IIB: – Asn – Thr – Thr – Ile – Cys – Ala – Gly – Tyr – Cys – Pro –
```

Fig. 107. Sequence homology between two regions in the luteinizing hormone (LH) β-component (the hormone specific component) and two regions in the B-chain of thrombin
IA: The sequence 154–168 in the B-chain of thrombin
IB: The sequence 43–57 of bovine LH (β).
IC: The sequence 43–57 of human LH (β).
IIA: The sequence 178–184A–186 of the B-chain of thrombin.
IIB: The sequence 31–40 of human LH (β). Identical amino acid residues in thrombin and LH have been underlined. In thrombin Cys-168 is disulphide-bridged to Cys-182
CHO stands for carbohydrate.

stretches in thrombin which it involves are connected by a disulphide bridge (Cys-168 to Cys-182). The disulphide bridges in LH and in the hormones that are related to LH structurally, namely TSH (thyroid stimulating hormone), CG (chorionic gonadotrophin) and FSH (follicle stimulating hormone) are not known with certainty. The part of thrombin that is homologous with LH constitutes so to speak the 'floor' in the tertiary structure model of the thrombin B-chain that can be constructed with the aid of the coordinates from the chymotrypsin structure. The sequence which is most similar to that of angiotensin also constitutes part of the surface of the tertiary structure model, running almost vertically through the entire 'height' of the molecule and is located in the 'left part' of the model, 'behind' the prosthetic carbohydrate group (all relative positions in space are based on the orientation usually used to present the tertiary structure of chymotrypsin with its active centre in 'front' and His-57 'to the left of' and slightly 'below' Ser-195). The significance and possible physiological importance of these structural similarities between thrombin on the one hand and angiotensin and LH (and its congeners) on the other hand is not clear. However, it does appear that these similarities are too extensive to have evolved purely by chance. Whether they are due to partial homology, i.e. the result of an evolutionary relationship, or due to analogous evolution of 'binding sites' in the thrombin molecule which would enable it to bind to structures with an affinity for angiotensin or LH, respectively, remains to be investigated. It stands to reason that the special affinities of thrombin (as compared to other serine proteases) for platelets, fibroblasts, heparin, and for hirudin, a thrombin-specific protease inhibitor, must be reflected in the thrombin structure as a specific binding site on the thrombin surface for each of these structures. Each of these 'binding sites' must involve structural elements additional to or different from those of the catalytic site.

D. Prothrombin—structure and activation

1. Specific cleavage by factor X_a and by thrombin. Nomenclature

The prothrombin concentration in blood plasma is approximately 90 mg per litre. On electrophoresis prothrombin moves to a position between those of α_1- and α_2-globulins. Its isoelectric point is approximately 4.2–4.3. Structurally prothrombin consists of a single polypeptide chain with N-terminal Ala-(Fig. 108, line 1). Incubation with thrombin leads to the formation of the A-fragment (or fragment 1) with N-terminal Ala- and of neoprothrombin-S (or intermediate I) with N-terminal Ser- (Fig. 108, line 2). Activation catalysed by Factor X_a leads to the formation of active thrombin, consisting of an A-chain and a B-chain as mentioned above. The A-chain has N-terminal Thr- and the B-chain N-terminal Ile-. Provided the thrombin activity formed is immediately inhibited with hirudin (Kiziel and Hanahan) or with DFP at a low concentration, which inhibits thrombin but not Factor X_a (Owen, Esmon and Jackson), a profragment (or fragment 1, 2) is formed, which has N-terminal Ala- (Fig. 108, line 4). Thrombin-catalysed cleavage of the profragment leads to the formation of A-fragment and S-fragment (or fragment 2). The latter has N-terminal Ser-. Neoprothrombin-T (or intermediate II) with N-terminal Thr- can also be isolated from prothrombin activation mixtures (Fig. 108, line 3). Neither neoprothrombin-S nor neoprothrombin-T has thrombin activity (measured as clotting of fibrinogen or cleavage of small substrates).

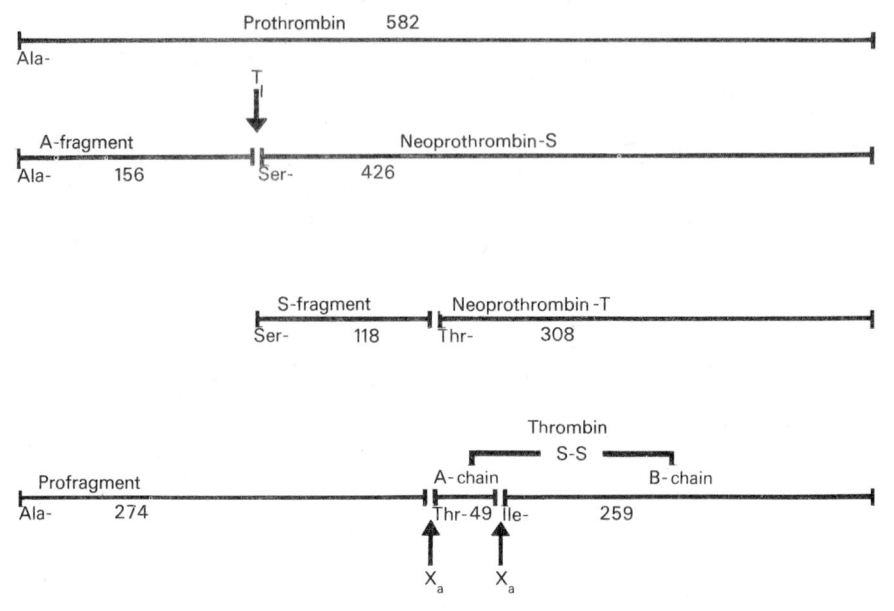

262 *Proteins taking part in coagulation and fibrinolysis*

Fig. 108. The polypeptide chain of bovine prothrombin (amino acid residues 1–582, with Ala- as N-terminal; see line 1) is cleaved by thrombin (T) at the arginyl bond in position 156. The two products are the A-fragment (amino acid residues 1–156, with Ala- as N-terminal) and neoprothrombin-S (amino acid residues 157–582, with Ser- as N-terminal; see line 2) Activation of prothrombin with Factor X_a (X_a) involves cleavage of the two arginyl bonds at positions 274 and 323. The two products are the 'pro'-fragment (amino acid residues 1–274, with N-terminal Ala-) and thrombin (the A-chain with amino acid residues 275–323 disulphide-bridged to the B-chain with amino acid residues 324–582 and with N-terminal Thr- and Ile, respectively; see line 4). Two other products, namely, the S-fragment (amino acid residues 157–274, with N-terminal Ser-) and neoprothrombin-T (amino acid residues 275–582, with N-terminal Thr-; see line 3) has also been isolated from prothrombin activation mixtures

They contain all the elements of primary structure that constitute the structure of thrombin and can be activated to thrombin. These modified zymogens or neozymogens don't have the same activation characteristics as prothrombin, the native zymogen.

2. The primary structure of prothrombin. Internal homology. 'Kringle' structures

The primary structure of bovine prothrombin has been known since 1974 (Magnusson et al., 1975). That part of the prothrombin structure which becomes thrombin on activation, constitutes about half of the prothrombin molecule and is placed as the C-terminal 'half' of the molecule (Fig. 108, line 4). The remainder of the prothrombin molecule, the so-called 'pro'-part, constitutes the N-terminal 'half' that is separated from thrombin on activation. As already mentioned thrombin can cleave the arginyl bond 156 giving rise to the A- and S-fragments. The amino acid sequence of both fragments contains an identical sequence of nine amino acid residues (-Glu-Asn-Phe-Cys-Arg-Asn-Pro-Asp-Gly-; see lines 9 and 10 in Fig. 109). In Fig. 109 the A- and S-fragment sequences have been aligned on the basis of these two identical non-apeptide

A: Ala-Asn-Lys-Gly-Phe-LEU-GLA-GLA-Val-Arg-Lys-Gly-Asn-LEU-GLA-Arg-GLA-Cys-LEU-GLA-
S:

A: -GLA-Pro-Cys-Ser-Arg-GLA-GLA-Ala-Phe-GLA-Ala-LEU-GLA-Ser-Leu-Ser-Ala-Thr-Asp-Ala-
S:

A: -Phe-Trp-Ala-Lys-Tyr-Thr-Ala-Cys-Glu-Ser-Ala-Arg-Asn-Pro-Arg-Glu-Lys-Leu-Asn-Glu-
S: Ser-Gly-Gly-Ser-Thr-Thr-Ser-Gln-Ser-

                                                    CHO
A: -Cys-Leu-Glu-Gly-Asn-Cys-Ala-Glu-Gly-Val-Gly-Met-Asn-Tyr-Arg-Gly-ASN-Val-Ser-Val-
         62
S: -Pro-Leu-Glu-Thr-Cys-Val-Pro-Asp-Arg-Gly-Arg-Glu-Tyr-Arg-Gly-Arg-Leu-Ala-Val-
         II

A: -Thr-Arg-Ser-Gly-Ile-Glu-Cys-Gln-Leu-Trp-Arg-Ser-Arg-Tyr-Pro-His-Lys-Pro-Glu-Ile-
S: -Thr-Thr-Ser-Gly-Ser-Arg-Cys-Leu-Ala-Trp-Ser-Ser-Glu-Gln-Ala-Lys-Ala-Leu-Ser-Lys-

       CHO
A: -ASN-Ser-Thr-Thr-His-Pro-Gly-Ala-Asp-Leu-Arg-Glu-Asn-Phe-Cys-Arg-Asn-Pro-Asp-Gly-
S: -Asp-Gln-Asp-Phe-Asn-Pro-Ala-Val-Pro-Leu-Ala-Glu-Asn-Phe-Cys-Arg-Asn-Pro-Asp-Gly-

A: -Ser-Ile-Thr-Gly-Pro-Trp-Cys-Tyr-Thr-Thr-Ser-Pro-Thr-Leu-Arg-Arg-Glu-Glu-Cys-Ser-
S: -Asp-Glu-Glu-Gly-Ala-Trp-Cys-Tyr-Val-Ala-Asp-Gln-Pro-Gly-Asp-Phe-Glu-Tyr-Cys-Asn-

A: -Val-Pro-Val-Cys-Gly-Gln-Asp-Arg-Val-Thr-Val-Glu-Val-Ile-Pro-Arg-
S: -Leu-Asn-Tyr-Cys-Glu-Glu-Pro-Val-Asp-Gly-Asp-Leu-Gly-Asp-Arg-Leu-Gly-Glu-Asp-Pro-

A:
S: Asp-Pro-Asp-Ala-Ala-Ile-Glu-Gly-Arg

Fig. 109. The amino acid sequences of the A-fragment (A:) and the S-fragment (S:) from the 'pro'-part of bovine prothrombin. In the A-fragment the ten Glu-residues in positions 7, 8, 15, 17, 20, 21, 26, 27, 30, and 33 have an 'extra' carboxyl group in γ-position. These γ-carboxyglutamic acid residues have tentatively been given the three-letter code Gla. CHO stands for carbohydrate. The underlined amino acid residues indicate the 31 identical positions in the mutually homologous positions of the A- and S-fragments

264 *Proteins taking part in coagulation and fibrinolysis*

sequences. When the A- and S-fragments were compared in this way it turned out that they contain corresponding sequences of 83 residues (starting with position 62 in the A-fragment and position 11 in the S-fragment) with 31 residues that are identical in the two fragments. This constitutes a high degree of internal sequence homology, showing that these two parts of the prothrombin structure have evolved through a duplication and cross-over of the corresponding part of the ancestral prothrombin genes. Six of the 31 identical positions in the A- and S-fragments are half-cystine residues. The disulphide-bridge pattern is identical in the two homologous regions, namely 1–6, 2–4, 3–5 giving rise to the kringle*-like structures in the two-dimensional schematic drawing in Fig. 110 and making it highly probable that the three-dimensional structure is also basically the same for these two regions. The two oligosaccharide substituents in the A-fragment are attached in the kringle region, while the S-fragment is entirely lacking in carbohydrate. All the three asparagine residues of prothrombin which are glucosylated, namely Asn-77, Asn-101, and Asn-376, occur in a sequence that fits the recognized sequence characteristics of glycoproteins with glucosamine-based oligosaccharide substituents, namely Asn-X-Ser or Asn-X-Thr. Those parts of the S-fragment kringle that correspond to Asn-77 and Asn-101 in the A-kringle don't fit this criterion for substitution with a glucosamine-based oligosaccharide. The detailed covalent structures of the three oligosaccharide substituents in prothrombin are not yet known. The comparison between the A- and S-fragments also shows that the first part of the A-fragment sequence (residues 1–61) has no counterpart in the S-fragment.

3. γ-Carboxyglutamic acid, Ca^{2+} and phospholipid binding, vitamin K

Since the studies by Link and by Dam in the 1930s and 1940s it had been generally assumed that a lack of vitamin K or the administration of dicoumarol would cause a shut-down of the biosynthesis of prothrombin in the hepatic cells of the liver. When a

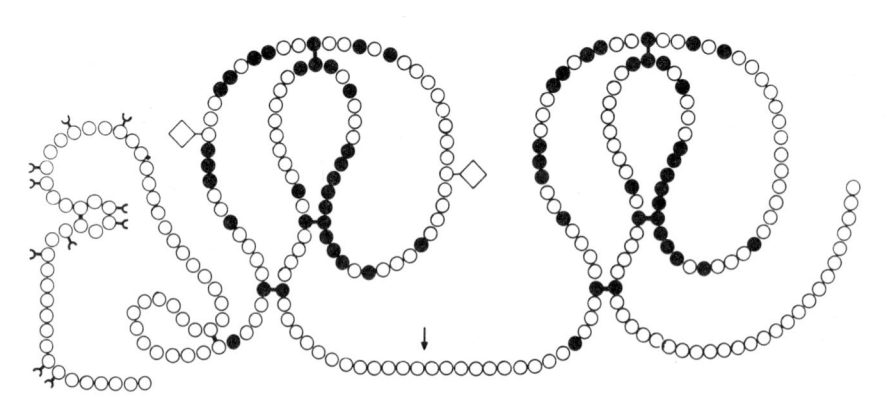

Fig. 110. The primary structure of the 'pro'-part (residues 1–274) of bovine prothrombin. Each circle represents one amino acid residue. The N-terminal is at the lower left-hand corner, the C-terminal in the middle on the right side. Circles with forks represent Gla-residues. The arrow points to the thrombin-sensitive arginyl bond 156–157. Cleavage of this bond gives the A- and the S-fragment (residues 1–156 and 157–274, respectively). Filled circles: sequence identities in the two mutually homologous kringle regions (residues 62–144 and 167–249). Joined circles: disulphide bridges. Diamonds: carbohydrate

*Shape of Scandinavian cake.

precipitin reaction was developed for the immunological determination of prothrombin in blood plasma (Josso et al., 1968; Ganrot and Niléhn, 1968) it turned out that patients on dicoumarol therapy had a protein in their plasma which cross-reacted with the prothrombin antiserum but could not be activated to thrombin in the usual Ca^{2+}, phospholipid-dependent test system. This 'dicoumarol' prothrombin differs from normal prothrombin not only in its activation properties but also by not being adsorbed to for example barium citrate and by not binding Ca^{2+}-ions (Ganrot and Niléhn, 1968). Stenflo (1972) developed a purification method for dicoumarol prothrombin and it was found (Stenflo, 1972; Nelsestuen and Suttie, 1972) that its amino acid and carbohydrate composition did not differ significantly from that of normal prothrombin. Ca^{2+}-binding studies using equilibrium dialysis indicate that normal prothrombin binds 3–4 Ca^{2+}-ions relatively strongly (Nelsestuen and Suttie, 1972; Stenflo and Ganrot, 1973). However, the affinity of prothrombin towards Ca^{2+}-ions is one or more orders of magnitude less than for most of the well-known Ca^{2+}-binding proteins, such as troponin C and parvalbumin.

The first indication that normal prothrombin contains an unusual structure was the isolation of the two tryptic peptides -Gly-Phe-Leu-Glx-Glx-Val-Arg- (residues 4–10) and -Gly-Phe-Leu-Glx-Glx-Val-Arg-Lys (residues 4-11) (Figs. 109 and 111). These peptides turned out to have electrophoretic mobilities at pH 6.5 that could not be explained unless the peptides had two negative charges in excess of those that could be accounted for by residues 7 and 8 being normal glutamic acid (Magnusson 1972, 1973), probably as a result of a vitamin-K-dependent substitution on Glu-7 and/or Glu-8 (Magnusson et al., 1973). Neither peptide contained carbohydrate. A different tryptic peptide (probably from position 12–35) was isolated (Nelsestuen and Suttie, 1973) by adsorption to barium citrate. Stenflo (1074) confirmed the presence of the extra negative charges on peptides 4–10 and 4–11. He also found that the corresponding peptides from dicoumarol prothrombin had electrophoretic mobilities indicating normal glutamic acid in positions 7 and 8. During the course of determining the primary structure of normal prothrombin by 'classical' sequence methods it turned out that at least six Glx-residues in positions 7, 8, 26, 27, 30, and 33 each carried one extra negative charge, and that acetylation and permethylation for mass spectrometry led to the formation of Glx-derivatives with an extra methyl group and showing a characteristic decarboxylation pattern (Magnusson et al., in Hemker and Veltkamp 1975). Stenflo et al. (1974) proposed the structure γ-carboxyglutamic acid for residues 7 and 8, on the basis of nuclear magnetic resonance measurements and mass spectrometry. By using either deuterated methanol in the 'acetylation' step or deuterated methyl iodide in the permethylation step for a complete mass spectrometric amino-acid sequence and structure investigation of the entire region 1–42 it turned out that all ten Glx-residues are in fact γ-carboxyglutamic acid residues, Gla (Magnusson et al., 1974; Morris et al., 1976) (Fig. 111). The two γ-carboxyl groups of each Gla-residue are esterified by methanol in the 'acetylation' step. In the permethylation step one methyl group reacts on the α-amino nitrogen as expected and an extra methyl group is added to the γ-carbon because of the malonic ester character of the structure. Thus, a total of *four* methyl groups are added in this derivation procedure (Magnusson et al., 1974; Morris et al., 1976), *not two* as was first claimed by Stenflo et al. (1974). These authors have later corrected their evidence for positions 7 and 8 (Fernlund et al., 1975). The structure has been confirmed by synthesis (Morris et al., 1975; several other groups).

The available evidence though not entirely conclusive, indicates that dicoumarol

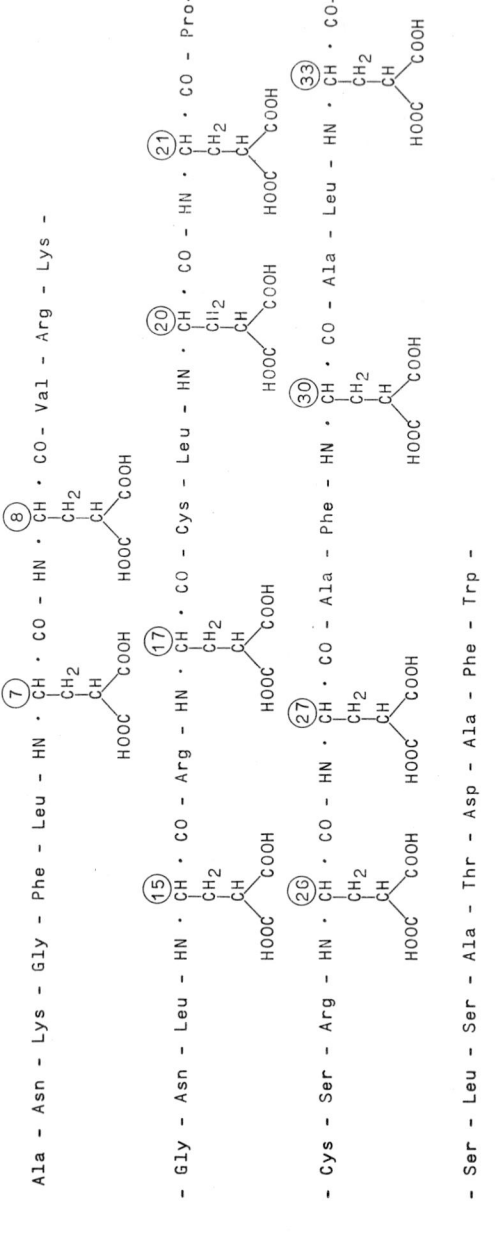

Fig. 111. Locations of the ten γ-carboxyglutamic acid residues in the primary structure of the vitamin-K-dependent, Ca^{2+}-binding region 1–42 of bovine prothrombin (Magnusson et al., 1974)

prothrombin has normal glutamic acid residues in all those ten positions that are γ-carboxylated in normal prothrombin. Until now no other difference has been found. Therefore, it seems logical to assume that the function of vitamin K in the biosynthesis of prothrombin is to make possible the γ-carboxylation of these glutamic acid residues. The stronger Ca^{2+}-binding of normal prothrombin can be accounted for by its content of γ-carboxyglutamic acid residues. Not only prothrombin itself (Ganrot and Niléhn, 1968) but also small peptides containing γ-carboxyglutamic acid change their electrophoretic mobility when Ca^{2+} is added to the buffer (Stenflo, 1974). Unless prothrombin can bind Ca^{2+}-ions it cannot interact normally with the phospholipids that stimulate its activation. The rapid activation of prothrombin to thrombin catalysed by Factor X_a in the presence of Factor V and phospholipids involves the formation of a Ca^{2+}-dependent complex of prothrombin and phospholipids (Bull et al., 1972; other groups). Three main lines of evidence imply the A-fragment (or fragment 1) and particularly the γ-carboxyglutamic acid residues as playing a decisive role in this complex formation. One is the fact that the neoprothrombin-S (intermediate I), which lacks the entire A-fragment (Magnusson 1962, 1965; Magnusson et al., 1975) cannot be activated (Magnusson 1962, 1965) in phospholipid-dependent test systems. The second line of evidence is that dicoumarol prothrombin which does contain the A-fragment (fragment 1) but without the extra carboxyl groups (Stenflo, 1974; Stenflo et al., 1974) also cannot be activated (Josso et al., 1968; Ganrot and Niléhn, 1968) in the phospholipid-dependent test systems. However, it can be activated by a specific snake venom enzyme (Echis carinatus) to form active thrombin. The third line of evidence comes from studies of the binding of metal ions and phospholipids to isolated prothrombin activation products (mainly by the groups of Jackson, Mann and Furie). These studies indicate that the Ca^{2+}-phospholipid binding characteristics of the A-fragment are very similar to those of native prothrombin, indicating that the A-fragment is the domain responsible for these properties of prothrombin. The detailed mechanism of the Ca^{2+}-phospholipid binding in structural terms will have to await a solution of the tertiary structure of the A-fragment or of prothrombin itself. X-ray crystallography of the A-fragment and of its Ca^{2+}-complex is going on in two different laboratories but the structure has not yet been solved. One can suggest different possibilities to describe the interactions in structural terms. None of the following three hypotheses can be ruled out at present.

1. The Ca^{2+}-ions form bridges between γ-carboxyl groups in the vitamin-K-dependent region of prothrombin and phosphate groups in phospholipids.
2. The Ca^{2+}-ions connect γ-carboxyglutamyl residues in prothrombin changing the conformation of the region 1–42 such that hydrophobic, normally internal parts of the structure are exposed and a lipid-binding site is formed.
3. It is conceivable that the conformational change in 2 leads to exposure of a hydrophobic lipid-binding site in a part of the prothrombin structure outside the region 1–42. Although this may appear to be a far-fetched hypothesis, it does offer a way out of the apparent paradox that a structure that does not bind phospholipid would become phospholipid-binding by the addition of ten extra negative charges. The question whether Ca^{2+}-ion binding is the only function of γ-carboxyglutamic acid cannot yet be answered. The carboxyl groups of normal aspartyl and glutamyl residues cannot be esterified under the 'acetylation' conditions that lead to esterifi-

cation of γ-carboxyglutamyl residues. However, at present there is no evidence to indicate that this higher reactivity of the γ carboxyl groups of the Gla-residues is of biological significance.

4. Homology with plasminogen

In connection with the determination of the primary structure of the urokinase-sensitive region, which overlaps the C-terminal part of the potential heavy chain to the N-terminal part of the potential light chain of plasmin, the heavy chain was found to contain a sequence that is homologous with part of the two kringle structures in the 'pro'-part of prothrombin (Sottrup-Jensen et al., 1975). When this finding was followed up by determining the primary structure of the whole heavy chain it turned out to contain five complete kringle structures (Claeys et al., 1976), which show a high degree of sequence homology with the two in prothrombin and also the same pattern of kringle disulphides (12 of the 15 disulphide bridges in the kringles have been determined) (Magnusson et al., 1976; Fig. 112). The complete amino acid sequence and 19 of the 24 disulphide bridges of plasminogen (residues 1–790) had been determined by May 1977 (Sottrup-Jensen et al.). Since plasmin is a serine protease, it was predictable that the light chain (residues 561–790) would turn out to be homologous with the other members of the serine protease family, such as thrombin and the pancreatic serine proteases. The occurrence of the five kringle structures in the heavy chain was not predictable on this basis. It means that this part of the heavy chain in plasmin has evolved as a result of a partial gen-'quintuplication' (or four duplications) and also that the two kringle structures of prothrombin and the five of plasminogen have evolved from a common ancestor. The strong conservation of the kringle structures implies that they have essential biological functions in both prothrombin and plasminogen. The mutual sequence homology of the seven kringle structures is sufficiently extensive to imply that they have basically the same tertiary structure and mechanism of action. While the vitamin-K-dependent region in prothrombin is clearly related to the binding of Ca^{2+} and phospholipids the function of the kringle structures is far from clear. Recent work (Mann et al., 1975) indicates that the S-fragment may bind to thrombin. Limited proteolysis of plasminogen by elastase (Sottrup-Jensen et al., 1978) provided a means of separating kringle 4 of plasminogen as a separate fragment (residues 354–439) with its native structure intact. This fragment has been crystallized and contains a lysine-affinity site. It is conceivable that the common denominator of function in the kringle structures is to provide binding sites for specific structures with which the particular zymogen interacts during activation or, in the case of plasminogen, perhaps after activation such that its proteolytic effect is prevented from spreading indiscriminately.

5. Homology with other vitamin-K-dependent proteins

The sequence determination of bovine Factor X_a has shown that the heavy chain (Titani et al., 1975) is strongly homologous with the B-chain of thrombin, which had been expected since it contains the active site with the DFP-reactive serine residue (Fig. 113). The light chain (Enfield et al., 1975) contains 144 amino acid residues. There is a high degree of homology with the A-fragment of prothrombin (75 per cent of the first 32–33 positions, 62 per cent in the first 44–45) in the N-terminal region but the

III. Thrombin and prothrombin   269

```
      1                                                        20
Glu-Pro-Leu-Asp-Asp-Tyr-Val-Asn-Thr-Gln-Gly-Ala-Ser-Leu-Phe-Ser-Val-Thr-Lys-Lys-
-Gln-Leu-Gly-Ala-Gly-Ser-Ile-Glu-Glu-Cys-Ala-Ala-Lys-Cys-Glu-Glu-Asp-Glu-Glu-Phe-
-Thr-Cys-Arg-Ala-Phe-Gln-Tyr-His-Ser-Lys-Glu-Gln-Glu-Cys-Val-Ile-Met-Ala-Glu-Asn-
-Arg-Lys-Ser-Ser-Ile-Ile-Arg-Met-Arg-Asp-Val-Val-Leu-Phe-Glu-Lys-Lys-Val-Tyr-Leu-
-Ser-Glu-Cys-Lys-Thr-Gly-Asp-Gly-Lys-Asn-Tyr-Arg-Gly-Thr-Met-Ser-Lys-Thr-Lys-Asn-
-Gly-Ile-Thr-Cys-Gln-Lys-Trp-Ser-Ser-Thr-Ser-Pro-His-Arg-Pro-Arg-Phe-Ser-Pro-Ala-
-Thr-His-Pro-Ser-Glu-Gly-Leu-Glu-Glu-Asn-Tyr-Cys-Arg-Asn-Pro-Asp-Asn-Asp-Pro-Gln-
-Gly-Pro-Trp-Cys-Tyr-Thr-Thr-Asp-Pro-Glu-Lys-Arg-Tyr-Asp-Tyr-Cys-Asp-Ile-Leu-Glu-
-Cys-Glu-Glu-Glu-Cys-Met-His-Cys-Ser-Gly-Glu-Asn-Tyr-Asp-Gly-Lys-Ile-Ser-Lys-Thr-
-Met-Ser-Gly-Leu-Glu-Cys-Gln-Ala-Trp-Asp-Ser-Gln-Ser-Pro-His-Ala-His-Gly-Tyr-Ile-
-Pro-Ser-Lys-Phe-Pro-Asn-Lys-Asn-Leu-Lys-Lys-Asn-Tyr-Cys-Arg-Asn-Pro-Asp-Arg-Glu-
-Leu-Arg-Pro-Trp-Cys-Phe-Thr-Thr-Asp-Pro-Asn-Lys-Arg-Trp-Glu-Leu-Cys-Asp-Ile-Pro-
-Arg-Cys-Thr-Thr-Pro-Pro-Pro-Ser-Ser-Gly-Pro-Thr-Tyr-Gln-Cys-Leu-Lys-Gly-Thr-Gly-
-Glu-Asn-Tyr-Arg-Gly-Asn-Val-Ala-Val-Thr-Val-Ser-Gly-His-Thr-Cys-Gln-His-Trp-Ser-
                                CHO
-Ala-Gln-Thr-Pro-His-Thr-His-Asn-Arg-Thr-Pro-Glu-Asn-Phe-Pro-Cys-Lys-Asn-Leu-Asp-
-Glu-Asn-Tyr-Cys-Arg-Asn-Pro-Asp-Gly-Lys-Arg-Ala-Pro-Trp-Cys-His-Thr-Thr-Asn-Ser-
-Gln-Val-Arg-Trp-Glu-Tyr-Cys-Lys-Ile-Pro-Ser-Cys-Asp-Ser-Ser-Pro-Val-Ser-Thr-Glu-
                      CHO
-Glu-Leu-Ala-Pro-Thr-Ala-Pro-Pro-Glu-Leu-Thr-Pro-Val-Val-Gln-Asp-Cys-Tyr-His-Gly-
-Asp-Gly-Gln-Ser-Tyr-Arg-Gly-Thr-Ser-Ser-Thr-Thr-Thr-Thr-Gly-Lys-Lys-Cys-Gln-Ser-
-Trp-Ser-Ser-Met-Thr-Pro-His-Arg-His-Gln-Lys-Thr-Pro-Glu-Asn-Tyr-Pro-Asn-Ala-Gly-
-Leu-Thr-Met-Asn-Tyr-Cys-Arg-Asn-Pro-Asp-Ala-Asp-Lys-Gly-Pro-Trp-Cys-Phe-Thr-Thr-
-Asp-Pro-Ser-Val-Arg-Trp-Glu-Tyr-Cys-Asn-Leu-Lys-Lys-Cys-Ser-Gly-Thr-Glu-Ala-Ser-
-Val-Val-Ala-Pro-Pro-Pro-Val-Val-Leu-Leu-Pro-Asn-Val-Glu-Thr-Pro-Ser-Glu-Glu-Asp-
-Cys-Met-Phe-Gly-Asn-Gly-Lys-Gly-Tyr-Arg-Gly-Lys-Arg-Ala-Thr-Thr-Val-Thr-Gly-Thr-
-Pro-Cys-Gln-Asp-Trp-Ala-Ala-Gln-Glu-Pro-His-Arg-His-Ser-Ile-Phe-Thr-Pro-Glu-Thr-
-Asn-Pro-Arg-Ala-Gly-Leu-Glu-Lys-Asn-Tyr-Cys-Arg-Asn-Pro-Asp-Gly-Asp-Val-Gly-Gly-
-Pro-Trp-Cys-Tyr-Thr-Thr-Asn-Pro-Arg-Lys-Leu-Tyr-Asp-Tyr-Cys-Asp-Val-Pro-Gln-Cys-
-Ala-Ala-Pro-Ser-Phe-Asp-Cys-Gly-Lys-Pro-Gln-Val-Glu-Pro-Lys-Lys-Cys-Pro-Gly-Arg-
 Val-Val-Gly-Gly-Cys-Val-Ala-His-Pro-His-Ser-Trp-Pro-Trp-Gln-Val-Ser-Leu-Arg-Thr-
-Arg-Phe-Gly-Met-His-Phe-Cys-Gly-Gly-Thr-Leu-Ile-Ser-Pro-Glu-Trp-Val-Leu-Thr-Ala-
-Ala-His-Cys-Leu-Glu-Lys-Ser-Pro-Arg-Pro-Ser-Ser-Tyr-Lys-Val-Ile-Leu-Gly-Ala-His-
-Gln-Glu-Val-Asn-Leu-Glu-Pro-His-Val-Gln-Glu-Ile-Glu-Val-Ser-Arg-Leu-Phe-Leu-Glu-
-Pro-Thr-Arg-Lys-Asp-Ile-Ala-Leu-Leu-Lys-Leu-Ser-Ser-Pro-Ala-Val-Ile-Thr-Asp-Lys-
-Val-Ile-Pro-Ala-Cys-Leu-Pro-Ser-Pro-Asn-Tyr-Val-Val-Ala-Asp-Arg-Thr-Glu-Cys-Phe-
-Ile-Thr-Gly-Trp-Gly-Glu-Thr-Gln-Gly-Thr-Phe-Gly-Ala-Gly-Leu-Leu-Lys-Glu-Ala-Gln-
-Leu-Pro-Val-Ile-Glu-Asn-Lys-Val-Cys-Asn-Arg-Tyr-Glu-Phe-Leu-Asn-Gly-Arg-Val-Gln-
-Ser-Thr-Glu-Leu-Cys-Ala-Gly-His-Leu-Ala-Gly-Gly-Thr-Asp-Ser-Cys-Gln-Gly-Asp-Ser-
-Gly-Gly-Pro-Leu-Val-Cys-Phe-Glu-Lys-Asp-Lys-Tyr-Ile-Leu-Gln-Gly-Val-Thr-Ser-Trp-
-Gly-Leu-Gly-Cys-Ala-Arg-Pro-Asn-Lys-Pro-Gly-Val-Tyr-Val-Arg-Val-Ser-Arg-Phe-Val-
-Thr-Trp-Ile-Glu-Gly-Val-Met-Arg-Asn-Asn
```

Fig. 112A–D. Comparison between the primary structures of prothrombin and plasminogen
Fig. 112A. Complete amino acid sequence of human plasminogen (residues 1–790). Heavy chain region (first 28 lines, residues 1–560). Light chain or serine protease region (Past 12 lines residues 561–790). The latter is homologous with the B-chain of thrombin and the other serine proteases

270 Proteins taking part in coagulation and fibrinolysis

```
PAP:                                        Glu-Pro-Leu-Asp-Asp-Tyr-Val-Asn-Thr-Gln-Gly-Ala-Ser-Leu-Phe-Ser-Val-
                                                           10                            20
A:   Ala-Asn-Lys-Gly-Phe-Leu-Gla-Gla-Val-Arg-Lys-Gly-Asn-Leu-Gla-Arg-Gla-Cys-Leu-Gla-Gla-Pro-Cys-Ser-Arg-
PAP: -Thr-Lys-Lys-Gln-Leu-Gly-Ala-Gly-Ser-Ile-Glu-Glu-Cys-Ala-Ala-Lys-Cys-Glu-Glu-Asp-Glu-Glu-Phe-Thr-Cys-
                     30                            40                            50
A:   -Gla-Gla-Ala-Phe-Gla-Ala-Leu-Gla-Ser-Leu-Ser-Ala-Thr-Asp-Ala-Phe-Trp-Ala-Lys-Tyr-Thr-Ala-Cys-Glu-Ser-
PAP: -Arg-Ala-Phe-Gln-Tyr-His-Ser-Lys-Gln-Glu-Glu-Cys-Val-Ile-Met-Ala-Glu-Asn-Arg-Lys-Ser-Ser-Ile-Ile-Arg-
                                   60                            70
A:   -Ala-Arg-Asn-Pro-Arg-Glu-Lys-Leu-Asn-Glu-Cys-Leu-Glu-Gly-Asn-Cys-Ala-Glu-Gly-Val-Gly-Met-Asn-Tyr-Arg-
S:             Ser-Gly-Gly-Ser-Thr-Thr-Ser-Gln-Ser-Pro-Leu-Leu-Glu-Thr-Cys-Val-Pro-Asp-Arg-Gly-Arg-Glu-Tyr-Arg-
1:   -Met-Arg-Asp-Val-Val-Leu-Phe-Glu-Lys-Lys-Val-Tyr-Leu-Ser-Glu-CYS-Lys-Thr-GLY-Asp-GLY-Lys-ASN-TYR-ARG-
2:                                                             CYS-Met-His-Cys-Ser-GLY-Glu-ASN-TYR-Asp-
3:                                                             CYS-Leu-Lys-GLY-Thr-GLY-Glu-ASN-TYR-ARG-
4:                                                             CYS-Tyr-His-GLY-Asp-GLY-Gln-Ser-TYR-ARG-
5:                                                  -Glu-Asp-CYS-Met-Phe-GLY-Asn-GLY-Lys-Gly-TYR-ARG-
             CHO       80                                2             90                            100
A:   -Gly-Asn-Val-Ser-Val-Thr-Arg-Ser-Gly-Ile-Glu-Cys-Gln-Leu-Trp-Arg-Ser-Arg-Tyr-Pro-His-Lys-Pro-Glu-Ile-
S:   -Gly-Arg-Leu-Ala-Val-Thr-Thr-Ser-Gly-Ser-Arg-Cys-Leu-Ala-Trp-Ser-Ser-Glu-Gln-Ala-Lys-Ala-Leu-Ser-Lys-
1:   -GLY-Thr-Met-SER-Lys-THR-Lys-Asn-GLY-ILE-Thr-CYS-GLN-Lys-TRP-SER-SER-Thr-Ser-PRO-HIS-Arg-PRO-Arg-Phe-
2:   -GLY-Lys-Ile-SER-Lys-THR-Met-SER-GLY-Leu-GLU-CYS-GLN-ALA-TRP-Asp-SER-Gln-Ser-PRO-HIS-ALA-His-Gly-Tyr-
                                                                                                     CHO
3:   -GLY-ASN-VAL-ALA-VAL-THR-Val-SER-GLY-His-Thr-CYS-GLN-His-TRP-SER-Ala-Gln-Thr-PRO-HIS-Thr-His-Asn-Arg-
4:   -GLY-Thr-Ser-SER-Thr-THR-THR-Thr-GLY-Lys-Lys-CYS-GLN-Ser-TRP-SER-SER-Met-Thr-PRO-HIS-Arg-His-Gln-LYS-
5:   -GLY-Lys-Arg-ALA-Thr-THR-Val-Thr-GLY-Thr-Pro-CYS-GLN-Asp-TRP-Ala-Ala-Gln-Glu-PRO-HIS-Arg-His-SER-ILE-Phe-

             CHO              110                    3              120
A:   -Asn-Ser-Thr-Thr-His-Pro-Gly-Ala-Asp-Leu-Arg-Glu-Asn-Phe-Cys-Arg-Asn-Pro-Asp-Gly-Ser-Ile-Thr-Gly-Pro-
S:   -Asp-Gln-Asp-Phe-Asn-Pro-Ala-Val-Pro-Leu-Ala-Glu-Asn-Phe-Cys-Arg-Asn-Pro-Asp-Gly-Asp-Glu-Glu-Gly-Ala-
1:   -Ser-Pro-Ala-THR-HIS-PRO-Ser-Glu-Gly-LEU-Glu-GLU-ASN-Tyr-CYS-ARG-ASN-PRO-ASP-Asn-ASP-Pro-Gln-GLY-PRO-
2:   -Ile-Pro-Ser-Lys-Phe-PRO-Asn-Lys-Asn-LEU-Lys-Lys-ASN-Tyr-CYS-ARG-ASN-PRO-ASP-Arg-Glu-Leu-Arg- - -PRO-
3:   -Thr-Pro-Glu-Asn-Phe-PRO-Cys-Lys-Asn-LEU-Asp-GLU-ASN-Tyr-CYS-ARG-ASN-PRO-ASP-GLY-Lys-Arg-Ala- - -PRO-
4:   -Thr-Pro-Glu-Asn-Tyr-PRO-Asn-ALA-Gly-LEU-Thr-Met-ASN-Tyr-CYS-ARG-ASN-PRO-ASP-Ala-ASP-Lys- - -GLY-PRO-
5:   -Thr-Pro-Glu-THR-ASN-PRO-Arg-ALA-Gly-LEU-Glu-Lys-ASN-Tyr-CYS-ARG-ASN-PRO-ASP-GLY-ASP-Val-Gly-GLY-PRO-
           4        130                   5       140          6                    150
A:   -Trp-Cys-Tyr-Thr-Thr-Ser-Pro-Thr-Leu-Arg-Arg-Glu-Glu-Cys-Ser-Val-Pro-Val-Cys-Gly-Gln-Asp-Arg-Val-Thr-
S:   -Trp-Cys-Tyr-Val-Ala-Asp-Gln-Pro-Gly-Asp-Phe-Glu-Tyr-Cys-Asp-Leu-Asn-Tyr-Cys-Glu-Glu-Pro-Val-Asp-Gly-
1:   -TRP-CYS-TYR-THR-THR-ASP-PRO-Glu-Lys-ARG-Tyr-Asp-TYR-CYS-ASP-Ile-Leu-Glu-CYS-Glu-Glu-Glu-  cont. in 2
2:   -TRP-CYS-Phe-THR-THR-ASP-PRO-Asn-Lys-ARG-Trp-GLU-Leu-CYS-ASP-Ile-PRO-Arg-CYS-Thr-Thr-Pro-Pro-Pro-Ser-
3:   -TRP-CYS-TYR-THR-Asn-Ser-Gln-Val-ARG-Trp-GLU-TYR-CYS-Lys-Ile-PRO-Ser-CYS-Asp-Ser-Ser-Val-Ser-
4:   -TRP-CYS-PHe-THR-THR-ASP-PRO-Ser-Val-ARG-Trp-GLU-TYR-CYS-Asn-LEU-Lys-Lys-CYS-Ser-Gly-Thr-Glu-Ala-Ser-
5:   -TRP-CYS-TYR-THR-THR-Asn-PRO-Arg-Lys-Leu-Tyr-Asp-TYR-CYS-ASP-VAL-PRO-Gln-CYS-Ala-Ala-Pro-Ser-Phe-Asp-

A:   -Val-Glu-Val-Ile-Pro-Arg
S:   -Asp-Leu-Gly-Asp-Arg-Leu-Gly-Glu-Asp-Pro-Asp-Pro-Asp-Ala-Ala-Ile-Glu-Gly-Arg
1:
2:   -Ser-Gly-Pro-Thr-Tyr-Gln-   cont. in 3.
                          CHO
3:   -Thr-Glu-Glu-Leu-Ala-Pro-Thr-Ala-Pro-Pro-Glu-Leu-Thr-Pro-Val-Val-Gln-Asp-   cont. in 4.
4:   -Val-Val-Ala-Pro-Pro-Pro-Val-Val-Leu-Leu-Pro-Asn-Val-Glu-Thr-Pro-Ser-Glu-   cont. in 5.
5:   -Cys-Gly-Lys-Pro-Gln-Val-Glu-Pro-Lys-Lys-Cys-Pro-Gly-Arg-   cont. in light chain.
```

Fig. 112B. An alignment of the amino acid sequence of residues 1–274 of bovine prothrombin (the 'pro'-fragment) with that of residues 1–560 (the heavy chain region) of human plasminogen. *A*: Amino acid residues 1–156 of prothrombin (the A-fragment). *S*: Amino acid residues 157–274 of prothrombin (the S-fragment). The A- and S-fragments have been aligned as in Fig. 110. *PAP*: The preactivation peptide region (residues 1–76) of plasminogen. 1–5: The heavy chain part of plasmin contains five regions of sequence that are both mutually homologous and homologous with the two kringle structures in prothrombin. Therefore, the heavy chain sequence 77–560 has been arranged as lines 1–5. Actually the first two residues Met–Arg on line 1 are residues 68–69

Figure 112B continued

of the PAP-region which ends with the sequence Glu–Lys (residues 75–76). The N-terminal of Lys-plasminogen is Lys-77 (aligned with Glu-60 of the A-fragment). The C-terminal of the heavy chain is Arg-560 at the end of line 5

The numbers 10, 20, 30, etc. refer to the residue numbers in the A-fragment of prothrombin. In addition, the six Cys-residues that are common to all seven kringle structures are numbered 1, 2, 3, 4, 5, and 6. Boxed residues are common to the two kringles in prothrombin, the five kringles in plasminogen, or to all seven kringles in both prothrombin and plasminogen. Twenty positions are identical in all seven kringle structures (25 per cent). Another ten are identical in only the two prothrombin kringles (a total of 38 per cent identity). Another eight are identical in only the five plasminogen kringles (a total of 35 per cent)

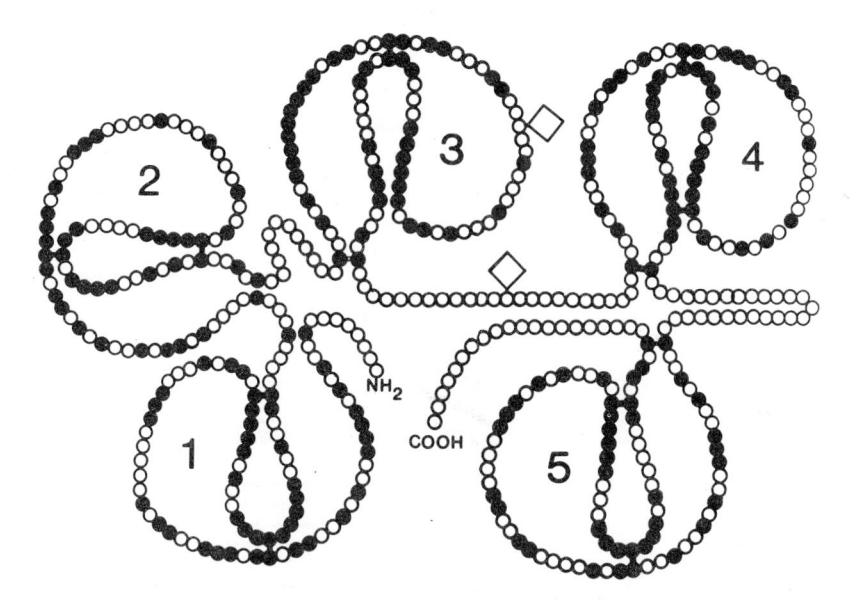

Fig. 112C. The primary structure of residues 75–560 of human plasminogen arranged the same way as that of the 'pro'-part of prothrombin in Fig. 110, and using the same symbols. Filled circles: Residues identical to the corresponding residues in the A-and/or S-fragment kringle of bovine prothrombin (the same residues that are written with three capital letters in Fig. 112B. Twelve of the fifteen kringle disulphide bridges have been established. NH_2: Glu-75 is the first residue shown. *COOH*: Arg-560 the C-terminal of the heavy chain. 1, 2, 3, 4, and 5: The five kringles, corresponding to the sequence stretches Cys-1 to Cys-6 for each of the five kringles in Fig. 112B. *Diamonds*: The two oligosaccharide groups. The glucosamine-based oligosaccharide is attached to Asn-288 (kringle 3) and is present in about half of the plasminogen molecules. The galactosamine-based oligosaccharide is attached to Thr-345 (connecting strand between kringles 3 and 4)

remainder of the two structures shows little or no sequence homology. This means that the vitamin-K-dependent Ca^{2+}-binding region has been strongly conserved during evolution and probably functions almost identically in the two proteins, and also that this structure comprises only the regions 1–45. This type of structure occurs also in Factor IX, Factor VII, and protein C, as indicated by the fact that all these proteins

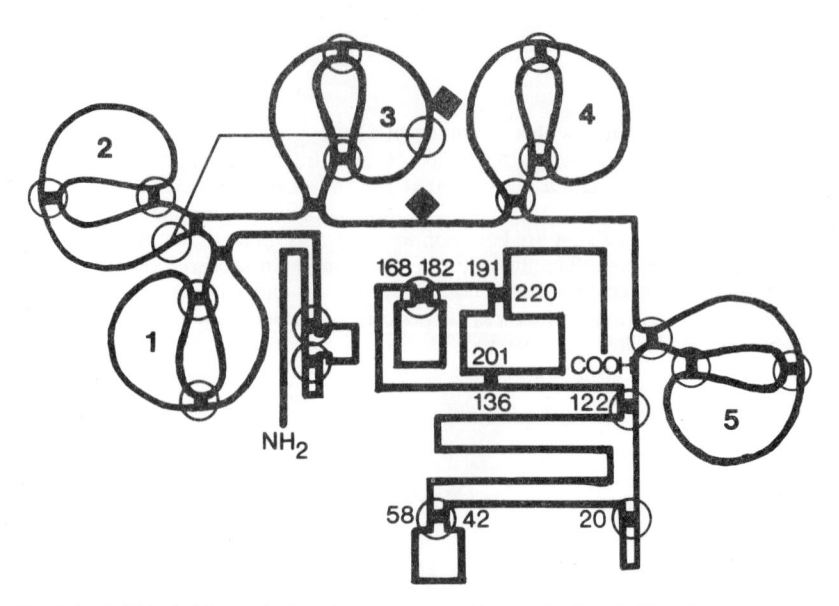

Fig. 112D. Disulphide bridges of plasminogen. NH_2: N-terminal end (Glu-1). *COOH*: C-terminal end (Asn-790). *Numbers 1 to 5*: The five kringle structures of the heavy chain part. *Circles*: Disulphide bridges that have been established (19 bridges). Bridges not circled (5 bridges) have been predicted on the basis of homology with prothrombin and the pancreatic serine proteases. *Thin line*: The inter-(2 to 3)-kringle disulphide bridge. *Numbers 20 to 220*: Cys-residues of light chain part using chymotrypsin numbering

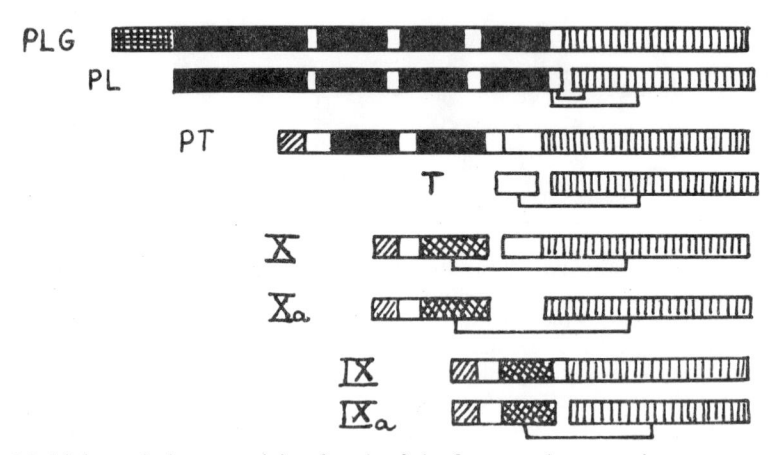

Fig. 113. Multiple evolutionary origin of each of the four regulatory serine protease zymogens; plasminogen (PLG), prothrombin (PT), Factor X (X), and Factor IX (IX). The corresponding activated enzymes are plasmin (PL), thrombin (T), Factor X_a (X_a) and Factor IX_a (IX_a). (Data on Factors X and IX from works by Enfield *et al.* and Titani *et al.* in laboratories of E. Davie and H. Neurath, Seattle.) Mutually homologous sequence regions marked identically in the different proteins. Thus, *vertical hatching* indicates serine protease region common to all four; *full black*: kringle structures common to plasminogen (5) and prothrombin (2); *rhombic cross-hatching*: 'pseudo-kringle' regions common to Factors X and IX; *squared cross-hatching*: N-terminal (PAP)-region unique to plasminogen; '*half*' *cross-hatching*: N-terminal (vitamin-K-dependent) regions common to prothrombin, Factors X, and IX. Each of these five types of structure represents one protein/'miniprotein' family from the evolutionary point of view. *White areas* have not been considered in this comparison.

show sequence homology with prothrombin and Factor X in their first 10–14 positions (Davie et al.; Nemerson et al.; Stenflo et al.).

The schematic comparison in Fig. 113 shows that activation of prothrombin to thrombin leads to the separation of the vitamin-K-dependent Ca^{2+}-phospholipid binding region and the serine protease into two different molecules, namely thrombin and the A-fragment, whereas in Factors X and IX the inter-chain disulphide bridge still connects the serine protease chain and the Ca^{2+}-phospholipid binding chain even after activation. Therefore it is possible that whereas Factors X_a and IX_a stay bound to the surface on which they are activated, thrombin probably doesn't. The overall effect of vitamin K on the clotting system appears to be that it provides the structural means (γ-carboxyglutamyl residues) by which Factors IX, IX_a, X, X_a, and prothrombin can be concentrated on an activating surface thus allowing a much more rapid activation than could otherwise take place, considering the low concentrations of these factors in plasma. Theoretically a 'long' thrombin (residues 1–323 disulphide-bridged to residues 324–582) containing all of the original prothrombin structure (analogous with Glu-plasmin) could be produced if only the second of the two Factor-X_a-sensitive bonds were split. So far there is no good evidence that such a 'long' thrombin is formed either in physiological or in pathological conditions. Such a thrombin molecule could be expected to stay bound to an activating surface and cause local precipitation of fibrin, for example on endothelial membranes.

Outside of the coagulation system γ-carboxyglutamic acid has been found in a bone protein (Hauschka et al., 1975). This protein, osteocalcin, has been sequenced (Price et al., 1976). Of its 49 residues three are γ-carboxyglutamic acid and one is an hydroxyproline. The protein has a high affinity for hydroxyl-apatite but not for other calcium phosphates. Its sequence shows no homology with prothrombin. Gallop et al. have found that this protein is also vitamin-K-dependent. A few other proteins have been reported to contain γ-carboxyglutamic acid but in the absence of supporting mass spectrometric evidence they must be regarded with scepticism. A large number of known Ca^{2+}-binding proteins have been found not to contain γ-carboxyglutamic acid.

6. Partial homology with the pancreatic secretory trypsin inhibitor (Kazal's inhibitor) and with hirudin

It was mentioned above that thrombin catalyses the cleavage of arginyl-156 in prothrombin, releasing the A-fragment. A comparison of the amino acid sequence of this region with sequences from other thrombin-sensitive or thrombin-binding proteins showed that part of the sequence of hirudin (positions 40–48: -Val-*Thr*-Gly-*Glu*-Gly-Thr-*Pro*-*Lys*-*Pro*) (Petersen et al., 1975) resembles the sequence in prothrombin (positions 149–157: -Val-*Thr*-Val-*Glu*-Val-Ile-*Pro*-*Arg*-Ser-) which is cleaved by thrombin. Hirudin from the leech *Hirudo medicinalis* is a specific inhibitor of thrombin (Markwardt, 1970) and Factor IX_a (Davie et al., 1975), which forms a very stable 1:1 complex with thrombin or Factor IX_a. The primary structure of hirudin doesn't particularly resemble those of previously known trypsin inhibitors. Therefore, it is not clear which part of its structure binds to thrombin. It is possible that the sequence 40–48 constitutes at least part of its thrombin-binding site. A synthetic peptide based on this sequence in hirudin showed no inhibitory activity against thrombin (Magnusson et al., 1976).

Another sequence near the C-terminal end of the A-fragment (positions 142–150: *-Pro-Val-Cys-Gly*-Gln-*Asp*-Arg-*Val-Thr*) is homologous with part of the sequence (positions 22–30: *-Pro-Val-Cys-Gly*-Thr-*Asp*-Gly-*Val-Thr-*) in the secretory inhibitor from the bovine pancreas. The significance of this homology is not clear.

7. Activation by limited proteolysis

The generally accepted view at present is that the Factor-X_a-catalysed activation of prothrombin which leads to cleavage at Arg-274 and Arg-323 (Fig. 108, line 4; Fig. 113, lines 3 and 4) occurs normally, not only in the *in vitro* systems that have been used so far in studies of the activation mechanism but also *in vivo*. As pointed out already the primary structure of prothrombin shows that a 'long' thrombin could be formed if Arg-323 were cleaved preferentially. Studies (particularly by Jackson *et al.*, 1975) indicate that Factor V has some affinity for the S-fragment part of the prothrombin structure. Thus, both prothrombin and neoprothrombin-S but not neoprothrombin-T bind to Factor V. The binding of Factor X_a to prothrombin seems to require rather small parts of the prothrombin structure. All three of the chymotryptic peptides -Ile-Glu-Gly-Arg-Ile-Val-Glu-Gly-Gln-Asp-Ala-Glu- (positions 320–331), Ile-Glu-Gly-Arg-Ile-Val-Glu-Gly-Gln-Asp- (positions 320–329) and 233–283 (the first two contain Arg-323, the third Arg-274) could be cleaved rapidly by Factor X_a but not by thrombin. Thus, rather short peptide sequences around the sensitive bonds are sufficient to define at least part of the substrate specificity towards Factor X_a. Since the sequences in the two Factor-X_a-sensitive regions around Arg-274 and Arg-323 are strikingly similar, namely -Ala-Ala-*Ile-Glu-Gly-Arg*-Thr-Ser-*Glu*- (269–277) and -Ser-Tyr-*Ile-Glu-Gly-Arg*-Ile-Val-*Glu* (318–326) and the sequence around the thrombin-sensitive Arg-156 (-Val-Thr-Val-Glu-Val-Ile-Pro-Arg-Ser-Gly-Gly-; 149–159) is considerably different, synthetic substrates have been developed for Factor X_a, e.g. Bz-Ile-Glu-Gly-Arg-pNA, which is cleaved 70–100 times faster by Factor X_a than by thrombin. A question that arises as a consequence of the thrombin-sensitive bond Arg-156 in a 'strategic' position between the Ca^{2+}-phospholipid-binding structure of the A-fragment region and the two Factor-X_a-sensitive bonds is whether thrombin-catalysed 'inactivation' of prothrombin to neoprothrombin-S (or intermediate I) (Fig. 108, line 2), which can no longer be activated rapidly in Ca^{2+}-phospholipid-dependent systems, because it has lost the A-fragment, is utilized as a means of regulation under *in vivo*-conditions thus avoiding conversion of all available prothrombin to thrombin. According to this concept thrombin would 'shut off' further generation of thrombin by converting not yet activated prothrombin to neoprothrombin-S. Studies of the activation mechanism in well-defined, pure systems in the absence of phospholipids have not indicated that such a thrombin-catalysed regulation mechanism is of essential importance, but such systems may lack the important surface which could adsorb Factor X_a leaving neoprothrombin-S in the 'plasma' phase, thus separating the two. Studies by Silberberg *et al.* (1975) of activation in the presence of phospholipid indicated that a large fraction of the total prothrombin is converted to neoprothrombin-S, not to thrombin. In human prothrombin Seegers *et al.* and Mann *et al.* recently found a second thrombin-sensitive Arg-bond, corresponding to position 287 of bovine prothrombin. This could be interpreted as an element in a back-up mechanism in the human system providing a second possibility for thrombin-catalysed feedback regulation of the amount of prothrombin that is converted to thrombin.

8. Activation by staphylocoagulase

An activation mechanism that does not seem to involve limited proteolysis of prothrombin is the activation by staphylocoagulase. This activation involves the formation of a 1:1 complex between staphylocoagulase and prothrombin. The N-terminals of the complex were found to be one Ala- and one Asp- as in intact prothrombin and staphylocoagulase, respectively. The apparent molecular weight on gel electrophoresis as well as the amino acid composition of the complex were found to correspond to the values expected from a 1:1 complex when adding the molecular weights and compositions of the two proteins. The complex which is called staphylothrombin, has thrombin activity (Hemker et al., 1975). The mechanism of this activation is not known, but a clue to a possible explanation might be provided by the recent finding (Delbaere et al., 1975) of a salt-bridge connecting Asp-194 to Arg-169 instead of to the usual Ile/Val-16. The enzyme with this structure is the serine protease B from *Streptomyces griseus*. It is conceivable that staphylocoagulase activation of prothrombin can lead to the formation of a corresponding alternative salt-bridge in prothrombin obviating the need for cleavage at Arg-323. It is not clear if the non-proteolytic formation of a streptokinase–plasminogen complex with plasminogen activator activity proceeds by a similar mechanism.

A third example of apparently non-proteolytic activation of a regulatory serine protease zymogen is the activation of the complement factor Clr by the formation of a 1:1 complex with Clq.

9. Multiple evolutionary origin of the larger serine protease zymogen structures

A comparison of the amino acid sequences of the three zymogens prothrombin, plasminogen, and Factor X show that each of these zymogen structures contains regions of structure evolved from at least three different protein families. In prothrombin the N-terminal, vitamin-K-dependent region is homologous with that in Factor X, but different from the so-called preactivation peptide region that constitutes the N-terminal region of plasminogen. The two kringle structures in prothrombin and the five in plasminogen belong to a common family of protein structures, whereas the corresponding structure in Factor X (and apparently Factor IX) belongs to a different family. The third major region, the serine protease part has the same origin in all three zymogens. Thus, from the evolutionary point of view each of these zymogens can be regarded as a 'multiprotein' consisting of three (Factor X) to seven (plasminogen) 'miniproteins' fused together to a single (plasminogen and prothrombin) or two-chain (Factor X) protein. The exact mechanisms at the gene level by which this evolution has occurred have not been explained.

E. Biosynthesis

The details of the vitamin-K-dependent reaction which leads to γ-carboxylation of the ten Glu-residues in the region 1–42 are not completely understood but it is clearly a postribosomal modification occurring after the completion of the synthesis of the polypeptide chain. It has been shown that the reaction requires a carboxylase, either vitamin K plus NADH or reduced vitamin K. Precursors of prothrombin and synthetic peptides mimicking part of the vitamin-K-dependent region in prothrombin (residues 3–9) have been used as substrates. It has been shown that both $^{14}CO_2$ and $H^{14}CO_3^-$ can be incorporated. In the presence of diamox (an inhibitor of carbonic anhydrase) $^{14}CO_2$ is incorporated 5–10 times faster than $H^{14}CO_3^-$. There is no requirement for biotin or for ATP. It is likely that prothrombin is synthesized as a preprothrombin, like most other proteins which are secreted through the cell membrane, but since synthetic peptides can be used as substrates in the carboxylation reaction, this pre-sequence is apparently not part of the recognition site for the carboxylase. Most of the work on the carboxylation reaction and the purification of the carboxylase has been carried out by Suttie et al. and by Olson et al., and more recently by Hemker et al.

F. Inhibition of thrombin by antithrombin-III (heparin cofactor)

The most important thrombin inhibitor in blood plasma is antithrombin-III (or heparin cofactor). The reaction between antithrombin-III and thrombin leads to the formation of a 1:1 complex, which lacks thrombin activity in the thrombin fibrinogen reaction and towards synthetic substrates for thrombin. The complex is very strong and it cannot be dissociated in sodium dodecylsulphate under reducing conditions. The reaction between thrombin and antithrombin-III is relatively slow. However, if antithrombin-III has first been complexed to heparin, the reaction with thrombin is very fast. Antithrombin-III is a single chain glycoprotein with approximately 430 amino acid residues, 4 prosthetic glucosamine-based oligosacharides, and 3 disulphide bridges. Thus, it is considerably larger than the structurally and functionally well-known small trypsin inhibitors. At present 98 per cent of the sequence is known (Petersen et al., 1978). So far no homologies have been found with the small trypsin inhibitors, hirudin or soya bean trypsin inhibitor. We have recently found that the first major CNBr fragment from human α_1-antitrypsin that has been sequenced (Owen et al., 1978) corresponds to the sequence 264–377 (tentative numbering) of antithrombin-III. A homology with 36 identical residues in the two proteins extends through 108 residues of antithrombin-III and 103 residues of α_1-antitrypsin. Two of the identical residues are the two Glu-residues that have been exchanged for Val and Lys, respectively, in the genetically abnormal α_1-antitrypsins S and Z, respectively. This homology is sufficiently extensive (35 per cent) that the two proteins must have a common evolutionary origin and a common basic mechanism of inhibition. For neither of them is the mechanism clear. Antithrombin-III is not specific for thrombin but also inhibits the other coagulation proteases (with one possible exception), plasmin, plasma kallikrein, and complement factor C1s.

IV. AHF and von Willebrand factor
LARS HOLMBERG

Patients with classical sex-linked haemophilia (haemophilia A) lack a factor which has been called antihaemophilic factor A (AHF) or Factor VIII. It has long been known that this factor is present in plasma and is linked to a protein. According to the classical coagulation theory factor VIII acts in the first phase of coagulation leading to the formation of activated Factor X.

Methods for exact quantitation of Factor VIII coagulant activity (VIII:C) have existed since the 1950s. Haemophilia A plasma is used as the test substrate and the test sample is compared with normal plasma in its ability to normalize the clotting defect of the haemophilic plasma. Several such one-stage clotting assays have been described with or without addition of a partial thromboplastin and/or kaolin. There are also so-called two-stage systems which are based on thromboplastin generation test.

Factor VIII coagulant activity is decreased not only in haemophilia A but also in von Willebrand's disease. This disease, which was first described on the Åland islands, is autosomally inherited and is characterized also by a prolonged bleeding time in contrast to haemophilia A. The prolonged bleeding time can be normalized by a plasma factor which is present in normal and haemophilic plasma and which is termed the von Willebrand factor (Nilsson et al., 1957).

Several Factor VIII concentrates for treatment of haemophiliacs are now available. In 1956, Blombäck and Blombäck produced fraction I-0 which was stable and had a high Factor VIII activity. Equally therapeutically important was the discovery by Pool et al. (1964) that Factor VIII could be cryoprecipitated when freshly frozen human plasma was slowly thawed in the cold. Brinkhous et al. (1968) obtained a high-potency concentrate by precipitating fibrinogen from cryoprecipitate and then precipitating Factor VIII with glycine. Newman et al. (1971) cryoprecipitated freshly frozen plasma with 3 per cent ethanol during thawing, absorbed the extracted precipitate with Al(OH)$_3$ and precipitated most of the fibrinogen with polyethylene glycol. However, all these concentrates for therapeutic use also contain other proteins. Methods for further purification of Factor VIII are, however, not available.

Table 47. AHF concentrates for clinical use

Preparation	Units of Factor VIII[a] per ml	Package purification factor	Volume (ml)	Units of Factor VIII per bottle
Fraction I-O (Blombäck's glycine method)				
a (KI-AHF)	3–8	13–30	100	300–800
b (Kabi-AHF)	2–4	7–15	100	300
Cryoprecipitate (Pool's method)	3–16	8–20	5–20	100–150
Profilate (Abbott)	8–10	c. 15	25	250
			20	250
(Immuno) Kryobulin	10–13	c. 15	50	500
			100	1 000
Hemofil[R] (Hyland)	25–30	c. 100	10	250–300
			30	c. 800

[a] 1 unit (U) of Factor VIII = the activity of Factor VIII which is present in 1 ml of fresh normal human plasma.

Fig. 114. SDS acrylamide electrophoresis of AHF following reduction of the disulphide bonds

Factor VIII coagulant activity (VIII:C) elutes near or at the void volume in columns of agarose at physiologic ionic strength and thus behaves as a very large molecule under these conditions. A protein associated with VIII:C has been extensively purified in this way and termed Factor VIII related protein (VIII:RP). This protein can be measured quantitatively in plasma as Factor VIII related antigen (VIII:RAG) with Laurell electroimmunoassay or immunoradiometric methods. It is composed of subunits of a molecular weight of about 200 000, held together probably by both covalent and non-covalent bonds. There is some evidence that VIII:RP in plasma is present in various molecular forms with a varying number of subunits and that the molecular forms are in a state of equilibrium with each other but others have claimed that the aggregation of subunits is only an *in vitro* artefact.

VIII:RP fractions purified from normal plasma have VIII:C activity. An VIII:RP can also be isolated from haemophilic plasma. Haemophilic VIII:RP is devoid of VIII:C activity. However, no structural difference between normal and haemophilic VIII:RP has so far been demonstrated. Several workers have shown that VIII:C may be a separate molecule, as it is possible to dissociate it from the VIII:RP isolated from normal plasma by increasing the ionic strength especially with 0.25 mol/l $CaCl_2$. The molecular weight of the separate VIII:C has been estimated from 25 000 to 240 000. It cannot, however, be excluded that the VIII:C obtained in this way is the result of some proteolytic activity contaminating the preparations. The effect of thrombin, for example, is similar to that of high ionic strength (Cooper et al., 1975). It is thus unclear whether VIII:C is a separate molecule with a tendency to associate with VIII:RP or whether VIII:C resides in VIII:RP itself.

The bulk of evidence is in favour of VIII:RP being some kind of carrier protein for a separate VIII:C. However, VIII:RP has a second biological function. In von Willebrand's disease platelet adhesiveness and the ability of plasma to aggregate platelets in the presence of the antibiotic ristocetin are decreased. VIII:RP can normalize the decreased platelet adhesiveness in von Willebrand's disease and can normalize the prolonged bleeding time in dogs with von Willebrand's disease. It thus seems as if VIII: RP is the protein responsible for the von Willebrand factor activity of normal and haemophilic plasma. VIII:RP is also involved in platelet aggregation in the presence of ristocetin. This activity of VIII:RP is termed ristocetin cofactor activity (VIII:RCoF). VIII:RCoF is easily measured *in vitro* and is somehow related to the von Willebrand factor effect of the protein.

VIII:RP measured immunologically as VIII:RAG is present in at least the same amount in haemophiliacs as in normals and there is no difference in this respect in haemophiliacs with a circulating antibody to Factor VIII. However the majority of patients with von Willebrand's disease have decreased amounts of VIII:RAG in plasma and thus of the protein with von Willebrand factor activity (Fig. 115). The patients with low levels of VIII:RAG also have decreased levels of VIII:RCoF and VIII:C but they are able to produce VIII:C after stimulation by an infusion of a Factor VIII concentrate (containing VIII:RP), indicating that their low VIII:C is only secondary to the deficiency of VIII:RP. This observation provides clinical evidence that VIII:RP and VIII:C are separate entities (Fig. 116).

Von Willebrand's disease is genetically heterogeneous, as the patients from some families have a normal level of VIII:RAG measured with electroimmunoassay (Holmberg and Nilsson, 1972). These patients seem to have a structurally abnormal VIII:RP as VIII:RCoF is decreased and the electrophoretic mobility of the protein is abnormally anodic (Kernoff *et al.*, 1974; Peake *et al.*, 1974). In some patient plasmas the gel filtration elution pattern of Factor VIII is abnormal.

VIII:RP is present in the endothelial cells of the vascular intima. There is experimental evidence suggesting that VIII:RP but not VIII:C is produced by endothelial cells. This view is strengthened by the fact that patients with severe typical von Willebrand's disease lack VIII:RAG in their vessels as well as in their plasma. Even after infusion of Factor VIII concentrates to such patients the endothelial cells lack VIII:RAG, suggesting that the presence of VIII:RAG in vessels is not due to simple adhesion of the protein to the endothelial surface.

VIII:RP is also present in megakaryocytes and in platelets. In platelets there are possibly two pools of the protein, one of which is associated with the membrane and

Table 48. Immunological studies performed on 44 patients suffering from haemophilia A

Type	Number of patients	AHF related protein %	Neutralizing ability U
Severe, AHF activity <1%	27	73–225	0.00–0.06
Moderate, AHF activity 1–3%	9	45–145	0.00–0.06
Mild, AHF activity 6–28 %	8	69–144	0.00–0.26

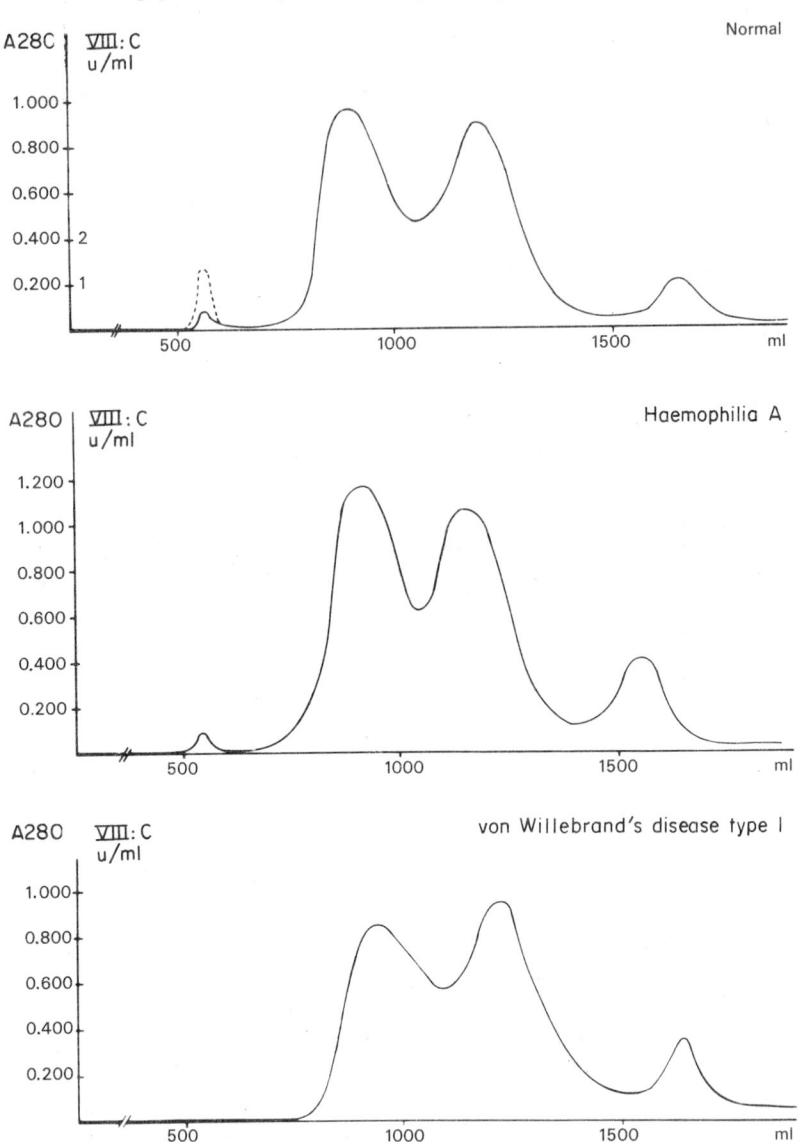

Fig. 115. Gel chromatography on Sepharose 6B of cryoprecipitate obtained from a normal individual, a patient having haemophilia A, and a patient having von Willebrand's disease

one which is contained in the granules. In patients with von Willebrand's disease, platelet VIII:RP is sometimes decreased VIII:RP has not been found with certainty in any other cells. It is still unknown where or how VIII:C is generated.

VIII:RP seems to be necessary for the initial events in primary haemostasis: the adhesion of platelets to a damaged vascular endothelium (Weiss et al., 1975). It is not known which of these localities: plasma, endothelium, or platelets, is most important. It

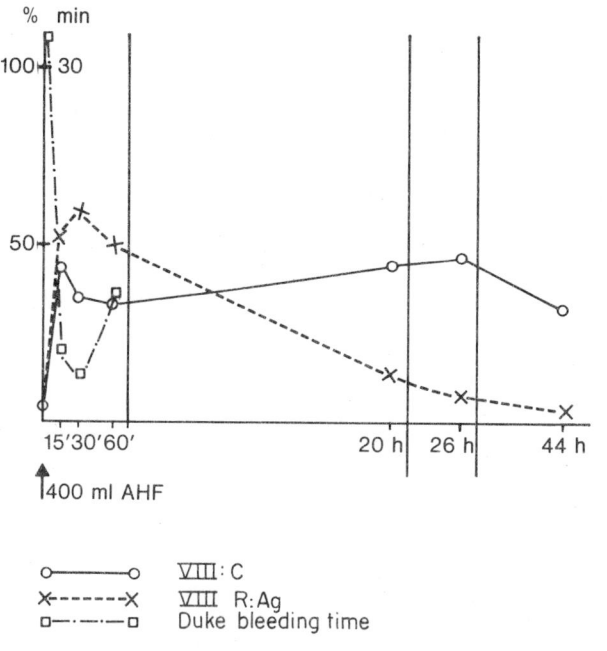

Fig. 116. The effect of transfusion of 400 ml of AHF (Kabi) in a patient suffering from von Willebrand's disease

may be the presence in plasma is most important since the bleeding time in von Willebrand's disease can be normalized by increasing plasma Factor VIII. The mechanism of the interaction between platelets and VIII:RP is not known either but it would appear that there exist receptors for VIII:RP on the platelets.

V. Haemophilia B-factor (Factor IX)

LARS-OLOV ANDERSSON

Bleeding disorders, haemophilia, have been known since the nineteenth century. It was thought that the illness was homogeneous but at the end of the 1940s Pavlovsky discovered that the coagulation defect in the blood of a certain haemophilia patient could be normalized by adding blood from another haemophilia patient. Similar results were obtained by other workers and it was agreed that there must be at least two types of haemophilia. One of these is the classical haemophilia, haemophilia A, which is due to an inherited deficiency of functionally active Factor VIII (AHF). The other form is caused by a hereditary deficiency of functionally active Factor IX. More recently, cases of haemophilia have been reported where the coagulation defect is due to a deficiency of functionally active Factor XI. This latter form of the disorder has been called haemophilia C.

Factor IX is often called B-factor or *Christmas factor*. Factor IX is normally measured as a biological activity. Haemophilia B plasma is used as the basis of the test. Studies are made to determine to what extent the test sample can normalize coagulation in the haemophilia B plasma. This is the so-called one stage method and exists in several modifications (Veltkamp *et al.*, 1968). In addition, there are so-called two stage methods which are based on the 'thromboplastin generation test'. Antiserum against Factor IX has recently been prepared, making possible the immunological determination of this factor (Orstavik *et al.*, 1975).

The demand for clinically applicable preparations for the treatment of haemoplilia B has resulted in the development of several methods for the preparation of Factor IX concentrates. Soulier and co-workers (1964, 1969) used adsorption to calcium phosphate followed by elution with citrate buffer as the basic separation step. Using this method, they obtained a preparation which was roughly 100 times more potent than normal plasma. A preparation which had similar activity was obtained by Tullis and co-workers (1965, 1970) by using adsorption to DEAE–cellulose as the basic separation step. The concentration of Factor IX protein in these concentrates was approximately 1 per cent. Since Factors II, VII, and X have adsorption characteristics which are similar to those of Factor IX, these preparations contained appreciable amounts of these factors. Both concentrates have provided good clinical results.

It was only recently that a method for the isolation of pure Factor IX was developed (Andersson *et al.*, 1975; Osterud and Flengsrud, 1975). The problems of isolation were difficult since factor IX is present in plasma in such small quantities (less than 10 mg/l) and since its properties are very similar to those of Factors II, VII, and X. The matter is further complicated by the activation of the factor which takes place during the purification procedure. Andersson and co-workers have used affinity chromatography on heparin–Sepharose, chromatography on DEAE–Sephadex and gel filtration on Sephadex 200 to purify Factor IX. The purified preparation was homogeneous according to various criteria and the activity demonstrated a purification factor of 12 000 compared to plasma. The purification procedure of Osterud and Flengsrud included barium sulphate adsorption, DEAE–cellulose fractionation, preparative polyacrylamide electrophoresis, and immunosorption. While the two preparations are similar in many respects, there is one significant difference: the NH_2-terminal amino acids are not the same. Andersson *et al.* found tyrosine in this position while Osterud and Flengsrud found glycine. Tyrosine is the NH_2-terminal amino acid in bovine Factor IX (Fujikawa *et al.*, 1973) and recent sequence studies on human Factor IX (Fryklund *et al.*, 1976) which was prepared according to Andersson *et al.*, have shown that the sequence of the first eight amino residues is almost identical with that of the bovine material. This suggests that the preparation of Factor IX which has tyrosine as NH_2-terminal is a native Factor IX while the other preparation probably contains a partially activated form of this factor. Thus the discussion which follows concerns that form of Factor IX which has tyrosine as NH_2-terminal amino acid.

Factor IX is a protein having a molecular weight of 55 000. The carbohydrate content is 22.8 per cent of which sialic acid makes up one-third. Its electrophoretic mobility is the same as that of an alphaglobulin (Fig. 117). The protein focuses isoelectrically between pH 4.1 and pH 4.5. The amino acid composition (Andersson *et al.*, 1975) is similar to that of human prothrombin but the lysine content is higher in Factor IX. The protein consists of one polypeptide chain containing approximately 13

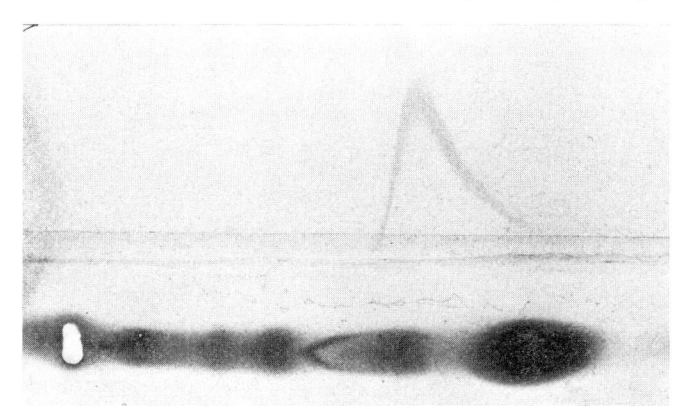

Fig. 117. Cross-immunoelectrophoresis of Factor IX compared with the corresponding agarose electrophoresis of plasma

disulphide bridges. The NH_2-terminal amino acid sequence was recently determined (Fryklund et al., 1976) and is given below together with that of bovine prothrombin. The GlA residues of positions 7 and 8 consist of γ-carboxyglutamic acid.

Human Factor IX H_2N-Tyr-Asn-Ile-Gly-Lys-Asn-GlA-GlA-
Bovine prothrombin H_2N-Ala-Asn-Lys-Gly-Phe-Leu-GlA-GlA-

It is thought that Factor IX can appear in several forms. Preparations of the factor which are obtained from various individuals show different isoelectric points and characteristics of adsorption to hydroxyapatite (Suomela, 1975). One possible explanation for this may be in the sialic acid content.

The clotting Factors II, VII, IX, and X are vitamin-K-dependent. This implies that in the absence of vitamin K there is no synthesis of the functionally active forms of these factors. Studies on prothrombin have shown that this protein contains ten residues of an unusual amino acid, γ-carboxyglutamic acid, which are located in the NH_2-terminal portion of the molecule and are necessary for the binding of calcium and phospholipid (platelet Factor 3). In the biosynthesis of prothrombin, γ-carboxyglutamic acid is introduced by a vitamin-K-dependent carboxylation of certain glutamic acid residues in the finished peptide chain. Recent data show that Factor IX also contains residues of γ-carboxyglutamic acid in its NH_2-terminal portion (Fryklund et al., 1976). The biosynthesis of Factor IX takes place in the liver.

Immunological studies on various patients suffering from haemophilia B have shown that more than half of these were devoid of Factor IX antigen (Orstavik et al., 1975). The remainder had an antigen which resembled the Factor IX antigen but this was often present in reduced concentration. Fig. 117 shows a cross-immunoelectrophoresis of Factor IX. In the early days of coagulation research, the possibility that Factors II, IX, and X were the same protein was often discussed. The isolation and characterization of the various factors has now shown this hypothesis to be without substance. In Fig. 118, an immunological technique has been employed to demonstrate this point. The precipitation lines with prothrombin and Factor IX cross each other without interference. Thus prothrombin and Factor IX have different antigenic structures.

The function of Factor IX in the coagulation system is to activate Factor X. To be

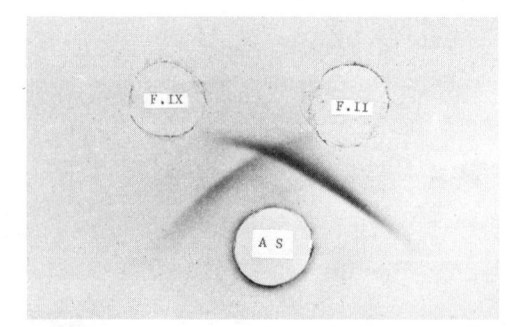

Fig. 118. Double immunodiffusion of Factor IX and prothrombin against a mixture containing antisera against Factor IX and prothrombin. AS = antiserum, F.II = prothrombin, F.IX = Factor IX

capable of doing this, Factor IX must itself become activated. This is brought about by the action of activated Factor XI in the presence of calcium to cleave off a portion of the peptide chain of Factor IX. The activated form of Factor IX has a molecular weight of approximately 47 000. It is a hydrolytic enzyme, a serine protease, and is inhibited by several protease inhibitors such as antithrombin III. The protein–lipid complex which normally activates Factor X consists of platelet Factor 3 (a phospholipoprotein of high molecular weight), Factor VIII in the activated form, the activated form of Factor IX, and calcium ions. A schematic representation of this complex is given in Fig. 119. Only in the presence of calcium ions will Factor IX bind to platelet Factor 3. The calcium ions probably act as bridges since these bind to the γ-carboxyglutamic acid residues in Factor IX and to the phosphate groups in the phospholipid of platelet Factor 3. The activation of Factor X takes place by activated Factor IX, which is bound in the complex, cleaving some peptide bonds within Factor X. Factor VIII acts

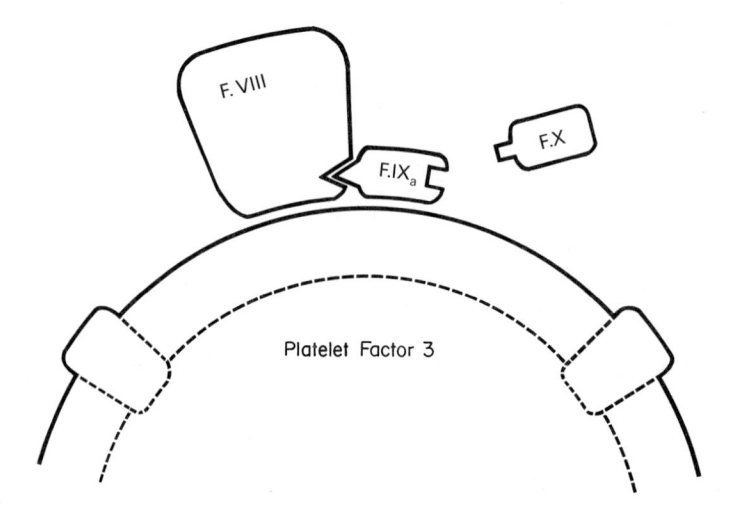

Fig. 119. Schematic representation of the protein–lipid complex containing activated Factor IX which converts Factor X into the active form

as an effector and probably does not take part in the modification of Factor X. The prime function of platelet Factor 3 is to bind and bring together the various factors. This is necessary since the participating factors are present in blood in very low concentrations.

The concentration of Factor IX in normal plasma is 6–8 mg/l and the half-life *in vivo* is between 20 and 40 hours (Menache, 1964).

VI. Additional coagulation factors
RAGNAR LUNDÉN

In the previous section, some of the proteins of the coagulation system were presented in detail by specialists within the respective fields. The remaining coagulation factors are less well known chemically. Factor III, thromboplastin, is a complex of coagulation factors, lipid, and calcium ions and has not been treated separately (see coagulation scheme, page 222). The entire field is at present undergoing a tremendous development. The following account is intended only to give a brief survey. The reader who wishes more detailed information is referred to the original literature. Recently published survey articles by Davie and Fujikawa (1975) and Baugh and Hougie (1977) are recommended.

1. Factor V

In order to obtain a fast conversion of prothrombin into thrombin, a protein (Factor V) is required which is capable of accelerating the thrombin generation and is therefore also called accelerator globulin (Ac-globulin).

Together with phospholipid, Factor X_a and calcium ions, Factor V forms a complex which causes the activation of prothrombin to produce thrombin. In contrast to prothrombin, Factor X, and Factor VIII, the synthesis of Factor V is not vitamin K dependent and so its ability to bind calcium ions and phospholipid is believed to be due to structural properties other than the presence of γ-carboxyglutamic acid. The factor is used up during coagulation and is not present in serum. In addition, the protein is particularly unstable which has caused great difficulty in its purification. As with several of the coagulation factors which are dealt with here, the starting material for the isolation of Factor V has mostly been bovine plasma and consequently less is known of the factor in human blood. Kandell *et al.* (1975) have published a method for the purification of bovine Factor V using adsorption on barium sulphate and TEAE–cellulose. The final stage consists of chromatography on cellulose–phosphate. The preparation obtained was free from Factors I, II, VIII, X, XI and was devoid of proteolytic activity. The molecule consists of a heavy peptide chain, which contains carbohydrate, and two light peptide chains. The molecular weights of the heavy and light chains are 125 000 and 75 000 respectively. This is in good agreement with an earlier report of the molecular weight of Factor V to be approximately 300 000. The activation of the factor by thrombin results in cleavage of the heavy chain down to a molecular weight of 87 000. The factor has been observed in several high molecular weight forms which probably arise from aggregation during the purification procedure.

2. Factor VII

Factor X can be activated by two separate mechanisms. The first has already been mentioned and the second is via the influence of a factor present in most tissues, the so-called tissue thromboplastin. This factor is released following tissue damage and requires for full activity the presence of yet another plasma protein, which is called proconvertin or Factor VII.

Several of the chemical properties of Factor VII are similar to those of prothrombin and the protein can be isolated from plasma or serum using procedures which are similar to those for prothrombin. Gladhaug, Berre (1970) and Prydz (1971) have described a method for the purification of Factor VII from human material by performing chromatography on Sephadex G-25 which contains barium sulphate followed by chromatography of DEAE–Sephadex. The protein was purified further by gel filtration and preparative gel electrophoresis. The Factor VII which was obtained from plasma had a molecular weight of 60 000 as opposed to a molecular weight of 45 000 for the material which was obtained from serum. The purified preparation of Factor VII had neither proteolytic nor esterolytic activity when tested by itself or in combination with tissue thromboplastin and calcium.

Factor VII which was isolated and purified according to earlier procedures has been shown to consist of two polypeptide chains joined together by disulphide bridges. A form of bovine Factor VII was isolated recently (Radcliffe et al., 1975) which consists of a single polypeptide chain having a molecular weight of 53 000. The synthesis of Factor VII takes place in the liver and is vitamin-K-dependent.

3. Factor X

Factor X, which is also called Stuart factor, takes part in its active form (X_a) together with Factor V, phospholipid, and calcium ions in the proteolytic conversion of prothrombin into thrombin. The active form of Factor X is a serine protease which is evident from the fact that its enzymatic activity is inhibited by DEP, diisopropylfluorophospate.

Most of the studies which have been performed on Factor X have made use of bovine material for which there are several available methods of purification. It has been shown that the molecule is composed of two polypeptide chains which have molecular weights of about 40 000 and 15 000. These are held together by disulphide bridges. The protein exists in two immunologically identical forms (X_1 and X_2) which seem to differ only in the carbohydrate composition of the heavy chains.

Factor X was isolated from human plasma by Aronson et al. (1969) who found the molecular weight of the human material to be 86 000. When compared with human prothrombin it is evident that the two proteins have quite different amino acid sequences. This makes it unlikely that Factor X is a portion of the prothrombin molecule as was previously suggested. Bovine Factor X contains γ-carboxylated glutamic acid, which has recently been shown to be a prerequisite for the ability of the molecule to bind calcium ions and phospholipid. Thus it belongs to the vitamin-K-dependent coagulation factors (II, VII, IX, and X).

4. Factor XI

The chemistry of Factor XI, haemophilia C factor (PTA), is not yet fully established. Partial purification of the protein has been described by several authors. One method of approach is to remove the proteins of the prothrombin complex (Factors II, VII, IX, and X) by adsorption on tricalcium phosphate. Factor XI is thereafter adsorbed on Celite and subsequently eluted with saline solution (2 mol/l) containing tris(hydroxymethyl)-amino-methane. The eluate is purified further by chromatography on CM- and DEAE–cellulose and a final gel filtration. The active form of Factor XI is obtained by this procedure. Like activated Factor XII, this form of activated Factor XI is a proteolytic enzyme. Factor XI is a glycoprotein having a molecular weight of approximately 160 000. The protein consists of two equally large polypeptide chains held together by disulphide bridges.

5. Factor XII

Factor XII, Hageman factor, is the protein in blood which together with Factor XI takes part in the initial step of blood coagulation. Both factors adsorb to foreign surfaces such as glass, kaolin, Celite, and barium carbonate. The adsorption causes an activation of the factors by a mechanism which has not yet been closely elucidated. In the presence of calcium ions, the activated Factor XII can activate Factor IX which finally results in the generation of thrombin.

Several attempts to isolate Factor XII from plasma have been made. Cochrane and Wuepper (1971) described a method where Factor XII is fractionally precipitated from plasma by ammonium sulphate and further purified by chromatography on DEAE–Sephadex A-50. The procedure was repeated and the resulting material was gel filtered through Sephadex G-200. Finally the active fractions were chromatographed on CM-Sephadex C-50. The purified protein was shown to be identical with the preactivator of kallikrein and had a molecular weight of approximately 100 000. The molecule consists of three polypeptide chains held together by disulphide bridges.

The experimental evidence suggests that activated Factor XII can convert prekallikrein into its active form, kallikrein. It is believed that Factor XII may even be important in the activation of the fibrinolytic system of blood and it is also physiologically connected with the complement system.

6. Factor XIII

The final stage in the coagulation process consists of a stabilization of the precipitated fibrin. This is brought about by a transamidating enzyme which is normally present in blood as the inactive form and is called *fibrin stabilizing factor* (FSF) or Factor XIII. The conversion into the active form takes place under the influence of thrombin and calcium ions. In the stabilization of the fibrin clot, new amide bonds are formed between the γ-carboxyl group of glutamic acid residues and ε-amino groups of lysine in adjacent chains of fibrin. The final stabilized clot is more resistant to proteolytic degradation and has a higher physical stability. Factor XIII also exists in high concentration in thrombocytes.

The method of purification of the proenzyme has been described by Lorand and Gotoh (1970) using methods such as chromatography on DEAE–cellulose, gel chromatography, and density gradient centrifugation.

Schwartz et al. (1973) have studied Factor XIII obtained from plasma and thrombocytes. The material isolated from plasma had a molecular weight of 320 000 and consisted of two subunits, a and b, of molecular weights 75 000 and 88 000 respectively. The molecule consists of two a- and two b-chains linked together by non-covalent bonds.

Factor XIII from thrombocytes contains two a-peptides which have a composite molecular weight of 150 000. All the evidence so far indicates that these peptides are identical with the a-peptides of the plasma factor. The activation of Factor XIII by thrombin consists in the release of a peptide from each of the a-chains to expose the active centre of the enzyme. Dissociation of the a- and b-chains by the influence of calcium ions then gives rise to enzymically active a_2-dimer.

The first stage in the cross-linking reaction consists of acylation of the SH-group of the active centre. This is followed by amidation of a lysin residue and the simultaneous reformation of the free SH-group. The enzyme is relatively unspecific and several different types of compounds containing amino groups have been shown to function as substrates for the enzyme.

VII. Plasminogen and fibrinolysis
PER WALLÉN

1. Introduction

Fibrinolysis is the dissolution of fibrin clots. The phenomenon has been known since the latter half of the eighteenth century when it was discovered that blood from corpses, especially when death was sudden, could not be made to coagulate. This was later demonstrated to be due to the total lack of fibrinogen in this blood. In 1893, Dastre showed that the blood clots which were obtained from dogs which had experienced haemorrhagic shock underwent spontaneous dissolution. In addition, he found that this was due to a proteolytic degradation of fibrin and he named the process 'fibrinolysis'. During the 1930s it was demonstrated that certain strains of β-haemolytic streptococci had a strong tendency to dissolve coagulated blood and that this characteristic was due to the release of an exotoxin, streptokinase, which in plasma had a fibrinolytic activity. At the beginning of the 1940s, it became known that a serum factor cooperated with streptokinase in the fibrinolytic reaction. Shortly afterwards, Christensen (1945) published some work which showed that the serum factor was a proenzyme of proteolytic enzyme and that streptokinase was the activator of this proenzyme. The proenzyme was christened 'plasminogen' and the enzyme which was obtained on activation of this was called 'plasmin'. Through the work of Christensen an understanding of the fibrinolytic system was available at the beginning of the 1950s. The fundamental features of this picture remain unchanged (Fig. 120). The central reaction is the conversion of plasminogen into plasmin. This reaction, like the activation of several other proenzymes to produce proteolytic enzymes such as trypsinogen into trypsin and prothrombin into thrombin, is a specific proteolytic reaction. The reaction causes a conformational change (change in the three-

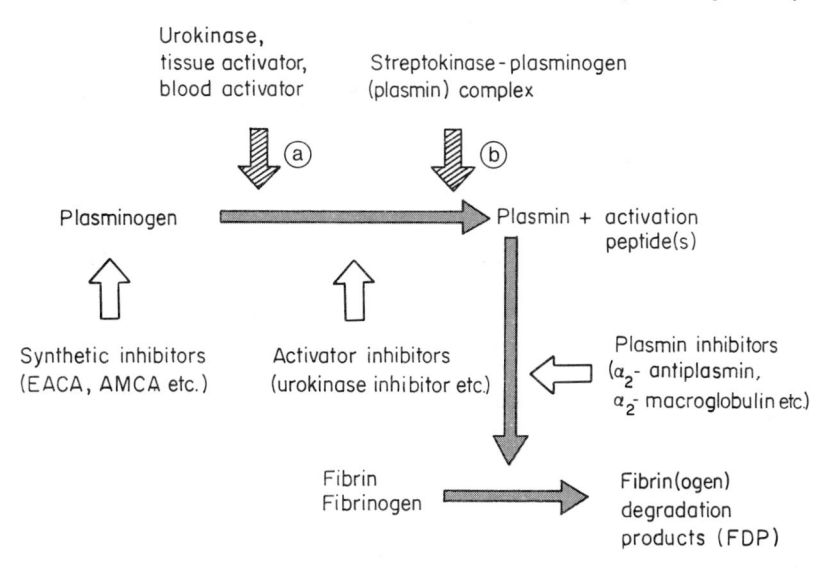

Fig. 120. Schematic representation of the fibrinolysis system. The conversion of plasminogen into plasmin takes place probably in two stages (see Fig. 123). Of the activities, streptokinase occupies a position of special importance. This enzyme is active only when it exists in a complex with a plasma factor, proactivator, which appears to be plasminogen or plasmin

dimensional structure) of the proenzyme so that the amino acids which compromise the 'active centre' are arranged in a definite relationship to one another.

The proteolytic effect of pure plasmin is reminiscent of that of trypsin. In other words, it is an enzyme which has a general proteolytic activity and as such should be capable of degrading several plasma proteins. That plasmin in its physiological environment of circulating blood appears to attack mainly *one* protein, fibrin, can probably be attributed to the presence of a regulation system which encompasses a cooperative play between specific activator mechanisms and an effective system of inhibitors.

2. Plasminogen: purification and properties

The discovery that fibrinolysis was caused by a proteolytic enzyme which was produced from a proenzyme created interest in the isolation of this proenzyme to enable studies to be performed on the mechanism of the activation process. The isolation of well-characterized preparations of plasminogen which are probably identical with the native plasminogen, has taken place within the last few years. The purification and characterization of plasminogen has been complicated mainly by two of its properties: (1) a marked tendency to become adsorbed to other proteins and (2) a strong tendency to become modified by proteolysis resulting from the action of trace amounts of contaminating protease (plasmin).

The early attempts to purify plasminogen were made problematic by the tendency of the protein to form complexes with other proteins. An early method used dilute sulphuric acid, which dissociates such complexes, for the extraction of plasminogen. Kline (1953) obtained a preparation of high specific activity by fractionating the extract. This type of plasminogen was used well into the 1960s in studies of fibrinolysis. However, the extremely acid conditions which are employed for the extraction cause irreversible alteration of some of the physicochemical properties of the protein. Preparations of this type are insoluble in neutral buffers.

The finding that certain amino acids such as lysine and ε-aminocaproic acid which have basic groups in the ω-position could dissociate the complex of plasminogen with other proteins was of great significance for the purification work which followed. The same amino acids have a marked effect on the fibrolytic system. Two such acids, ε-aminocaproic acid and later AMCHA (4-aminomethylcyclohexane carbonic acid) have found wide use as inhibitors of fibrinolysis in clinical work (Kjellman, 1971). Because of the use of the purification of plasminogen, this has become a relatively simple procedure. The first application of these amino acids for purification purposes was in ion exchange chromatography where an almost pure plasminogen could be obtained from an impure plasma fraction in a few steps (Wallén and Bergström, 1959). During the 1960s, several methods making use of ω-amino acids for the purification of plasminogen were developed (Heberlein and Barnhart, 1971; Wallén and Wiman, 1970). One method which is especially worthy of mentioning here is that developed by Deutsch and Mertz (1970) which involves affinity chromatography and because of its simplicity and efficiency has become widely used in all fields where purified plasminogen is required. The key reagent is lysine which has been coupled primarily via its α-amino group to a solid support, which is normally Sepharose. In this way an 'insoluble' ε-aminocaproic acid is obtained which can specifically adsorb plasminogen (Fig. 121). By passing plasma or serum through a column of lysine–Sepharose, practically all of the plasminogen can be adsorbed. Following a wash with a suitable buffer, the plasminogen can be eluted by using a solution of ε-aminocaproic acid. Plasminogen which is obtained by this simple technique is practically pure (80–90 per cent of the protein content) and can be used without further purification for several purposes in the clinical or biochemical laboratory.

Plasma and fractions of plasma which contain plasminogen contain trace amounts of plasmin and the activator of fibrinolysis. These components together with plasminogen become concentrated during the purification. Plasmin is easily partially degraded by even small amounts of plasmin. This degradation takes place largely in the NH_2-terminal portion of the molecule, but can be avoided by including plasmin inhibitors in crucial stages during the preparation. This proteolysis had been responsible for the

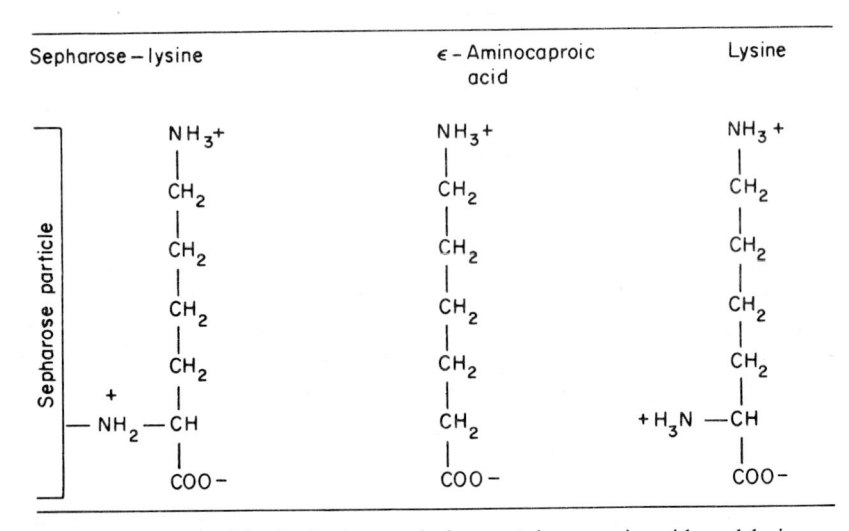

Fig. 121. Similarities in Sepharose–lysine, ε-aminocaproic acid, and lysine

isolation and characterization of two types of highly purified plasminogen. One of these, which is believed to be identical with native plasminogen, has glutamic acid as the NH_2-terminal amino acid while the other form, which results from a partial degradation, has mainly lysine in this position. These two types are hereafter termed 'Glu-plasminogen' and 'Lys-plasminogen'. The reader who wishes further information on this point is referred to a publication by Wallén and Wiman (1975). Each of these forms of plasminogen is converted by activation into a largely identical form of plasmin. However, the two forms show considerable dissimilarities in their physicochemical properties, their activation kinetics, and their behaviour *in vivo*. Thus, it is important that the quality of the plasminogen preparation be known prior to its use in experiments which are aimed at elucidating the physiological relationships in fibrinolysis.

Plasminogen is present in blood at a concentration of about 0.2 g/l and can be practically quantitatively precipitated in an euglobulin fraction which is obtained by diluting citrated plasma with 9 volumes of distilled water and acidifying the diluted plasma to pH 5.5. A precipitate which is obtained in this manner and which contains fibrinogen and possibly activators is used for the screening of the fibrinolytic activity in plasma samples. When subjected to electrophoresis in the usual way, plasminogen is found in the β-globulin fraction of plasma.

By using electrophoretic systems which have high resolution powers, it has been shown that plasminogen appears in several electrophoretically distinct forms. Native plasminogen can be separated into two fractions on starch gel or polyacrylamide gel electrophoresis in weakly acidic conditions (pH 4.5). This separation can also be obtained by chromatographing on CM–cellulose (Wallén, 1962) and on Sepharose-lysine (Brockway and Castellino, 1972). When subjected to electrophoresis in starch gel or polyacrylamide gel, at pH 8.5, each of these fractions can be separated into a further six fractions. Thus, it would appear that plasma contains at least twelve different forms of plasminogen. A similar heterogeneity is found in the plasminogen of other animal species. Studies performed on rats and rabbits on the turnover of plasminogen which had been radioactively labelled *in vivo* and which was then isolated have shown that at least those forms which can be separated during electrophoresis at pH 4.3 are not interconvertible in the bloodstream (Siefring and Castellino, 1974). Thus, it would appear that these are released as separate components from liver cells and do not represent different levels of degradation. The chemical background to the microheterogeneity is not known in detail but differences in carbohydrate composition and especially in content of sialic acid seem to be of importance. For references and discussion see Collen and Maeyor (1975) and Sottrup-Jensen *et al.* (1978).

It is now generally held that Glu-plasminogen represents the native form of the proenzyme as it occurs in plasma. The other form, Lys-plasminogen, which arises from partial degradation is interesting since it is almost identical with an intermediate form of plasminogen which may be formed during activation. Thus, a comparison of the physicochemical properties of these two forms is of value. As can be seen in Fig. 122, Glu-plasminogen is identical with the plasminogen of fresh serum in terms of their electrophoretic mobility in starch gel while the mobility of the Lys-form suggests that this plasminogen has a markedly higher isoelectric point. These two forms differ in many other aspects. Some of the physicochemical characteristics of these two forms are given in Table 49. It is interesting to note that the conversion of Glu-plasminogen into

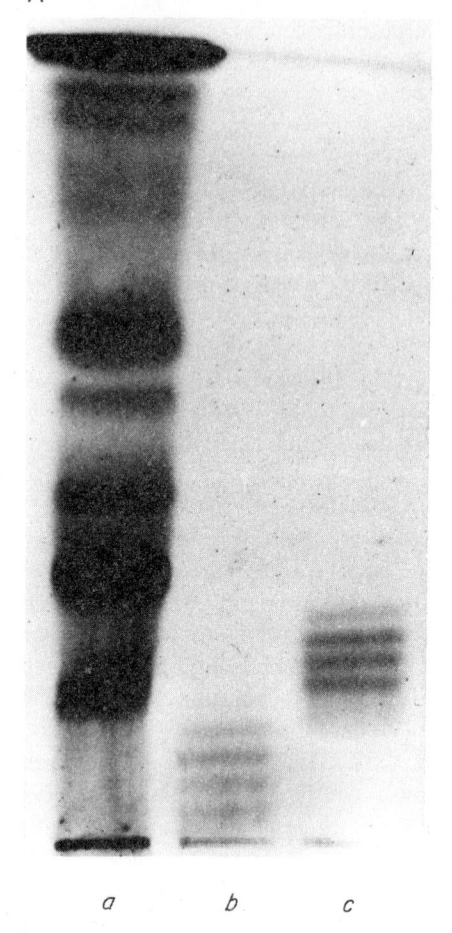

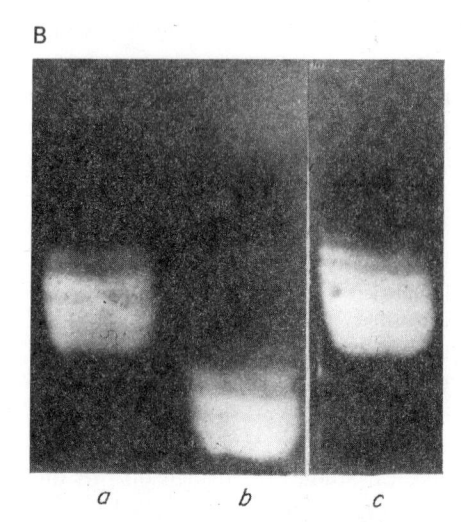

Fig. 122. Starch gel electrophoresis of plasminogen in plasma and in purified preparations (Wallén and Wiman, 1970). Buffer = 75 mmol/l ε-aminocaproic acid, 75 mmol/l Tris, pH 8.65.
The following preparations were used: (a) human serum, (b) Lys-plasminogen, (c) Glu-plasminogen.
A. Location of the protein components by staining with amidoblack.
B. Location of plasminogen in the same gels by using an enzymographic technique (fibrin film saturated with activator).

Lys-plasminogen entails an alteration in the molecule of plasminogen which is reflected in an increased Stokes's radius and an increased friction ratio. These findings are further supported by the observed differences in their circular dichroic spectra and the fact that Lys-plasminogen, in spite of its lower molecular weight, is eluted in a smaller volume on gel filtration. Further details and references can be obtained in an article by Sjöholm et al. (1973). The conformational changes observed on conversion of Glu-plasminogen into Lys-plasminogen seem to be due to a dissociation of a non-covalent interaction between a specific site (Ala 45–Lys 51) in the NH_2-terminal part of Glu-plasminogen and a lysine binding site (vide infra: 'structure of plasminogen ...') in the A-chain part of plasminogen (Wallén and Wiman, 1975, Wiman and Wallén, 1975).

Table 49. Physicochemical properties of plasminogen. The conversion of Glu-plasminogen (native form) into Lys-plasminogen (intermediate form of plasminogen, formed during activation) entails conformational changes which are probably of significance in the activation process

	NH$_2$-terminal amino acids[a]	Isoelectric point	Molecular weight[b]	Sedimentation constant	Frictional ratio	Stokes radius, nm
Glu-plasminogen	*Glutamic acid*	6.2–6.6	93 000	5.10	1.50	4.34
Lys-plasminogen	*Lysine* Valine Methionine	7.3–8.5	86 000	4.80	1.56	4.51

[a] Major amino acid in italics.
[b] Determined by polyacrylamide gel electrophoresis in the presence of sodium dodecylsulphate.

The determinations of molecular weight by ultracentrifugation (Table 49) show less difference between Glu-plasminogen and Lys-plasminogen than would be expected from differences in amino acid composition. As determined from the primary structure (*vide infra*) the molecular weight of Glu-plasminogen and Lys-plasminogen are about 91 000 and 82 000, respectively, after correction of a carbohydrate content of about 3 per cent.

3. Activation of the fibrinolytic system

The activation of the fibrinolytic system, i.e. the conversion of the proenzyme, plasminogen, into plasmin, is a proteolytic process whereby a few sensitive peptide bonds in the plasminogen molecule are cleaved. Both plasmin and trypsin can give rise to *in vitro* cleavage of these same bonds but, since both of these proteases have a highly general proteolytic activity, an increasingly unspecific degradation is obtained which soon results in the inactivation of the plasmin. The *in vivo* activation is carried out by special activators, proteolytic enzymes, which cause specific cleavage in plasminogen which results in its conversion into the proteolytic enzyme.

The structure of plasminogen and structural changes during activation

Plasminogen, both the native (Glu-plasminogen) and the partially degraded type (Lys-plasminogen), is composed of a single polypeptide chain, which is made up of 791 and 714 amino acid residues, respecitvely (Fig. 123). On activation, Glu-plasminogen is subjected to cleavage at two sites. Cleavage in the NH$_2$-terminal part will release peptide material (part marked III in Fig. 123) whereas the cleavage at the second site (Arg$_{561}$–Val$_{562}$) results in the generation of plasmin composed of two chains, A-(heavy)-chain (part marked I in Fig. 123) and B-(light)-chain (part marked II in Fig. 123) consisting of 484 and 230 amino acid residues respectively. The chains are connected by two disulphide bonds. The activation of Lys-plasminogen is effected by cleavage at one site only (Arg$_{561}$–Val$_{562}$) since the NH$_2$-terminal part has already been removed. The plasmins obtained in both cases are identical. The active centre of plasmin is situated in the B-chain (Robbins *et al.*, 1967). Like trypsin and chymotrypsin, plasmin belongs to the so-called serine proteases in which a certain serine residue, a certain histidine residue, and a certain aspartic acid residue are all three situated in the B-chain and play the leading parts in the catalytic process.

One of the greatest recent advancements in the field of fibrinolysis is the determination of the complete primary structure of plasminogen. (For references see Sottrup-Jensen *et al.*, 1978;

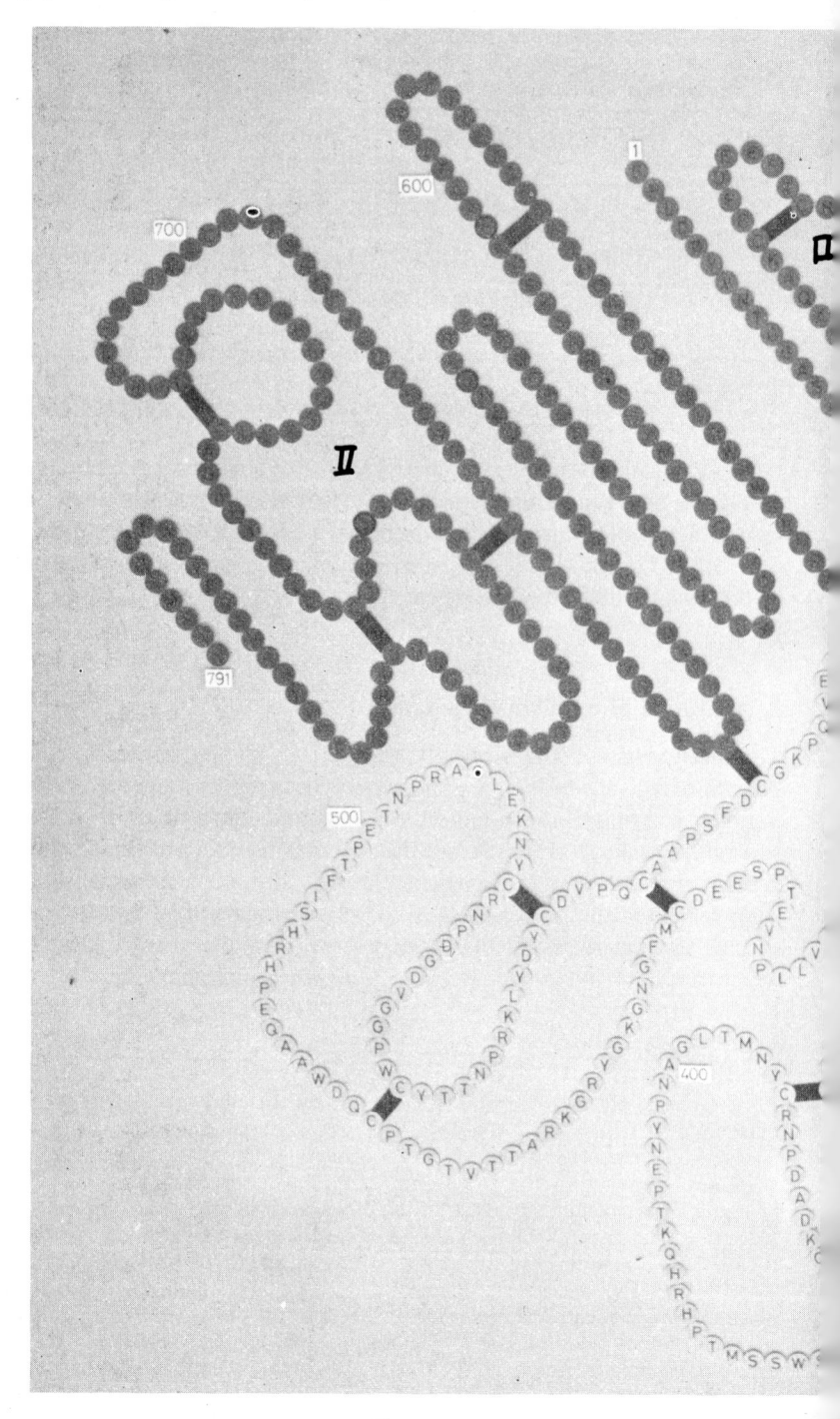

294 *Proteins taking part in coagulation and fibrinolysis*

Fig. 123. The primary structure of Glu-plasm
(cf. *European J. Biochem.*, **5** (1968) p. 151). Th
chain, I; The B-(light)-chain, II; The activati
acti

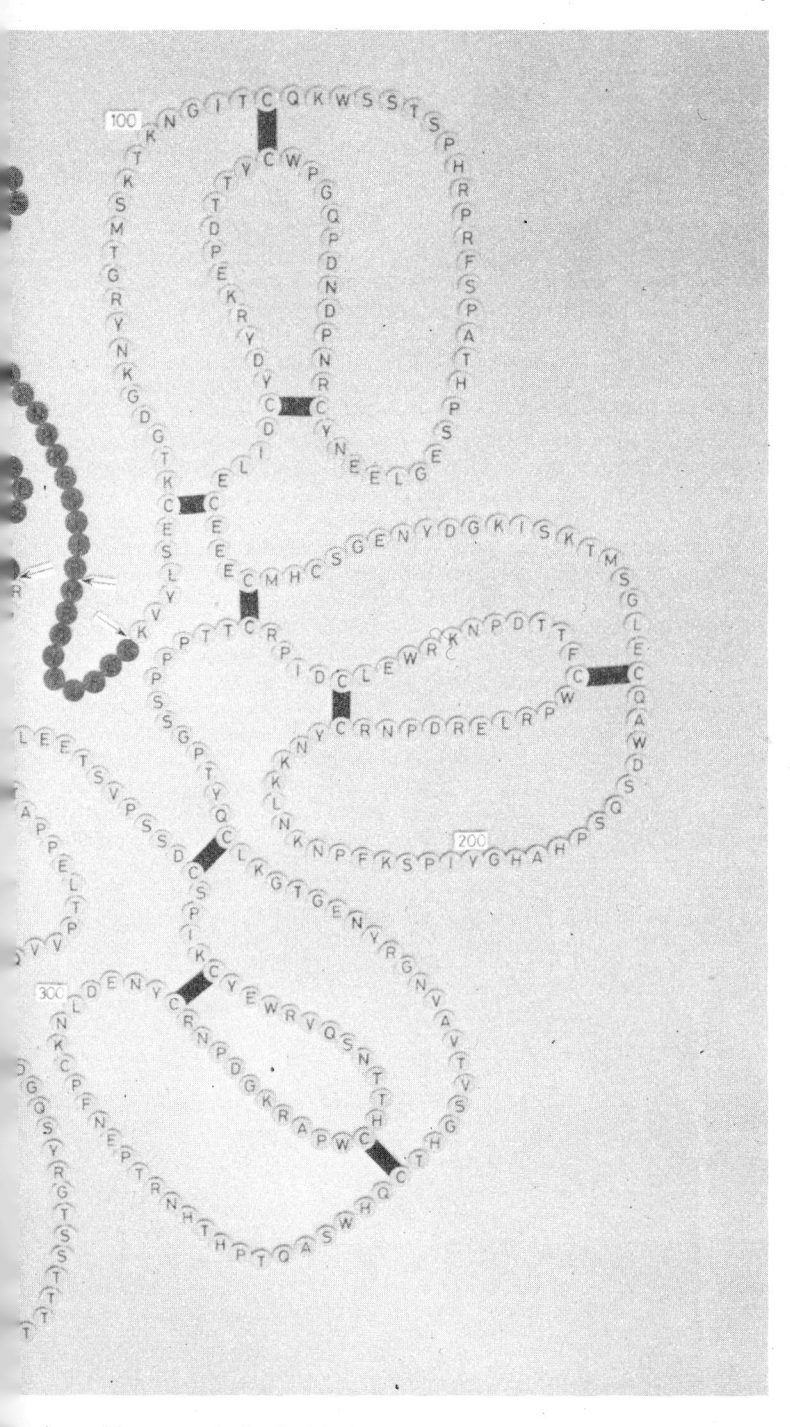

amino acids are symbolized with the 'One-Letter Notation'
obtained on activation are indicated I–III: The A-(heavy)-
, III. The arrows indicate peptide bonds cleaved during
Wiman, 1978.)

Wiman, 1977 and 1978; Magnusson this book page 254.) The sequence is shown in Fig. 123 in which the one letter code for amino acids has been used. The (different) chains in which plasminogen is cleaved during the activation are shown by marking I–III. The sequence of the B-chain (II) shows extensive homologies with chymotrypsin and other serine proteases. The amino acids constituting the active site are encircled with heavy lines (Wiman, 1978). The A-chain (I) originating from the NH$_2$-terminal two-thirds of the plasminogen molecule contains characteristic triple-disulphide loops, called kringles by Magnusson *et al.*, who discovered this type of structure first in prothrombin (cf. page 264), which contains two such structures and later in plasminogen, which contains five triple disulphide loops. These findings indicate a phylogenetic relationship between prothrombin and plasminogen and that a partial gene duplication and quintuplication have occurred during the development of prothrombin and plasminogen respectively. The connection between the A-chain and B-chain in plasmin occurs by two disulphide bonds. One of these bonds (Cys$_{548}$–Cys$_{666}$) is homologous with the interchain bond in chymotrypsin whereas the other bond (Cys$_{558}$–Cys$_{566}$) is specific for plasmin. In plasminogen the latter bond forms a disulphide loop containing the peptide bond sensitive to plasminogen activators (Arg$_{561}$–Val$_{562}$). It is very likely that this loop is a specific structure recognizable by the activators of plasminogen. This view is supported by the fact that synthetic *p*-nitroanilide substrates derived from the sequence Pro–Gly–Arg$_{561}$ are rather poor substrates for activators of plasminogen (Göran Claesson, unpublished results).

As mentioned above the generation of plasmin from Glu-plasminogen is accomplished by selective proteolysis at two different parts of the molecule. There has been some discussion as to the sequence of events leading to the generation of plasmin from Glu-plasminogen. According to present views two pathways, described in Fig. 124, are possible. In one pathway the first step is the cleavage of the Arg$_{561}$–Val$_{562}$ bond, which leads to the generation of a plasmin with a large heavy chain containing glutamic acid in NH$_2$-terminal position (Glu-plasmin). The second step is a release of NH$_2$-terminal peptides from the heavy chain, which gives rise to the final product, Lys-plasmin. The other pathway (Fig. 124B) starts with the generation of Lys-plasminogen by the release of NH$_2$-terminal peptides (the part marked III in Fig. 123), Lys-plasmin is then obtained by cleavage of the Arg$_{561}$–Val$_{562}$ bond. Analysis of the fragments isolated from activation mixtures at different times shows that the latter pathway (Fig. 124B) is clearly predominating. Lys-plasminogen formed as an intermediary component in this pathway differs in many properties from the native plasminogen, Glu-plasminogen. Thus, the intermediary plasminogen is considerably more sensitive to activator attack (*vide infra*). This is probably connected with the difference in conformation observed between Glu- and Lys-plasminogen as demonstrated for instance by circular dichroism studies (Sjöholm *et al.*, 1973). The marked changes in properties of plasminogen in the first step of this pathway, suggest that it is a

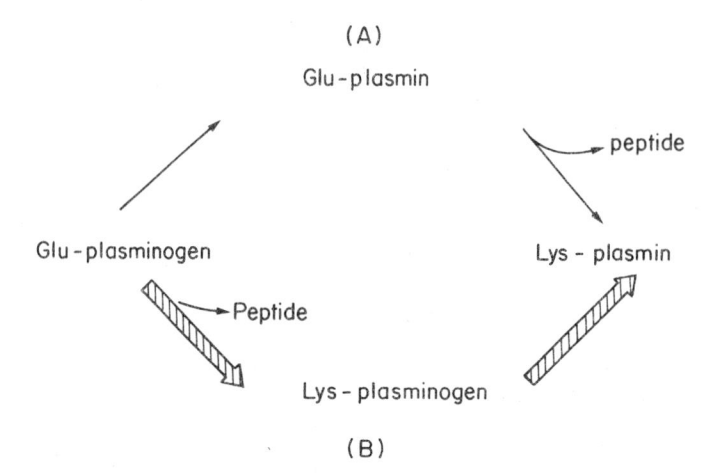

Fig. 124. Two possible pathways for activation of Glu-plasminogen to Lys-plasmin. Pathway B seems to be the most probable

regulatory step possibly of physiological importance in fibrinolysis. There has been some uncertainty as to which enzymes participate in the proteolytic reactions leading to the generation of plasmin. It now seems clear that urokinase and probably also tissue activator only cleave the Arg_{561}—Val_{562} bond of plasminogen, which is then transformed to Glu- or Lys-plasminogen. The release of NH_2-terminal peptides in plasminogen is probably effected by plasmin since two bonds Arg_{68}–Met_{69} and Lys_{77}–Lys_{78} (arrows Fig. 123) are extremely sensitive to plasmin. Thus, plasmin may stimulate the activation of plasminogen by a feedback mechanism. It is also possible that one function of Glu-plasmin is to cleave these bonds. (For further references and discussion see Violand and Castellino, 1976; Wallén, 1978; Wiman, 1978).

An interesting property of plasminogen and plasmin, which also is of practical use is the specific interaction with amino acids such as *trans*-4-aminomethylcyclohexase acid (AMCHA), ε-aminocaproic acid, and lysine. These amino acids have as common characteristic a basic group situated at a distance of about 0.7 nm from the carboxylic group. According to investigations by Abiko *et al.* (1969) AMCHA forms a 1:1 stoichiometric complex with plasminogen. The dissociation constants for the complexes formed with AMCHA, ε-aminocaproic acid, and lysine are 8×10^{-4}, 4.5×10^{-4}, and 6.8×10^{-2} respectively (Brockway and Castellino, 1972). The sites in plasminogen and plasmin participating in these interactions, the so-called lysine binding sites, have been localized to the A-chain (Rickli and Otavsky, 1975). Studies on fragments of an A-chain indicate that more than one site can interact with lysine and that the triple disulphide loops (kringles) are involved in these interactions (for further discussion and references see: Sottrup-Jensen *et al.*, 1978 and Wiman, 1978). These interactions bring about a marked change in the physicochemical properties of plasminogen such as a lowering of the sedimentation constant, an increase in Stokes's radius as well as changes in the circular dichromatic spectrum. The results suggest that marked conformational changes take place within the molecule of plasminogen and that these are similar to those seen on the release of the activation peptides (Sjöholm *et al.*, 1973).

The fibrinolytic system is affected *in vivo* by the presence of ε-aminocaproic acid and AMCHA. Apart from this antifibrinolytic effect (for references see Kjellman, 1971) it has been noticed that a marked increase in the turnover of plasminogen takes place during therapy with AMCHA (Collen *et al.*, 1972). *In vitro* studies have also shown that these amino acids have a marked effect on the activation kinetics. Several of these phenomena may be explained on the basis of the conformational changes which take place within the molecule of plasminogen.

Kinetics of activation of plasminogen

The two-stage model of the activation which was presented in the previous section provides a possibility of regulating the course of this activation if the first stage is rate determining and can be controlled. Work in several laboratories has shown that native plasminogen which has the intact NH_2-terminal sequence (Glu-plasminogen) has a rate of activation which is considerably lower than that of the partially degraded plasminogen (Lys-plasminogen) which has lost the NH_2-terminal portion containing the activation peptides. This is clearly demonstrated in Fig. 125 which shows the time course for the urokinase activation of native Glu-plasminogen and Lys-plasminogen. This figure also shows that the presence of lysine in a concentration of 0.01 mol/l has a strong accelerating effect on the activation of Glu-plasminogen. Lysine at the same concentration has no effect on the activation of Lys-plasminogen. Figure 126 shows that ε-aminocaproic acid in a concentration of up to about 2.5×10^{-3} mol/l has a stimulative effect on

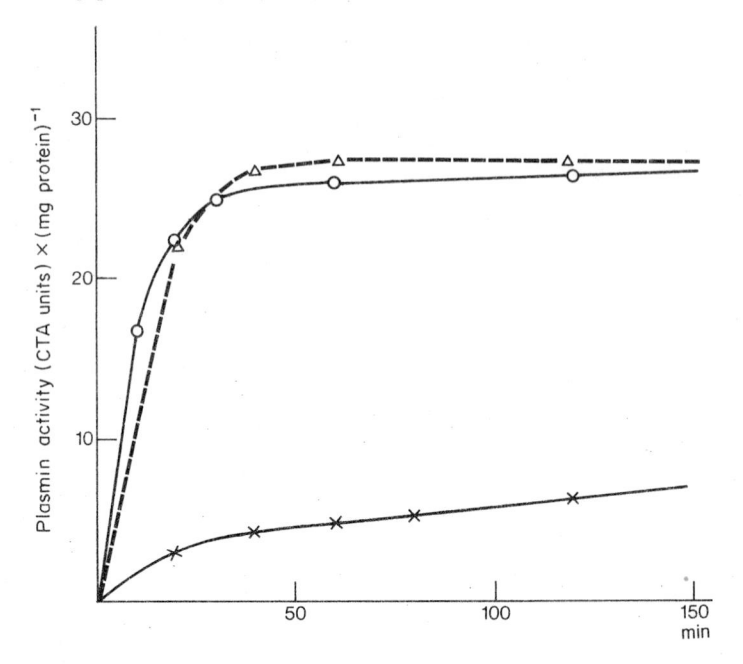

Fig. 125. Time course of the activation of Glu-plasminogen (x—x) and Lys-plasminogen (O—O) by urokinase at 25°C. (Incubation mixture: 0.5 ml plasminogen, 1 250 Ploug units urokinase and 0.25 ml glycerol/ml phosphate buffer, pH 7.5.) The effect of lysine (0.01 mol/1) on the activation of Glu-plasminogen is also shown (△+ +△). CTA units are in respect of the standard which was accepted by 'the Committee on Thrombolytic Agents', National Heart Institute

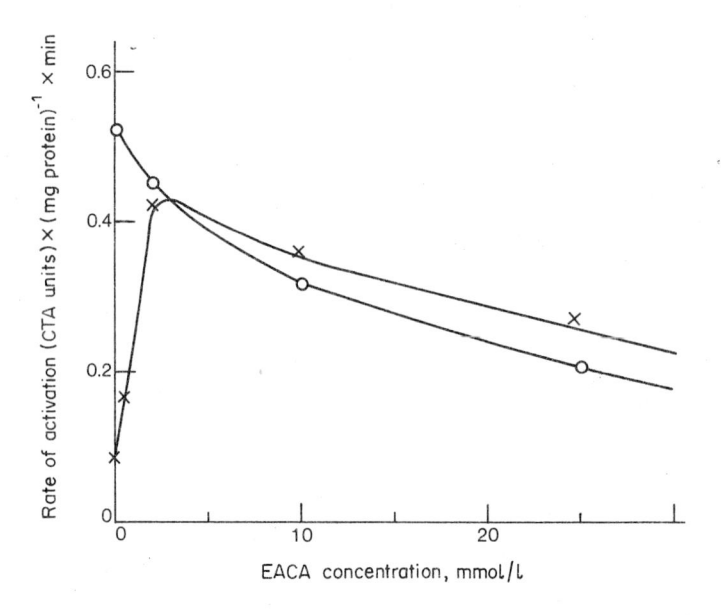

Fig. 126. Effect of EACA concentration on the rate of activation of Glu-plasminogen (x—x) and Lys-plasminogen (O—O)

the activation of Glu-plasminogen, whereas increasing inhibition is observed in concentration over this value. Corresponding experiments using Lys-plasminogen have not shown any tendency to stimulation but instead increased inhibition with increasing concentration of ε-aminocaproic acid. Studies of the activation of plasminogen thus indicate that the change of conformation induced in the plasminogen by dissociation of the non-covalent interaction between the NH_2-terminal part of Glu-plasminogen and a lysine binding site within the molecule brings about an increased sensitivity in plasminogen towards attack by activators. This dissociation may occur either by release of NH_2-terminal peptides or by reaction with substances which interact with the lysine binding sites in plasminogen like lysine, ε-aminocaproic acid, or analogous compounds. In this sense the conversion of Glu-plasminogen to Lys-plasminogen may function as a regulatory step in which a 'stockform' plasminogen is transformed into a 'standby form'. (For references and further discussion see Wallen, 1978 and Wiman, 1978.)

It should be pointed out that all of the studies on the mechanism of activation have been carried out in an artificial, pure system and should be considered as models. It remains to be seen if these models are relevant to physiological fibrinolysis. Furthermore, urokinase has been used in the majority of these investigations. These enzymes probably do not occur in blood but appear only in urine. Some experiments have been carried out using the tissue activator, which is probably the activator in blood. The results of these studies have shown a different mechanism (Thorsen and Astrup, 1974).

4. Activators

Urokinase

Several research workers showed independently at the beginning of the 1950s that urine contained an activator of plasminogen. This activator became known as urokinase. (For references see Astrup, 1977.) Urokinase is a proteolytic enzyme which, judging by its effect on synthetic substrates, cleaves only lysyl and arginyl bonds. The enzyme causes the specific cleavage in plasminogen thereby converting this protein into plasmin. However, its general proteolytic activity towards substrates such as casein is very low. One obvious function of urokinase is to maintain the canals of the kidney by dissolving blood clots. Studies have shown that there is a correlation between the increase in the fibrinolytic activity in blood and that in urine. This is taken to mean that the activator in urine originates from activators which are found in circulating blood. Despite the fact that specific antisera against urokinase are effective inhibitors of the fibrinolytic activity in urine, they are without effect on the blood activator. The idea of using urokinase as a thrombolytic agent is quite old and so it became important to purify the enzyme. Two groups of workers, Lesuk *et al.* and White *et al.* have independently prepared the enzyme which is homogeneous according to physicochemical analysis. However, these preparations appear to contain two types of urokinase. One form has a molecular weight of 54 000 and has been crystallized. The second form of urokinase has a molecular weight of 32 000 and has a specific activity which is almost double that of the first form. This second form is believed to arise from the first form by proteolytic cleaving of the inert portion of the molecule. Recently affinity chromatography on agmatine–Sepharose was applied to separate the two types of urokinase in a highly purified state (Soberano *et al.*, 1976, this article contains several references to the recent studies on the purification and characterization of urokinase).

Tissue activators

At the end of the 1940s, Astrup and co-workers showed that various tissues contained plasminogen activators, which explains the observation that certain tissues often contain a lot of fibrinolytic activity (Astrup and Permin, 1947). The activity is strongly connected with cell material which is difficult to dissolve. Some of this activity can be extracted with physiological saline. However, for a complete extraction effective solvents such as 2 mol/l KSCN must be used. A difference has also been observed in the stability of the activity in these two different types of extract. The activity extracted with physiological saline is easily destroyed by acidic pH and heat while the other extract is very stable. This has been interpreted to mean that there are two different tissue activators. The two types of extract are thought to differ considerably in their purities and protein compositions and conclusions concerning the identity of the activators must await purification of them. Astrup and co-workers have carried out a detailed examination of the concentration of the activator activity in the KSCN extract from various tissues and from various animals and man. They have found large differences in this concentration. Some tissues such as uterus, ovary, lymphatic glands, adrenal glands, prostate gland, thyroid gland, and the lungs contain high concentrations of this activator activity while other tissues such as testicles, spleen, and liver contain very low levels. The distribution of the tissue activator between the various organs has shown that the concentration of activator is related to the vascularization in the organ. One exception is liver tissue which normally contains only very small quantities of the activator (Astrup, 1966). The activator(s) are localized to the blood vessels. This has been demonstrated by a technique (Todd, 1959) where thin histological slices are covered with plasminogen-containing fibrin and are incubated at 37°C. The preparations are then fixed and stained at various times. The fibrinolytic activity is observed as unstained spots in the film of fibrin and the activator can be localized in this way to the various structures in the slices. By standardizing this method carefully, semiquantitative determinations of the activator concentration in various tissues and vessels can be carried out (Pandolfi, 1972). Investigations of this type which have been carried out by several research groups have shown that the highest activity is present in the small veins and capillaries as well as in the endothelium of the larger veins while the arterioles are relatively poor in the activators. The adventitia of the large blood vessels is very rich in the activators, a finding which can be attributed to the abundance of small vessels (*vasa vasorum*) in this region. The concentration of activator in the various parts of the human body is not uniform. Arm veins contain higher levels than leg veins. Additional details and references are given in a publication by Nilsson and Pandolfi (1970).

Relatively few attempts have been made to purify tissue activator. The starting material is generally porcine heart-muscle tissue. The ovaries of pregnant pigs is a second rich source of starting material. On a weight basis, this tissue contains 10–20 times more activity than heart tissue or the ovaries of non-pregnant pigs (Kok and Astrup, 1969). The best results have been obtained by Cole and Bachmann (1977), who extracted acetone-dried heart tissue with potassium acetate, pH 4.2, subjected this to fractionation with ammonium sulphate and zinc acetate and finally carried out a gel filtration step. The final product had a high specific activity (about 150 000 CTA units/mg protein). Polyacrylamide gel electrophoresis revealed one major component. A preparation of similar purity has been obtained by affinity adsorption on fibrin and affinity chromatography on Sepharose–arginine (Wallén et al., 1978).

Aoki (1974) has isolated an activator from human material by perfusing the network of blood vessels in legs obtained from corpses. The perfusion was carried out using a barbiturate buffer, pH 7.4, and the liquid which was recovered was fractionated to yield a partially purified product (3 000 CTA units/mg). These preparations lose their activity easily in a slightly acidic environment and when warmed and are therefore different from the preparations obtained from tissue homogenates which are remarkably stable. In this respect, Aoki's activator is similar to the activator in blood.

It has been possible to determine only some of the chemical characteristics of the tissue activators. Preliminary studies on the molecular weight using gel filtration have shown this to be between 60 000 and 80 000. Polyacrylamide gel electrophoresis of reduced activator shows that the activator is composed of two disulphide linked subunits of about equal size, about 30 000 daltons (Wallén et al., 1978).

Activators in blood

As with urine, other body fluids such as blood, milk, saliva, and tears contain activators of plasminogen. Since the activator which is present in blood is supposed to be responsible for the thrombolytic activity in blood, this activator has been devoted most attention. Because of the presence of various types of inhibitors, it is practically impossible to demonstrate the presence of fibrinolytic activity in whole blood or plasma. Apart from plasminogen and fibrinogen, the euglobulin fraction of citrated plasma contains activators but low concentrations of inhibitors. Thus, the determination of the lysis time for euglobulins (Nilsson, 1971) is a simple and relatively sensitive method for estimating the fibrinolytic activity in blood. An increase in the fibrinolytic activity is normally seen following vein stasis or the injection of vasoactive drugs such as adrenaline or nicotinic acid and in physical or mental stress.

Speculation surrounds the question of the origin of the blood activator. The earlier theory that this activator was identical with urokinase is no longer accepted. This is supported by the facts that the blood activator is not inhibited by antibodies against urokinase (Kucinski et al., 1968) and that patients who have undergone bilateral nephrectomy do not show any disorders of the fibrinolytic activity in blood even as late as one year after the operation. There is much in favour of the idea that the vessels are a source of activator. Thus, individuals who have a tendecy to develop thrombosis often have considerably lower levels of the activator in the vessel wall than the normal person (Nilsson and Pandolfi, 1970). How the activator activity of blood is related to that of tissue is not known since preparations having purity sufficient to permit comparative analysis are not available. Attempts to purify the acrivity have been complicated by the lability of the material in slightly acid or alkaline environments or at increased temperatures.

There is also evidence for an endogenous mechanism for generation of fibrinolytic activity within the blood, triggered by contact with foreign surfaces. This intrinsic fibrinolysis is mediated by the Hageman factor (Factor XII), kininogens, and prekallikrein indicating a close relationship with blood coagulation and kinin release. The detailed mechanism and the physiological significance of the intrinsic fibrinolysis are still unclear (for references and discussion see Saito et al., 1974.)

Streptokinase

Tillett and Garner showed in 1933 that all 28 cultures of *Streptococcus haemolyticus* which they had isolated from infected patients could dissolve human plasma clots. The active factor, an exotoxin which was released by the bacteria, was detectable in the filtrate of the culture. Christensen demonstrated that the streptococcal factor was an activator of plasminogen. The factor was consequently called streptokinase. This enzyme can now be isolated in the pure from as well as on an industrial scale and is the most widely used thrombolytic agent. Information concerning the purification and properties of streptokinase is rather scanty. A pure preparation has been isolated and charactrtized by de Renzo et al.(1967) who used chromatography on DEAE-cellulose and preparative electrophoresis. The molecular weight of the molecule has been determined to be 47 000. The amino acid analysis shows that cysteine and cystine are both missing. Thus, the molecule of streptokinase is thought to be a long polypeptide chain which does not contain any disulphide bridges. This lack of disulphide bridges in such a large protein molecule is particularly remarkable.

The mechanism of action of streptokinase is peculiar in that it differs from the other known activators. In contrast to these activators which exercise their proteolytic powers, streptokinase is without peptidase activity. A second peculiarity of streptokinase is its selective reactivity towards the plasminogen of various mammals. Of all plasminogens, human plasminogen is activated particularly rapidly while that which is isolated from the dog or the rabbit is activated considerably more slowly. The plasminogen of certain species, e.g. cow and pig does not react at all with streptokinase. However, these refractory types of plasminogen are activated quickly by streptokinase in the presence of small amounts of human serum. Early attempts to explain this suggested the presence of a cofactor in human blood, the so-called proactivator of streptokinase which together with streptokinase should give rise to a plasminogen activator. However, attempts to isolate the proactivator from the plasminogen activity in human plasminogen have been fruitless. Furthermore, it has been found that catalytic amounts of streptokinase can convert practically all plasminogen into plasmin while equimolar amounts of streptokinase and plasminogen form a complex which has primarily an activator function (Barg et al., 1965). It is clearly established that a proactivator function is inbuilt in the plasminogen molecule. It was suggested earlier that the streptokinase–plasmin complex was the true activator. By virtue of the fact that a certain amount of plasminogen exists in the active form as plasmin, the activator complex would rapidly activate the remaining plasminogen to plasmin and this would then form more activator complex. By studying the reaction between streptokinase and human plasminogen in the presence of p-nitrophenylgunidinobenzoate (NPGB)*, McClintock and Bell (1971) showed that a complex is formed which has a working active centre and that this is due to the induction of a conformational change in plasminogen by streptokinase. It has also been shown that the active centre in this complex is identical with that in plasmin (Schick and Castellino, 1974). McClintock and co-workers have recently presented the following theory for the course of events in the interaction of streptokinase and plasminogen. First, a complex is formed which has peptidase activity and in which plasminogen appears in an unchanged form. During the few stages which follow, streptokinase and plasminogen both undergo partial degradation until in the final stage, the plasminogen-streptokinase complex has been converted into a plasmin-streptokinase complex. It is not known which of the various derivatives is the prime activator. Recently Summaria and Robbins 1976) made the interesting finding that the site in human plasminogen and plasmin participating in the

---

*NPGB is a so-called *active site titrant* which blocks the active site with the consequent release of an equivalent amount of p-nitrophenol.

complex with streptokinase is situated in the B-(light)-chain of plasmin. They also demonstrated that B-chain isolated from plasmin after partial reduction still has the ability to form complex with streptokinase. On a molar basis this complex activates bovine plasminogen almost as fast as the plasmin streptokinase complex.

5. Inhibition of fibrinolysis

There are primarily two different proteolytic processes taking part in the fibrinolytic system. These are the activation of plasminogen and the plasmin-catalysed proteolysis. The presence in plasma of inhibitory activity against both of these activities has been demonstrated. Blood has a high ability to inhibit proteolytic activity.

Early attempts to assay the antifibrinolytic capacity of serum showed that serum *in vitro* can inhibit 30 times its own potential amounts of plasmin (Norman, 1958). With regard to the rate of reaction with plasmin two types of plasmin inhibitors were suggested, immediate and slow inhibitors. Until a few years ago four well characterized protease inhibitors, α_1-antitrypsin, α_2-macroglobulin, CT-inactivator, and antithrombin III were recognized as plasmin inhibitors (Heimburger et al., 1971). On a molar basis, there is 25 times more α_1-antitrypsin and 1.5 times more α_2-macroglobulin than plasminogen. It was originally thought that these two inhibitors represented the main part of the plasmin-inhibiting capacity of blood. Based on studies on the rate of their reactions *in vitro* it was suggested that α_2-macroglobulin was the immediate inhibitor and α_1-antitrypsin the slow inhibitor. Of the above named inhibitors, it is probable that only α_2-macroglobulin is of any physiological significance. During the extensive activation of plasminogen which is obtained by the use of urokinase or streptokinase in fibrinolytic therapy a marked reduction in the level of α_2-macroglobulin is seen while that of α_1-antitrypsin remains unaltered (Niléhn and Ganroth, 1967; Arnesen and Fagerhol, 1972).

An interesting observation was made by Müllertz in 1972. While examining fibrinolytic *post mortem* plasma, two compounds with plasminogen (plasmin) antigeneicity but without enzymic or proenzymic activity towards casein were demonstrated. One of them was identified as the plasmin–α_2-macroglobulin complex. The other compound, which had a higher molecular weight than plasminogen, showed no immunological relationship with plasmin inhibitors known at that time. On the basis of his findings Müllertz suggested the existence in plasma of a new inhibitor with high affinity for plasmin.

Subsequent studies by Aoki, Collen, Müllertz, Wiman, and others have resulted in the isolation and characterization of this inhibitor, which has been named antiplasmin, α_2-plasmin inhibitor, or primary plasmin inhibitor. According to current general opinion plasmin formed *in vivo* is mainly bound to antiplasmin. Binding of plasmin to α_2-macroglobulin occurs to a greater extent only if the capacity of antiplasmin is exceeded. The properties of antiplasmin and α_2-macroglobulin are more extensively discussed in other parts of this book (Andersson, Einarsson, and Lundén page 305).

Nilsson and co-workers found in 1961 that the serum of a patient with a strong tendency to develop thrombosis had a powerful inhibitor of fibrinolysis in normal plasma. Since the ability to inhibit plasmin was normal it was concluded that the effect was due to the inhibition of activation. On electrophoresis the inhibitor migrated in the α_2-region. Other studies have been performed which show that there may be several types of activator inhibitors. Brakman and co-workers have shown that increased inhibition of the tissue activators was present in a group of patients where urokinase-induced fibrinolysis was unaffected. Very few attempts have been made to isolate and characterize the activator inhibitors of plasma. This is probably due to the facts that these substances are particularly labile and as such can easily become inactive during the isolation procedure and that accurate activation assaying is difficult. A method for the preparation of a highly pure activator inhibitor has been published recently (Hedner, 1973). By using a special adsorption technique, Hedner has prepared a specific antiserum against the inhibitor. Using this she had been able to eliminate the possibility that this inhibitor was α_2-macroglobulin, antiplasmin, C-T-inactivator, or inter-α-inhibitor. Gel filtration studies have estimated the molecular weight to be 75 000. Because of its behaviour on gel filtration and electrophoresis, it is supposed that this substance is identical with the inhibitor which was previously described by Nilsson et al., 1961. It has recently been shown that this inhibition is an effective inhibitor of activated Hageman factor (Factor XIIa) and it may therefore mainly act within the endogenous fibrinolytic system of blood (Hedner and Martinsson, 1978).

The early investigations of fibrinolytic inhibitors were generally studies using well-characterized inhibitors, the effects of which are directed primarily against other proteolytic enzymes. With the exception of α_2-macroglobulin, it would appear that these inhibitors are of little importance in the inhibition of fibrinolysis. During recent years interest has grown in inhibitors which are specific for fibrinolysis. These substances are surely of great importance for the regulation of the fibrinolytic activity in blood.

6. Interactions between fibrin and the fibrinolytic system

It has been known for a long time that fibrin promotes fibrinolysis. The specific adsorption of components in the fibrinolytic system is probably of considerable importance for this effect. Thus, it has been shown that plasminogen activators, especially the tissue activator, are adsorbed to fibrin (Thorsen et al., 1972; Wallén, 1978). A site in fibrin for interaction with tissue activator has been localized to an A-chain (Wallén et al., 1978). Studies on the interaction between fibrin and plasminogen have shown that Lys-plasminogen is strongly adsorbed to fibrin. Also Glu-plasminogen has an affinity to fibrin although much weaker. The complex between plasminogen and fibrin is dissociated by ε-aminocaproic acid, lysine, and their analogues in low concentrations (Thorsen, 1975). The site in plasminogen responsible for this interaction seems therefore to be a lysine binding site, presumably the one which is related to the triple disulphide loop ('kringle') situated in the NH_2-terminal part of plasminogen (Wiman and Wallén, 1977). Fibrin has a strong potentiating effect on the activator of plasminogen by tissue activator. This effect of fibrin is neutralized by ε-aminocaproic acid in the concentration range 10^{-2} to 10^{-3}. Epsilon aminocaproic acid does not dissociate the complex between tissue activator and fibrin and nor does it inhibit the activity of the activator as measured by synthetic substrates. The effect of ε-aminocaproic acid and its analogues is probably due to the dissociation of the fibrin–plasminogen complex, which should therefore also be the background to its antifibrinolytic effect in vivo. Recent studies on fibrinolysis thus indicate that the fibrinolytic process is a rather complicated interplay between fibrin, plasminogen, and the activator, which may serve the purpose to localize the process to regions with fibrin deposits and to accelerate the reaction between the activator and plasminogen (for references and further discussion see Astrup, 1978 and Wallén, 1978).

Inhibitors of proteolysis in plasma

LARS-OLOV ANDERSSON, MONICA EINARSSON, and RAGNAR LUNDÉN

There exists in plasma an important system of protease inhibitors with the function to protect the protein in blood against unspecific proteolytic breakdown. Six such inhibitors have received special attention: α_1-antitrypsin, α_1-antichymotrypsin, inter-α-trypsin inhibitor, antithrombin III, cholinesterase inhibitor, α_2-macroglobulin, and recently α_2-antiplasmin. Of these, α_2-antiplasmin, α_1-antitrypsin, and α_2-macroglobulin are responsible for the major portion of the antiproteolytic activity in plasma. The role of these inhibitors in regulating the fibrinolytic activity of blood has been discussed in detail by Wallén (page 303). The following is a summarized account of their chemical properties.

1. α_1-Antitrypsin

This inhibitor was isolated, characterized, and named by Schultze et al. (1962).

The molecular weight is 54 000 and the concentration in plasma varies between 2 and 5 g/l (40–100 μmol/l). Thus, of all the protease inhibitors α_1-antitrypsin has the highest molar concentration in blood. It is a so-called acute phase reacting protein which implies that the concentration in plasma increases in infection and in inflammatory conditions. The inhibitor is a glycoprotein having 12 per cent carbohydrate and containing galactose, mannose, acetylglucosamine, and sialic acid. The protein is heat labile and can be irreversibly inactivated at low pH (<5). Purification of the inhibitor has been complicated by the difficulty in removing contaminating proteins, especially albumin.

The purification method of Schultze makes use of fractionation with ammonium sulphate in combination with precipitation with Rivanol and methanol. More recent procedures have employed various types of preparative electrophoresis and chromatography. A recent method of Liener et al. (1973) makes use of solid phase concanavalin A for the specific adsorption of α_1-antitrypsin following fractionation with ammonium sulphate and chromatography on DEAE–Sephadex.

Pannell et al. (1974) used plasma which had been freed of albumin by treating with Sephadex–Blue Dextran as starting material. Following fractionation with ammonium sulphate and chromatography at both high and low pH on DEAE–cellulose an immunologically pure preparation was obtained in a 60 per cent yield. The specific activity of this material was 125 times higher than of plasma.

C-B Laurell (1975) has published a method which is based on the binding of α_1-antitrypsin to a solid carrier via a disulphide exchange reaction. The procedure provides a preparation which is fully active immunologically and the yield of inhibitor activity is very high.

The inhibitor can exist in a large number of genetic variants of which the so called MM type is the form found in normal individuals. In cases of extensive genetically determined deficiency, a slowly migrating component called ZZ is seen on electrophoresis. Cases of total lack of α_1-antitrypsin have been described (Talamo et al.,1973; Eriksson, 1972). Patients who suffer from a severe deficiency of α_1-antitrypsin are often affected by lung emphysema in their early years but a small proportion of these patients, especially women, may reach old age without showing any clinical signs of lung disease. Even cases of juvenile liver cirrhosis have been shown to be connected with a deficiency of α_1-antitrypsin (Eriksson, 1972). In spite of its name, α_1-antitrypsin has a broad spectrum of interaction and inhibits enzymes such as chymotrypsin and plasmin (Table 50, page 314). As has been suggested by Pannell et al. (1974), a more appropriate name for this inhibitor would be α_1-protease inhibitor.

The clinical aspects of a deficiency of α_1-antitrypsin are discussed on page 343.

2. α_2-Protease inhibitor, antiplasmin

In 1976 a new protease inhibitor which efficiently inhibits the plasminogen activator induced lysis of fibrin clots was found in human plasma. The inhibitor is chemically and immunologically distinct from the hitherto known inhibitors and has been described independently by several investigators. It has been named antiplasmin (Collen, 1976), α_2-plasmin inhibitor (Moroi and Aoki, 1976), or primary plasmin inhibitor (Müllertz and Clemmensen, 1976).

A protein which inhibits the activation of plasminogen by urokinase and streptokinase has been partially purified from plasma by Hedner. Immunochemical evidence has been provided for the non-identity of this inhibitor and the novel protease inhibitor (Hedner and Collen, 1976).

The new α_2-plasmin inhibitor is a glycoprotein, consisting of a single polypeptide chain with a molecular weight of about 70 000. The sedimentation constant is estimated to 3.45 S and the partial specific volume to 0.72 cm^3/g. The total carbohydrate content is approximately 13 per cent. The NH$_2$-terminal amino acid sequence is found to be: Asn–Gln–Glu–Gly–. The absorptivity ($A_{280}^{1\%}$) is estimated to be about 6.7–7.0. The inhibitor is found to be stable above pH 6. Lyophilization is reported to destroy the activity of the purified protein (Moroi and Aoki, 1976). Other data have shown (Wiman and Collen, 1977), however, that the inhibitor is completely stable during lyophilization.

The concentration of the inhibitor in plasma is about 0.07 g/l. For purification various techniques have been utilized, such as chromatography on plasminogen–Sepharose after removal of plasminogen, DEAE–Sephadex, hydroxylapatite, and concanavalin-A–Sepharose. The protease inhibitor forms almost instantaneously a very stable complex with plasmin even at low temperature (0°C). Reduction of the complex α_2-protease inhibitor–plasmin shows that the B-chain of the plasmin molecule is covalently linked to the inhibitor. Plasminogen activation by urokinase or urokinase-induced clot lysis is inhibited by the α_2-protease inhibitor mainly through a mechanism of instantaneous development of a complex with the plasmin formed and not through the inhibition of urokinase. Furthermore the inhibitor also appears to inhibit trypsin.

The effects of purified inhibitor upon various proteases participating in human blood coagulation and kinin regeneration have been studied (Saito et al., 1977). Their results suggest that the protease inhibitor is an inhibitor of broad specificity that may play an important role in regulation of blood coagulation, fibrinolysis, and kinin regeneration.

3. α_2-Macroglobulin

Shultze has also been responsible for the isolation and characterization of α_2-macroglobulin. This inhibitor is the quantitatively predominant protein of the α_2-region and is present in plasma at a concentration of 2–4 g/l (2.5–5 µmol/l). The molecular weight is 725 000 which in plasma is surpassed only by certain lipoproteins, Factor VIII, and IgM.

Many different methods for the purification of α_2-macroglobulin have been published. These are dealt with at length in an article by Bourrillon and Razafimahaleo (1972). Hamberg et al. (1973) have recently described a method which provides an immunologically homogeneous preparation. This purification procedure involved fractionation with ammonium sulphate, gel chromatography, ultracentrifugation, and preparative electrophoresis on polyvinylchloride.

The inhibitor is capable of forming complexes with endopeptidases of various origins. The complex formation, which is probably irreversible, partly covers the active centre of the enzyme and thereby greatly reduces the activity of the enzyme towards high molecular weight substrates. A total inactivation may often result. However, the more general activity towards low molecular weight substrates and esters is practically unaltered.

The question of how many molecules of an enzyme bind to one molecule of α_2-macroglobulin has been examined using several different proteases. Ganroth (1966) found two molecules of trypsin bound per molecule of inhibitor. This result was later verified by a number of different investigators. However, more recent investigations (Barrett et al., 1973; Hamberg, 1974) have shown that the complex consists of one molecule of each of the two components. Uncertainty still surrounds this question. The report by Barrett et al. contains a table which summarizes the results of the experiments which have so far been carried out using proteases.

The physiological function of α_2-macroglobulin is clearly to quickly eliminate the free proteolytic activity in plasma. When dogs were injected intravenously with the complex ^{125}I-trypsin-α_2-macroglobulin, 80–85 per cent of the radioactivity was located in the liver, spleen, and bone marrow within a period of 30 minutes (Ohlsson, 1971). Ohlsson has also shown that the time for elimination of the complex in humans is likewise short. However, in the case of plasmin it is conceivable that the remaining proteolytic activity of its complex with α_2-macroglobulin may be of physiological significance in for example the activation of the fibrinolytic system (Fig. 120, page 289).

4. Antithrombin

The presence in plasma of an inhibitor of the coagulation process was insinuated as early as the turn of the century. Morawitz called this inhibitor antithrombin. The inhibitor is described at length in his famous work of 1905. Despite the fact that it was observed at such an early date, the inhibitor was not isolated until the end of the 1960s and even then it was obtained only in trace amounts (Abildgaard, 1967). A method for the isolation of material which was sufficient to permit proper characterization was not developed until the 1970s (Miller-Andersson et al., 1974).

Antithrombin III is a protein having a molecular weight of 65 000. It is an α_2-

globulin of which 15 per cent is carbohydrate. The molecule consists of one peptide chain which has three disulphide bridges. Histidine is the NH_2-terminal amino acid and the concentration of the inhibitor in plasma is 0.2 g/l.

Much work has been devoted over the years to the purification of antithrombin III. The problem has been complicated by the fact that the protein has approximately the same molecular size and electrical charge as albumin. Among the conventional methods which have been used in the purification of the inhibitor are: adsorption to aluminium hydroxide, chromatography on DEAE–Sephadex, gel filtration, and preparative polyacrylamide electrophoresis.

The discovery that antithrombin can be purified by chromatography on a heparin–agarose gel (Miller-Andersson et al., 1974) is an important development. This step gives a purification factor of over 200 and the yield is high. The method can be applied on the large scale to permit the purification of gram quantities of the inhibitor.

Antithrombin III is a protease inhibitor which has a broad specificity. Not only does it inhibit thrombin but also the activated forms of Factors IX, X, and XI (Rosenberg et al., 1975) as well as plasmin and trypsin. The reactions are relatively slow in the absence of heparin. Heparin binds to antithrombin III to give a more active form of the inhibitor. Antithrombin is identical with heparin cofactor, i.e. the plasma protein which causes heparin to have a high inhibition effect on blood coagulation.

Plasma proteins as diagnostic aids. Methods and clinical applications

BENGT G. JOHANSSON

I. Introduction

The possibility of analysing plasma proteins as a means of providing clinical information has increased rapidly during the last few decades. The only assay of this type which was available in the middle 1940s was the determination of the total protein content of plasma or serum. This was often a rough estimation based on the specific weight of serum or determinations by the Biuret method. The electrophoretic separation introduced at this time was a great advantage since it permitted at least a group separation of plasma proteins. Nowadays, specific assays can be performed on practically all known plasma proteins and these assays can be carried out with high precision and certainty. The development of immunological methods has contributed greatly to this favourable situation. The amount of clinical information which can be obtained through the multitude of different assays which can be performed can not today be conclusively evaluated. It is likely that more systematic studies of the plasma proteins will provide more definite clinical information than is presently available.

The remainder of this book will be devoted to a summary of the methods which are available for the separation of plasma proteins and assays of individual proteins as well as an attempt to interpret the data which are obtained through these methods.

II. Chemical methods

1. Determination of total protein

The simplest method for the quantitative determination of protein is in fact a purely physical method and entails the measuring of the light absorption of a solution of protein at 280 nm. This absorption is due to the presence of aromatic amino acids such as tyrosine and tryptophan and, to a less extent, phenylalanine. This procedure is complicated by two phenomena which are noteworthy: the ultraviolet absorption of a protein varies with the amino acid composition and the analysis is perturbed by the presence of turbidity in the solution. The latter complication, which arises during all measurements carried out in the ultraviolet region, can be checked by performing the measurement at two wavelengths, e.g. 280 and 260 nm, where the absorption at 280 nm should be greater than that at 260 nm. The simplicity of the method makes it suitable for the analysis of the fractions which are obtained from the column chromatography of proteins. This can be achieved by employing a continuous recording of the absorption of the column effluent. The method can be used also for the determination of the concentration of isolated proteins, where absolute values can be recorded if the absorption value for a certain concentration of the protein is known. However, the method is not recommended for the determination of the total protein concentration in plasma, cerebrospinal fluid, or other biological fluids since interference can arise from turbidity or the presence of other substances which absorb in the ultraviolet region.

The biuret reaction is based on the formation of a red–violet complex between copper(II) ions and the amide (peptide) bonds of proteins. Since at least three peptide bonds are required per molecule for the characteristic biuret colour, a tetrapeptide is the smallest molecule required for this reaction. The reaction mechanism is rather complicated and not fully understood for proteins. However, because of the simplicity and reproducibility of the reaction it has become widely used in several manual or automatic versions. The biuret method is without doubt the most commonly used method for the determination of total protein in plasma or serum. On the other hand, the method is not sufficiently sensitive to permit the determination of proteins which are present in low concentrations, e.g. in cerebrospinal fluid.

A much more sensitive method than the conventional biuret method was developed by Lowry, using a combination of biuret reagent and the Folin–Ciocalteu phenol reagent. The increase in the colour which is developed in this technique is due to the presence of tyrosine and tryptophan in the analysed protein. The mechanism of the reaction is poorly understood. Despite some differences in colour formation between various proteins and the interference from many substances, the Lowry method has become the standard method in protein chemistry because of its simplicity and high sensitivity. In Scandinavia, this method has become the standard method for the determination of total protein in cerebrospinal fluid. Due to the interference mentioned above, however, the Lowry method has been replaced in many laboratories by techniques employing binding of the dye Ponceau S to cerebrospinal fluid proteins.

Among other methods for protein determination the classical Kjeldahl method deserves attention. This is a reference method in analytical protein chemistry and despite the fact that it is not used as often as before, the method is still very useful. An exact protein determination with the Kjeldahl method requires knowledge of the nitrogen content of the protein in question. In most cases this lies between 12 per cent and 18 per cent. The determination can be complicated by the presence of bound ligands and may be such that the determination is rendered impossible. In many cases of mixtures of proteins, a conversion factor of 6.25 (corresponding to a nitrogen content of 16 per cent) has been used. This can give rise to significant errors. The conventional Kjeldahl method, which is based on the titration of ammonium ions following combustion of the sample with sulphuric acid, requires a rather large amount of sample material. The sensitivity of the method can be increased by using colorimetric methods such as the ninhydrin method for the determination of the ammonia formed. The ninhydrin reaction can also be used following hydrolysis of the protein with hydrochloric acid but the results obtained with this method are somewhat influenced by the amino acid composition of the protein.

Several methods employing fluorescence can be used for determination of protein concentrations. Direct measurements of the proteins may be performed, but it is more simple to couple fluorescent components to the free amino groups within the protein, e.g. fluorescamine (fluram). This reagent can easily be coupled to primary amino groups in weakly alkaline solutions. While the coupled fluorescamine exhibits a strong fluorescence, excess reagent is rapidly converted to non-fluorescent compounds in water solution. The high sensitivity of fluorescence measurements is an obvious advantage but so far these methods have not been widely used for protein determinations. The fluram technique may also be used for the detection and quantitation of proteins after electrophoretic separation in polyacrylamide gels.

2. Determination of individual plasma proteins

Only a few plasma proteins have special properties which allow them to be assayed specifically without prior separation of the protein in question. To this group of proteins belong certain molecules which have enzymic activity or have enzyme-inhibiting properties, many proteins which are involved in coagulation, and proteins which can bind other proteins or low molecular weight ligands. However, most of the methods based on such properties which were used earlier have been replaced by the simple immunological methods now available. As examples of enzyme determinations can be mentioned the assay of *ceruloplasmin* by measurement of the oxidase activity of this protein. *Lysozyme* can be assayed by measuring its enzymic ability to dissolve certain strains of bacteria such as *Micrococcus lysodeicticus*. Immunological assay methods are now available for both of these two proteins. Many of the proteins which take part in coagulation are enzymes and can thus be determined by assaying their enzyme activity. An indication of the serum level of α_1-*antitrypsin* can be obtained by measuring the total trypsin-inhibiting activity in serum.

A well-known example of determination of plasma proteins with a ligand-binding method is the determination of the total iron-binding capacity of serum, which is a measure of the level of *transferrin* in serum. This anlysis plays an important role in addition to serum iron determinations in the diagnosis of iron deficiency.

Haptoglobin is another protein which can be determined on the basis of its binding capacity. The protein forms stable complexes with haemoglobin (see page 102) and this phenomenon is used in the determination of haptoglobin expressed as the haemoglobin-binding capacity of serum (HbBC). The earliest methods for the assay of this protein were semiquantitative and involved the use of a series of plasma samples to which were added various amounts of free haemoglobin. The free and bound haemoglobin were then separated by electrophoresis to give an idea of the concentration of haptoglobin in plasma. Quantitative methods, which were based on the greater peroxidase activity (or stability) of haptoglobin-bound haemoglobin compared with free haemoglobin were later developed.

Analysis of haptoglobin by measurement of its capacity to bind haemoglobin has been replaced more and more by immunochemical methods. Because of the differences in molecular size distribution of the different genetic variants of haptoglobin radial immunodiffusion may give erroneous results but electroimmunoassay or immunonephelometry are useful methods for haptoglobin determinations.

Albumin was earlier determined by electrophoretic techniques. The more recent methods which have become widely used are based on the ability of this protein to bind indicator dyes. The substance most commonly used is bromocresol green which binds comparatively firmly to albumin with a simultaneous change in colour. This principle has lead to the development of simple spectrophotometric methods for the assay of albumin which can easily be automated. The method is not influenced by increases in the serum bilirubin levels or by certain drugs which also bind to albumin.

By the dye-binding techniques the determination of albumin has become readily available and in some hospitals the older approach of determining the total protein content has been replaced by the determination of the level of albumin in plasma as a measure of the patient's protein situation. Recent investigations have shown, however, that the use of colour-binding techniques for the assay of albumin may give rise to serious errors. This complication is particularly noticeable at low concentrations of albumin and since the error is not systematic it can not be corrected for satisfactorily. The error arises mainly from the binding of bromocresol green to some other proteins which increase in inflammatory conditions (see page 35) sometimes giving rise to a considerable overestimation of the albumin values in such conditions. The dye-binding techniques for albumin are therefore not completely reliable, but a sastisfactory accuracy can be obtained if the measurements are performed immediately (within 8–10 seconds) after the addition of bromocresol green to the samples, since there is a considerable difference in the time necessary for colour development by albumin and the interfering proteins. The dye-binding technique employing bromocresol green can also be used for measurements of urinary albumin. Immunochemical methods like electroimmunoassay and immunonephelometry are also useful for analysis of albumin and electroimmunoassay has in fact been recommended as a reference method for albumin determinations.

III. Physicochemical methods

1. Analytical ultracentrifugation

This method is based on the fact that protein molecules sediment at different rates when they are subjected to fast centrifugation (approximately 60 000 revs/min). The rate of sedimentation is dependent primarily on the molecular weight and molecular size of the protein. In the analytical ultracentrifuge, the sedimentation takes place radially in sector formed cells and can be followed by optical registration where the peaks represent proteins of various sedimentation rates (Fig. 127). The area under the peaks is a measure of the concentration in a solution of the corresponding protein fractions. Analytical centrifugation is an important technique in physicochemical studies of individual proteins such as the determination of molecular weight. On the other hand, the method does not have the resolution required in the examination of complicated solutions of proteins such as plasma or serum. Serum can be divided into three distinct fractions: a 19 S fraction which corresponds to macroglobulins, a 7 S fraction which contains mostly IgG (and IgA) and a 4.5 S fraction in which albumin is the major component. Despite the relatively poor resolution and the complicated apparatus which is required for analytical centrifugation, the method has been of great value in the past for the analysing of plasma when an alternative method for the investigation of molecular size was not available. This situation changed completely after the introduction of gel filtration techniques.

The designation by sedimentation coefficients is still used to some extent for the characterization of proteins of differing molecular size, e.g. the immunoglobulins. Thus the pentameric form of IgM is called 19 S IgM while the monomeric form is known as 7 S IgM. Such notations are also used in an inappropriate manner to describe immunoglobulin fractions, separated by gel filtration and not by ultracentrifugation. It should be mentioned that preparative ultracentrifugation can also be used as an analytical tool. The method is important, e.g. in the analysis of lipoproteins of different density classes.

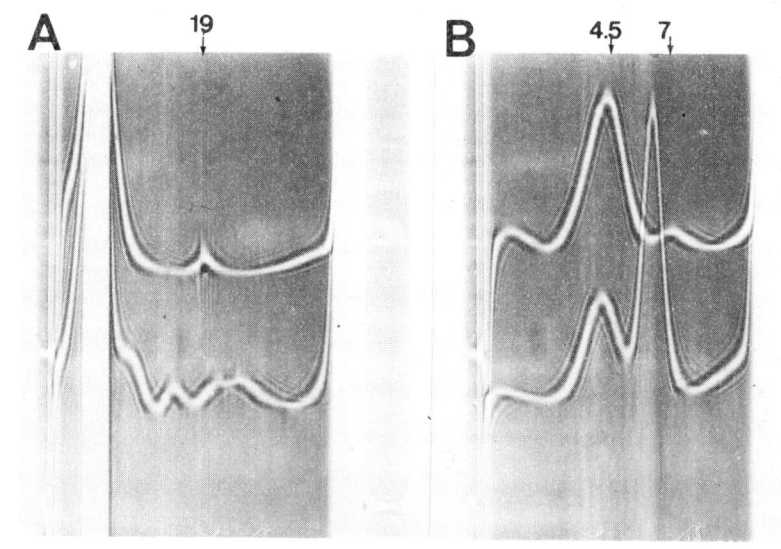

Fig. 127. Analytical ultracentrifugation of serum proteins. Two samples have been analysed in the same run; the upper trace is of normal serum while the lower is of serum from a patient suffering from an 'immunocomplex disease'. The sedimentation takes place from left to right in the picture. The picture on the left (A) was taken early in the analysis and shows the separation of the 19 S component in the normal sample and the presence of several macroglobulin components in the lower sample. The picture on the right (B) was taken later in the analysis and shows components having sedimentation coefficients of 7 S and 4.5 S, where IgG dominates in the former and albumin in the latter. In special cases such as this, good resolution of certain components of pathological serum can be achieved

2. Gel filtration

The gel filtration technique was developed at the beginning of the 1960s mainly through the contributions of Porath and Flodin. The technique has been of tremendous importance in preparative protein chemistry as a simple preparation procedure with high recovery. The method is based on the separation of substances according to their molecular size on a column of gel particles of dextran which has been rendered insoluble by the introduction of cross-links between the carbohydrate chains. Molecules which are larger than a certain size are not capable of penetrating into the porous gel particles and consequently migrate fast through the column in the solvent phase outside the gel particles while smaller molecules which can penetrate more or less into the interior of the gel particles become retarded. This gives rise to a separation of the molecules according to their molecular size. Various types of Sephadex gel are available and the choice of one of these is determined by the molecular size of the substances which are to be separated (Table 50). Sephadex G-75 or G-100 is most suitable for the separation of low molecular weight proteins while plasma proteins are best separated on Sephadex G-200 which has the lowest degree of cross-linking and permits the separation of globular proteins which have molecular weights in the region of 25 000 30 000 (Fig. 128). It should be noted here that the separation is dependent on the molecular *size* which is not necessarily strictly proportional to molecular

Table 50. Gels which can be used in protein separation which is dependent on molecular size. The volume of the gel-bed per gram of dry gel is an indirect measure of the porosity of the gel. Each gel is available in various particle sizes

Gel type	Bed volume (ml/g dry gel)	Separation range for globular proteins (daltons)
Dextran[a]		
Sephadex G-50	9–11	1 500–30 000
Sephadex G-75	12–15	3 000–70 000
Sephadex G-100	15–20	4 000–150 000
Sephadex G-150	20–30	5 000–400 000
Sephadex G-200	30–40	5 000–800 000
Polyacrylamide[b]		
Bio-Gel P-30	11	2 500–40 000
Bio-Gel P-60	14	3 000–60 000
Bio-Gel P-100	15	5 000–100 000
Bio-Gel P-150	18	15 000–150 000
Bio-Gel P-200	29	30 000–200 000
Bio-Gel P-300	36	60 000–400 000
Agarose		
8 % agaros	—	<10 000–1 500 000
6 % agaros	—	10 000–5 000 000
4 % agaros	—	40 000–15 000 000

[a] Information on properties supplied by manufacturer (Pharmacia Fine Chemicals, Uppsala Sweden).
[b] Information on properties supplied by manufacturer (BioRad Laboratories, Richmond, California, USA).

weights. However, in the case of globular proteins the molecular size is usually closely correlated to the molecular weight except for glycoproteins which have a high content of carbohydrate.

While gel filtration can not compete with the electrophoretic methods in the clinical analysis of plasma proteins, it has served as a useful method for obtaining additional information, e.g. concerning the molecular size distribution of pathological immunoglobulins.

For analytical purpose, the normal column technique for performing gel filtration can be replaced by thin-layer gel filtration. This procedure gives better separation of proteins than the column method and permits the simultaneous analysis of several samples containing microgram quantities of material. Using this technique, which is labour-saving in comparison to the column technique, it was possible to demonstrate the presence of some cases of half molecules of immunoglobulin in an investigation of a large number of plasma samples containing M-components. The combination of thin-layer gel filtration and immunodiffusion (immunogelfiltration) has produced very interesting results, especially in studies of immunoglobulins, e.g. the aggregation and fragmentation of IgG. It is also quite possible to combine thin-layer gel filtration with crossed immunoelectrophoresis. However, thin-layer gel filtration has not become of more general use in the field of plasma proteins.

During more recent years new gels such as polyacrylamide and agarose have become available for use in gel filtration. The agarose gels are of particular interest since they

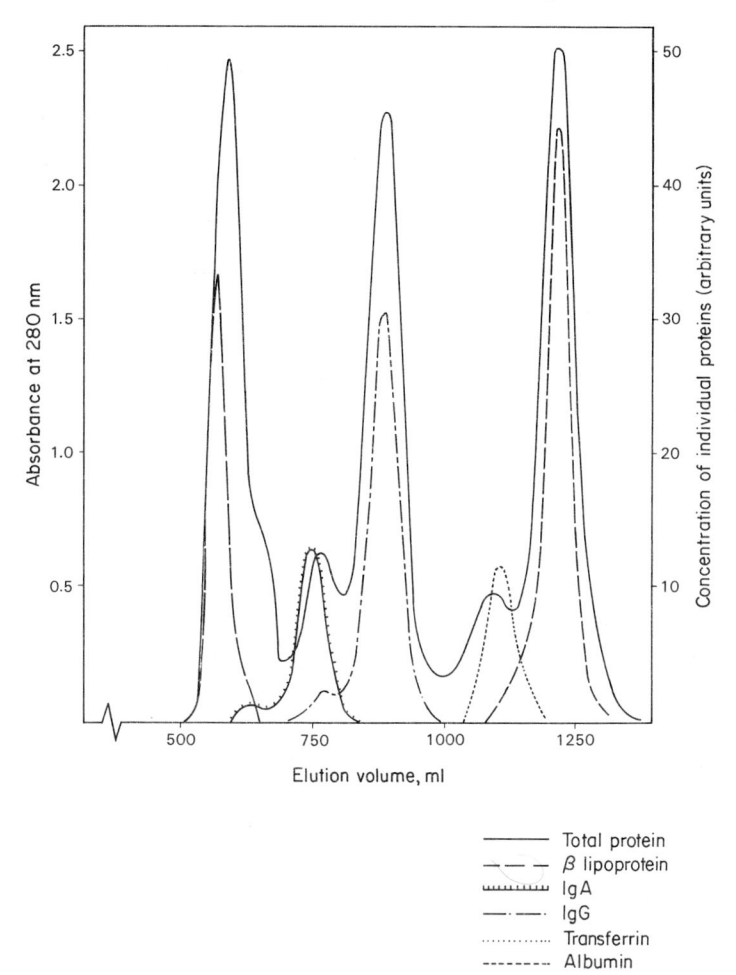

Fig. 128. Example of protein separation carried out by gel filtration. Protein in 10 ml plasma was separated on a column (5+90 cm) of Sephadex G-200. The distribution of protein was measured spectrophotometrically at 280 nm while the localization of some individual proteins was estimated by immunochemical analyses. The good separation is due to the use of Sephadex with a fine particle size (20–30 μm)

permit the separation of molecules of a higher molecular weight than those which can be separated by Sephadex.

The macroglobulin fraction obtained by Sephadex G-200 filtration can be separated into several fractions by filtration through agarose gels. This gives an opportunity to obtain separations of lipoproteins with large particle sizes, e.g. very low density lipoproteins (VLDL) from low density lipoproteins (LDL). No evaluation of the usefulness of such separations in clinical routine has so far been made.

Other gels have recently been introduced which combine a comparatively high resolution power with high flow rates, e.g. Ultrogels[R] which consist of a mixture of polyacrylamide and agarose and Sephacryl[R] which is a dextran gel with better flow properties and higher resolution than the corresponding Sephadex gels.

3. Electrophoresis

Because of its simplicity and good resolution power, electrophoresis is undoubtedly the most important technique in the clinical routine laboratory for the separation of proteins. Paper electrophoresis was the predominant method in earlier days but this technique has now been replaced by electrophoresis in other stabilizing media with increased resolution and less interfering phenomena e.g. adsorption.

Several electrophoretic methods giving a very high resolution have been developed during the past few years. This is most evident in the technique of polyacrylamide gel electrophoresis (Davis and Ornstein, 1964) where electrophoretic separation is combined with separation according to molecular size. The high resolution allows the separation of more than 20 protein components of plasma. While the technique is extremely useful for protein chemistry in general, the high resolution does not quite match the demands of the clinical chemistry laboratory, since the interpretation of the patterns is often difficult, not least due to the many genetic variants which can complicate the patterns. Similar difficulties arise in other methods where the resolution is very high, e.g. isoelectric focusing.

There are several alternatives, however, to the highly resolving electrophoretic methods. Cellulose acetate membranes e.g. have become widely used but the resolution provided by this method is not always quite satisfactory. Agar gel electrophoresis is a second alternative which appears to give very satisfactory results. Despite the good separations obtained by agar gel electrophoresis, the earlier methods had significant disadvantages such as low capacity. This disadvantage has been eliminated in the technique developed by Laurell and co-workers. In this method the agar is replaced by agarose, a fraction of agar which contains a considerably lower content of charged groups (sulphate and carboxyl). By using agarose instead of agar, interfering phenomena are considerably reduced, e.g. the adsorption of certain components to the gel matrix and the so-called electroendosmosis. The latter phenomenon gives rise to a flow of solvent towards the cathode during electrophoresis due to by the presence of negatively charged groups in the agar gel. A comparatively low degree of electroendosmosis is especially important in immunoelectrophoretic methods such as electroimmunoassay, which will be described later.

The electrophoretic separation is performed on thin glass plates (10×20 cm) or plastic films (Mylar) on which has been layered a 1 mm thick layer of agarose. The 15 samples which can be analysed simultaneously are applied in thin slits along one of the long sides of the plate. The electrophoresis is run until a serum albumin reference dyed with bromophenol blue has migrated 5 cm which takes about one hour. After rapid precipitation of the separated protein components with picric acid, the gel is dried to a thin film and the proteins are stained with amido black or, if higher sensitivity is required, with Coomassie Brilliant Blue, R-250. The technique requires a simple apparatus where the most important part is a water-cooled thin glass plate to support the agarose film (Fig. 129).

Agarose electrophoresis which is carried out according to this procedure provides results which meet the requirements of a clinical laboratory in respect of the resolution of the protein components (Fig. 130). The method is rapid and has a high capacity which makes it useful as a routine method. The electrophoresis plates can also be stained with sudan black to visualize the lipoproteins or with other suitable reagents in

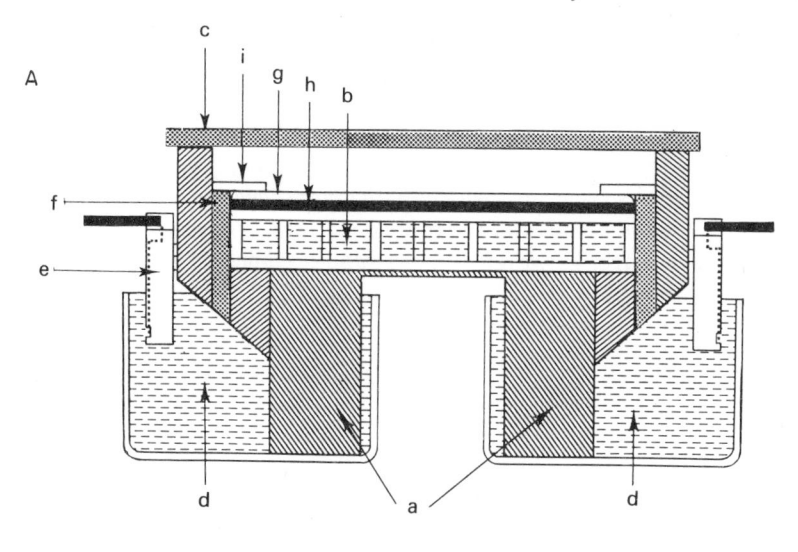

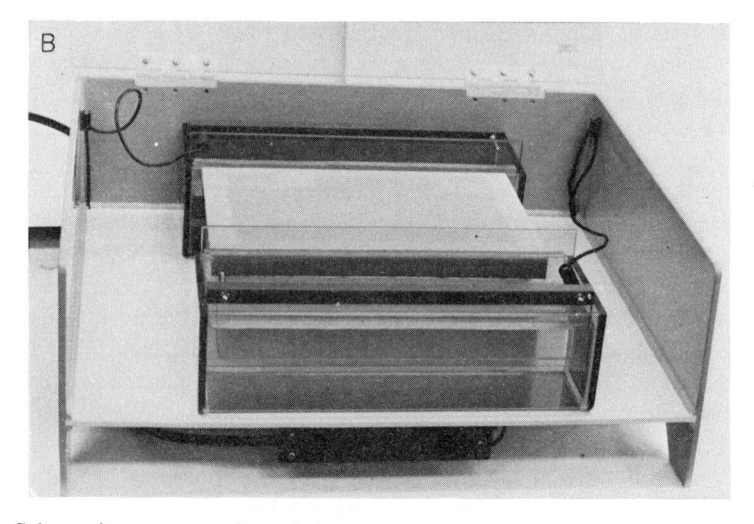

Fig. 129A. Schematic representation of the apparatus used in agarose gel electrophoresis. (*a*) perspex frame, (*b*) water-cooled support plate, (*c*) glass cover, (*d*) electrophoretic buffer solution, (*e*) electrode plate with electrodes, (*f*) connecting bridges between buffer and gel (*g*) agarose gel layer on thin glass plate (*h*). (Johansson, 1972) B. Apparatus for agar gel electrophoresis (Analysteknik, Vallentuna, Sweden)

the separation of isoenzymes such as lactate dehydrogenase, amylase, or alkaline phosphatase (Fig. 131). One further advantage is that the method forms the basis of the rapid immunochemical assays of proteins which have been developed during recent years. These methods are described later in this chapter.

Agarose gel electrophoresis can also be used in research work and in many cases provides information which is comparable to that of the considerably more complicated technique of polyacrylamide gel electrophoresis. It should be noticed that agarose gel electrophoresis does not produce separations which are dependent on molecular size. Thus, this technique can not be used for the determination of molecular size of proteins. This parameter can be determined by carrying out electrophoresis in polyacrylamide gels in the presence of sodium dodecylsulphate, which forms complexes with various proteins so that they all obtain the same negative charge. The technique has been suggested for the analysis of the proteins in urine to distinguish between different types of kidney damage. However, it is doubtful if clinical information which can not be provided by the more simple agarose gel electrophoresis can be obtained in this way.

IV. Immunochemical methods

1. Introduction

Because of their high specificity and sensitivity, immunochemical methods have become important tools in analytical protein chemistry. A prerequisite for immunochemical analysis is that the protein in question must be a good immunogen, i.e. capable of eliciting an antibody response in a suitable laboratory animal. In addition, there must be available a suitable detection system for measuring the antigen–antibody reaction. These two requirements are met in the case of most of the plasma proteins. All plasma proteins which have so far been isolated have been found to have good immunogenic properties, giving rise to precipitating antibodies. Antibodies for the methods described are often produced in rabbits but goats and sheep are also suitable animals. Horse antisera on the other hand are often less useful. Certain difficulties can arise in the production of strictly monospecific antibodies. However, this is no great problem since a variety of useful methods is available for the purification of proteins and since antibodies against impurities can be removed from the antiserum by immunoabsorption. The absorption is carried out using plasma or plasma protein fractions which do not contain the antigen concerned. In suitable cases, such absorptions can be effected by using patient serum which contains a very low level of the antigen in question. The absorption of unwanted antibodies in an antihaptoglobin antiserum can be effected by addition of plasma from a patient who has increased haptoglobin elimination due to haemolysis. In other cases, the absorption can be achieved by using fractions which are obtained as a by-product in the preparation of a specific protein used for immunization. These fractions must of course not contain the protein in question. The absorption process may be performed by addition of the antigen in the soluble form or insolubilized, e.g. by polymerization with glutaraldehyde or by coupling to agarose. The use of insolubilized antigens eliminates the risk of having an excess of antigens in the antiserum after absorption, which may complicate the results of certain immunochemical analyses. The antiserum can be used directly after appropriate absorption. However, it is advantageous not to use whole antiserum in immunoprecipitation methods but instead to prepare the immunoglobulin fraction, which can be easily prepared from serum by removal of the main lipoprotein and subsequent salting out of immunoglobulins.

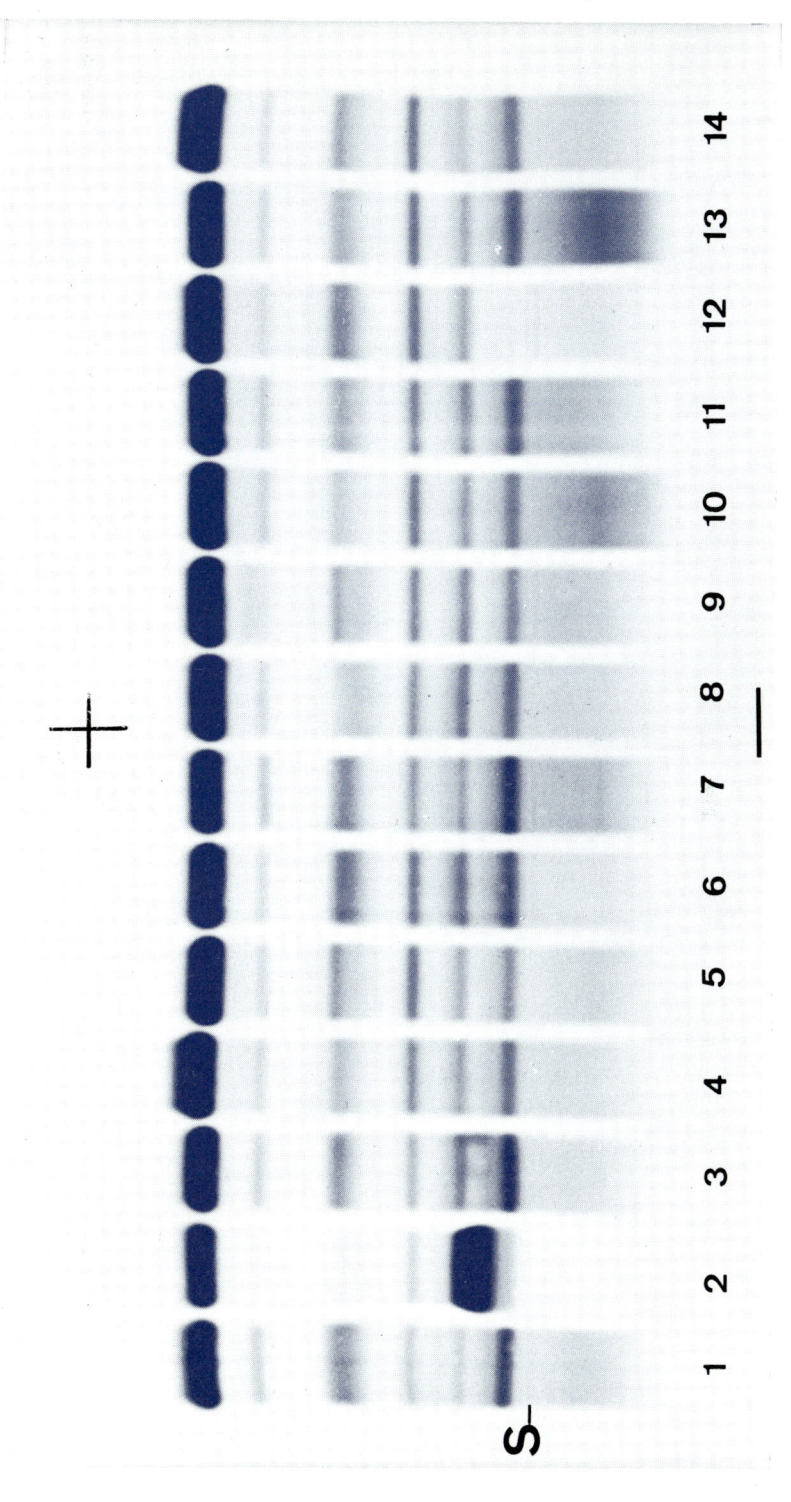

Fig. 130. Plasma protein patterns obtained in agarose gel electrophoresis. Samples were applied at the position marked with 'S'. The original size of the electrophoresis plate was 10 × 20 cm

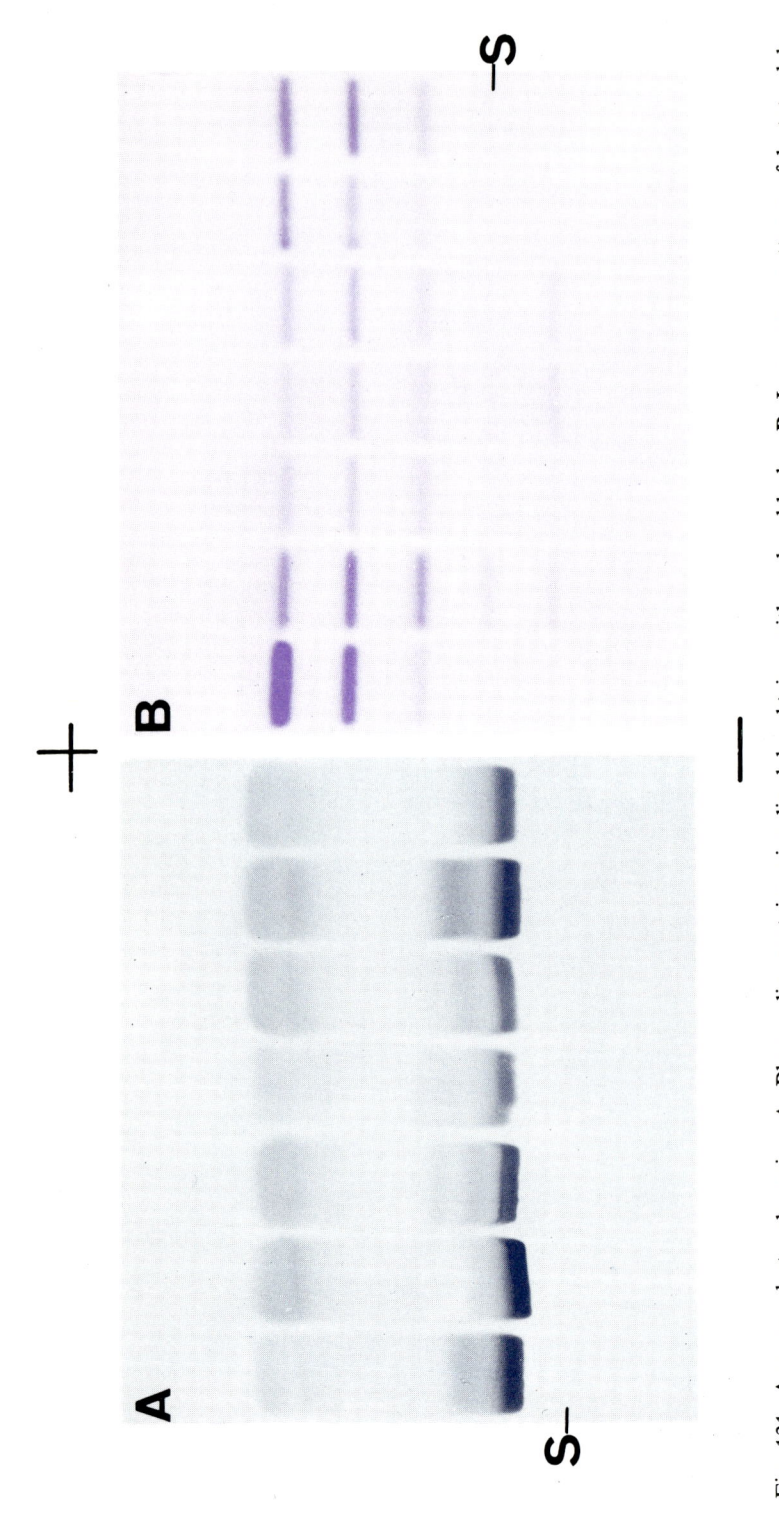

Fig. 131. Agarose electrophoresis. **A.** Plasma lipoproteins visualized by dyeing with sudan black. **B.** Isoenzyme patterns of lactate dehydrogenase. Samples were applied at the position marked with 'S'

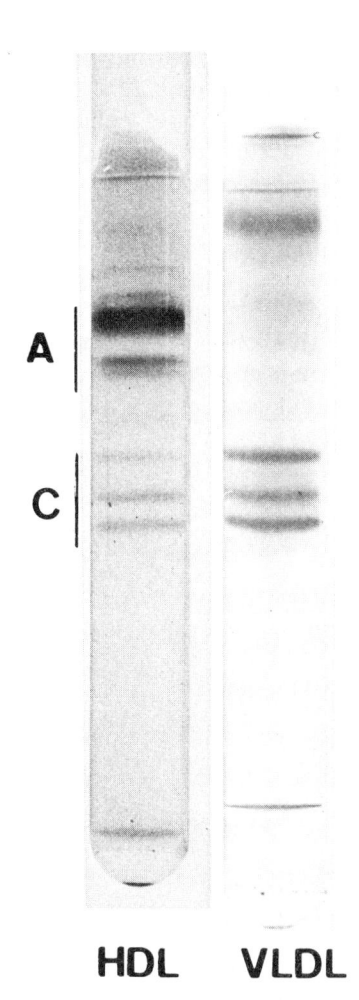

Fig. 132. Separation of apolipoproteins by polyacrylamide gel electrophoresis in urea (8 mol/l). Apolipoproteins obtained by delipidation of *high density lipoprotein* (HDL) and *very low density lipoprotein* (VLDL) with chloroform–methanol were used as sample. 'A' indicates the so called A-family of apoproteins which is dominant in HDL and 'C' indicates the C-family which is dominant in VLDL. An additional component (C.I.) of the C-family is seen in the upper part of the VLDL gel

The immunological reaction which can be recorded by measuring the *primary* reaction which takes place between the antigen and the antibody or by using some *secondary* manifestation such as precipitation reaction is by far the most common means of assaying plasma proteins.

2. Quantitative precipitation in solution

This method, which was introduced by Heidelberger and Kendall in the 1930s, is a useful but rather laborious method for the quantitative determination of proteins. Even if the method is not used for plasma protein analyses in its original form, it is worth while describing the technique to illustrate the principles of the immunoprecipitation reaction. The analysis is carried out by adding a constant volume of antibody solution to a series of test tubes. Various known amounts of antigen are then added to some of the tubes so that a standard series is obtained. The samples to be assayed are added to the remaining tubes. Following incubation for several days, the tubes are centrifuged and the immunoprecipitate formed is recovered, washed effectively, and its nitrogen

322 *Plasma proteins as diagnostic aids. Methods and clinical applications*

content is determined. The method is illustrated by Fig. 133. As seen in this figure, the amount of precipitate increases with increasing antigen concentration until a maximum is reached. A further increase in the antigen concentration causes reduction in the amount of precipitate formed. On the addition of a sufficiently high concentration of antigen, no precipitation at all is formed. This is not caused by an inhibition of the primary antigen–antibody reaction in the presence of an excess of antigen but is due to the fact that *secondary* precipitation does not appear in antigen excess. Under these conditions, each divalent antibody is saturated with two molecules of the antigen to form low molecular weight complexes of the type Ag–Ab–Ag. A prerequisite for the precipitate formation is that the antigen contains at least two determinants per molecule so that large antigen–antibody complexes can form. In the analysis of unknown samples it should be noticed that a certain amount of precipitate formed corresponds to two possible concentrations of antigen (in antibody or antigen

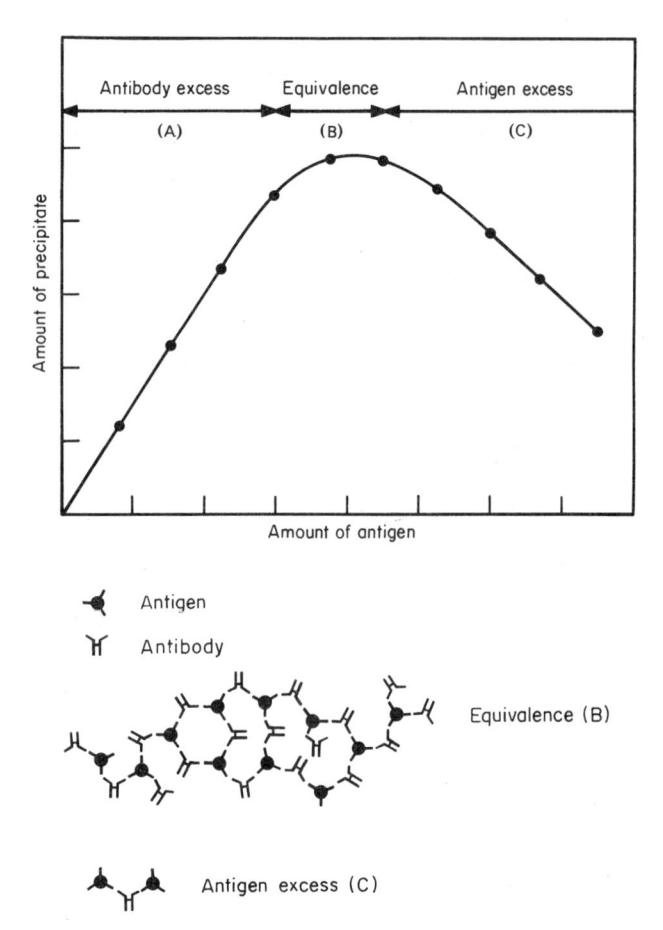

Fig. 133. Quantitative immunoprecipitation. The lower part of the figure shows a very schematic representation of the composition of the precipitate obtained in the region of equivalence (B) and the formation of low molecular weight complexes of antigen and antibody when the former is in excess (C)

excess). To elucidate which of these concentrations is correct, the analysis must be carried out at a different dilution. Thus the method in its original form is time-consuming and is hardly suitable for routine analysis of proteins.

3. Double diffusion in agar gel

Significant advances in analytical immunochemistry resulted from the techniques which were developed at the end of the 1940s by Oudin, Ouchterlony, and others where the immunoprecipitation reaction was carried out in transparent agar gels. In the so-called double-diffusion technique, the antigen and the antibody are allowed to diffuse towards each other from separate pools in a gel of agar. A precipitate is obtained where the reactants are present in optimal concentrations. This technique provides the possibility of distinguishing several immunoprecipitations by performing studies of antigen mixtures with polyvalent antisera. Furthermore, the technique affords a simple and reliable method for studying the immunological relationships between various antigens and antibodies, although great caution is demanded in the interpretation of results. The technique of double diffusion is mainly a qualitative method and is therefore not suitable for determination of plasma protein concentrations.

4. Immunoelectrophoresis

This technique, which might be described more correctly as gel electrophoresis followed by immunodiffusion, was introduced in 1953 by Grabar and Williams. The principle of the technique is represented in Fig. 134. Much valuable information concerning the plasma proteins has been obtained by using this method. As with double diffusion, modification of this technique has enabled a comparison of an antigen in a complex mixture with standard antigens so that the antigens can be separated and hence identified by electrophoresis (Wadsworth and Hanson, 1960). The technique of immunoelectrophoresis is very simple and permits many parallel analyses to be performed. However, there are some important disadvantages. The method is not quanti-

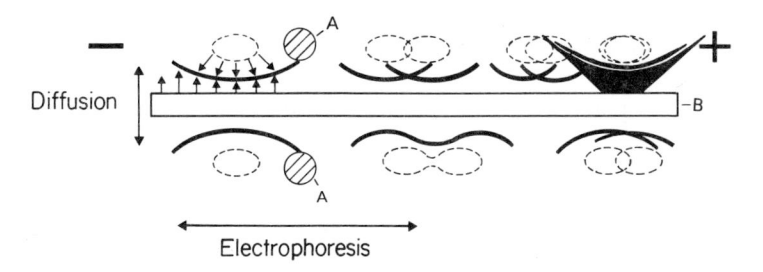

Fig. 134. The principle of immunoelectrophoresis. The proteins to be separated are placed in the circular basins (A). Following electrophoresis, the long antiserum well (B) is cut out of the gel and is filled with antiserum containing antibodies against the separated proteins. The separated proteins are indicated by the dashed oval zones. The antigens and antibodies meet following diffusion (arrows) and give rise to an immunoprecipitate. Proteins which are related immunologically but which have different electrophoretic mobilities produce double arches of the type shown in the lower portion of the figure

tative and the separation of immunologically related material which maybe obtained in the first step (electrophoresis) can be lost during the subsequent immunodiffusion step. These disadvantages are overcome by the move recently introduced *crossed immunoelectrophoresis.*

5. Quantitative gel immunodiffusion

The first useful technique for *quantitative* determinations of proteins by gel immunodiffusion was developed by Oudin. The technique, which should be characterized as a one-dimensional single immunodiffusion, is carried out in columns filled with antibody-containing agar gels. The antigen is applied to the surface of the gel and is allowed to diffuse into the gel. A precipitate is formed which migrates into the gel. After a period of 24–72 hours, the distance from the surface of the agar to the front edge of the immunoprecipitate is measured. This distance is proportional to the logarithm of the concentration of the antigen. Thus the concentration of antigen in the sample can be obtained from a standard curve which is normally plotted on semilogarithmic paper.

The procedure is laborious, however, especially in large series and for this reason the development of the single radial immunodiffusion technique (Mancini et al., 1965) was an important contribution. This method employs glass plates onto which have been layered 1–2 mm thick films of antibody-containing gel. Circular antigen wells are punched in the gel and are filled with a known volume of sample or of standard solution. The antigen diffuses into the gel and a ring of immunoprecipitate is formed around the well. The diameter of the rings increases over a period of 7–14 days and thereafter remains constant. The area which is then enclosed by the immunoprecipitate is proportional to the concentration of the antigen. This long diffusion time can be considerably reduced and in practice the antigen is allowed to diffuse for only 24 hours or, if it is a high molecular weight protein, 48–72 hours. Under these conditions, a strict linear relationship between antigen concentration and the area of the precipitation ring is not always obtained but by using a series of standard solutions of antigen, accurate determinations can be made. The error of the method can be maintained as low as 1–2 per cent (CV) and the sensitivity of the method is considerable. Extremely weak precipitation rings can be visualized by staining with Coomasie Brilliant Blue and by this means the method can be applied to determinations of low concentrations of antigen. The sensitivity limit of the technique after protein staining of the immunoprecipitate is around 0.5–1 mg/1 (Fig. 135). This means that a large number of plasma proteins can be assayed quantitatively by this method.

The radial immunodiffusion procedure is very simple to perform and there is no demand for expensive equipment. It has the disadvantage, however, of being comparatively time-consuming especially for high molecular weight proteins. This is sometimes unsatisfactory in clinical routine, and also when the method is used as an assay system in the preparation of labile proteins. It should also be noted that molecular size heterogeneity of the assayed protein may give inaccurate results, since the method is based on diffusion of the antigen. Especially if short diffusion times (1–2 days) are used considerable errors can arise if the samples and standards differ in molecular size distribution.

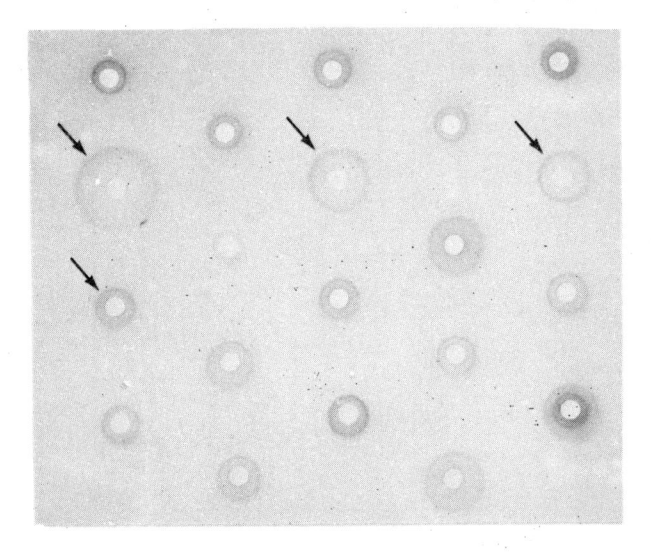

Fig. 135. Simple radial immunodiffusion (Mancini et al., 1965) of β_2-microglobulin in the concentration region 1–5 mg/l. The arrows indicate standard samples and the remaining wells contained samples of human serum. The very faint precipitates were stained with Coomassie Brilliant Blue

6. Electroimmunoassay (rocket immunoelectrophoresis)

This technique, which was developed by Laurell (1966, 1972) should be considered as a true immunoelectrophoresis in the proper sense of the word, more so than the 'classical' immunoelectrophoresis. The method is very well suited for rapid, quantitive determination of proteins and is also used as the second step in crossed immunoelectrophoresis, which will be described later in this chapter. In American literature the method is sometimes referred to as electroimmunodiffusion; this term should be abandoned since the principle does not involve diffusion. In fact, diffusion of the antigen should be avoided since it may cause erroneous results.

The technique, which is schematically described in Fig. 136, is based on electrophoresis of charged antigens, e.g. proteins, into an antibody-containing agarose gel, under such conditions (pH, ionic strength, etc.) that the antibodies do not migrate in the electric field. Furthermore the concentrations of antigen and antibody must be balanced in such a way that the antigen is in excess when migrating into the gel from the start basins. Under these conditions low molecular weight antigen–antibody complexes of the type AgAb and Ag$_2$Ab are initially formed and these migrate further in the electrical field due to the charge of the antigen. During the continued migration of the complexes they encounter new antibody molecules, which are bound to accessible determinants of the antigen. The complexes grow successively in size and finally reach such dimensions that they precipitate in the gel. In this way a continuous 'consumption' of precipitating antigen takes place and the final result is a closed immunoprecipitate which a rocket shape (cf. the designation 'rocket immunoelectrophoresis). The area enclosed by the immunoprecipitate is proportional to the antigen

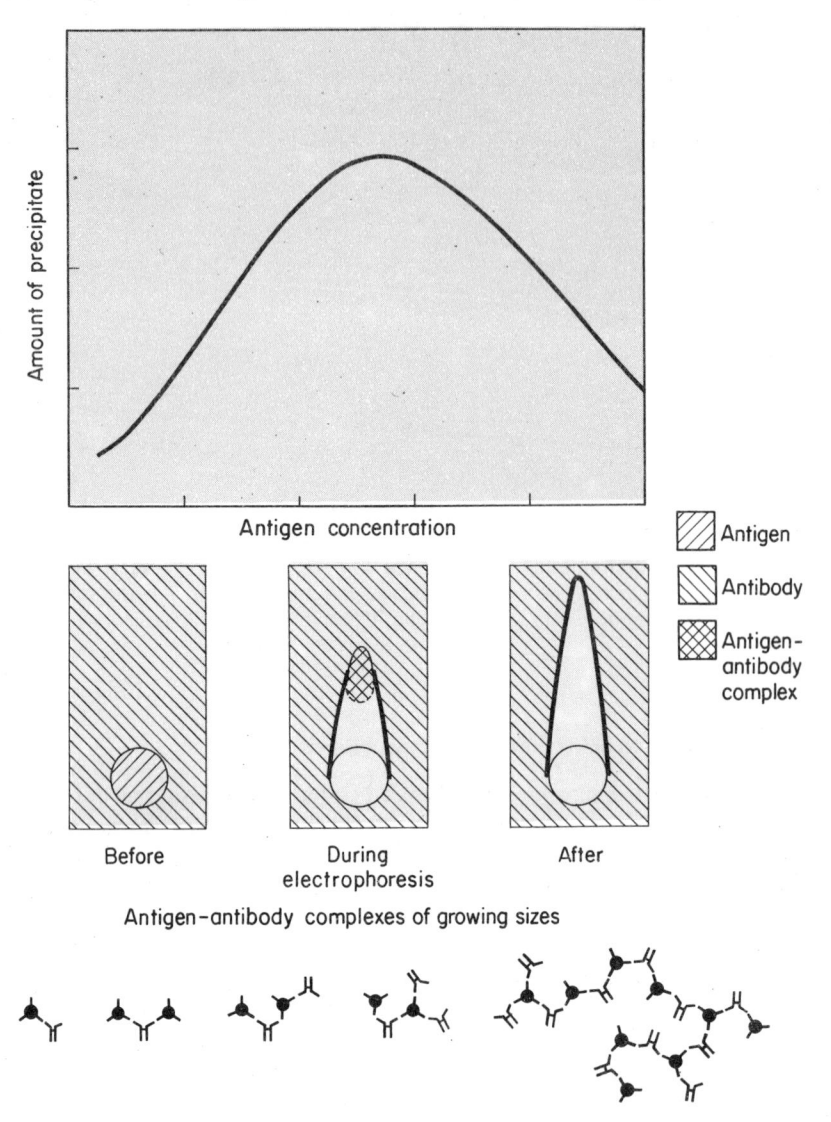

Fig. 136. Principle of electroimmunoassay (EIA). The upper portion of the figure shows a diagram of quantitative immunoprecipitation (cf. Fig. 133). Below this is shown the formation of the immunoprecipitate during electrophoresis. This involves the formation of antigen–antibody complexes of growing size which are demonstrated in the lower portion

concentration in the sample. In practice, the heights of the precipitates are measured rather than the area and these are compared with the corresponding heights obtained for the antigen applied in various known concentrations.

Apart from being somewhat more technically complicated than radial immunodiffusion, electroimmunoassay has several advantages. First it is less time-consuming. The results may be obtained in less than 2 hours if antigens with high migration rate are analysed. However, runs of 10–12 hours may be required for slowly migrating antigens.

A second advantage is the possibility to assay two or even more proteins simultaneously, since the immunoprecipitates are often distinguishable by differences in morphology (cf. Fig. 137). The two methods have roughly the same sensitivity, but small, very faint precipitates are easier to recognize in electroimmunoassay. Because of the application of an electrical field in electroimmunoassay, the avidity of the antibody preparations used in this technique must be greater than in radial immunodiffusion.

Whereas radial immunodiffusion may give rise to misleading results on analysis of proteins with molecular size heterogeneity, analyses by electroimmunoassay are more affected by electrophoretic (charge) heterogeneity of the proteins. However, differences in molecular size may sometimes affect the results of electroimmunoassay, i.e. in determinations of immunoglobulins.

One prerequisite in electroimmunoassay is that the antigen has an electrophoretic mobility, which is different from that of the antibodies, i.e. the antigen should migrate into the gel under conditions where the antibodies remain essentially stationary. This is a major problem in immunoglobulin determinations, which are further complicated by the pronounced electrophoretic heterogeneity of these molecules. Clinically useful information on IgG concentrations can be obtained, however, by measuring the immunoprecipitates formed on both the anode and cathode sides of the antigen basins, provided that the proportions of the heights of the anode and cathode precipitates be the same for the unknown sample and standards of serum with a normal distribution of IgG. Unproportional increases of the anodic precipitate observed in some serum samples might indicate the presence of selectively increased levels of IgG subclasses. IgA causes less difficulties in this respect since the main part of this Ig class migrates anodically under suitable conditions, whereas IgM cannot be satisfactorily determined by direct application of electroimmunoassay.

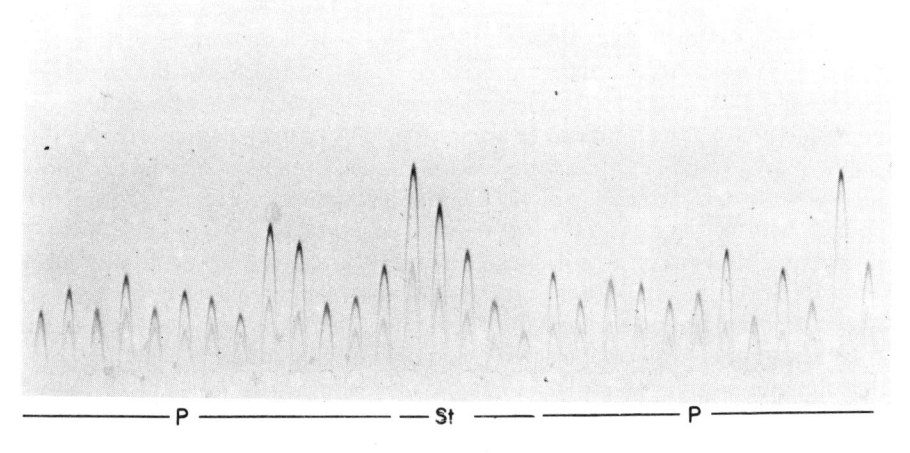

Fig. 137. The simultaneous assay of two proteins, orosomucoid and ceruloplasmin using electroimmunoassay. The longest precipitation lines are due to orosomucoid. These can be distinquished from those of ceruloplasmin by easily observable differences in appearance. Standard samples are indicated by 'St' and plasma samples by 'P'

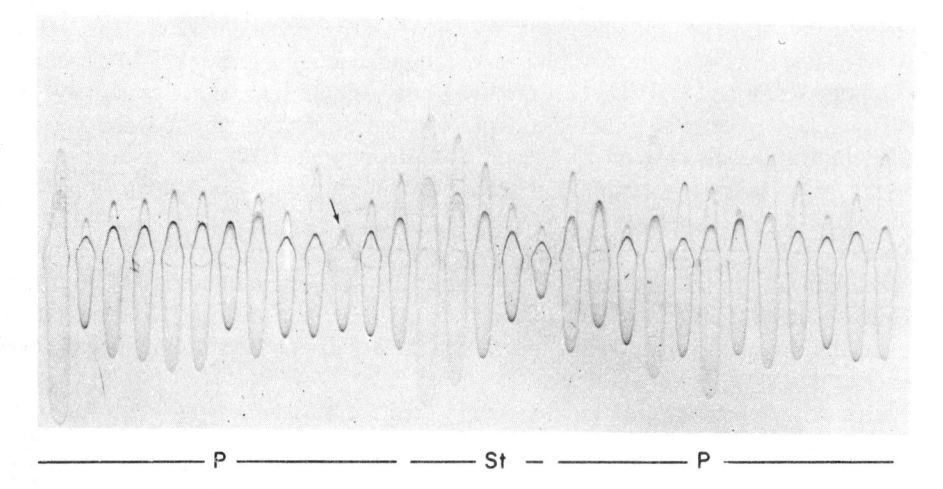

Fig. 138. Electroimmunoassay of IgG and IgA. The picture shows the migration of IgG towards both anode and cathode as opposed to the migration of IgA almost entirely towards the anode under the conditions used (pH 8.6, ionic strength 0.07, agarose with medium electroendosmosis). The anode is towards the top of the picture. Standard samples are denoted by 'St' and unknown plasma samples by 'P'. Note the abnormal appearance of the sample which is marked with an arrow. This is due to the presence of an M-component of IgG class

The problem concerning determination of antigens with electrophoretic migration rates which are similar to that of the antibody can be solved by altering the electrical charge of either the antigen or the antibody. This can easily be accomplished by modifying the amino groups e.g. by carbamylation:

$$-\overset{|}{\underset{|}{C}}-NH_3^+ + CNO^- \rightarrow -\overset{|}{\underset{|}{C}}-NH-CO-NH_2$$

This treatment converts the charged amino groups into neutral amido groups and the protein antigen acquires an increased negative net charge without causing any noticeable change in the immunoreactivity (Weeke, 1969). This procedure must be performed with each antigen sample. An alternative procedure would be to change the charge of the antibodies and then perform the electrophoresis at a pH value where the modified antibodies do not migrate. This can be accomplished by carbamylation of the antibodies to a suitable degree and performing the electroimmunoassay at a comparatively low pH (pH 5) as described by Axelsen et al. (1973). Modifications of the carboxyl groups of the antibodies, with a decrease of their negative charges is also possible. The electroimmunoassay is then performed at high pH (pH 10) in agarose gels essentially devoid of endosmosis (Grubb, 1974). Both these modifications of the original electroimmunoassay have been used for the determination of immunoglobulins, which migrate exclusively towards the cathode or the anode at pH 5 and pH 10, respectively.

Electroimmunoassay like radial immuno-diffusion has a lower limit of sensitivity in the order of 1 mg antigen per litre. This limit can be reduced to about 0.2 mg/l by using larger, rectangular antigen basins. A considerable increase of the sensitivity can be obtained by *radioelectroimmunoassay* (Kindmark and Thorell, 1972; Nørgaard-Pedersen, 1973). In such procedures either the antigen or the antibody is labelled with ^{125}I and the very faint precipitates visualized by autoradiography. Antibodies conjugated with enzymes (e.g. peroxidase) are also useful in the detection of very faint precipitates. The sensitivity limit, which seems to be determined by the immunoprecipitation reaction rather than the detection principle, is about 10–20 µg/l both with radioelectroimmunoassay and enzyme detection.

7. Crossed immunoelectrophoresis

The principle of crossed immunoelectrophoresis is shown in Fig. 139. The high resolution power of the technique and its ability to give at least semiquantitative results have made it useful for several purposes. Thus, the method is of value in the study of genetically determined protein polymorphism and in the analysis of the microheterogeneity of proteins (Fig. 140). The technique may also be used in the demonstration of abnormal components, e.g. M-components in plasma, as well as in studies of protein–protein interactions. Even protein degradation processes can be studied advantageously by using the technique of crossed immunoelectrophoresis. The method can also be used to reveal changes which may occur during the isolation of a protein. This can be achieved by comparing the immunoprecipitation pattern of the starting material with that of the protein after different preparative steps.

Even if some quantitative information can be obtained, the original technique is not suitable for quantitative determinations of plasma proteins. A modified method introduced by Clarke and Freeman (1971) with a considerably lower electrophoretic resolution is better suited for such work. By using an antiserum against human total

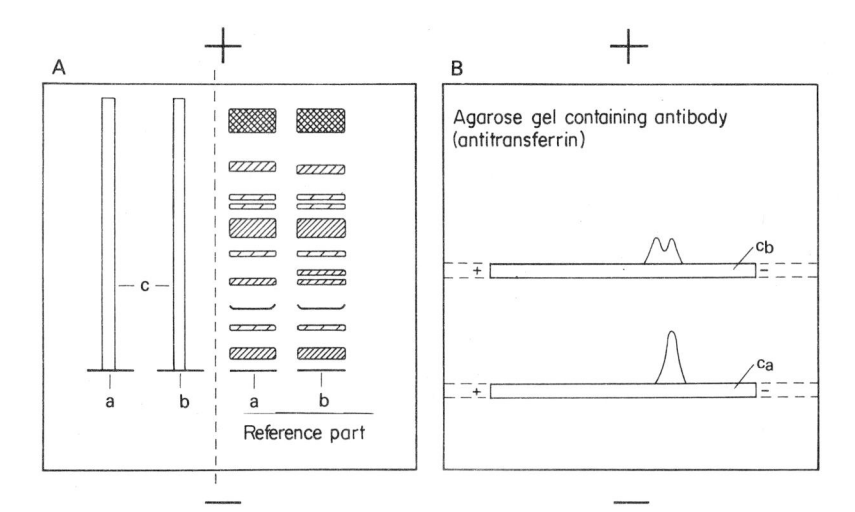

Fig. 139. Principle of crossed immunoelectrophoresis. During the first electrophoretic step (A) the proteins in the samples of plasma (a) and (b) are separated. The strips of agarose (c) are cut out immediately after the electrophoresis and are transferred to a new gel (B) which contains antibody and in which troughs to fit the strips have been cut. The electrophoresis is repeated and immunoprecipitates are formed in the same manner as for the electroimmunoassay. The electrophoretic positions of these precipitates can be located by comparing with the stained electrophoretic pattern in the reference portion of the first plate where the same samples of plasma have been applied. The example shown here illustrates the possibility of demonstrating the presence of a double band for transferrin in the electrophoretic pattern of sample (b)

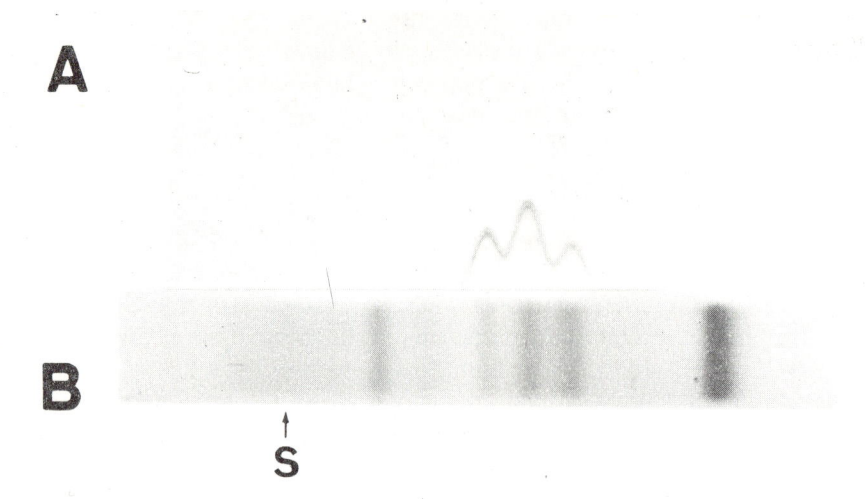

Fig. 140. Example of crossed immunoelectrophoresis. The urine proteins of a patient excreting low molecular weight protein are separated electrophoretically. The electrophoretic pattern is shown in the lower part of the picture (B). On the completion of the electrophoresis in the second dimension (A) against anti retinol-binding protein (anti-RBP) three immunoprecipitation peaks can be located. These peaks correspond to three bands in the electrophoretic pattern. The anode is to the right of the picture. Samples were applied in the first electrophoresis at the position marked by 'S'.

plasma proteins, the technique can provide the quantitative analysis of a large number of plasma proteins (Fig. 141). However, detailed studies (Weeke, 1969) of the composition of plasma proteins in various diseases have demonstrated that the method gives only restricted clinical information in relation to the work involved.

The modified crossed immunoelectrophoresis method of Clarke and Freeman has been used successfully as a basic method for the development of several other techniques which permit detailed analyses of complicated antigen–antibody systems (Axelsen et al., 1973). One such technique is crossed immunoelectrophoresis with intermediate gels, which can be used for the demonstration and identification of antibodies in human plasma. The principle of this technique is illustrated in Fig. 142.

8. Other gel immunoprecipitation techniques

The most direct way to perform immunoprecipitation reactions after agarose gel electrophoresis is by simply coating with an antiserum preparation over the gel surface immediately after the electrophoretic run. This procedure, called *immunofixation* (Alpers, 1969) is very useful, for example in studies of genetic polymorphism and for the identification of abnormal electrophoretic bands, e.g. M-components. Classification of M-components with regard to heavy and light chain types is easily performed with immunofixation. The technique is very simple to perform, but requires a good quality agarose gel electrophoresis procedure, as described earlier in this chapter. The samples applied in the electrophoretic run should be suitably diluted in order to avoid antigen excess, which gives results that may be difficult to interpret.

Counter immunoelectrophoresis is another gel immunoprecipitation technique

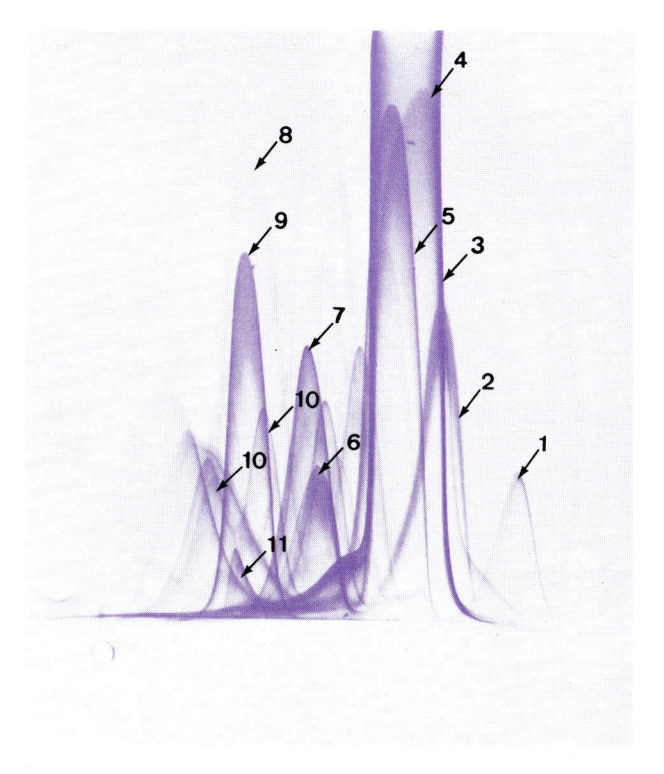

Fig. 141. Crossed immunoelectrophoresis of human serum according to the modified procedure of Clarke and Freeman (1966). The agarose gel of the second dimension contains an antiserum against human serum proteins. Some of the immunoprecipitates have been marked with arrows: (1) prealbumin (TBPA), (2) orosomucoid, (3) albumin, (4) α-lipoprotein, (5) α_1-antitrypsin, (6) α_2-macroglobulin, (7) haptoglobin, (8) haemopexin, (9) transferrin, (10) complement factor C3, separated into two electrophoretic components because of changes undergone in serum on storage, (11) β-lipoprotein. The immunoglobulins, which are not indicated in the picture, are not well suited to this type of analysis on account of their low mobility

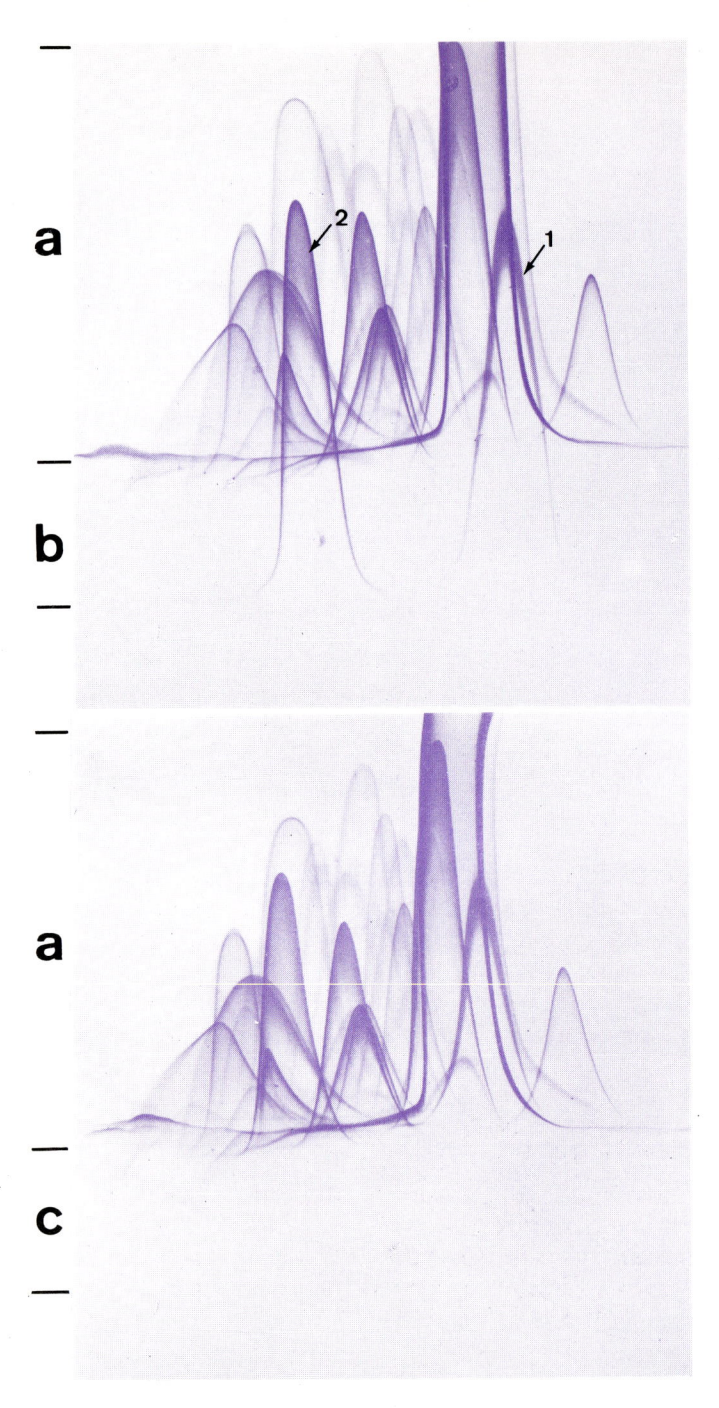

Fig. 142. Crossed immunoelectrophoresis with intermediate antibody gel (Axelsen, 1973). This example shows the separation of human serum (upper pattern) against a reference serum in the part of the agarose gel which is denoted by (a). The antiserum which is to be compared with the reference antiserum is situated in the region denoted by (b). In this case, the antiserum in (b) contains antibodies against orosomucoid (1) and transferrin (2). The lower pattern shows a control experiment where normal rabbit Ig has been added to the gel in region (c). The method is valuable in the demonstration and identification of antibodies in antiserum preparations and in biological fluids

which is sometimes useful for rapid semiquantitative determinations of proteins. In this procedure two parallel rows of circular wells are punched in a 1–2 mm thick agarose gel at a distance of 5–10 mm. After filling one row of basins with antigen samples and the other one with antiserum preparation the agarose plate is placed in an electrophoresis apparatus with the antibody basins localized towards the anode. By using agarose with a comparatively high electroendosmosis the antibodies will migrate towards the cathode in the electric field applied and will then meet antigen(s) with anodic migration and precipitate(s) will be formed. The localization of the precipitate is determined by the antigen concentration if the amount of antibody is kept constant and this forms the basis for the semiquantitative estimations of protein concentrations. Counter immunoelectrophoresis has a considerable degree of sensitivity; the detection limit for some antigens is as low as 0.05 mg/l. The method is useful in the detection of increased levels of α-fetoprotein in serum and has also gained a widespread use in the detection of HBAg$_s$.

9. Nephelometric determinations of immunoprecipitates

As was mentioned previously, immunoprecipitation in free solution has not been employed in routine determinations of plasma proteins. However, the development of automated methods made such analyses possible on a large scale. By using a continuous flow system (Technicon Auto Analyser) equipped with a nephelometric detection unit for the recording of turbidity which arises in the precipitation reaction, immunochemical analysis of plasma proteins can be performed with high precision at a rate of 90 samples per hour. From the chart recording of the continuous system the samples containing an excess of antigen can be identified and rerun at a more suitable dilution (Fig. 143). The procedure requires comparatively large amounts of highly specific antisera. However, the consumption of antiserum can be decreased with a simultaneous increase in sensitivity by adding water-soluble polymers such as polyethylene glycol to the reaction mixture. Such reagents accelerate the formation of the aggregates and decrease the solubility of the antigen–antibody complex (Hellsing, 1973). This form of analysis is an important complement or alternative to radial immunodiffusion and quantitative immunoelectrophoresis in the analysis of plasma proteins in the clinical chemistry laboratory. An important difference between this method and the gel immunoprecipitation techniques is the fact that the immunonephelometric determinations are less dependent on variations in molecular size and charge of the antigens.

Immunonephelometry can also be performed with equipment other than the continuous flow system and several specially designed immunonephelometers have been introduced on the market. Turbidimetric determinations of immunoprecipitates are also possible and can be performed with ordinary spectrophotometers, but the sensitivity of such determinations is naturally inferior to that of nephelometry. It should be noted that in contrast to the discrete analysers the continuous flow system allows differentiation between precipitates in antigen and antibody excess (cf. Figs. 133 and 143).

10. Radioimmunoassay

The sensitivity limit of the immunoprecipitation techniques described restricts their application to determination of plasma proteins occurring in concentrations above 0.5–

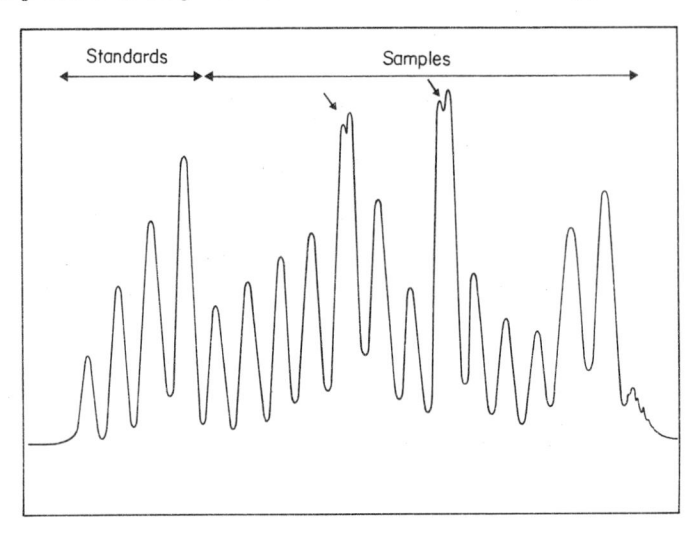

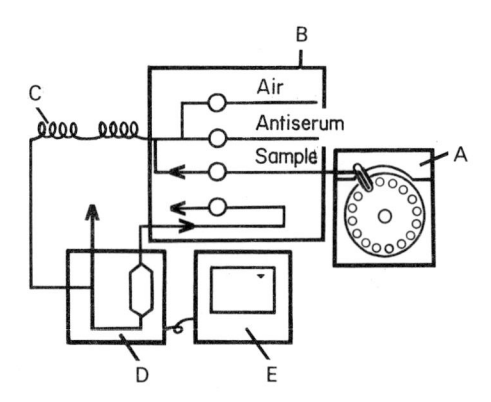

Fig. 143. Principle of protein determination used in nephelometric immunoprecipitation assay. A, sampler; B, peristaltic pump; C, mixing coils. D, nephelometer; E, recorder. The upper part of the figure shows a typical curve obtained in this assay. The arrows indicate abnormal peaks formed in antigen excess. Such samples should be reassayed at suitable dilutions

1 mg/l. Beyond this limit more sensitive techniques must be used. The most useful technique in this respect is radioimmunoassay (RIA) where a fixed amount of labelled antigen (usually ^{125}I) is allowed to compete with standard or sample antigen for added antibody. Following separation of antibody-bound antigen from free antigen, the proportions of these can be calculated from measurements of radioactivity in a γ-counter. The concentration of unlabelled antigen in the unknown samples can then be estimated from a standard curve. Radioimmunoassay, which is now used for the determination of a vast number of immunogenic substances, including protein hormones in plasma such as insulin, growth hormone and thyroid stimulating hormone, is also applied in the assay of other proteins occurring in trace amounts in plasma, e.g. α-fetoprotein, carcinoembryonic antigen. IgE etc. A reverse technique, immunoradiometric assay (IRMA), in which ^{125}I-labelled purified antibody is used has also been

developed. This technique is employed in several methods for the determination of ferritin in plasma.

Radioimmunological techniques have certain inherent disadvantages, i.e. work with radioactive isotopes and a limited shelf-life of the radioactively labeled substances. For this reason such methods should not be used for determinations where it is possible to use the simpler immunoprecipitation techniques. An attractive alternative to the radioimmunological analyses may be to replace the radiolabelled antigen with other detectors, e.g. enzymes, fluorescent or even chemiluminiscent compounds. Enzyme immunoassays (e.g. ELISA enzyme linked immunosorbent assay; Engvall and Perlman, 1971), have gained widespread use for detection of antibodies and titre determinations, and are also useful for antigen determinations. Fluorescein-labelled antigens have also been introduced recently in the determination of plasma proteins e.g. immunoglobulins.

V. Diagnostic use of plasma protein analyses

1. The normal agarose electrophoresis pattern

Despite the development of simple procedures for determinations of specific plasma proteins, electrophoresis is still of importance as a supplementary method, providing valuable information about 'qualitative' changes of the plasma protein, which is not obtained from the quantitative analysis of individual proteins. By reasons mentioned earlier agarose gel electrophoresis is a very suitable method for this purpose.

The use of EDTA plasma is recommended for plasma protein analyses. The EDTA reagent complexes calcium ions, which leads to an increased stability of certain proteins, e.g. complement factor C3, which is rapidly converted to other components in serum samples. Also the plasma lipoproteins are apparently more stable, as judged from their unchanged electrophoretic migration rates in EDTA plasma stored for several days in the refrigerator. Furthermore by using plasma a visual estimation of the appearance and concentration of fibrinogen can be obtained. On the other hand M-components migrating together with the rather intense fibrinogen band may escape detection if plasma samples are used. If the presence of such components is suspected the sample can be rerun after removal of fibrinogen by adding thrombin.

Although the presence of calcium ions in the plasma samples is undesirable, it is advantageous to include small amounts of calcium ions in the electrophoresis buffer. Certain plasma proteins e.g. complement factor C3 and C-reactive protein form complexes with calcium, which are not dissociated in the electrical field. The binding of calcium changes the migration rate of these proteins, which improves the resolution.

Agarose gel electrophoresis is a comparatively sensitive technique, visualizing protein components with a concentration of as little as 0.2 g/l. The composition of the protein bands obtained by agarose electrophoresis of plasma has been studied immunochemically by crossed immunoelectrophoresis. A compilation of the results is shown in Fig. 144, demonstrating the electrophoretic distribution and the relative concentration of the proteins, contributing to the electrophoretic pattern.

The normal pattern can be described as follows (cf. also Fig. 130). Nearest the anode is a very faint band corresponding to thyroxin-binding prealbumin (TBPA). Next comes the dominating broad albumin band. The width of this band is not entirely due to the high concentration of albumin in plasma, but is also caused by an

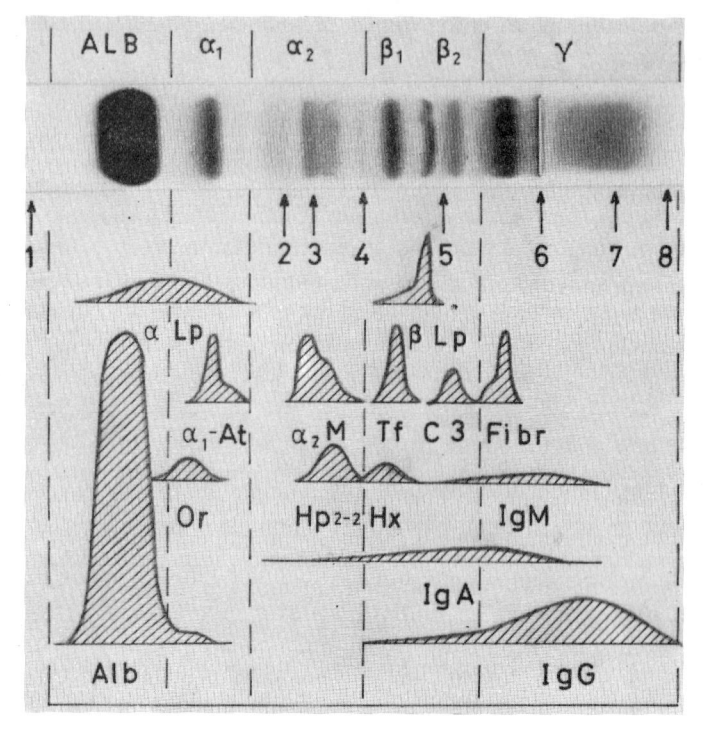

Fig. 144. The plasma protein pattern in agarose gel electrophoresis (Laurell, 1972). The diagram shows the distribution in crossed immunoelectrophoresis of the quantitatively dominant plasma proteins. The following notation has been used: Alb, albumin; α-Lp, α-lipoprotein; Or, orosomucoid; $α_1$-At, $α_1$-antitrypsin; $α_2$-M $α_2$-macroglobulin; Hp, haptoglobin; Hx, haemopexin; Tf, transferrin; β-Lp, β-lipoprotein, Fibr, fibrinogen. Small components which can be seen in pathological conditions have been indicated: 1, prealbumin; 2, antichymotrypsin, inter-α-trypsin inhibitor, and Gc-components; 3, ceruloplasmin; 4, cryoprecipitating protein; 5, C4; 6, sample application; 7, C-reactive protein, 8, γ-trace protein

electrophoretic heterogeneity induced by binding of ligands. The next distinct band (or bands) is due to $α_1$-antitrypsin. The diffusely staining zone between albumin and $α_1$-antitrypsin comes from electrophoretically heterogeneous α-lipoprotein (practically synonymous with high density lipoprotein, HDL). Orosomucoid is also present in this region, but does not contribute to the pattern because of its low concentration in combination with its poor stainability.

A few faint bands, corresponding to antichymotrypsin, inter-α-trypsin inhibitor, and group specific proteins (Gc) can be seen following the $α_1$-antitrypsin band. The more intense broad zone in the $α_2$-region contains mainly $α_2$-macroglobulin and haptoglobin. Ceruloplasmin is also found here. A faint, narrow band corresponding to a cryoprecipitable protein (fibronectin) follows the main $α_2$-zone.

The distinct zone in the $β_1$-area contains mainly transferrin, but also haemopexin is present in this band with a slightly more anodic localization than transferrin. The contribution of haemopexin to the intensity of the $β_1$-band is small. In stored samples, especially if serum is used, a conversion product of C3, called C3c, appears just in front of the ordinary $β_1$-band. The thin irregular band which comes next corresponds to β-lipoprotein (low density lipoprotein, LDL). The position of the β-lipoprotein band varies with the agarose quality, concentration of β-lipoprotein in the samples, and the age of the sample. High content of charged groups in the agarose gel, low lipoprotein concentration and old samples are factors which tend to increase the migration rate of β-lipoprotein.

The regularly shaped band in the β_2-region consists of the complement factor C3 with a small contribution of C4 in the anodal edge of the band. The fibrinogen band appears just in front of the application line. A faint but distinct band on the anodic side of the fibrinogen band is also immunologically related to fibrinogen as revealed by crossed immunoelectrophoresis.

On the cathode side of the application line a broad zone appears which consists mainly of IgG. As seen in Fig. 144 a small portion of IgG is also present on the anode side of the application slit. Other immunoglobulins which are present in plasma in a lower concentration cannot be detected in the normal plasma protein pattern, except IgA which contributes to a small increase of the background colour in front of the application line.

2. Normal variants of the electrophoretic plasma protein pattern

A number of variants of the normal patterns can be recognized depending upon age, sex and the genetic polymorphism of several plasma proteins (Fig. 145). Knowledge of such variants is very important in the correct interpretation of plasma protein patterns.

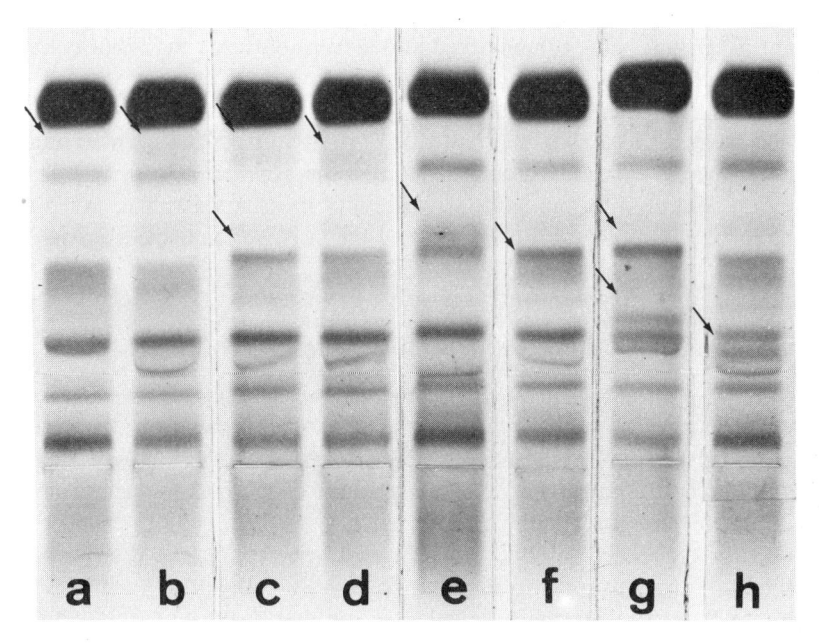

Fig. 145. Examples of normal variants of plasma protein patterns obtained in agarose gel electrophoresis. The arrows indicate the variations in question. Difference in the concentrations of α-lipoproteins of adult male and female (a, b); α_1-antitrypsin with high electrophoretic mobility and heterozygous in α_1-antitrypsin deficiency (c); double band for α_1-antitrypsin (d); haptoglobin of genetic type 1-1 (e) and 2-2 (f); genetically determined transferrin variants with double bands and different electrophoretic mobilities (g, h). In addition, the difference in the appearance of α_2-macroglobulin can be seen, the marked front on the anode side can be seen best in (c) and (g)

Albumin is separated into two bands in the very rare cases of bisalbuminaemia, but more commonly the albumin zone is abnormally broad, usually with a cathodal extension. The structural basis for the last mentioned genetically determined variants is not known.

The very heterogeneous α-lipoprotein shows no genetic variations detectable by electrophoresis, but the distinct sex-dependent concentration differences are easily seen with more intensely stained α-lipoprotein zones in the plasma protein patterns from women in fertile ages. Oestrogen influence, e.g. from contraceptive pills or pregnancy, further increases the intensity of the α-lipoprotein. Genetically determined $α_1$-antitrypsin variants are very common and appear as double bands or as single bands with slightly changed position (cf. $α_1$-antitrypsin deficiency page 343).

A faint band corresponding to α-fetoprotein is sometimes observed in the new-born especially in cases of premature delivery. This band is situated closer to albumin than commonly seen $α_1$-antitrypsin variants, which facilitates a correct interpretation.

$α_2$-Macroglobulin has no known genetic variation, but the appearance of the electrophoretically heterogeneous zone varies with age. In children and adolescents the $α_2$-macroglobulin zone has a distinct narrow band in its anodal front. This pattern can also be seen in aged individuals.

Haptoglobin appears as three genetically determined variants. Haptoglobin, type 1-1 (page 102) occurring in about 15 per cent of the population gives rise to a band on the anode side of $α_2$-macroglobulin, covering the faint bands appearng in this region. Haptoglobulins 2-1 and 2-2 are found in the major $α_2$-zone together with $α_2$-macroglobulin. In infants with low levels of haptoglobin the $α_2$-zone is rather faintly stained on the cathode side of the marked anode front of the $α_2$-macroglobulin.

Genetic variants of transferrin and complement factor C3 are occasionally observed as double bands located close to each other. The C3 bands cannot always be separated and in such cases a broad single zone of C3 is obtained. The transferring band is usually more marked in children than in adults; the apposite is true of β-lipoprotein. The immunoglobulins show no normal variability in its appearance, except the faint zone in the IgA regon in new-born infants and the likewise faint IgG zone in infants 3–12 months old.

3. Pathological variations in the electrophoretic patterns

Several types of patholological changes are recognized: (1) absence of normal components, (2) change of position and/or distribution of components, (3) changes of the concentration of components, and (4) appearance of extra bands. The following description does not attempt to give a full account of these changes but merely gives some examples of the most prominent changes.

Albumin can be reduced in concentration or its electrophoretic distribution can be altered. Slight reductions of the albumin levels are difficult to estimate from the electrophoretic pattern. Hyperbilirubinaemia is commonly associated with a shift of the albumin position towards the anode. A similar change of the albumin distribution is seen in plasma from patients treated with large doses of penicillin, probably due to binding of acid metabolites of this antibiotic to albumin.

Very faint α-lipoprotein zones are a common finding in the plasma patterns from patients with acute hepatocellular damage or long-standing biliary obstruction.

Increased levels of α-lipoprotein are often noted in subjects with a heavy alcohol consumption, and may occasionally be found in patients with *anorexia nervosa* after a prolonged period of starvation.

The α_1-antitrypsin band is missing in α_1-antitrypsin deficiency (page 343) and is often intensified in inflammatory conditions. An extra band between albumin and α_1-antitrypsin may be observed in the new-born. This band which corresponds to α-fetoprotein is occasionally seen also in adults, suffering from primary liver cancer. The faint inter-α bands are also often increased in inflammatory processes due to high levels of antichymotrypsin.

The α_2-zone can vary considerably in appearance and intensity in pathological conditions. These variations may be due to changes of haptoglobin and/or α_2-macroglobulin levels, which make the interpretation of alterations in the α_2-zone rather uncertain.

The intensity of the β_1-band is subject primarily to the concentration of transferrin in plasma and hence provides a means of a rough visual estimation of this protein. The β-lipoprotein level can be estimated not only from the band intensity, but also from its position, as mentioned earlier. In plasma from patients with obstructive jaundice the β-lipoprotein is regularly increased and sometimes a β-lipoprotein band with a reduced electrophoretic mobility can be seen, which probably represents lipoprotein X, regularly present in cholestatic plasma. Changes of the C3 levels can be roughly estimated from the intensity of the β_2-band. Patterns with decreased C3 should always be inspected for the presence of conversion products formed *in vitro*, e.g. C3c appearing in front of the transferrin band. The use of plasma makes possible the revelation of changes in the fibrinogen concentration; in some cases with acute pancreatitis the fibrinogen band exhibits a changed appearance with diffuse outlines.

A changed background colour on the anode side of the application slit is often indicative of altered IgA levels. The intense staining of this region in many cases of alcohol liver cirrhosis may serve as an example, Changes of the IgG levels are easier to estimate. Increases of IgG can be polyclonal with a diffuse increase of the entire IgG zone; sometimes the increase is oligoclonal with the appearance of several small distinct bands. A single faint band can also be seen in the cathodal part of the IgG zone in inflammatory conditions. This should not be mistaken for a small monoclonal IgG band, but corresponds to C-reactive protein (CRP) which migrates cathodically when calcium is included in the electrophoresis buffer. The CRP band often appears as a narrow, irregular band due to its strong tendency to adsorb to the agarose.

Monoclonal immunoglobulin components (M-components) can appear in the electrophoretic regions corresponding to the distribution of the immunoglobulins, e.g. from the α_2-region to the extreme cathodal part of the γ-region. Monoclonal light chains may be found occasionally even in the α_1-region.

4. Normal variations in the concentrations of individual plasma proteins

Age- and sex-dependent variations of the concentration appear for many plasma proteins as seen in Table 51. It should be noted that the concentrations in this table, given in absolute values (g/l) may be inaccurate for several proteins due to difficulties in standardization. There is an obvious, urgent need for more work in this field.

The largest sex-dependent concentration difference is shown by α-lipoprotein (high

340 *Plasma proteins as diagnostic aids. Methods and clinical applications*

Table 51. Sex- and age-related concentrations of some plasma proteins (g/l). The values which are based partly on work by Ganrot (1972) and Weeke (1973) are given in the form of reference intervals covering 95% of the population

Protein	Adult women	Men	New-born	Changes with age
Prealbumin	0.20–0.36	0.24–0.36	0.04–0.12	Approx. 60 % of adult value in children.
Albumin	38–51	40–52	28–41	Approx. 10 % lower value in old age.
α_1-Antitrypsin	0.95–1.85	0.85–1.85	0.60–1.60	Approx. 70 % of adult value in infants.
α_1-Lipoprotein Orosomucoid	0.50–1.00	0.55–1.15	0.10–0.40	
α_2-Macroglobulin	2.05–4.30	1.80–3.40	2.35–5.30	Highest values obtained in first two years of life (3 × adult value).
Haptoglobin	0.50–2.70	0.55–3.20	<0.20	Subnormal values usual in children between 0 and 12 years.
Ceruloplasmin	0.25–0.55	0.20–0.45	0.05–0.25	Slight increase during childhood.
Transferrin	1.65–2.90	1.54–2.75	0.90–1.90	Slight increase can appear during childhood.
Haemopexin	0.60–0.95	0.65–0.95	0.05–0.30	
C3 complement factor	0.80–1.85	0.90–1.90	0.70–1.15	
C4 complement factor	0.20–1.00	0.30–1.25		
Fibrinogen	1.90–4.70	1.80–4.50		
IgG	7.2–15.5	6.7–14.7	5.5–12.7	See Fig. 146 concerning IgM, IgG, and IgA.
IgA	0.5–3.0	0.5–3.0	<0.1	
IgM	0.20–2.10	0.15–1.20	0.02–0.12	

density lipoprotein) which is markedly higher in women than in men. Females have also higher levels of IgM, α_2-macroglobulin, and ceruloplasmin, while β-lipoprotein and haptoglobins are higher in males.

Concerning age variations of the plasma protein levels, the new-born baby has concentrations of many plasma proteins which are considerably lower than those found in adults (Table 51). Only the α_2-macroglobulin level is higher in children than in adults. In premature infants the differences are even more pronounced.

The immunoglobulin levels undergo marked changes during the first year of life (Fig. 146). The reduction of the IgG levels after delivery is due to catabolism of the IgG, received by the foetus from the mother *via* placental transfer, without the infant being able to compensate this by own IgG synthesis. Changes of a number of other proteins also occur during the first year, e.g. haptoglobin which increases from values near zero during the first weeks of life. Subnormal levels of haptoglobin are a common finding in childhood, occurring in about one-third of apparently healthy children under 12 years.

Changes in the concentrations of individual plasma proteins take place also in old age, but our knowledge of such changes is limited. The albumin concentration is about 10 per cent lower in 70-year-olds than in individuals who are between 20 and 40. The

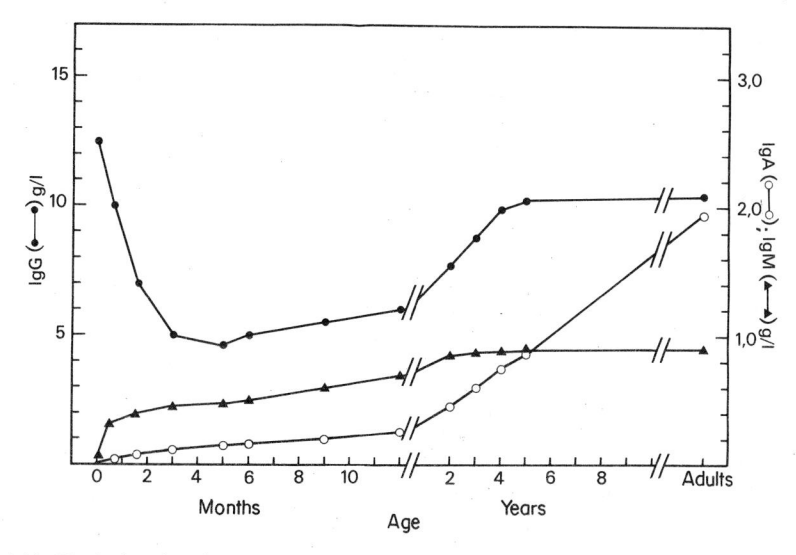

Fig. 146. Variation in plasma concentration of immunoglobulins G, A, and M with age

Ig levels seem to remain unchanged in advanced age, with the possible exception of IgA which has been reported to be about 15 per cent higher at the age of 70 than at the age of 40.

5. Influence of steroid hormones on the plasma protein pattern

Women taking oestrogen-containing oral contraceptives show marked changes in their plasma protein patterns (Fig. 147). As can be seen, the proteins react in many different ways from the considerable reduction in the level of orosomucoid to the marked elevation of ceruloplasmin. Other studies with contraceptive pills which did not contain the oestrogen component showed only insignificant changes in the plasma protein pattern. Thus, this change which is observed when the combined preparation is used and which returns to normal about four weeks after withdrawal, is most likely due to the oestrogen component. A comparison of the changes which are induced by contraceptive pills containing oestrogen and those which are observed during pregnancy have shown that these changes are very similar but are not identical, suggesting that factors other than oestrogen may also play a role in the plasma protein-alterations in pregnancy.

For a correct interpretation of the plasma protein pattern of a woman of fertile age, there is an obvious need to know if she is taking oral contraceptives. Since such information is seldom furnished by the clinicians, determination of ceruloplasmin is routinely included in all plasma protein analyses to give a warning about changes induced by oral contraceptives. The use of oestrogen in the treatment of prostatic cancer of course give similar problems. However, some oestrogen-containing drugs with long-term effects, have been shown to exert a minimal effect on the plasma protein pattern.

Androgens have a less pronounced influence on the plasma protein profiles (Table 52). The administration of 17 α-alkylated anabolic steroids has been shown to increase

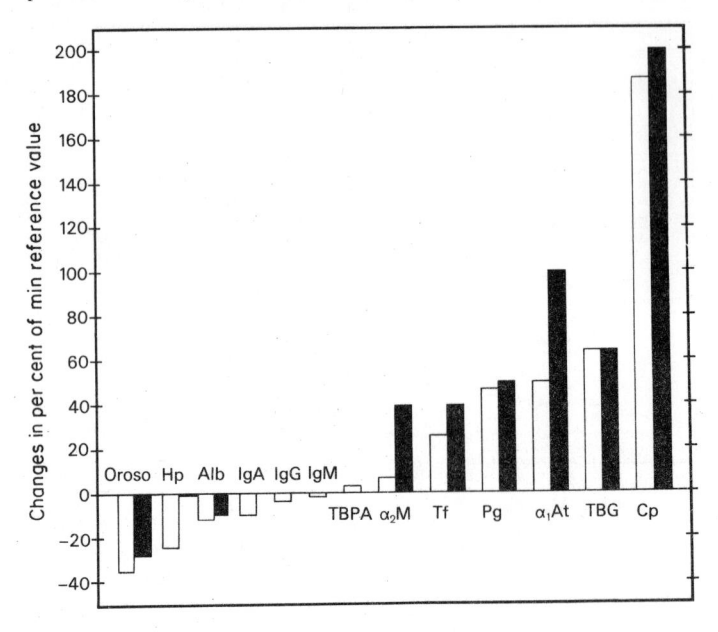

Fig. 147. Changes in the levels of plasma proteins following a six month administration of peroral contraceptive (mestranol–megestrol, unfilled columns) as compared with the corresponding values obtained during the latter part of pregnancy (filled columns). Oroso, orosomucoid; Hp, haptoglobin; TBPA, thyroxine-binding prealbumin; α_2M, α_2-macroglobin; Tf, transferrin; Pg, plasminogen; α_1At, α_1-antitrypsin; TBG, thyroxine-binding globulin; Cp, ceruloplasmin (data from Laurell et al., 1968)

Table 52. Effect of administration of androgen on the concentration of some plasma proteins (Barbosa et al. 1971)

Protein	Testosterone[a]	17 α-Alkylated anabolic steroids	Non 17 α-alkylated anabolic steroids
Albumin	0[b]	+	
α_1-Antitrypsin	–	+	
Orosomucoid		+	
Haptoglobin	0	+	
Transferrin	–	0	0
Ceruloplasmin	0	0	
TBG	–	–	0
TBPA		+	0
Transcortin	–	+	0
Fibrinogen	–	–	0

[a] Testosterone cyclopentylproprionate (parental supply).
[b] 0, –, + signify no change, significant reduction, and increase respectively.

the levels of prealbumin, albumin, α_1-antitrypsin, haptoglobin, and transcortin while fibrinogen and thyroxin-binding globulin decreased. No changes were noted for transferrin and ceruloplasmin. Testosterone administration seems to give other changes with decrease of α_1-antitrypsin, transferrin, thyroxin-binding globulin, transcortin, and fibrinogen. Increased levels were not found with testosterone.

Administration of corticosteroids is mainly reflected by a reduction of the IgG levels in plasma. A selective increase of orosomucoid but not of other acute phase proteins may also be noted in some cases.

VI. Deficiency states—α_1-antitrypsin deficiency

Genetically determined deficiencies have been reported for a considerable number of plasma proteins. Analbuminaemia and atransferrinaemia appear to be extremely rare conditions. Other more or less rare deficiencies of immunoglobulins complement factors, coagulation factors, lipoproteins, etc. are discussed in other sections.

The deficiency of α_1-antitrypsin is a genetically determined condition which is interesting in several respects and will be treated in more detail here. α_1-Antitrypsin is a glycoprotein, which contains 12 per cent carbohydrate and has a molecular weight of 50 000 to 55 000. With a concentration of 1.5 g/l α_1-antitrypsin is next to α_2-macroglobulin the quantitatively dominating protease inhibitor in plasma. In contrast to α_2-macroglobulin, which is a more general protease inhibitor reacting with most types of proteases, α_1-antitrypsin is an exclusive inhibitor of serine proteases.

As mentioned earlier there are a great number of genetic variants of α_1-antitrypsin; to date 23 alleles have been recognized in the *Pi* (protease inhibitor) system. Some of these can be detected in agarose gel electrophoresis by differences in electrophoretic mobility compared to the most common phenotype *PiMM*, but a correct phenotyping requires more sophisticated techniques including electrophoresis at acid pH or isoelectric focusing.

Only a few alleles, Pi^z and Pi^s, produce phenotypes with a reduced concentration of α_1-antitrypsin in plasma. On the average the plasma concentration of α_1-antitrypsin in homozygotes of types *ZZ* and *SS* is only 15 per cent and 60 per cent, respectively, of that in individuals of phenotype *MM*. This corresponding values for the heterozygotes *SZ*, *MZ*, and *MS* are 37.5 per cent, 57.5 per cent, and 80 per cent. The very rare *Pi*−, representing a gene deletion, gives homozygotes in which no α_1-antitrypsin can be detected in plasma. The frequency of *PiZZ* homozygotes and *PiMZ* heterozygotes in the Swedish population is 0,07 per cent and 4 per cent, respectively.

α_1-Antitrypsin deficiency is associated with the development of obstructive pulmonary disease (*pulmonary emphysema*) in most of the deficient individuals. The lung disease is often observed clinically in patients between 30 and 40 years. The deficiency is also associated with liver disease. Individuals with α_1-antitrypsin deficiency regularly have histological liver changes with the presence of inclusion bodies in the hepatocytes and some patients develop clinically manifest liver cirrhosis already in infancy or early childhood. Less than one-third of α_1-antitrypsin deficient infants develop liver disease. Hepatic cirrhosis in association with α_1-antitrypsin deficiency has also been reported in adults.

The mechanisms for the development of liver and pulmonary tissue damage in α_1-antitrypsin deficiency are so far not completely understood. The low level of α_1-antitrypsin ZZ in plasma is obviously due to a decreased synthesis since this protein is eliminated from plasma with the same rate as α_1-antitrypsin *MM*. Microscopic examination of liver tissue from patients with α_1-antitrypsin deficiency has revealed the presence of hyaline inclusion bodies in the endoplasmatic network of the hepatocytes, consisting of aggregated α_1-antitrypsin. The carbohydrate composition of this liver antitrypsin and that of the ZZ type, isolated from plasma are both different from that of type M α_1-antitrypsin, with two sialic acid residues less in the ZZ α_1-antitrypsin. The accumulation of the deficient α_1-antitrypsin in the liver might possibly be related to a defective transportation of the protein through the hepatocyte into plasma; such a defective transportation might in turn be connected with the differences in carbohydrate composition between normal and deficient α_1-antitrypsin. It should be noted, however, that the *primary* difference in structure between α_1-antitrypsins M and Z resides in the peptide part, in which a glutamic acid residue in the M proteins is replaced by a lysine residue in the Z protein.

The progressive wasting of pulmonary elastic tissue, which develops independent of liver damage is obviously associated with the protease inhibiting properties of α_1-antitrypsin. In fact 'α_1-antitrypsin' is a rather unfortunate designation, since the trypsin-inhibiting property of this protease inhibitor may play a minor physiological role. On the other hand α_1-antitrypsin due to the high concentrations is a very important protease inhibitor in the extravascular space. Neutrophil granulocytes contain high amounts of the two serine proteases collagenase and protease, which are inhibited by α_1-antitrypsin. Release of these enzymes from active granulocytes in the lung tissue is normally followed by a rapid inhibitory action of α_1-antitrypsin. In α_1-antitrypsin deficiency, this inhibition will be incomplete and the enzymes can attack the elastic tissue of the lungs, with lung emphysema as a consequence.

α_1-Antitrypsin deficiency is easily detected by agarose gel electrophoresis (Fig. 148) and can be confirmed by immunochemical quantitation of the plasma α_1-antitrypsin level. It is reasonable to believe that the low concentration of α_1-antitrypsin in plasma of phenotypes *ZZ* and *SZ* is responsible for the lung tissue damage; no qualitative changes in inhibitory function of the *ZZ* type compared to *MM* have been found. Thus it is very doubtful whether heterozygous individuals of the types *MZ* (or *MS*) are more prone to develop pulmonary emphysema than *MM* individuals. Detection of heterozygotes may be of interest in certain situations; this can be accomplished by isoelectric focusing of plasma in polyacrylamide gels (Pierce et al., 1976).

VII. Immunoglobulin alterations in disease

1. Decrease in the level of immunoglobulin

Reduced levels of one or several immunoglobulin classes appear in a number of primary immunoglobulin deficiency conditions (see page 168). Acquired, secondary forms of immunoglobulin deficiencies which are much more common can be caused by a reduced synthesis, which is often the case in lymphoproliferative disorders such as lymphoma, lymphatic leukaemia, and myelomatosis or by an increased metabolism and/or loss of immunoglobulins into the intestine in protein-losing enteropathies, in the urine in nephrotic syndrome, and in the exudate in cases of burns. In these conditions there is often a reduction in the level of IgG while levels of IgM and IgA may remain normal or even increase. This pattern can be explained partly by the difference in the molecular size of these molecules. It should be mentioned that the IgA

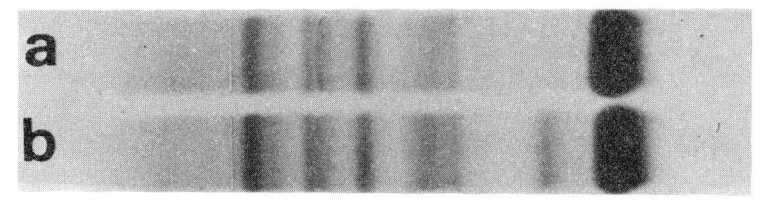

Fig. 148. Agarose electrophoresis of plasma from a patient showing α_1-antitrypsin deficiency, type *ZZ* (a), compared with plasma having normal α_1-antitrypsin type *MM* (b)

molecule is larger than that of IgG although both are present in plasma mainly as monomers (see Fig. 128, page 315).

A similar pattern is also seen in conditions with a preferential reduction in the level of IgG, not uncommon in diabetes, bone marrow hypoplasia, certain intoxications, and in the overproduction or administration of corticosteroids. A slight drop in the levels of IgA and IgM may be seen in some other forms of intoxications and sometimes in uraemia.

Low levels of immunoglobulin are also found in the infant whose own production of immunoglobulin has not yet started. Premature new-borns show low levels of IgG already at birth since the placental supply of this immunoglobulin takes place primarily during the last trimester of the pregnancy. Such newborns may present a comparatively pronounced hypoimmunoglobulinaemia. A few full-term infants show a delayed start of their immunoglobulin production after delivery. In some cases the IgG does not reach normal levels until the child is 3–4 years old.

2. Monoclonal increase of immunoglobulins

An increased synthesis of immunoglobulins can lead to monoclonal or polyclonal increase of Ig in plasma. The monoclonal increase is revealed by the presence of an M-component, in plasma and/or urine, due to a greatly increased immunoglobulin synthesis by the proliferation of *one* immunoglobulin-producing cell clone. Structurally, the immunoglobulin is homogeneous and consists of heavy chains of a certain class or subclass and identical light chains of the κ- or λ-type (page 119). The characteristic narrow band which is produced by the M-component on electrophoresis is an expression of this homogeneity. The M-components are normal immunoglobulins and should therefore have a specific antibody activity, which has also been demonstrated in many M-components. Because of the enormous variability in structure and thereby widespread electrophoretic mobility of the immunoglobulins, the M-components can appear in the electrophoretic patterns from the α_1-region to the most cathodic part of the γ-region.

The M-components do not always represent complete immunoglobulin molecules, but can sometimes consist of different Ig subunits, e.g. light chains, heavy chains, or even half-molecules. The most common of these are monoclonal light chains ('Bence Jones protein') which most often appear simultaneously with M-components, consisting of whole Ig molecules. In 10–20 per cent of patients with multiple myeloma, however, a monoclonal light chain is the only M-component present (*light chain disease*).

The light immunoglobulin chains, which have a molecular weight of only 20 000 (40 000 for dimers), readily pass through the glomerular membrane and appear in the urine. The excretion can sometimes be very high (20–40 g/l). Because of the rapid elimination from the blood, M-components consisting of light chains are difficult to detect in plasma, although the concentration may rise considerably in cases with impaired kidney function (reduced glomerular filtration rate). Thus, it is important to analyse both plasma and urine from suspected cases of myeloma for the presence of M-components. The urine analysis is best accomplished by electrophoresis of concentrated urine. It should be noted that Albustix and other tests based on the same principle do not give positive reactions for M-components.

In *heavy chain disease*, which is much less common than *light chain disease*, M-components are present which are structurally related but not identical with heavy chains. The first M-components of this type described were related to γ-chains (i.e. related to IgG) but since then, γ- and μ-components have been described. However, the latter components appear to be very rare. The *γ-chain disease* has usually a marked localization to soft tissues with little or no involvement of the bone. The γ-chain components can be difficult to detect on electrophoresis and only small amounts are excreted in the urine. The clinical picture of *α-chain disease* shows predominant gastrointestinal symptoms with chronic diarrhoea and intractable malabsorption (Seligmann, 1968). The proliferation of plasma cells is limited to the intestine. The disease, which is rare, has so far been found only in individuals from the Middle East. Also a few cases with μ-chain disease have been recognized, presenting clinical features of chromic lymphocytic leukaemia or splenomegaly. No cases with ∂- or ε-heavy chain disease have so far been found.

The classification of a newly detected M-component can be accomplished by 'classical' immunoelectrophoresis, which is the main application of this methodology in clinical chemistry. The immunoelectrophoresis is carried out with antisera specific to various Ig chains (Fig. 149). This classification provides information on the Ig class and also on the type of the light chain (κ or λ). The latter information is most often of a limited clinical value, but can sometimes be of use to confirm the monoclonal nature of bands in the Ig region. In addition, immunoelectrophoresis with anti-light chain antisera may reveal the presence of monoclonal free light chains in plasma. During recent years immunofixation has been introduced as a method which is very well suited for classification of M-components. (Fig. 150), provided that a good resolution is obtained by the electrophoretic technique used.

The quantitative determination of M-components may be achieved by immunochemical methods or by densitometric determination of the M-component after electrophoresis. Immunochemical methods should be used very cautiously, since the M-component may differ considerably in immunological and physicochemical behaviour from the polyclonal Ig commonly used as standard.

Apart from differentiation of myeloma and macroglobulinaemia, the classification in combination with quantitative determination of M-components offers the possibility of estimating roughly the mass of the cells producing the M-component. In this connection, it should be realized that the rates of elimination of the various classes of immunoglobulin are not identical. Because of the higher turnover rate of IgA, an M-component of this type, in general corresponds to a significantly greater cell mass than IgG component of the same size. Determination of the subclass specificity of IgG

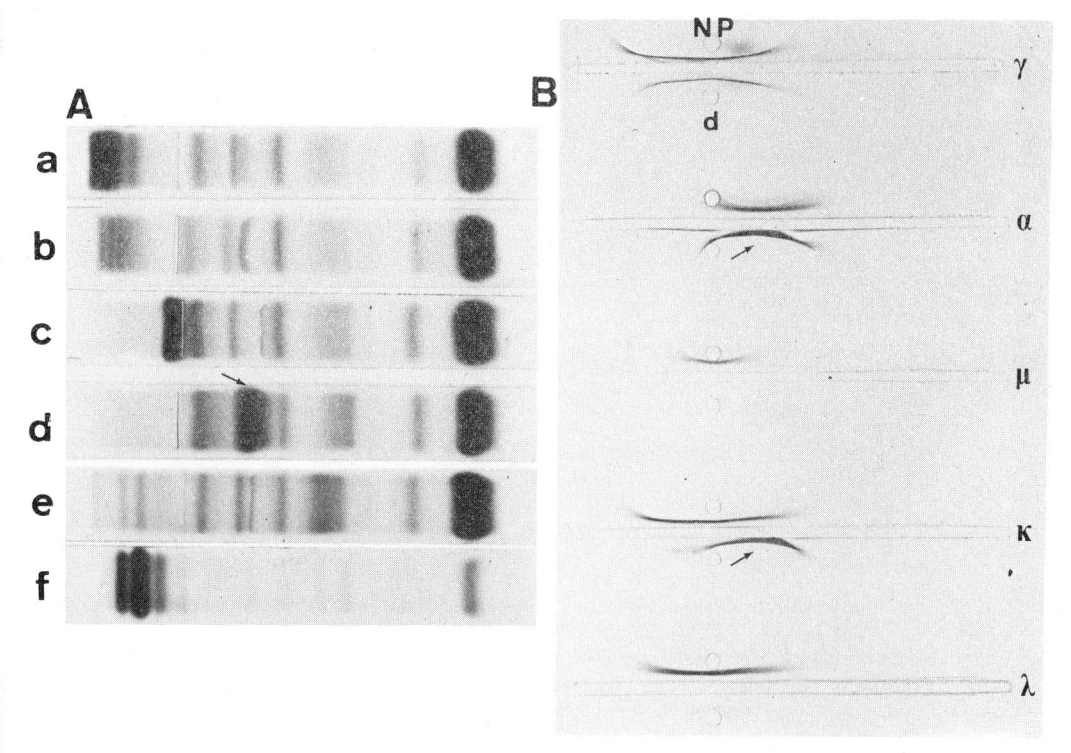

Fig. 149. A. Examples of M-components in plasma and urine. M-components of class IgG (A, b), IgM (c), IgA (d) monoclonal light chains of κ-type in plasma (e) and the corresponding urine (f) B. Classification of the M-component which is marked with an arrow in the electrophoresis pattern (d). The classification has been performed by electrophoresing sample (d) and normal plasma (NP) against class-specific antiserum (anti-γ, anti-α, and anti-μ) as well as antiserum against the light chains of type κ and λ. The arrows indicate the abnormal immunoprecipitates against anti-α and anti-κ. Thus the M-component is of the type IgA (kappa)

components may also be of value in selected cases. Immunoelectrophoresis of urine can be used to verify if extra bands observed in urine are due to M-components. Once classified the M-component can be monitored by quantitative determination, in order to follow the progress or to measure the effect of clinical trials.

The occurrence of M-components is a characteristic finding in multiple myeloma and Waldenström's macroglobulinaemia where they are present in high concentrations (10–100 g/l). They can also occur in other lymphoproliferative disorders, e.g. lymphoma of various kinds and in solitary plasmocytoma. However, the detection of an M-component in plasma does not necessarily indicate the presence of a lymphoproliferative disorder. This should be kept in mind especially since the improved electrophoretic techniques now available enable the detection of very small M-components. Population studies have shown that the frequency of occurrence of M-components is approximately 1/100 in adults. The majority of these patients are apparently healthy (benign monoclonal gammopathy), (Axelsson et al., 1967). In most cases the concentration of the M-components was low and in only 20 per cent of the cases was the concentration greater than 10 g/l. The frequency of M-components increases with age, and could be demonstrated in 5 per cent of individuals, who were

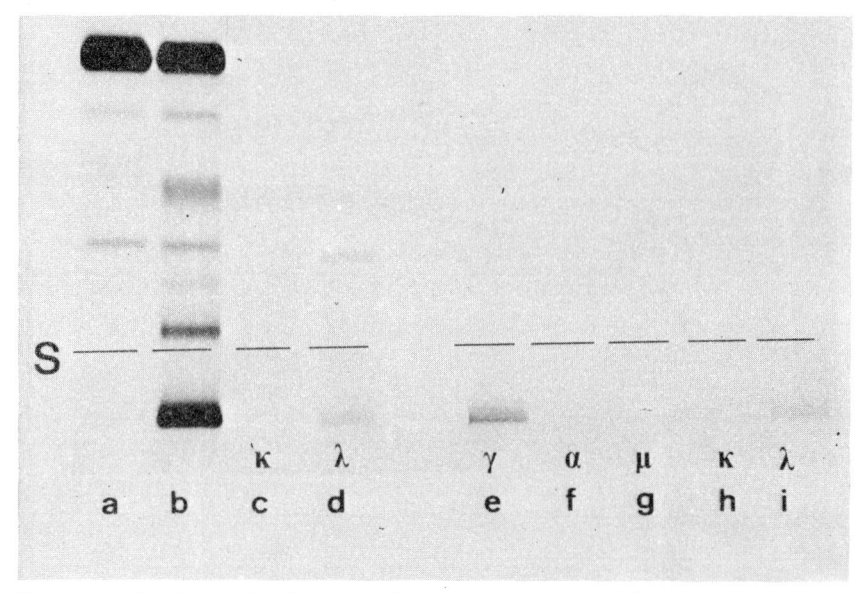

Fig. 150. Immunofixation in the detection of M-components. The left part shows electrophoretic patterns of urine (a) and plasma (b) from a patient with a large M-component in plasma. Immunofixation (right part) shows that the plasma component is of the type IgG (lambda) as judged from the precipitates in (f) and (i). Immunofixation of urine proteins against light chains shows besides the excretion of the main plasma M-component reaction with anti-λ also a monoclonal lambda chain (d) hidden by the transferrin band in (a)

over 80 years old. The clinical significance of an observed M-component should be judged in the light of several factors such as the patient's age and clinical history, the size and Ig class of the M-component, the concentration of the polyclonal 'background immunoglobulin', and the appearance of monoclonal free light chains in urine. Detection of monoclonal light chains gives strong evidence of malignancy. Follow-up of patients with benign gammopathy at yearly intervals for control of progress is recommended, especially if large M-components are present (>5 g/l). However, the risk for malignant development of benign gammopathy seems to be rather small.

Cytological examination should be carried out, although this is unfortunately of limited value in the prediction of malignancy. The following features may indicate the presence of malignant gammopathies: (1) M-component level >10 g/l for IgG and IgM components, or >5 g/l for IgA components. (2) Progressive increase of the M-component concentration. (3) Reduced concentration of the polyclonal background immunoglobulin. (4) Presence of light chains in the urine.

3. Oligoclonal and polyclonal immunoglobulin increase

Polyclonal increase comprising one or several immunoglobulin classes may be observed in a wide range of clinical disorders. The polyclonal increase of the Ig levels can be measured with various immunochemical methods, for example electroimmunoassay, radial immunodiffusion, or immunonephelometry.

The polyclonal immunoglobulin reactions can be divided into various types depending on the relative increases in the concentrations of the different classes of immunoglobulin (cf. Hobbs, 1971). A simplified summary of the characteristics of the immunoglobulin changes occurring in various diseases is given in Table 53. The first group covers conditions with a major increase in IgG. The IgG level may sometimes increase to a considerable extent (more than 25 g/l). The IgA concentration remains normal and that of IgM is normal or only slightly increased. In other conditions, the increase of IgG is more moderate and is accompanied by slight increases in the levels of IgG and IgA. The highest concentrations of IgG are seen in cases of SLE where they may exceed 50 g/l. Marked increased in the level of IgG can sometimes indicate the presence of abscesses.

In the second group there is a predominant increase in IgA while IgG and IgM remain normal or are only slightly increased. Completely selective increases in IgA are not uncommon and may occur, for example in the early phase of alcohol-induced liver damage, in rheumatoid arthritis, and not infrequently in malignant tumors. In the third group there is a predominant increase in the level of IgM while those of IgG and IgA are normal or only slightly increased. Virus diseases, e.g. viral hepatitis, some diseases caused by protozoa (malaria, toxoplasmosis), and primary biliary cirrhosis dominate this group. Acquired intrauterine infections in the new-born can often give rise to a selective increase in the level of IgM.

A large number of disorders with Ig reactions cannot be comprised in this scheme, but are included in the fourth group with more or less harmonic increases of all three Ig classes (Table 53).

Table 53. Outline of the increase in concentration of immunoglobulin in various diseases

Group I (dominant increase in IgG)	Group II (dominant increase in IgA)	Group III (dominant increase in IgM)	Group IV (harmonic increase in IgG, IgA, IgM)
SLE	Lung diseases	Malaria (initial)	Most infections (bacteria, virus, protozoa)
Chronic aggressive hepatitis	Inflammatory intestinal diseases	Trypanosomiasis	Liver cirrhosis
Abscesses	Alcohol-induced liver disease	Filaria	Sarcoidosis
Advanced malignant tumours	Rheumatoid arthritis	Mycoplasma infections	Rheumatoid arthritis
Malaria (non-initial)	Malignant tumours	Primary biliary cirrhosis	
Hashimoto's thyroiditis		Infectious hepatitis (A and B)	
		Mononucleosis	
		Cytomegal virus infections	
		Coxackie infections	
		Rubella	
		Intrauterine, congenital, and neonatal infections (rubella, lues, toxoplasmosis, or bacterial infections)	

Oligoclonal IgG reactions, which are not infrequently seen on agarose gel electrophoresis, are characterized by the presence of several small, but distinct bands in the IgG region. The reaction is most probably the result of a restricted antibody response on antigen stimulation. An oligoclonal reaction can be present in spite of normal levels of total IgG and in some conditions can be observed in conjunction with reduced concentration of IgG, for example in chronic lymphatic leukaemia, in which a few small bands often appears in the IgG region. For this reason it is of value that agarose gel electrophoresis be carried out in addition to quantitative Ig determinations in order to reveal Ig alterations. Oligoclonal patterns may occur in acute infections, especially if these are induced by viruses. The oligoclonal IgG response in infection is often changed into polyclonal patterns. Oligoclonal patterns may also be found in connection with various other conditions giving changes of IgG, for example collagen disease, chronic liver disease, and malignant tumors. Unlike the infectious processes, the oligoclonal patterns remain more stationary in the last-mentioned conditions. The clinical significance of oligoclonal IgG reaction is not explored in detail.

While determinations of IgD in plasma have so far not provided any useful clinical information, analysis of IgE is of interest in the diagnosis of certain allergic conditions, for example atopic disease. However, the diagnostic sensitivity of determinations of total IgE, seems to be limited, since only one-half of the cases with known atopic disease show increased IgE levels. The situation may be somewhat improved by the introduction of more precise reference values. It is also known that the IgE levels are often increased in diseases caused by parasites, e.g. *Ascaris lumbricoides* etc. This increase, which may sometimes be extreme, can be of diagnostic help in the diagnosis of such diseases. Detection of specfic IgE antibodies of reagin type is discussed on page 179.

Determinations of changes in concentration of IgG subclasses (IgG1–IgG4) may be a further aid in the diagnosis of IgG alterations. Changes of the electrophoretic distribution of IgA sometimes observed in electrophoresis or in electroimmunoassay of IgG may be due to changes in the concentrations of one or more subclasses. Figure 151 shows an extreme example of such an abnormal IgG distribution with huge amounts of fast migrating IgG, due to increase of apparently polyclonal IgG4. Systematic studies on changes in the concentration of IgG subclasses in disease, have so far been seriously

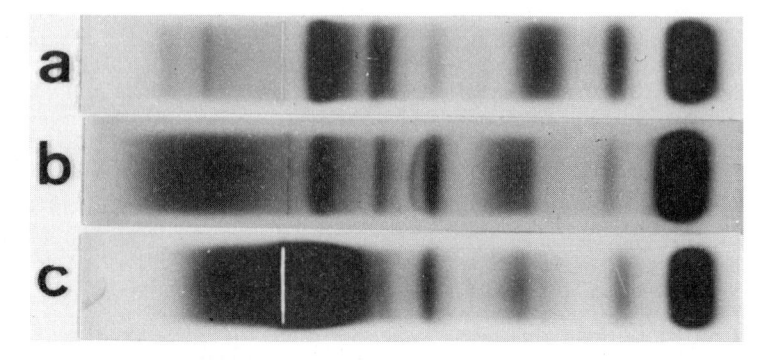

Fig. 151. Agarose gel electrophoresis of plasma samples which have various types of IgG abnormalities: (a) oligoclonal in IgG reaction, (b) polyclonal increase in IgG, (c) massive increase in IgG mainly affecting IgG4, as demonstrated by using a specific antiserum against IgG4

hampered by the difficulties encountered in the production of subclass-specific antibodies of high quality. In a few cases, selective deficiencies of IgG subclasses have been revealed in plasma from individuals with increased susceptibility to infections. A disproportionate decrease of IgG subclasses has also been described in patients with nephrotic syndrome. No reports on polyclonal, selective increase of IgG subclasses have been published as yet.

VIII. The plasma protein profile in inflammatory conditions

It has long been known that a large number of disorders in the acute or active phase give rise to characteristic changes in the electrophoretic serum protein pattern. A large number of plasma proteins appear to undergo changes in their concentration during this so-called acute-phase reaction. This seems to be dependent on a general reaction which is caused by an inflammatory response independent of the genesis of the process.

Studies performed on a large number of proteins have provided a survey of the changes of various proteins during the course of an inflammatory reaction. Such studies have been performed with the aid of crossed immunoelectrophoresis (Weeke, 1972) or with electroimmunoassay (Laurell et al., 1972). In the latter studies, two conditions were used as models: surgical trauma (cholecystectomy, mastectomy) and myocardial infarction. These and other similar studies have shown that the proteins may be divided into four main groups with respect to the changes in concentration during the course of the illness.

The first group of proteins show a rapid increase in their concentration to reach a maximum level about 5–7 days after the onset of the inflammatory process. Return to normal levels occurs within 4–6 weeks if the process is uncomplicated. Included in this group of proteins are: C-reactive protein, antichymotrypsin, fibrinogen, haptoglobin, orosomucoid and α_1-antitrypsin. The course of the concentration changes of these proteins is shown in Fig. 152 and 153. The increase in concentration is given in percentage of the initial value with the exception of C-reactive protein which shows a particularly pronounced increase to reach a level which is 20 times the original very low level. The protein having the next highest increase in antichymotrypsin where the level increases 3 times (not shown in the figures). The lowest increase in this group is shown by α_1-antitrypsin. Both C-reactive protein and antichymotrypsin differ from the other proteins in this group in the initial phase of the inflammatory process: the increase of these two proteins can be registered as early as 5–10 hours after the onset of the reaction.

The second group of proteins shows a slight to moderate *decrease* in concentration which follows essentially the same course as the proteins of group I (Fig. 152). A few proteins with comparatively low molecular weight such as albumin, transferrin, and prealbumin (TBPA) belong to this group, but also some larger proteins such as α-lipoprotein show the same principal course. The reduction of prealbumin concentration is especially marked: decreases to 20–30 per cent of the normal levels may be observed in intense inflammation.

The third group, which contains proteins such as the complement factors C3 and C4, haemopexin, prothrombin, and ceruloplasmin, exhibits a moderate increase with

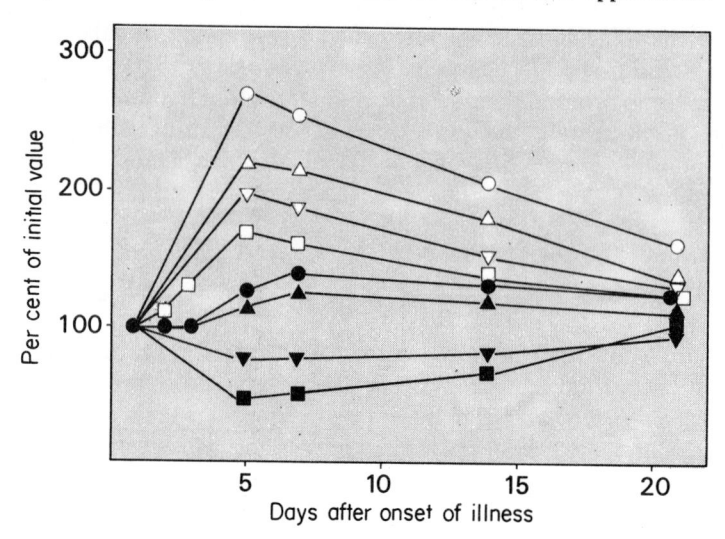

352 *Plasma proteins as diagnostic aids. Methods and clinical applications*

Fig. 152. Average changes in concentration of some plasma proteins in an acute inflammatory process (uncomplicated myocardial infraction). The following proteins have been assayed: ○ haptoglobin, △ fibrinogen, ▽ orosomucoid, □ α_1-antitrypsin, ● ceruloplasmin, ▲ C3 complement factor, ▼ albumin, ■ prealbumin (TBPA). Transferrin (not shown in the diagram) shows the same changes as albumin

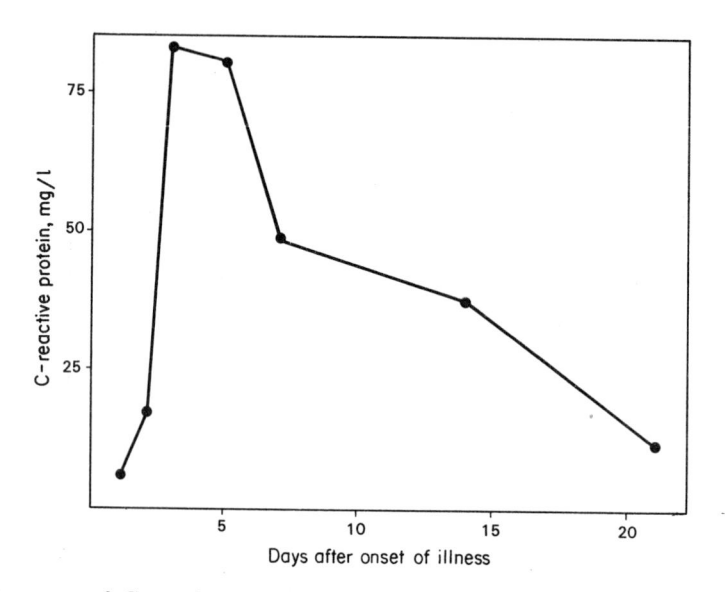

Fig. 153. Response of C-reactive protein in an acute inflammatory process (uncomplicated myocardial infarction). Note the rapid, extremely high increase in CRP in comparison with the other acute-phase reactants. A comparatively rapid, but less pronounced increase is also seen in plasma antichymotrypsin

maximal levels reached after 1–2 weeks and then slowly returns to normal. The increase is seldom particularly pronounced. The course of this group is represented in Fig. 153 by C3 and ceruloplasmin in uncomplicated myocardial infarction.

The fourth group, finally, characterized by virtually unaltered levels of protein in plasma during the course of an acute inflammatory process. Members of this group are α_2-macroglobulin, and probably also the immunoglobulins. Although slight decreases of IgG have been observed.

The changes in the pattern of the plasma proteins described here can of course vary in different pathological conditions, especially in the presence of complicating factors. The most reliable indicators of inflammatory processes seem to be orosomucoid, antichymotrypsin, and C-reactive protein, which are seldom unaffected in such conditions. It should be pointed out however, that inflammatory processes, for example some viral infections, may proceed without increases in CRP concentration. Normal levels of orosomucoid may occasionally be found in intestinal inflammatory diseases. Increased orosomucoid values without any further indications of inflammatory reaction are a common finding in kidney insufficiency, probably due to a decreased renal elimination of the relatively low molecular weight orosomucoid (page 366). An increase in the level of orosomucoid can also be seen after administration of corticosteroids.

Other indicators of inflammatory reactions such as fibrinogen, haptoglobin, α_1-antitrypsin, C3, and C4 are more variable in their behaviour. No increase of fibrinogen or haptoglobin in inflammatory reactions is due to an increased breakdown (elimination) in processes complicated by intravascular coagulation and fibrinolysis in the first case and increased consumption of haptoglobin in the presence of haemolysis or increased ineffective erythropoiesis in the second case. A slight increase in the elimination of haptoglobin in inflammatory processes can easily be detected by comparison of the concentrations of orosomucoid and haptoglobin. In uncomplicated cases, the increase in haptoglobin is usually larger than that in orosomucoid, while the rise in the level of haptoglobin is reduced or is non-existent in inflammatory reactions complicated by haemolysis, for example. Similarly, activation of complement can result in normal or even reduced levels of C3 (and C4) despite the appearance of an intense inflammatory reaction.

The α_1-antitrypsin levels often fail to increase in inflammatory reactions. The reasons for this are incompletely understood. Genetic variants, like α_1-antitrypsin *MZ*, with normally reduced levels, and present in about 5 per cent of the population should always be taken into account as an explanation for the observation of apparently normal α_1-antitrypsin levels in inflammatory conditions. It is known that these variants similar to the deficient *ZZ* protein show a percentage increase of the same order as the common variants of type *MM*. The localization and type of the inflammatory process may also play a role for α_1-antitrypsin response. Normal or only slightly increased α_1-antitrypsin levels are common findings in processes mainly restricted to mesenchymal tissues, for example rheumatoid arthritis and polymyositis. On the other hand marked increases have been found in advanced malignant tumors, especially those with liver metastases, α_1-Antitrypsin is also increased in inflammatory liver diseases.

The mechanisms which lie behind the changes in the plasma protein pattern described here are poorly understood. The concentrations of individual proteins in plasma are determined by the rate of symthesis, the rate of elimination (catabolism and possible losses), and the intra- extravascular distribution. A better understanding of the mechanisms causing the changes in concentration should be gained by detailed studies of plasma protein metabolism in disease. For those proteins which drop in level, there is a redistribution of the proteins between the intravascular and the extravascular space. This primarily affects low molecular weight proteins and can partly explain the reduction in the levels of albumin, prealbumin, and transferrin. It is more uncertain if the corresponding drop in α-lipoprotein concentration can be explained in this way. The fact that the reduction of prealbumin is more pronounced in prealbumin than in albumin despite the similarity in molecular size indicates that other mechanisms contribute to the reduction. Such mechanisms may be reduced rate of synthesis or catabolism but the role played by these factors is not clear.

Similarly, little is known about the causes of the increase in concentrations of a number of proteins. There is no doubt that the raised levels are due to increases synthesis of these proteins, but it is not known which factors are responsible for the stimulation of the synthesis. More than one mechanism may be involved. It is reasonable to believe that haptoglobin, orosomucoid, and fibrinogen have a common stimulant while other mechanisms may be operating in the cases of the rapidly increasing CRP and the moderate or slow increase of several other proteins.

Despite the observations of a considerable variance of the '*acute phase*' patterns in different kinds of conditions with inflammatory response, there is an obvious need for more systematic studies to evaluate the ultimate diagnostic potentials of plasma protein profiles in such conditions. Recent studies of plasma protein patterns in infectious diseases caused by bacteria or viruses did not reveal any qualitative differences between these groups, but merely a difference in intensity of the inflammatory reaction, being less pronounced in viral infections. On the other hand liver diseases are associated with a very peculiar constellation of acute phase proteins. In general the diagnostic information obtained from the patterns of acute phase proteins is so far restricted to the detection of inflammatory conditions and estimation of the extent and/or intensity of the process. Complicating factors such as haemolysis, complement activation etc. can also be detected. Furthermore, determinations of one or a few acute phase proteins are of great value in following the natural history of inflammatory diseases or the response to treatment. CRP analyses may turn out to be very suitable for this purpose, since the CRP levels closely parallel the clinical activity due to its short biological half-life.

IX. Plasma protein changes in gastrointestinal diseases

The most pronounced changes of the plasma protein patterns occur in intestinal inflammatory diseases, e.g. Crohn's disease and ulcerative colitis, which are characterized in the active phases by intense inflammatory reaction often in combination with protein losses. There are no noticeable differences in the inflammatory plasma protein patterns of the two diseases. Orosomucoid and haptoglobin levels are often markedly raised in both diseases in active stages. Very high haptoglobin concentrations have

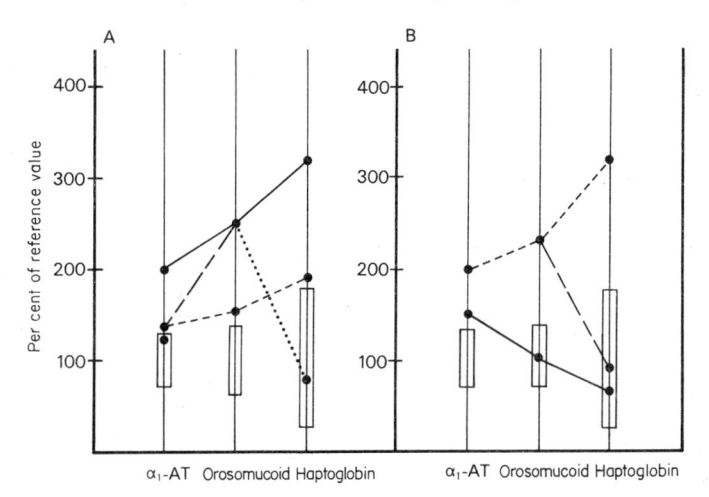

Fig. 154. The pattern of some acute-phase proteins in various types of inflammatory reactions. A. Mild inflammatory reaction ●--●--●. Pronounced inflammatory reaction: without special characteristics ●—●—●, in a patient with α_1-antitrypsin of the type MZ (heterozygous for α_1-antitrypsin deficiency). ●——●—●, with simultaneously increased elimination of haptoglobin ●—●···●. B. Inflammatory reaction patterns in jaundice of various origins. Inflammatory liver disease ●-●-●. Extrahepatic cholestasis with inflammatory reaction. ●--●--●. Liver cancer (primary or secondary) generally displays the same picture as extrahepatic processes; the haptoglobin level may be reduced ●---●— —●.

been observed in Crohn's disease, complicated by intestinal fistulas and/or abcesses. In clinically inactive periods plasma protein patterns indicating liver engagement may be seen in ulcerative colitis. In Crohn's disease a peculiar pattern, characterized by normal levels of CRP and orosomucoid but slightly elevated α_1-antitrypsin and haptoglobin concentrations, often appears after treatment.

Protein losses are a common feature in gastrointestinal diseases (*protein-losing enteropathy*) and occur in a number of different conditions (exemplified in Table 54). Enteric plasma protein leakage, which may be caused by damage of the mucosa or disorders of the intestinal lymphatics, is a non-selective process, and the losses of

Table 54. Examples of diseases associated with protein-losing enteropathy

Primary intestinal lymphangiectasia
Colonic lymphangiectasia
Crohn's disease
Ulcerative colitis
Hypertrophic gastritis
Whipple's disease
Gastrointestinal tract carcinoma
Tropical and non-tropical sprue
Coeliac disease
Acute gastrointestinal infections
Megacolon

various proteins are proportional to their concentration in the extracellular fluid. Protein-losing enteropathy may be suspected in subjects with a marked generalized hypoproteinaemia not caused by nephrosis or advanced liver disease. In chronic inflammatory bowel diseases in active stages, the losses are mirrored by a low plasma albumin level, while the IgG concentration is most often normal, owing to compensation of the losses by increased synthesis rate.

The immunoglobulins show considerable variations in appearance in gastrointestinal diseases. Apart from the reduced levels of Ig in protein-losing gastroenteropathy, selective deficiencies of plasma IgA are found in an increased frequency in certain intestinal diseases such as gluten-sensitive enteropathy, nodular lymphatic hyperplasia, and lactase deficiency. Selectively *increased* IgA levels which are a comparatively common finding in gastrointestinal disease, for example in malabsorption states, Crohn's disease, and ulcerative colitis, are of limited diagnostic importance. Various other patterns of polyclonal Ig increase may also occur.

Malnutrition or malabsorption states demonstrate in severe cases a hypoalbuminaemia, which may give rise to oedema if the albumin levels fall below 20–25 g/l. However, the serum albumin level is an insensitive indicator of inadequate supply or poor intestinal absorption of amino acids. Attempts have been made to find more sensitive protein indicators in these cases but so far no plasma protein has been found really suitable for this purpose. It has been suggested that transferrin should be used but the interpretation of transferrin levels must be made with due regard to iron deficiency which is often present in such cases. Similarly, decreases in the level of prealbumin (TBPA) have been observed in malnutrition or malabsorption. Studies in our laboratory have shown that one week of strict fasting is sufficient to produce a distinct decrease of the plasma prealbumin in plasma from healthy volunteers. Also in the case of prealbumin, the interpretation is complicated by the fact that the prealbumin level is considerably reduced in inflammatory processes, which are often present in malnourished individuals or patients with malabsorption. Liver damage must also be taken into consideration in the interpretation of reduced prealbumin levels.

Determination of retinol-binding protein (RBP) in plasma has been suggested as a method for detection of vitamin A deficiency in conditions with malabsorption. This protein transports retinol which is the active form of vitamin A, from the liver to the target organs (cf. page 111). After delivery of the retinol, RBP is rapidly eliminated from plasma through the kidneys. Since RBP is secreted from the liver cells as a retinol–protein complex exclusively, deficiency of vitamin A leads to a reduced concentration of RBP in plasma, which has been established in experimental animals and in patients with known vitamin A deficiency. A good correlation was found between reduction of plasma RBP level and impairment of dark adaption, which is a functional estimate of vitamin A deficiency. Unfortunately, however, low concentrations of RBP are encountered in inflammatory conditions and in liver disease; in both cases the RBP changes parallel those of prealbumin. Thus conclusions from RBP analyses about vitamin A deficiency due to deficient resorption in malabsorption are restricted to non-inflammatory conditions or at least conditions in an inactive stage. For this reason it is advisable to determine for example orosomucoid simultaneously with RBP to exclude inflammation as a cause of RBP reduction. It should also be noted that kidney insufficiency gives high RBP levels due to decreased elimination (page 366).

X. Plasma protein alterations in liver and biliary diseases

1. Hepatitis and liver cirrhosis

A variety of plasma protein changes occur in acute and chronic liver inflammatory processes. Earlier analysis by using paper electrophoresis revealed only small changes in the plasma protein in acute hepatitis. The most characteristic alteration was an increase α_1-globulin without concomitant rise in the α_2-globulin, usually found in inflammatory reaction. This pattern, which was called α_1-α_2-discrepancy, involves characteristic changes of the acute phase proteins in acute hepatitis (hepatitis B), for example a slight to moderate increase in α_1-antitrypsin, normal levels of orosomucoid and normal or reduced haptoglobin concentrations (Fig. 155). Other acute phase proteins: CRP, fibrinogen, and α_1-antichymotrypsin are normal or slightly increased, but

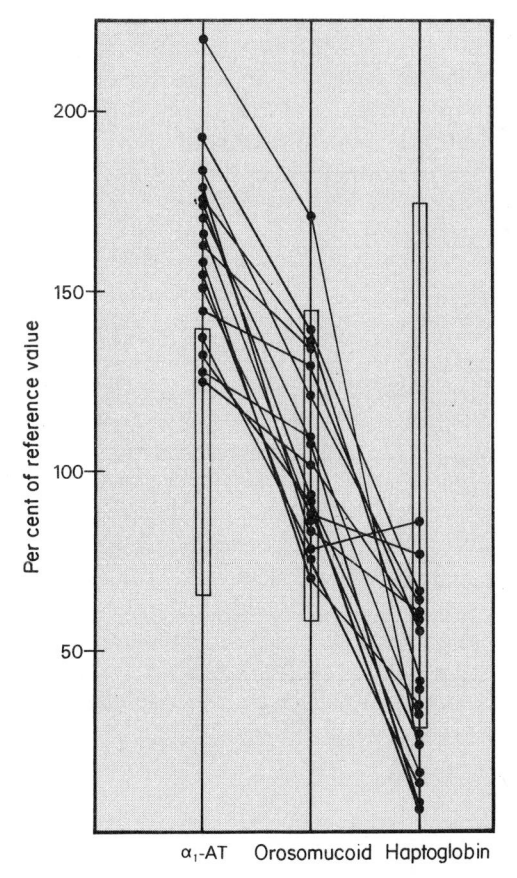

Fig. 155. Concentrations of α_1-antitrypsin, orosomucoid, and haptoglobin in the plasma of 17 patients during the course of hepatitis B. All samples were taken during the first week in hospital. The diagram shows the divergent inflammatory response in all of these patients (data from Kindmark and Laurell, 1972)

to a lesser degree than α_1-antitrypsin. However, high concentrations of ceruloplasmin is a common finding.

It is not known what causes these changes. The rise of α_1-antitrypsin is most probably due to an increased rate of synthesis. The discrepancy in orosomucoid and haptoglobin levels indicate that increased elimination of haptoglobin is an important factor; this assumption is supported by evidence of increased red cell destruction in hepatitis possibly due to changes in the hepato–splanchnic blood flow. The increase in ceruloplasmin seems to be associated with the presence of cholestasis.

Other plasma protein changes in acute hepatitis involve a marked decrease in prealbumin and to a less extent in prothrombin levels while albumin is normal in practically all cases. Transferrin is also normal or increased in concentration. The α-lipoprotein (high density lipoproteins) shows marked alterations with reduced concentrations, combined with changes in immunoreactivity, this behaviour is not specific for hepatitis, but is also found in long-standing extrahepatic cholestasis. The changes of α-lipoprotein are caused by a deficiency of the cholesterol esterifying enzyme in plasma lecithin cholesterol acyl transferase (LCAT) in these two conditions.

The immunoglobulin levels are within the normal limits in the majority of patients with hepatitis B. Increase of IgM is the most frequent finding and occurs in about 50 per cent of the cases. Raised levels of IgG are occasionally found, whereas IgA concentration is normal in practically all cases.

The changes described are most pronounced during the first 3–4 weeks after admission and then return to normal within 2–3 months. Similar changes as described

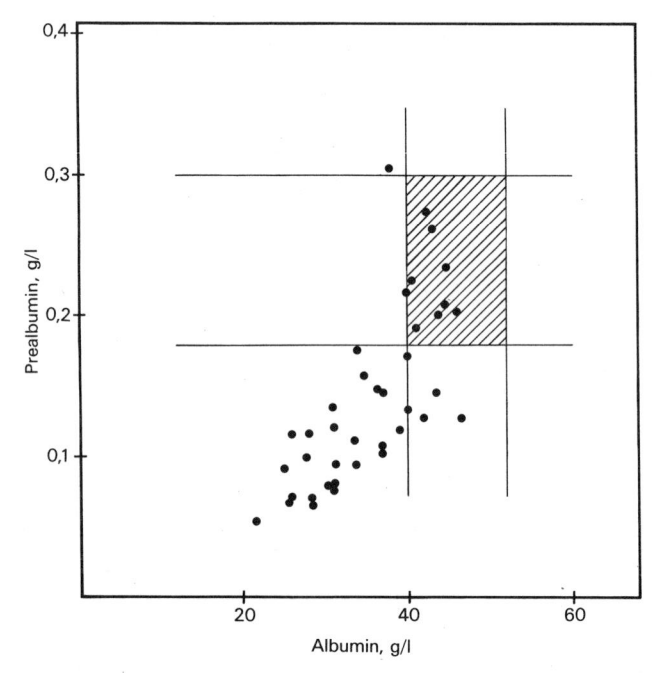

Fig. 156. Levels of prealbumin and albumin in plasma in cirrhosis of the liver. The hatched region is the reference region ($\pm$2SD) for these two proteins (from Hállén and Laurell, 1972)

for hepatitis B, occur in other types of acute hepatitis and also in exacerbations of chronic liver disease, except for immunoglobulins which show considerable variations. The peculiar profiles formed by the changes in concentrations of α_1-antitrypsin, orosomucoid, and haptoglobin in the first place and prealbumin and ceruloplasmin in the second place are thus very characteristic of active inflammatory liver disease. It should be mentioned however, that with the exception of decrease in prealbumin levels, patients under increased influence of oestrogen have the same patterns (page 341). Furthermore the apparent absence of elevated levels of α_1-antitrypsin in patients with phenotypes MZ (and MS) may give misleading information. The presence of extrahepatic inflammatory processes also renders the detection of liver inflammatory processes more difficult. Hepatitis of type A is often characterized by a rather 'conventional' inflammatory plasma protein pattern; this might possibly indicate inflammation outside the liver. Immunoglobulin determinations are of limited diagnostic value in acute liver disease, but are of importance in following the course of disease since persistently high or rising immunoglobulin values are a sign of development of chronic hepatic disease.

The chronic liver diseases show wide variations of the plasma proteins dependent upon the stage and activity of the disease. In active phases the acute phase proteins, i.e. α_1-antitrypsin, orosomucoid, and haptoglobin, display the same pattern as in acute hepatitis. The haptoglobin levels are sometimes very low in liver cirrhosis, which is at least partly explained by increased consumption in connection with impaired hepatosplenic circulation leading to increased red cell destruction. Distinct increase of CRP and/or orosomucoid concentrations in chronic liver disease indicates the presence of inflammatory processes outside the liver.

Decreases of prealbumin and prothrombin are sensitive indicators in liver disease. Since *accurate* measurements of prothrombin concentrations are usually difficult to obtain we prefer to determine prealbumin levels. The drop in prealbumin, which might occasionally be the only pathological finding in the plasma protein profile in liver disease, usually precedes decrease of albumin, which is a comparatively late event in chronic liver disease. Pronounced decreases of albumin are especially found in patients with ascites. Although prealbumin determinations are very valuable in the diagnosis of liver disease it must be remembered, however, that low prealbumin levels are also a very common part of plasma protein profile obtained in various inflammatory conditions.

The patterns of immunoglobulin increase, most often present in chronic liver disease, are very variable as shown in the examples given below. The most peculiar pattern is found in *primary biliary cirrhosis* with a predominant or selective increase of IgM, a finding of considerable diagnostic importance. Secondary forms of biliary cirrhosis have Ig increases of mixed types.

Dominant increase of IgG is seen in chronic aggresive hepatitis and in lupoid hepatitis. Massive increase of IgG (up to 50 g/l), may be found often associated with low levels of complement factors C3 and C4. The IgG concentrations in these cases seem to mirror well the progress/regress of disease, for example in connection with administration of steroids. The increase is sometimes distinctly oligoclonal. Increase of IgA is very common in alcohol-induced liver disease. In early stages isolated elevation of IgA is not uncommon. With progress of the liver damage increase in IgG is also encountered, but still the IgA elevation is most pronounced, sometimes reaching levels of 10–15 g/l in advanced alcohol cirrhosis. The same pattern may be found in cirrhosis of other aetiology.

2. Liver tumours

In contrast with inflammatory liver disease and cirrhosis tumours in the liver are not associated with a specific 'liver profile' in the plasma protein pattern. Malignant tumours with liver metastases show more or less pronounced inflammatory pattern, sometimes with absence of haptoglobin elevation. A characteristic feature of *primary* liver cancer is the presence of high levels of α-fetoprotein. This protein is synthesized in foetal liver cells and gives rise to a band in the α-region of the electrophoretic pattern of foetal plasma. Very low levels of this protein (in the order of 10 μg/l) have been detected in the plasma of adults by using radioimmunoassay. Increased levels can be demonstrated in cases of *primary* liver cancer. In roughly one-half of the cases the increase is so great that simple immunoprecipitation techniques are sufficient for the detection and quantitation of the protein. Values of α-fetoprotein exceeding 0.5 mg/l in plasma are with few exceptions diagnostic of primary liver cancer. By using more sensitive radioimmunological methods it has been shown that 80–90 per cent of the cases of primary liver cancer show increased levels of α-fetoprotein. However, since other liver diseases also display slight elevations of this protein the diagnostic value of the more sensitive methods is doubtful. On the other hand, these sensitive techniques for the determination of α-fetoprotein can be used in the control of the course of primary liver cancer.

3. Protein and lipoprotein changes in cholestasis

Biliary obstruction without liver damage does not present any special features of the plasma protein profiles. If the obstructive jaundice is due to stones in the common duct without concomitant inflammatory processes essentially normal patterns are obtained, while biliary obstruction caused by, for example, malignant tumour often shows a conventional inflammatory pattern with increase of the acute phase proteins. However, marked β-lipoprotein bands are most often seen on electrophoresis of cholestatic plasma. This is not only due to a rise of normal β-lipoprotein but also to the appearance of a unique cholestatic low density lipoprotein called lipoprotein X (LP-X). In *agar* gel electrophoresis this lipoprotein, in contrast to other plasma lipoproteins, acquires a cathodic migration and can easily be detected after electrophoresis by precipitation with manganese–heparin. Lipoprotein X is detected in about 90 per cent of all cases with biliary obstruction either of extra- or intrahepatic origin. However, except in special cases, the diagnostic importance of detecting this lipoprotein seems to be very limited.

Additional lipoprotein changes can easily be revealed in cholestasis of longer duration (3–4 weeks), involving a marked reduction of the α-lipoprotein level seen on agarose electrophoresis of cholestatic plasma. This change appears to be of the same nature as the α-lipoprotein changes seen in acute hepatitis (page 358).

XI. Kidney disease

Renal diseases are accompanied by a variety of plasma protein changes, including inflammatory patterns, plasma protein losses, immunoglobulin responses, and complement activation. The most marked alterations of the plasma protein profile are seen in nephrotic syndrome, characterized by considerable losses of comparatively low molecular weight proteins, such as albumin, α_1-antitrypsin, transferrin, and often also IgG, while high molecular weight proteins (α_2-macroglobulin, haptoglobin polymers, β-lipoprotein, and fibrinogen) are distinctly increased. Although low levels of IgG are a common finding in nephrosis the IgA concentration is usually normal or even raised. The reason for this is unknown, but one explanation might be differences in molecular size of IgG and IgA, due to polymerization of IgA or complex formation with other proteins. It should also be noted that a hypercatabolism of proteins is added to the urinary losses in nephrosis, complicating the interpretation of the plasma protein profile. The plasma protein pattern in nephrosis is of restricted diagnostic value, but on the other hand protein analyses may be of value in order to determine the decrease in plasma of functionally important proteins. The estimation of the urinary protein losses will be discussed in Section XIII, 1.

In acute glomerulonephritis a more or less pronounced inflammatory pattern is observed with harmonic increase of most acute phase reactants except C3, due to complement activation with decrease of the C3 levels in most cases of acute glomerulonephritis. While the C3 level can be roughly estimated from the agarose gel electrophoretic patterns, quantitative determinations of this and other complement factors are achieved by immunochemical methods. Elctroimmunoassay seems to give reliable values at least for C3 and C4. The complement system is described in detail on page 147.

The most pronounced drop in C3 levels is seen in lupus erythematosus with active nephritis and during the first week after the onset of acute glomerulonephritis. Also during active periods in chronic glomerulonephritis a decrease of C3 is seen. Measurements of C3 levels are thus valuable for estimation of disease activity. In membranoproliferative glomerulonephritis low C3 levels occur together with normal or even increased concentrations of complement factor C4. This combination suggests that the activation takes place via the alternate pathway and with participation of the so-called nephritic factor, a protein occurring in this disease and possibly also in normal plasma. In membranoproliferative disease the C3 level is decreased for long periods; no obvious relation between C3 levels and activity of the disease is found.

In uraemic patients no constant changes of the plasma protein profiles are present. Inflammatory patterns may occur, but it should be pointed out that in uraemia increased levels of orosomucoid may occur without any signs of inflammatory process. The cause of this increase is not quite clear but it is reasonable to assume that orosomucoid, which has a comparatively low molecular weight (40 000), is normally in part filtered through the glomerular membrane and reabsorbed and catabolized in the tubular cells. This normal elimination route should be less effective with decreasing glomerular filtration rate, resulting in an increased plasma level. The same mechanism for elimination has been proposed for a number of low molecular weight proteins in plasma. Because of the efficient elimination such proteins are normally present in plasma in only very low concentration. A considerable increase in the plasma levels of low molecular weight proteins (β_2-microglobulin, retinol-binding protein, and others) is found in uraemic patients (see also Urinary proteins, page 364).

XII. Blood and bone marrow diseases

As was mentioned previously, the reduction in the level of haptoglobin is a very sensitive indicator of disorders in the turnover of the erythron. The reduction is caused by the forming of complexes between haptoglobin and the released haemoglobin in plasma or in the extracellular fluid. This complex is rapidly eliminated from the circulation by uptake into hepatocytes and subsequent degradation.

Consumption of haptoglobin occurs of course in intravascular haemolysis, e.g. in sepsis, immunohaemolytic conditions, paroxysmal nocturnal haemoglobinuria, and in serious valvular disorders of the heart, especially following an operation for the installation of prosthetic valve. Disseminated intravascular coagulation may also be associated with haptoglobin elimination due to haemolysis. However, bone marrow haemolysis and so-called ineffective erythropoiesis are also common causes of reduced levels of haptoglobin. Under normal conditions, it is estimated that roughly one-half of the synthesized haptoglobin is eliminated by the formation of a complex with haemoglobin from that fraction of the erythrocytes which normally die during the maturation process in the bone marrow. Thus a doubling of the ineffective erythropoiesis will cause a reduction in the plasma level of haptoglobin to undetectable levels.

Patients with deficiencies of vitamin B_{12} or folic acid, which causes a considerable increase of the ineffective erythropoiesis, show an apparent absence of haptoglobin in their plasma unless there is increased synthesis brought on by the simultaneous presence of a severe inflammatory reaction. Reduced levels of haptoglobin are often present also in hepatosplenomegaly. These may be caused by defective sinus function or a retarded passage through the spleen or liver causing damage to the erythrocytes. In liver diseases, a reduced rate of synthesis may also contribute to the low levels of haptoglobin. Low levels of haptoglobin are often seen in normal children, without any evidence of increased red cell destruction.

Haptoglobin levels in plasma, should always be interpreted with regard to the balance between synthesis and elimination. Haptoglobin is an indicator of acute inflammatory reactions and a high rate of synthesis in such conditions can mask a slight to moderate consumption. Additional information can be obtained in such cases by simultaneously assaying the concentration of orosomucoid, since the rate of synthesis of this protein appears to parallel that of haptoglobin. The presence of an inflammatory reaction with an increased level of orosomucoid and normal or decreased levels of haptoglobin (orosomucoid–haptoglobin discrepance) can indicate intravascular haemolysis or abnormal function of the liver or bone marrow and may appear in sepsis, in the active phase of LED, *endocarditis lenta* as well as in cancer with liver or bone marrow metastases.

As mentioned previously, the level of haptoglobin drops rapidly towards undetectable levels in haemolysis or increased ineffective erythropoiesis. Thus the level of haptoglobin is not a good indicator of the *degree* of haemolysis. This is more easily obtained by assay of the concentration of *haemopexin* (page 106), which together with albumin is the protein which can bind free haem in plasma. The concentration of haemopexin is an inverse measure of the accumulation of haem in plasma which in turn is a reflection of the degree of haemolysis and/or accumulation of haem in the tissues. It should be pointed out that, similar to haptoglobin, the level of haemopexin increases in inflammatory processes although the increases are very moderate, and seldom reach a doubling of the normal levels. Low levels of haemopexin can also be found in the absence of haemolysis in patients with glomerulur damage since haemopexin being of the same molecular size as albumin is readily lost in the urine. Low values of haemopexin, 10–40 per cent of the normal value found in adults, are also seen in new-borns.

In severe haemolysis or pronounced ineffective erythropoiesis, with increased elimination of haemopexin, a temporary complex is formed between haem and albumin (*methaemalbumin*), which gives plasma a characteristic brownish tint. The binding is reversible and the haem is successively transferred to newly synthesized haemopexin, replacing that eliminated after complexing with haem. Analysis of methaemalbumin is of little clinical value. Determinations have been suggested to be helpful in the diagnosis of acute haemorrhagic pancreatitis, but the practical use of such analyses remains to be proved.

Finally it should be noted that free haemoglobin appears in plasma in haemolysis when the capacity of haptoglobin to bind haemoglobin has been exceeded. The haemoglobin is partially dissociated to $\alpha\beta$-dimers, which are filtered through the glomerular membrane and eventually appear in the urine (haemoglobinuria), when the tubular reabsorption capacity is exceeded. Determination of free haemoglobin in plasma is only of value in special situations, for example measurement of erythrocyte destruction in connection with heart surgery.

While it is generally accepted that haptoglobin is an indicator of an increase in ineffective erythropoiesis, transferrin is used as an indicator of iron deficiency. A typical finding in iron deficiency is an increased level of transferrin with an iron saturation of less than 15 per cent. Increases in the level of transferrin without iron deficiency are seen in pregnancy, during the use of contraceptive drugs which contain oestrogen, and often in liver diseases. In these conditions, however, the iron saturation is not reduced. The increases in the level of transferrin which normally occur in iron deficiency can be masked by inflammatory processes, loss of protein, and low protein intake. In advanced liver diseases the level of transferrin is reduced because of insufficient synthesis.

In recent years, another protein, *ferritin*, has become of interest as a possible measure of the iron stores in the organisms. This protein is present in plasma at a concentration of the order of 0.1 mg/l. Subnormal levels are found in iron deficiency. On the other hand increased values can be observed in the abnormal accumulation of iron and even in inflammatory diseases, liver diseases, and certain malignant tumours. Despite the fact that the low levels of ferritin require determinations by rather complicated radioimmunological techniques ferritin analyses seem to be of value in the assessments of the iron stores of the body, both in iron deficiency and especially in iron overloading.

Leukaemia does not give rise to any characteristic protein pattern. Reduced levels of immunoglobulin are often seen in lymphatic leukaemia. This is especially true of IgG where in many cases a few small bands (oligoclonal reaction) can be seen despite the reduced total concentration.

Increased levels of the enzyme lysozyme are found in plasma (and urine) from patients with myelocytic or myelomonocytic leukaemia; the latter disease especially shows considerable increase of lysozyme. The increase is a measure of the turnover of leukaemic cells, containing lysozyme.

XIII. Analysis of proteins in body fluids other than blood

1. Urinary proteins

In healthy individuals, the daily loss of protein via the urine is less than 0.1 g. Although the major part of this amount comes from plasma, normal urine also contains proteins which are synthesized locally in the urinary tract such as uromucoid (the protein of Tamm and Horsfall) and secretory IgA.

Many plasma proteins are normally passing to some extent through the glomeruli. The degree of filtration is related to the molecular size. Thus, proteins of small molecular sizes (molecular weight less than 10 000–12 000, Stokes's radius* approximately 1.5 nm) have a glomerular clearance approaching that of inulin. The degree of filtration decreases with increased molecular size. Serum albumin having a molecular weight of 66 000 (Stokes's radius approximately 3.5 nm) passes through the glomerular membrane only in trace amounts. Proteins which appear in the primary urine are reabsorbed almost completely by the cells in the proximal tubules where they are degraded by lysosomal enzymes and the amino acids are added to the amino acid pool. In this way the kidneys have an important function in the catabolism of low molecular weight plasma proteins.

Pathological increase of excretion of proteins into urine (proteinuria) may be caused by several mechanisms. A simple classification of proteinuria is given below (examples of urinary patterns are presented in Fig. 157).

1. *Prerenal proteinuria* is caused by insufficient capacity of normal tubules to reabsorb low molecular weight proteins filtered through the glomerular membrane, when such proteins are present in increased concentrations in plasma.
2. *Glomerular proteinuria* is caused by leakage of normally retained proteins through damaged glomerular membranes.
3. *Tubular proteinuria* is caused by impaired reabsorption of low molecular weight proteins due to damage of the proximal tubules.
4. *Postglomerular proteinuria* is caused by leakage of proteins from plasma of lymphatics in the kidney or urinary tract.

A *prerenal proteinuria* occurs in many conditions. In inflammatory reactions with marked increase of acute phase proteins, e.g. orosomucoid, this and other comparatively low molecular weight acute phase proteins can be found in urine. The proteinuria in febrile conditions can also partly be explained in this way, but a slightly increased glomerular permeability also contributes to the 'fever proteinuria'. The most clinically important prerenal proteinuria occurs in myeloma, involving excretion of

---

*Stokes's radius is a useful measure of the molecular size of proteins.

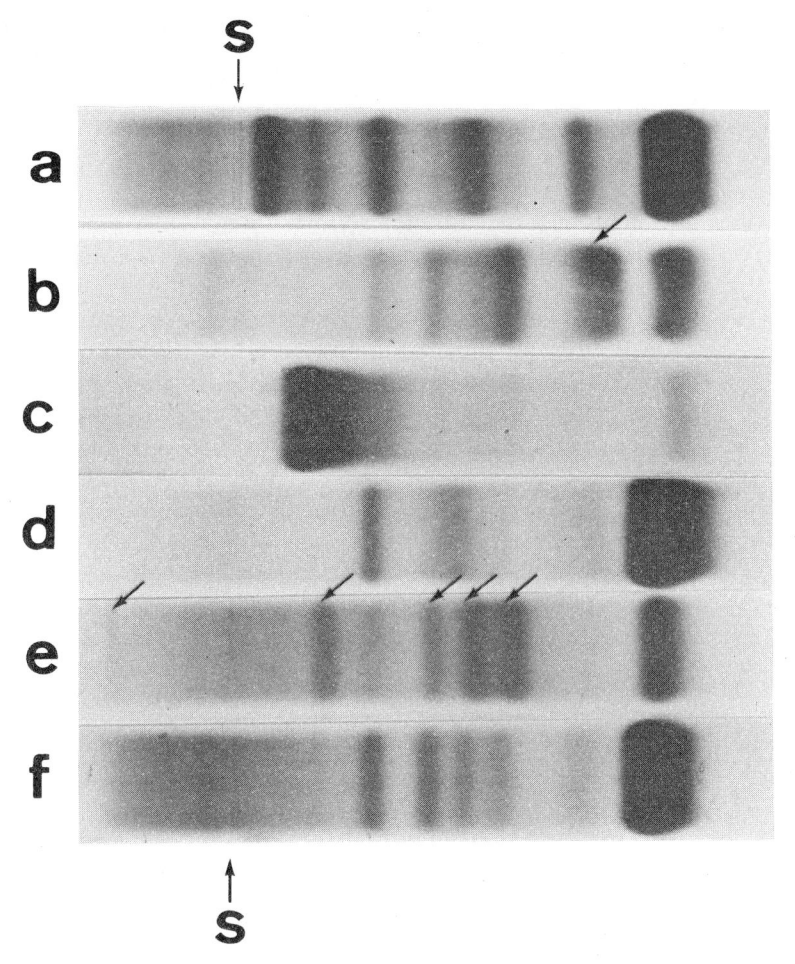

Fig. 157. Agarose electrophoresis of urine proteins in various types of proteinuria: (a) reference plasma, (b) proteinuria in an inflammatory condition with excessive excretion of orosomucoid, (c) excretion of monoclonal light chains in myeloma, (d) proteinuria in increased glomerular protein leakage, (e) proteinuria in injury to the tubules, caused by exposure to cadmium, (f) proteinuria in an uraemic patient with excretion of low molecular weight proteins in combination with plasma proteins of higher molecular weight. The samples were applied at 'S'. The arrows indicate orosomucoid (b), three bands which contain retinol-binding protein (e), β_2-microglobulin (e), and γ-trace protein (e)

monoclonal light chains (Bence Jones proteinuria), occurring in myeloma (page 345). In myelomonocytic leukaemia and to a lesser extent in chronic myelocytic leukaemia, there is an increase in the level of lysozyme in plasma and urine. This is caused by the increased destruction of leukaemic cells related to monocytes or neutrophilic granulocytes which contain this protein in considerable amounts. In myelomonocytic leukaemia, the lysozymuria can be very pronounced; values in excess of 1 g/l are not unusual. It should be noted that lysozymuria also occurs as part of the 'tubular proteinuria' described below. Further examples of prerenal proteinuria are myoglobinuria which arises in various types of damage to muscle and haemoglobinuria in haemolytic conditions where the capacity of plasma haptoglobin to bind haemoglobin is exceeded.

Glomerular proteinuria is dominated by albumin excretion, due to the moderate molecular size and high concentration. The glomerular damage may be of different kinds, giving rise to selective glomerular proteinuria with leakage of comparatively low molecular weight proteins (albumin and transferrin with molecular weights 66 000 and 76 000 respectively) or non-selective proteinuria with excretion of proteins with higher molecular weight such as IgG (molecular weight 150 000) or even α_2-macroglobulin (molecular weight 725 000). The degree of selectivity bears no correlation to the total excretion of proteins; even heavy proteinuria may be of the selective type.

It has been suggested that measurements of the degree of selectivity in glomerular proteinuria should be helpful as a guide to choice of therapy in glomerular disease. Although there is a correlation between histological findings in kidney biopsies and selectivity, measurements of selectivity at least in adults has little clinical value. In children with nephrotic syndrome such measurements might be of some use.

Tubular proteinuria arises from defective resorption of low molecular weight protein in the proximal tubules. In this form of proteinuria, which was first detected in connection with cadmium poisoning (Friberg, 1959; Piscator, 1966), the daily excretion of protein is usually less than 1 g and the electrophoretic pattern is dominated by a series of low molecular weight components. The properties of these components are listed in Table 55. The true form of tubular proteinuria with defective resorption and normal levels of low molecular weight protein in the primary urine is rare or even extremely rare. It is present in certain hereditary defects of the tubules such as Fanconi's syndrome. The demonstration of tubular proteinuria is of importance primarily to reveal kidney damage which has been caused by exposure to heavy metals such as cadmium.

However, the majority of cases of 'tubular' proteinuria are patients with reduced glomerular filtration. Since the proteinuria in these cases is at least partially due to 'overflow' this does not give a good measure of the degree of function of the tubules. The primary cause in these cases is probably a retarded elimination of low molecular weight proteins brought about by reduced glomerular filtration. This leads to an increased concentration in plasma and, in this way, a primary urine is produced in the remaining intact nephrons, which has a high concentration of low molecular weight proteins, exceeding the reabsorption threshold of the proximal tubules, even if these are normally functioning. For this reason the 'tubular proteinuria' in uraemic patients is in one sense 'prerenal', and the term tubular proteinuria should be replaced by the more neutral 'low molecular weight proteinuria' (LMW proteinuria). The proteinuria in uraemia is often of a mixed type with variable amounts of albumin and even IgG appearing in addition to the low molecular weight proteins.

There are few indications for electrophoretic analysis of proteinuria. The detection of the monoclonal light chains (Bence Jones proteinuria) in urine is naturally of great diagnostic value. This should be carried out using agarose gel electrophoresis and a urine sample which has been concentrated by for example ultrafiltration to give a protein concentration of approximately 50 g/l. In cases where the electrophoretic pattern is difficult to interpret, complementary immunoelectrophoretic analysis should be performed, preferentially with immunofixation.

Table 55. Properties of some low molecular weight proteins (less than 40 000) which can be isolated in patients having defective tubular resorption

Protein	Molecular size (Stokes's radius nm)	Molecular weight	Concentration in plasma (mg/l)	Properties (function)
α_1-Glycoprotein (HC protein)		25 000	30–60 (HC-protein, α_1-Microglobulin)	*Not* synonymous with orosomucoid. Present in cell membrane of most lymphocytes. Forms complexes with several other proteins in plasma.
Retinol-binding protein (RBP)	2.05	21 000	40–80	Transport of vitamin A. (retinol). Complexes with prealbumin in plasma.
β_2-Microglobulin	1.50	11 800	1–3	Part of HL-A antigen complex.
β-Trace protein		31 000		Glycoprotein. Heterogeneous on electrophoresis
Light Ig chains	2.30 (2.80)	22 000 (45 000)		Polyclonal distribution in patients with tubular defects. Monomer–dimer equilibrium.
γ-Trace protein		11 000		Contains hydroxyproline.
Lysozyme		14 300	1–4	Present in the granules of neutrophilic granulocytes and macrophages. Enzyme, which cleaves mucopeptides containing muramic acid.

It should be noted that the finding of a glomerular proteinuria in patients with suspected myeloma should always be followed by immunofixation, since the M-component might have caused a renal amyloidosis with a glomerular leakage.

In other situations electrophoresis of urine protein is of limited value. In patients with glomerular glomerular disease, the excretion of protein can best be measured by immunochemically determining the level of albumin in the urine. The most exact measure of the increased glomerular filtration of albumin and other proteins is obtained by calculation of the relative protein clearance. Here, consideration is given to the plasma concentration of the protein in question and to the patient's glomerular filtration.

$$\text{Albumin clearance} = \frac{\text{U-Albumin}}{\text{S-Albumin}} \times \frac{V}{T} \bigg/ \frac{\text{U-Creatinine}}{\text{S-Creatinine}} \times \frac{V}{T}$$

This implies the determination of albumin and creatinine in serum and urine, which can easily be carried out on a morning sample. As can be seen from the above formula, no measurements of urine volumes (V) and periods of collection (T) are necessary.

The degree of selectivity can be determined similarly by measuring the IgG clearance expressed as a percentage of the albumin clearance. Electrophoretic techniques are not sufficiently sensitive to permit accurate determination of the degree of selectivity.

The excretion of low molecular weight proteins such as β_2-microglobulin can also be suitably determined by using specific immunochemical analysis. This can be achieved by use of the simple radial immunodiffusion technique which not only detects normal levels of this protein in urine but which registers even very slight increases. The simultaneous measurement of protein in plasma and urine is essential in the diagnosis of damaged tubules. When β_2-microglobulin is used as an indicator of such damage, the instability of the protein in acidic urine (pH less than 6) can be a serious source of error. This can be avoided by giving the patient bicarbonate to produce a slightly alkaline urine. The diagnosis of damage to the tubules is considerably complicated if there is a simultaneous reduction of glomerular filtration. Finally, it should be mentioned that the determination of the excretion of lysozyme in urine has some value in the classification and therapeutic control of leukaemia. Such assays can be performed with immunochemical or enzymatic techniques. The immunochemical measurements of lysozyme may be more specific than the commonly employed measurements of bacterial lysis.

2. Cerebrospinal fluid proteins

Determinations of proteins in cerebrospinal fluid (CSF) are usually performed with electrophoresis of concentrated CSF and quantitative evaluation by densitometry or merely by visual inspection. In recent years immunochemical determinations of single proteins in CSF and plasma have also come into use.

The so-called blood–brain barrier gives a marked protein concentration gradient between plasma and CSF. The ease with which a plasma protein can pass from plasma to cerebrospinal fluid is generally dependent on its molecular size. Thus the distribution of protein in cerebrospinal fluid is somewhat different from that of plasma. While the concentration of albumin is roughly the same as that in plasma, proteins with higher molecular weights are present at lower concentrations. Certain proteins do not conform to this generalization. Thus, transferrin and especially prealbumin (TBPA) are present in cerebrospinal fluid at higher concentrations than would be expected from their molecular size. Prealbumin constitutes at least 5 per cent of the total protein in cerebrospinal fluid. The electrophoretic behaviour of prealbumin and especially of transferrin in cerebrospinal fluid are different from that of the corresponding proteins in plasma. Apart from the apparently normal transferrin, a transferrin component (τ-fraction) which has a lower mobility, can also be detected in CSF. The prealbumin in CSF has a slightly different mobility compared to plasma. The cause of these differences is not known. Certain low molecular weight proteins such as β-trace protein and γ-trace protein are present in CSF at concentrations which are considerably higher than those of the corresponding proteins in plasma.

There is often an increased passage of plasma proteins into cerebrospinal fluid in diseases of the central nervous system or of the membranes of the brain giving rise to

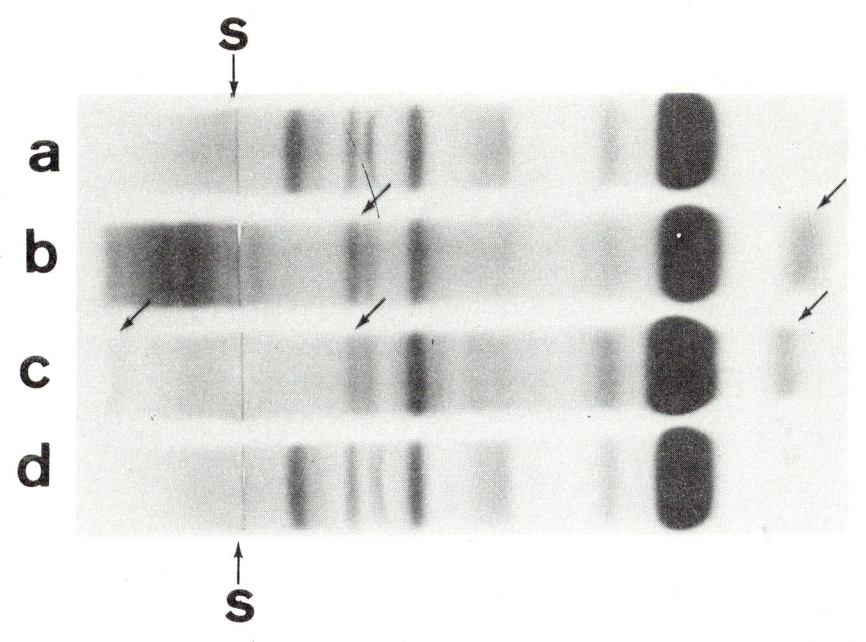

XIII. *Analysis of proteins in body fluids other than blood* 369

Fig. 158. Agarose electrophoresis of plasma (a) and cerebrospinal fluid (b) from a patient having multiple sclerosis and oligoclonal production of immunoglobulin. The normal protein pattern of cerebrospinal fluid is shown in (c) and that of plasma from the same individual in (d). Apart from the Ig pattern, note should be made of the distinct prealbumin band and the so called τ-fraction (b, c) and the weak band in (c), γ-trace protein, which is not caused by the immunoglobulins. The position of sample application is indicated by 'S'

inflammatory reactions or circulation disorders. This causes an increase in the concentration of total protein in CSF with an electrophoretic pattern which more resembles that of plasma. By determination of individual proteins in plasma and CSF, it has been shown that the ratio of the concentration of various proteins in plasma to that in CSF is correlated to the total protein concentration in CSF.

Thus, the information which can be obtained from the electrophoresis of cerebrospinal fluid and/or the quantitative determination of individual plasma protein components generally provides no more information than that obtained by simply determining the total protein content. The electrophoretic assay of the immunoglobins especially IgG, is an important exception. An increased local synthesis of IgG occurs in meningoencephalitis, tuberculous meningitis, syphilis, multiple sclerosis, and in some rare conditions such as subacute sclerosing panencephalitis (SSLE). The local synthesis is most often observed as an oligoclonal IgG pattern with distinct bands in agarose gel electrophoresis (Fig. 158). The possibility that the bands are due to a transfer of oligoclonal igG from plasma can be eliminated by performing a simultaneous protein electrophoresis of the patient's plasma. Oligoclonal IgG can be seen in 90 per cent of the cases of multiple sclerosis but it is not known how early the oligoclonal IgG appears in these cases. Oligoclonal IgG is present in the cerebrospinal fluid of less than half of those cases of primary opticus neuritis which can be suspected of later developing into multiple sclerosis.

The electrophoretic examination of cerebrospinal fluid on agarose gels requires a relatively large volume of this fluid which must be concentrated to 1/200 of its original volume before it can be used for analysis. An alternative and apparently simpler approach to the demonstration of locally produced IgG involves the quantitative immunochemical assay of CSF-IgG which, in these cases, is increased in comparison to the total protein concentration or the level of albumin. The levels of IgG and albumin in plasma are also assayed to correct for the influence of plasma levels of these two proteins. The local synthesis of IgG can be distinguished from an increase in the level of IgG resulting from leakage from plasma, occurring in inflammatory reactions, by comparing the fractions CSF-Ig/P-Ig and CSF-Alb/P-Alb, (P=plasma). If local IgG synthesis occurs the ratio CSF-IgG/P-IgG is elevated to a higher extent than the corresponding albumin ratio.

References

KAI O. PEDERSEN (1–15)

A Manual of Quantitative Immunoelectrophoresis. Methods and Applications. Ed. N. H. Axelsen, J. Kröll and B. Weeke. Universitets-förlaget, Oslo, Bergen, Tromsö (1973).
CLAESSON, S. and PEDERSEN, K. O.: The Svedberg 1884–1971. *Biographical Memoirs of Fellows of the Royal Society,* **18** (1972) p. 595.
Electrophoresis. Theory, Methods and Applications. Ed. M. Bier. Academic Press, New York (1959).
HARROW, B.: Emil Fischer. In: *Eminent Chemists of Our Time.* D. van Nostrand Company, New York (1920) p. 217.
HEIDELBERGER, M.: *Lectures in Immunochemistry.* Academic Press, New York (1956).
KEKWICK, R. A. and PEDERSEN, K. O.: Arne Tiselius 1902–1971. *Biographical Memoirs of Fellows of the Royal Society,* **20** (1974) p. 401.
MARTIN, A. J. P.: The principles of chromatography. *Endeavour,* **6** (1947) p. 21.
SCHULTZE, H. E. and HEREMANS, J. F.: *Molecular Biology of Human Protein with Special Reference to Plasma Proteins.* Elsevier Publishing Company, Amsterdam 1 (1966).
TISELIUS, A. Some recent advances in chromatography. *Endeavour* 11 (1952) p. 5.
TISELIUS, A., PORATH, J. and ALBERTSON, P. Å.: Separation and fractionation of macromolecules and particles. *Science,* **141** (1963) p. 13.

LARS-OLOV ANDERSSON and RAGNAR LUNDÉN (17–21)

KAWAI, T.: *Clinical Aspects of the Plasma Proteins.* Springer Verlag, Igaku Shoin Ltd., Tokyo (1973).
PUTNAM, F. W. (ed.): *The Plasma Proteins,* Academic Press, New York I–III (1975–77).
SCHULZE, H. E. and HEREMANS, J. F.: *Molecular Biology of Human Proteins.* Elsevier, Amsterdam, London, New York 1 (1969).
TURNER, M. W. and HULME, B.: *The Plasma Proteins.* Pitman Medical and Scientific Publishing Co. Ltd., London (1971).

JOHANNES A. G. RHODIN (23–27)

Capillary Permeability. Ed. C. Crone and N. A. Larson. Alfred Benson Symposium II. Academic Press, New York (1970).
RHODIN, J. A. G.: Ultrastructure of the microvascular bed. In: *The Microcirculation in Clinical Medicine.* Ed. R. Wells. Academic Press, New York (1973).
ZWEIFACH, B. W.: Microcirculation. *Ann. Rev. Physiol.,* **35** (1973) p. 117.

HENRIK BJÖRLING (29–37)

ANDRASSY, K., RITZ, E. and SANWALD, R.: Australia-Antigen-Nachweis in Fibrinogenkonzentraten und anderen gerinnungsaktiven Proteinen. *Dtsch. Med. Wochenschr.,* **95** (1970) p. 2467.

BARANDUN, S., KISTLER, P., JEUNET, F. and ISLIKER, H.: Intravenous administration of human γ-globulin. *Vox Sang.*, **7** (1962) p. 157.

BERG, R., BJÖRLING, H., BERNTSEN, K. and ESPMARK, Å.: Recovery of Australian antigen from human plasma products separated by a modified Cohn fractionation. *Vox Sang.*, **22** (1972) p.1.

BJÖRLING, H.: Concentration and purification of ceruloplasmin from human blood plasma fractions. *Vox Sang.*, **8** (1963) p. 641.

BLOMBÄCK, M.: Purification of antihemophilic globulin. I. Some studies on the stability of the antihemophilic globulin activity in fraction I-0 and a method for its partial separation from fibrinogen. *Ark. Kemi*, **12** (1958) p. 387.

COHN, E. J., STRONG, L. E., HUGHES, W. L. Jr, MULFORD, D. J., ASHWORTH, J. N., MELIN, M. and TAYLOR, H. L.: Preparation and properties of serum and plasma proteins. IV. A system for the separation into fractions of the protein and lipoprotein components of biological tissues and fluids. *J. Am. Chem. Soc.*, **68** (1946) p. 459.

COHN, E. J., GURD, F. R. N., SURGENOR, D. M., BARNES, B. A., BROWN, R. K., DEROAUX, G., GILLESPIE, J. M., KAHNT, F. W., LEVER, W. F., LIU, C. H., MITTELMAN, D., MOUTON, R. F., SCHMID, K. and UROMA, E.: A system for the separation of the components of human blood: Quantitative procedures for the separation of the protein components of human plasma. *J. Am. Chem. Soc.*, **72** (1950) p. 465.

DEUTSCH, H. F., GOSTING, L. J., ALBERTY, R. A. and WILLIAMS, J. W.: Biophysical studies of blood plasma proteins. III. Recovery of γ-globulin from human blood protein mixtures. *J. Biol. Chem.*, **164** (1946) p. 109.

DEUTSCH, D. G. and MERTZ, E. T.: Plasminogen: purification from human plasma by affinity chromatography. *Science*, **170** (1970) p. 1095.

ONCLEY, J. L., MELIN, M., RICHERT, D. A., CAMERON, J. W. and GROSS, P. M. Jr: The separation of the antibodies, isoagglutinins, prothrombin, plasminogen and β-lipoprotein into subfractions of human plasma. *J. Am. Chem. Soc.*, **71** (1949) p. 541.

POOL, J. G. and SHANNON, A. E.: Production of high-potency concentrates of antihemophilic globulin in a closed-bag system. Assay *in vitro* and *in vivo*. *New Engl. J. Med.*, **273** (1965) p. 1443.

SCHMID, K.: Preparation and properties of serum and plasma proteins. XXIX. Separation from human plasma of polysaccharides, peptides and proteins of low molecular weight. Crystallization of an acid glycoprotein. *J. Am. Chem. Soc.*, **75** (1953) p. 60.

SCHULTZE, H. E. and SCHWICK, G.: Über neue Möglichkeiten intravenöser Gammaglobulin-Applikation. *Dtsch. Med. Wochenschr.*, **87** (1962) p. 1643.

SGOURIS, J. T.: The preparation of plasmin treated immune serum globulin for intravenous use. *Vox Sang.*, **13** (1967) p. 71.

STEFÁNSSON, M., AAGESEN, G., LUNDSTRÖM, R. and ROSANDER, G.: Gamma globulin solution for intravenous administration. *Scand. J. Infect. Dis.* **4** (1972) p. 53.

STEFÁNSSON, M. and LUNDSTRÖM, R.: Intravenous administration of non-dissociated gamma globulin in infectous diseases. *VI. International congress of infections and parasitic diseases. Warszawa*, **3** (1974) p. 370.

WIMAN, B. and WALLEN, P.: Activation of human plasminogen by an insoluble derivative or urokinase. Structural changes of plasminogen in the course of activation to plasmin and demonstration of a possible intermediate compound. *Eur. J. Biochem.*, **36** (1973) p. 25.

HUGO NIHLÉN (37–41)

Chromatography, Electrophoresis and Membrane Technology. Bio-Rad Laboratories, Richmond, California, USA. Catalogue Z (1974–1975).

CUATRECASAS, P. and ANFINSEN, C. B.: Affinity chromatography. *Ann. Revue Biochem.*, **40** (1971) p. 259.

DIETZEL, E. and GEIGER, H.: Gewinnung und Eigenschaften therapeutisch wichtiger human Plasma Proteine. *Behringwerke Mitteilungen*, **43** (1964) p. 129.

EDSALL, J. T.: The plasma proteins and their fractionation. *Advances in Protein Chemistry*, **3** (1947) p. 383.

FISCHER, L.: *Introduction to Gel Chromatography. Laboratory Techniques in Biochemistry and Molecular Biology*. North Holland Publications, Amsterdam, London 1:2 (1969).
HOŘEJŠI, A. and SMETANA, R.: The isolation of γ-globulin by Rivanol. *Acta Med. Scand.*, **155** (1965) p. 65.
KECKWICK, R. A.: *Medical Research Council Report Series No 286*. Her Majesty's Stationery Office (1954).
PETERSON, E.: *Cellulosic Ion Exchangers, Laboratory Techniques in Biochemistry and Molecular Biology*. North Holland Publications, Amsterdam, London 2:2 (1970).
POLSON, A. POTGIETER, G. M. LARGIER, J. F., MEARS, G. E. F. and JOUBERT F. G.: The fractionation of protein mixtures by linear polymers of high molecular weight. *Biochem. Biophys. Acta*, **82** (1964) p. 463.
POLSON, A. and RUIZ-BRAVO, C.: Fractionation of plasma with polyethylenglycol. *Vox Sang.*, **23** (1972) p. 107.
SCHWICK, H. G.: A survey of the production of plasma derivatives for clinical use. *Vox Sang.*, **23** (1972) p. 82.
Sephadex, Gel Filtration in Theory and Practice. Pharmacia Fine Chemicals, Uppsala 1 (1973).
STEINBUCH, M.: Precipitation methods in plasma fractionation. *Vox Sang.*, **23** (1972) p. 92.

LARS-OLOV ANDERSSON (43–54)

ANDERSSON, L.-O.: The heterogeneity of bovine serum albumin. *Biochim. Biophys. Acta*, **117** (1066) p. 115.
ANDERSSON, L.-O.: Reduction and reoxidation of the disulfide bonds of bovine serum albumin. *Arch. Biochem. Biophys.*, **133** (1969) p. 277.
ANDERSSON, L.-O., BRANDT, J. and JOHANSSON, S.: The use of trinitrobenzenesulfonic acid in studies on the binding of fatty acid anions to bovine serum albumin. *Arch. Biochem. Biophys.*, **146** (1971b) p. 428.
ANDERSON, L.-O., REHNSTRÖM, A. and EAKER, D. L.: Studies on "nonspecific" binding. The nature of the binding of fluorescein to bovine serum albumin. *Eur. J. Biochem.*, **20** (1971a) p. 371.
BJERRUM, O. J.: Interaction of bromphenol blue and bilirubin with bovine and human serum albumin determined by gel filtration. *Scand. J. Clin. Lab. Invest.*, **22** (1968) p. 41.
BRADSHAW, R. A. and PETERS, T. Jr: The amino acid sequence of peptide (1–24) of rat and human serum albumins. *J. Biol. Chem.*, **244** (1969) p. 5582.
BRADSHAW, R. A., SHEARER, W. T. and GURD, F. R. N.: Sites of binding of copper (II) ion by peptide (1–24) of bovine serum albumin. *J. Biol. Chem.*, **243** (1968) p. 3817.
BROWN, J. R., LOW, T., BEHERNS, P., SEPULVEDA, P., PARKER, K. and BLAKENEY, E.: Amino acid sequence of bovine and porcine serum albumin. *Fed. Proc.*, **30** (1971) p. 1241.
CHEN, R. F.: Removal of fatty acids from serum albumin by charcoal treatment. *J. Biol. Chem.*, **242** (1967) p. 173.
DOUMAS, B. T., WATSON, W. A. and BIGGS, H. G.: Albumin standards and the measurement of serum albumin with bromcresol green. *Clin. Chim. Acta*, **31** (1971) p. 87.
FOSTER, J. F.: Plasma albumin. In: *The Plasma Proteins*. Ed. F. W. Putnam. Academic Press, New York 1 (1960) p. 179.
FOSTER, J. F., SOGAMI, M., PETERSEN, H. A. and LEONARD, W. J. Jr: The microheterogeneity of plasma albumins. I. Critical evidence for and description of the microheterogeneity model. *J. Biol. Chem.*, **240** (1965) p. 2495.
GOODMAN, D. S.: The interaction of human serum albumin with long-chain fatty acid anions. *J. Am. Chem. Soc.*, **80** (1958) p. 3892.
HUGHES, W. L. and DINTZIS, H. M.: Crystallization of the mercury dimers of human and bovine mercaptalbumin. *J. Biol. Chem.*, **239** (1964) p. 845.
JANATOVA, J., FULLER, J. K. and HUNTER, M. J.: The heterogeneity of bovine albumin with respect to sulfhydryl and dimer content. *J. Biol. Chem.*, **243** (1968) p. 3612.
KARUSH, F.: The role of disulfide bonds in the acquisition of immunologic specificity. *J. Pediat.*, **60** (1962) p. 103.

KING, T. P.: On the sulfhydryl group of human plasma albumin. *J. Biol. Chem.*, **236** (1961) p. PC5.
KING, T. P. and SPENCER, M.: Structural studies and organic ligand-binding properties of bovine plasma albumin. *J. Biol. Chem.*, **245** (1970) p. 6134.
KING, T. P. and SPENCER, E. M.: Amino acid sequences of the amino and the carboxyl terminal cyanogen bromide peptides of bovine plasma albumin. *Arch. Biochem. Biophys.*, **153** (1972) p. 627.
MCMENAMY, R. H. and LEE, Y.: Microheterogeneity in albumin: a contaminant. *Arch. Biochem. Biophys.*, **122** (1967) p. 635.
NIKKEL, H. J. and FOSTER, J. F.: A reversible sulfhydryl-catalyzed structural alteration of bovine mercaptalbumin. *Biochem.*, **10** (1971) p. 4479.
PEDERSEN, K. O.: Exclusion chromatography. *Arch. Biochem. Biophys.*, Suppl. 1 (1962) p. 157.
PETERS, T. Jr: Serum albumin. *Adv. Clin. Chem.*, **13** (1970) p. 37.
PETERSEN, H. A. and FOSTER, J. F.: The microheterogeneity of plasma albumins. II. Preparation and solubility properties of subfractions. *J. Biol. Chem.*, **240** (1965) p. 2503.
PETERSEN, H. A. and FOSTER, J. F.: The microheterogeneity of plasma albumins. III. Comparison of some physicochemical properties of subfractions. *J. Biol. Chem.*, **240** (1965) p. 3858.
PUTNAM, F. W.: Structure and function of plasma proteins. In: *The Proteins*. Ed. E. H. Neurath. Academic Press, New York 3 (1965) p. 153.
RODKEY, F. L.: Direct spectrophotometric determination of albumin in human serum. *Clin. Chem.*, **11** (1965) p. 478.
ROSSENEU-MOTREEF, M. Y., BLATON, V., DECLERQ, B. and PEETERS, H.: The contribution of bound fatty acids to the heterogeneity of BSA. In: *Protides of the Biological Fluids*. Ed. H. Peeters. Pergamon Press, Oxford 18 (1970) p. 503.
SALAMAN, M. R. and WILLIAMSON, A. R.: Isoelectric focusing of proteins in the native and denatured states. Anomalous behaviour of plasma albumin. *Biochem. J.*, **122** (1971) p. 93.
SPECTOR, A. A. and JOHN, K. M.: Effects of free fatty acid on the fluorescence of bovine serum albumin. *Arch. Biochem. Biophys.*, **127** (1968) p. 65.
SWANEY, J. B. and KLOTZ, I. M.: Amino acid sequence adjoining the long tryptophan of human serum albumin. A binding site of the protein. *Biochem.*, **9** (1970) p. 2570.
VALMET, E.: The heterogeneity of human serum albumin. In: *Protides of the Biological Fluids*. Ed. H. Peeters. Pergamon Press, Oxford 17 (1969) p. 443.
WATSON, D.: Albumin and 'total globulin' fractions of blood. *Adv. Clin. Chem.*, **8** (1965) p. 237.
WATSON, D.: Factors for calculating serum albumin and total protein from the nitrogen content. *Clin. Chim. Acta*, **16** (1967) p. 322.

GUNNAR BIRKE, STEN-OTTO LILJEDAHL and MARC ROTHSCHILD (54–71)

ANDERSEN, S. B. and JARNUM, S.: Gastrointestinal protein loss measured with ^{59}Fe-labelled iron-dextran, *Lancet*, **I** (1966) p. 1060.
BIRKE, G., JACOBSSON, F., LILJEDAHL, S.-O., PLANTIN, L.-O. and WETTERFORS, J.: Catabolism of albumin and gamma globulin after treatment with ionising radiation to the abdomen. *Acta Radiol. Ther. Phys. Biol.*, **6** (1967) p. 113.
BIRKE, G., ERICSSON, H., NORBERG, R., OLHAGEN, B., PLANTIN, L.-O. and WETTERFORS, J.: Proteinrubbningar och proteinterapi. *Läkartidningen*, **65** (1968) p. 4358.
BJØRNEBOE, M. and JARNUM, S.: The changes in serum proteins and blood volume during immunization. *J. Exp. Med.*, **113** (1961) p. 1005.
BRAUER, R. W.: Liver circulation and function. *Physiol. Rev.*, **43** (1963) p. 115.
COHEN, S. and HANSEN, J. D. L.: Metabolism of albumin and γ-globulin in kwashiorkor. *Clin. Sci.*, **23** (1962) p. 351.
DAVIES, J. W. L., LILJEDAHL, S.-O. and BIRKE, G.: Protein metabolism in burned patients treated in a warm (32°C) or cool (22°C) environment. *Injury*, **1** (1969) p. 43.
FREEMAN, T. and GORDON, A. H.: Metabolism of albumin and γ-globulin in protein deficient rats. *Clin. Sci.* **26** (1964) p. 17.

JENSEN, H., ROSSING, N., ANDERSEN, S. B. and JARNUM, S.: Albumin metabolism in the nephrotic syndrome in adults. *Clin. Sci.*, **33** (1967) p. 445.

KIRSCH, R., FRITH, L., BLACK, E. and HOFFENBERG, R.: Regulation of albumin synthesis and catabolism by alternation of dietary protein. *Nature*, **271** (1968) p. 578.

KOJ, A. and MCFARLANE, A. S.: Effect of endotoxin on plasma albumin and fibrinogen synthesis rates in rabbits as measured by the (^{14}C) carbonate method. *Biochem. J.*, **108** (1968) p. 137.

KUKRAL, J. C., KERTH, J. D., PANCNER, R. J., CROMER, D. W. and HENEGAR, G. C.: Plasma protein synthesis in the normal dog and after total hepatectomy. *Surg. Gynecol. Obstet.*, **113** (1961) p. 360.

LANDIS, E. M. and PAPENHEIMER, J. R.: Exchange of substances through the capillary walls. In: *Handbook of Physiology*. Sect. 2. Circulation. American Physiological Society 2 (1963) p. 961.

MCFARLANE, A. S.: Measurement of synthesis rates of liver produced plasma proteins. *Biochem. J.*, **89** (1963) p. 277.

MCFARLANE, A. S., TODD, D. and CROMWELL, S.: Fibrinogen catabolism in humans. *Clin. Sci*, **26** (1964) p. 415.

MILLER, L. L. and BALE, W. F.: Synthesis of all plasma protein fractions except gamma globulins by the liver. The use of zone electrophoresis and lysine-ε-C^{14} to define the plasma proteins synthesized by the isolated perfused liver. *J. Exp. Med.*, **99** (1954) p. 125.

MUNRO, H. N.: Evolution of protein metabolism in mammals. In: *Mammalian Protein Metabolism.* Ed. H. N. Munro. Academic Press, New York, London (1969) p. 133.

ORATZ, M., WALKER, C., SCHREIBER, S. S., GROSS, S. and ROTHSCHILD, M. A.: Albumin and fibrinogen metabolism in heat- and coldstressed rabbits. *Am. J. Physiol.*, **213** (1967) p. 1341.

REEVE, E. B. and CHEN, A. Y.: Regulation of interstitial albumin. In: *Plasma Protein Metabolism.* Ed. M. A. Rothschild and T. Waldmann. Academic Press, New York, London (1970) p. 89.

ROSENOER, V. M. and ROTHSCHILD, M. A.: The extravascular transport of albumin. In: *Plasma Protein Metabolism.* Ed. M. A. Rothschild and T. Waldmann. Academic Press, New York, London (1970) p. 111.

ROTHSCHILD, M. A., BAUMAN, A., YALOW, R. S. and BERSON, S. A.: The effect of large doses of dessicated thyroid on the distribution and metabolism of albumin–I^{131} in euthyroid subjects. *J. Clin. Invest.*, **36** (1957) p. 422.

ROTHSCHILD, M. A., ORATZ, M., EVANS, C. D. and SCHREIBER, S. S.: Role of hepatic interstitial albumin in regulating albumin synthesis. *Am. J. Physiol.*, **210** (1966) p. 57.

ROTHSCHILD, M. A., ORATZ, M., MONGELLI, J. and SCHREIBER, S. S.: Effects of a short-term fast on albumin synthesis studied *in vivo*, in the perfused liver, and on amino acid incorporation by hepatic microsomes. *J. Clin. Invest.*, **47** (1968) p. 2591.

ROTHSCHILD, M. A., ORATZ, M. and SCHREIBER, S. S.: Serum albumin. *Am. J. Dig. Dis.*, **14** (1969) p. 711.

SIDRANSKY, H., SARMA, D. S. R., BONGIORNO, M. and VERNEY, E.: Effect of dietary tryptophan on hepatic polyribosomes and protein synthesis in fasted mice. *J. Biol. Chem.*, **243** (1968) p. 1123.

STERNLIEB, I., MORELL, A. G., WOCHNER, R. D., AISEN, P. and WALDMANN, T. A.: Use of copper 67-labelled ceruloplasmin in the study of protein losing enteropathies. *Proc. Physiol. and Pathophysiol. of Plasma Protein Metabolism.* Proc 3rd Symp. held at Grindelwald, Switzerland, 1964. H. Huber, Bern, Stuttgart (1965) p. 34.

WASSERMAN, K. and MAYERSON, H. S.: Exchange of albumin between plasma and lymph. *Am. J. Physiol.*, **165** (1951) p. 15.

WETTERFORS, J.: Catabolism and distribution of serum-albumin in the dog. An experimental study with homologous ^{131}I-albumin. *Acta Med. Scand.*, **177** (1965) p. 243.

WILKINSON, P. and MENDELHALL, G. L.: Serum albumin turnover in normal subjects and patients with cirrhosis measured by ^{131}I-labelled human albumin. *Clin. Sci.*, **25** (1963) p. 281.

WILLIAMS, C. A. and GANOZA, M. C.: Identification of proteins made on microsomes and free ribosomes of rat liver. In: *Plasma Protein Metabolism.* Ed. M. A. Rothschild and T. Waldmann. Academic Press, New York, London (1970).

YOFFEY, J. M. and COURTICE, F. C.: Lymphatics, *Lymph and Lymphoid Tissue*. Edward Arnold, London (1956) p. 510.

GÖRAN CLAES (71-72)

BLOHMÉ, I. and CLAES, G.: Experimental studies on continuous perfusion for preservation. The 4th symposium on organ preservation. *Opuscula Medico-Technica Lundensia* XIV (1975) p. 9.

CLAES, G. and BLOHMÉ, I.: Clinical results of organ preservation in Gothenburg. The 4th symposium on organ preservation. *Opuscula Medico-Technica Lundensia* XIV (1975) p. 108.

ANDERS GUSTAFSON (72-94)

ALAUPOVIC, P.: Conceptual development of the classification systems of plasma lipoproteins. In: *Protides of the Biological Fluids.* 19th Coll. Proc. Bruges. 1971. Pergamon Press, Oxford (1972) p. 9.

BERG, K.: A new serum type system in man—the Lp system. *Acta Pathol Microbiol. Scand.*, **59** (1963) p. 369.

BILHEIMER, D. W., EISENBERG, S. and LEVY, R. I.: The metabolism of very low density lipoprotein proteins. In: *Preliminary in vitro and in vivo Observations. Biochim. Biophys. Acta,* **260** (1972) p. 212.

BJÖRNTORP, P., GUSTAFSON, A. and PERSSON, B.: Adipose tissue fat cell size and number in relation to metabolism in endogenous hypertriglyceridemia. *Acta Med. Scand.*, **190** (1971) p. 363.

BONDJERS, G., GUSTAFSON, A., KRAL, J., SCHERSTÉN, T., and SJÖSTRÖM, L.: Cholesterol content is arterial tissue in relation to serum lipoproteins in man. *Artery*, **2** (1976) p. 200.

BREWER, H. B. Jr, LUX, S. E., RONAN, R. and JOHN, K. M.: Amino acid sequence of human apoLp-Gln-II (apoA-II), an apolipoprotein isolated from the high-density lipoprotein complex. *Proc. Natl. Acad. Sci., USA*, **69** (1972a) p. 1304.

BREWER, H. B. Jr, SHULMAN, R., HERBERT, P., RONAN, R. and WEHRLY, K.: The complete amino acid sequence of an apolipoprotein obtained from human very low density lipoprotein (VLDL). *Adv. Exp. Med. Biol.*, **26** (1972b) p. 280.

BROWN, W. V., LEVY, R. I. and FREDRICKSON, D. S.: Further characterization of apolipoproteins from the human plasma very low density lipoproteins. *J. Biol. Chem.*, **245** (1970) p. 6588.

CAHLIN, E., JÖNSSON, J., PERSSON, B., STAKEBERG, H., BJÖRNTORP, P., GUSTAFSON, A. and SCHERSTÉN, T.: Sucrose feeding in man. Effects on substrate incorporation into hepatic triglycerides and phosphoglycerides *in vitro* and on removal of intravenous fat in patients with hyperlipoproteinemia. *Scand. J. Clin. Lab. Invest.*, **32** (1973) p. 21.

DAHLÉN, G. and ERICSON, C.: A new lipoprotein pattern in patients with angina pectoris. *Scand. J. Clin. Lab. Invest. Suppl.*, **118** (1971) p. 54.

ELLEFSON, R. D., JIMENEZ, B. J. and SMITH, R. C.: Pre-β (or α_2) lipoprotein of high density in human blood. *Mayo Clin. Proc.*, **46** (1971) p. 328.

FIELDING, C. J., SHORE, V. G. and FIELDING, P. E.: A protein cofactor of lecithin: cholesterol acyltransferase. *Biochem. Biophys. Res. Commun.*, **46** (1972) p. 1493.

GANESAN, D., BRADFORD, R. H., ALAUPOVIC, P. and McCONATHY, W. J.: Differential activation of lipoprotein lipase from human post-heparin plasma, milk and adipose tissue by polypeptides of human-serum apolipoprotein C. *FEBS Lett-*15 (1971) p. 205.

GLOMSET, J. A.: The plasma lecithin: cholesterol acyltransferase reaction. *J. Lipid Res.*, **9** (1968) p. 155.

GOFMAN, J. W., DeLALLA, O., GLAZIER, F., FREEMAN, K., LINDGREN, F. T., NICHOLS, A. V., STRISOWER, E. H. and TAMPLIN, A. R.: The serum lipoprotein transport system in health, metabolic disorders, atherosclerosis and coronary heart disease. *Plasma*, **2** (1954) p. 413.

GUSTAFSON, A.: Effect of training on blood lipids. In: *Coronary Heart Disease and Physical Fitness.* Ed. O. Andrée Larsen and R. O. Malmborg. Munksgaard, Köpenhamn (1971) p. 125.

GUSTAFSON, A., ALAUPOVIC, P. and FURMAN, R. H.: Studies of the composition and structure of serum lipoproteins: isolation, purification, and characterization of very low density lipoproteins of human serum. *Biochem.*, **4** (1965) p. 596.

GUSTAFSON, A., ELMFELDT, D., WILHELMSEN, L. and TIBBLIN, G.: Serum lipids and lipoproteins in men after myocardial infarction compared with representative population sample. *Circulation*, **46** (1972) p. 709.

HAMILTON, R. L., REGEN, D. M., GRAY, M. E. and LeQUIRE, V. S.: Lipid transport in liver. I. Electron microscopic identification of very low density lipoproteins in perfused rat liver. *Lab. Invest.*, **16** (1967) p. 305.

HAVEL, R. J. and KANE, J. P.: Primary dysbetalipoproteinemia: predominance of a specific apoprotein species in triglyceriderich lipoproteins. *Proc. Natl. Acad. Sci., USA*, **70** (1973) p. 2015.

HAZZARD, W. R., GOLDSTEIN, J. L., SCHROTT, H. G., MOTULSKY, A. G. and BIERMAN, E. L.: Hyperlipidemia in coronary heart disease. III. Evaluation of lipoprotein phenotypes of 156 genetically defined survivors of myocardial infarction. *J. Clin. Invest.*, **52** (1973) p. 1569.

KOSTNER, G. and HOLASEK, A.: Characterization and quantitation of the apolipoproteins from human chyle chylomicrons. *Biochem.*, **11** (1972) p. 1217.

KOSTNER, G. M.: Studies of the composition and structure of human serum lipoproteins. Isolation and partial characterization of apolipoprotein AIII. *Biochem. Biophys. Acta*, **336** (1974) p. 383.

LANGER, T., STROBER, W. and LEVY, R. I.: The metabolism of low density lipoprotein in familial type II hyperlipoproteinemia. *J. Clin. Invest.*, **51** (1972) p. 1528.

LEE, D. M. and ALAUPOVIC, P.: Studies of the composition and structure of plasma lipoproteins. Isolation, composition, and immunochemical characterization of low density lipoprotein subfractions of human plasma. *Biochem.*, **9** (1970) p. 2244.

LINDESKOG, G. R., GUSTAFSON, A. and ENERBÄCK, L.: Serum lipoprotein deficiency in diffuse 'normolipemic' plane xanthoma. *Arch. Dermatol.*, **106** (1972) p. 529.

LUX, S. E., LEVY, R. I., GOTTO, A. M. and FREDRICKSON, D. S.: Studies on the protein defect in Tangier disease. Isolation and characterization of an abnormal high density lipoprotein. *J. Clin. Invest.*, **51** (1972) p. 2505.

NILSSON, S.: Synthesis and secretion of biliary phospholipids in man. An experimental study with special reference to the relevance for gallstone formation. *Acta Chir. Scand. Suppl.*, **405** (1970) p. 38.

NORUM, K. R., GLOMSET, J. A., NICHOLS, A. V. and FORTE, T.: Plasma lipoproteins in familial lecithin: cholesterol acyltransferase deficiency: physical and chemical studies of low and high density lipoproteins. *J. Clin. Invest.*, **50** (1971) p. 1131.

POLLARD, H., SCANU, A. M. and TAYLOR, E. W.: On the geometrical arrangement of the protein subunits of human serum low-density lipoprotein: evidence for a dodecahedral model. *Proc. Natl. Acad. Sci., USA*, **64** (1969) p. 304.

QUARFORDT, S., LEVY, R. I. and FREDRICKSON, D. S.: On the lipoprotein abnormality in type III hyperlipoproteinemia. *J. Clin. Invest.*, **50** (1971) p. 754.

RIDER, A. K., LEVY, R. I. and FREDRICKSON, D. S.: 'Sinking' prebeta lipoprotein and the Lp antigen. *Circulation*, **42**, Suppl. 3 (1970) p. 10.

RUDMAN, D., GARCIA, L. A. and HOWARD, C. H.: A new method for isolating the nonidentical protein subunits of human plasma α-lipoprotein. *J. Clin. Invest.* **49** (1970) p. 365.

SCANU, A. M.: Structural studies on serum lipoproteins. *Biochim. Biophys. Acta*, **265** (1972) p. 471.

SCANU, A. M., TOTH, J., EDELSTEIN, C., KOGA, S. and STILLER, E.: Fractionation of human serum density lipoprotein in urea solutions. Evidence for polypeptide heterogeneity. *Biochem.*, **8** (1969) p. 3309.

SCHUMAKER, V. N. and ADAMS, G. H.: Circulating lipoproteins. *Ann. Rev. Biochem.*, **38** (1969) p. 113.

SCOW, R. O., HAMOSH, M., BLANCHETTEMACKIE, E. J. and EVANS, A. J.: Uptake of blood triglyceride by various tissues. *Lipids*, **7** (1972) p. 497.

SEIDEL, D., ALAUPOVIC, P. and FURMAN, R. H.: A lipoprotein characterizing obstructive jaundice. I. Method for quantitative separation and identification of lipoproteins in jaundiced subjects. *J. Clin. Invest.*, **48** (1969) p. 1211.

SIMONS, K., EHNHOLM, C., RENKONEN, O. and BLOTH, B.: Characterization of the Lp(a) lipoprotein in human plasma. *Acta Pathol. Microbiol. Scand. Sect. B.*, **78** (1970) p. 459.

SMITH, U.: Personal communication.
STANBURY, J. B., WYNGAARDEN, J. B. and FREDRICKSON, D. S.: *The Metabolic Basis of Inherited Disease*, McGraw-Hill, New York (1972).
WIKLUND, O., GUSTAFSON, A. and WILHELMSEN, L.: α-Lipoprotein cholesterol in men after myocardial infarction compared with a population sample. *Artery*, 1 (1975) p. 399.

GITTEN CEDERBLAD (94–96)

ASHWELL, G. and MORELL, A. G.: The role of surface carbohydrates in the hepatic recognition and transport of circulating glycoproteins. *Adv. Enzymol.*, 41 (1974) p. 99.
BOCCI, V.: Metabolism of plasma proteins. *Arch. Fisiol.*, 67 (1970) p. 314.
FREEMAN, T.: The function of plasma proteins. In: *Protides of the Biological Fluids*. Proc. 15th Coll. Bruges. Ed. H. Peeters, Elsevier. Amsterdam (1968) p. 1.
WEEKE, B.: *Humane serumproteiner identificeret og kvantiteret med Laurell's immunelektroforeser*. Kopenhamn (1973) p. 155.

GITTEN CEDERBLAD (96–99)

EVANS, G. W.: Copper homeostasis in the mammalian system. *Physiol. Rev.*, 53 (1973) p. 535.
FREEMAN, S. and DANIEL, E.: Dissociation and reconstitution of human ceruloplasmin. *Biochem.*, 12 (1973) p. 4806.
HSIEH, H. S. and FRIEDEN, E.: Evidence for ceruloplasmin as a copper transport protein. *Biochem. Biophys. Res. Comm.*, 67 (1975) p. 1326.
HOLMBERG, C. G. and LAURELL, C.-B.: Investigations in serum copper. II. Isolation of the copper containing protein, and a description of some of its properties. *Acta Chem. Scand.*, 2 (1948) p. 550.
HOLTZMAN, N. A. and GAUMNITZ, B. M.: Studies on the rate of release and turnover of ceruloplasmin and apoceruloplasmin in rat plasma. *J. Biol. Chem.*, 245 (1970) p. 2354.
JAMIESON, G. A.: Studies on glycoproteins. I. The carbohydrate portion of human ceruloplasmin. *J. Biol. Chem.*, 240 (1965) p. 2019.
LØWENSTEIN, H.: Immunochemical investigation on human ceruloplasmin. Partial explanation of the 'heterogeneity'. *Int. J. Peptide Protein Res.*, 7 (1975) p. 1.
MARCEAU, N. and ASPIN, N.: Distribution of ceruloplasmin-bound ^{67}Cu in the rat. *Am. J. Physiol.*, 222 (1972) p. 106.
MØLLEKAER, A. M. and RESKE-NIELSEN, E.: Case report. Kinky hair syndrome. *Acta Paediat. Scand.*, 63 (1974) p. 289.
RYDÉN, L.: Single-chain structure of human ceruloplasmin. *Eur. J. Biochem.*, 26 (1972) p. 380.
RYDÉN, L. and EAKER, D.: The amino-acid sequences of three tryptic glycopeptides from human ceruloplasmin. *Eur. J. Biochm.*, 44 (1974) p. 171.
SIMONS, K. and BEARN, A. G.: Isolation and partial characterization of the polypeptide chains in human ceruloplasmin. *Biochim. Biophys. Acta*, 175 (1969) p. 260.

GITTEN CEDERBLAD (99–102)

AISEN, PH., LEIBMAN, A., PINKOWITZ, R. A. and POLLACK, S.: Exchangeability of bicarbonate specifically bound to transferrin. *Biochem.*, 12 (1973a) p. 3679.
AISEN, PH. and LEIBMAN, A.: The role of the anion-binding site of transferrin in its interaction with the reticulocyte. *Biochim. Biophys. Acta*, 304 (1973b) p. 797.
BROWN, E. B., OKADA, S., AWAI, M. and CHIPMAN, B.: *In vivo* evidence for the functional heterogeneity of transferrin-bound iron. III. Studies of transferrin at high and low iron saturation. *J. Lab. Clin. Med.*, 86 (1975) p. 576.
BULLEN, J. J., ROGERS, H. J. and GRIFFITHS, E.: Iron binding proteins and infection. *Br. J. Haematol.*, 23 (1972) p. 389.

FLETCHER, J.: Iron transport in the blood. *Proc. R. Soc. Med.*, **63** (1970) p. 1216.
FLETCHER, J. and HUEHNS, E. R.: Function of transferrin. *Nature*, **218** (1968) p. 1211.
FRIEDEN, E.: The ferrous to ferric cycles in iron metabolism. *Nutr. Rev.*, **31** (1973) p. 41.
HAHN, D. and GANZONI, A. M.: Functional heterogeneity of the transport iron compartment. **Acta Haemat., 53** (1975) p. 321.
HARRIS, D. C. and AISEN, P.: Functional equivalence of the two iron-binding sites of human transferrin. *Nature*, **257** (1975) p. 821.
HEILMEYER, L., KELLER, W., VIVELL, O., KEIDERLING, W., BETKE, K., WÖHLER, F. and SCHULTZE, H. E.: Kongenitale Atransferrinämie bei einem sieben Jahre alten Kind. *Dtsch. Med. Wochenschr.*, **86** (1961) p. 1745.
JAMIESON, G. A., JETT, M. and DEBERNARDO, S. L.: The carbohydrate sequence of the glycopeptide chains of human transferrin. *J. Biol. Chem.*, **246**, (1971) p. 3686.
LANE, R. S.: Transferrin-reticulocyte binding: Evidence for the function importance of transferrin conformation. *Br. J. Haematol.*, **22** (1972) p. 309.
LEVINE, P. H., LEVINE, A. J. and WEINTRAUB, L. R.: The role of transferrin in the control of iron absorption: Studies on a cellular level. *J. Lab. Clin. Med.*, **80** (1972) p. 333.
MANN, K. G., FISH, W. W., COX, A. CH. and TANFORD, C. H.: Single-chain nature of human serum transferrin. *Biochem.*, **9** (1970) p. 1348.
PALMOUR, R. M. and SUTTON, H. E.: Vertebrate transferrins. Molecular weights, chemical composition, and iron-binding studies. *Biochem.*, **10** (1971) p. 4926.
SPIK, G., BAYARD, B., FOURNET, B., STRECKER, G., BOUQUELET, S. and MONTREUIL, J.: Studies on glycoconjugates. LXIV. Complete structure of two carbohydrate units of human serotransferrin. *FEBS Lett.*, **50** (1975) p. 296.
SULLIVAN, A. L., GRASSO, J. A. and WEINTRAUB, L. R.: Micropinocytosis of transferrin by developing red cells: An electron-microscopic study utilizing ferritin-conjugated transferrin and ferritin-conjugated antibodies to transferrin. *Blood*, **47** (1976) p. 133.
SUTTON, M. R., MACGILLIVRAY, R. T. A. and BREW, K.: The amino-acid sequences of three cystine-free cyanogen-bromide fragments of human serum transferrin. *Eur. J. Biochem.*, **51** (1975) p. 43.

GITTEN CEDERBLAD (102–106)

BARNETT, D. R., LEE, T.-H. and BOWMAN, B. H.: Amino acid sequence of the human haptoglobin β chain. I. Amino- and carboxyl-terminal sequences. *Biochem.*, **11** (1972) p. 1189.
BLACK, J. A. and DIXON, G. H.: Amino-acid sequence of alpha chains of human haptoglobins. *Nature*, **218** (1968) p. 736.
CHIAO, M. T. and BEZKOROVAINY, A.: Interaction of modified haptoglobin with hemoglobin. *Biochim. Biophys. Acta*, **263** (1972) p. 60.
FREEMAN, T.: Haptoglobin metabolism in relation to red cell destruction. In: *Protides of the Biological Fluids*, Proc. 12th Coll. Bruges. Ed. H. Peeters. Elseviér, Amsterdam (1965) p. 344.
FULLER, G. M., RASCO, M. A., MCCOMBS, M. L., BARNETT, D. R. and BOWMAN, B. H.: Subunit composition of haptoglobin 2-2 polymers. *Biochem.*, **12** (1973) p. 253.
GERBECK, C. M., BEZKOROVAINY, A. and RAFELSON, M. E. Jr: Glycopeptides obtained from human haptoglobin 2-1 and 2-2. *Biochem.*, **6** (1967) p. 403.
HERSHKO, C., COOK, J. D. and FINCH, C. A.: Storage iron kinetics. II. The upptake of hemoglobin iron by hepatic parenchymal cells. *J. Lab. Clin. Med.*, **80** (1972) p. 624.
JAVID, J. and LIANG, J. C.: The hemoglobin–haptoglobin bond. 1. Dissociation of the complex and recovery of the native haptoglobin in an affinity chromatography system. *J. Lab. Clin. Med.*, **82** (1973) p. 991.
KIRK, R. L.: The haptoglobin groups in man. In: *Monographs in Human Genetics*. Ed. L. Beckman and M. Harge, Karger, Basel (1968).
MAKINEN, M. W., MILSTIEN, J. B. and KON, H.: Specificity of interaction of haptoglobin with mammalian hemoglobin. *Biochem.*, **11** (1972) p. 3851.
MALCHY, B., RORSTAD, O. DIXON, G. H.: The half-molecule of haptoglobin: studies on the

obtained by the selective cleavage of a haptoglobin disulfide. *Can. J. Biochem.*, **51** p. 265.
R. L. & GIBSON, Q. H.: The binding of hemoglobin to haptoglobin and its relation to subunit dissociation of hemoglobin. *J. Biol. Chem.*, **246** (1971) p. 69.
SMITHIES, O., CONNELL, G. E. and DIXON, G. H.: Gene action in the human haptoglobins. I. Dissociation into constituent polypeptide chains. *J. Mol. Biol.*, 21 (1966) p. 213.

GITTEN CEDERBLAD (106–109)

LANE, R. S., RANGELEY, D. M., LIEM, H. H., WORMSLEY, S. and MULLER-EBERHARD, U.: Plasma clearance of ^{125}I-labelled haemopexin in normal and haem-loaded rabbits. *Br. J. Haematol.*, **25** (1973) p. 533.
MULLER-EBERHARD, U.: Hemopexin. *New Engl. J. Med.*, **283** (1970) p. 1090.
SCHULTZE, H. E., HEIDE, K. and HAUPT, H.: Charakterisierung von hochgereinigtem Hämopexin, *Naturwissenschaften*, **48** (1961) p. 696.
SEARS, D. A.: Disposal of plasma heme in normal man and patients with intravascular hemolysis. *J. Clin. Invest.*, **49** (1970) p. 5.
SEERY, V. L. and MULLER-EBERHARD, U.: Binding of porphyrins to rabbit hemopexin and albumin. *J. Biol. Chem.*, **248** (1973) p. 3796.
SMIBERT, E., LIEM, H. H. and MULLER-EBERHARD, U.: Studies on the induction of serum hemopexin by pentobarbital and polycyclic hydrocarbons. *Biochem. Pharmacol.*, **21** (1972) p. 1753.

GITTEN CEDERBLAD (109–111)

ALLEN, R. H. and MAJERUS, PH. W.: Isolation of bitamin B_{12}-binding proteins using affinity chromatography. III. Purification and properties of human plasma transcobalamin II. *J. Biol. Chem.*, **247** (1972) p. 7709.
BURGER, R. L., MEHLMAN, C. S. and ALLEN, R. H.: Human plasma R-type vitamin B_{12}-binding proteins. *J. Biol. Chem.*, **250** (1975) p. 7700.
CARMEL, R. and HERBERT, V.: Deficiency of vitamin B_{12}-binding alpha globulin in two brothers. *Blood*, **33** (1969) p. 1.
GRÄSBECK, R.: Intrinsic factor and the other vitamin B_{12} transport proteins. *Prog. Hematol.*, **6** (1969) p. 233.
HAKAMI, N., NEIMAN, P. E., CANELLOS, G. P. and LAZERSON, J.: Neonatal megaloblastic anemia due to inherited transcobalamin II deficiency in two siblings. *New Engl. J. Med.*, **285** (1971) p. 1163.
HALL, C. A. and FINKLER, A. E.: Isolation and evaluation of the various B_{12} binding proteins in human plasma. In: *Methods in Enzymology*. Academic Press, New York, London 18 (1971) p. 108.
HOM, B. L. and OLESEN, H. A.: Plasma clearance of ^{57}cobalt-labelled vitamin B_{12} bound *in vitro* and *in vivo* to transcobalamin I and II. *Scand. J. Clin. Lab. Invest.*, **23** (1969) p. 201.
SCOTT, C. R., HAKAMI, N., TENG, C. C. and SAGERSON, R. N.: Hereditary transcobalamin II deficiency: The role of transcobalamin II in vitamin B_{12}-mediated reactions. *J. Pediat.*, **81** (1972) p. 1106.

GITTEN CEDERBLAD (111–113)

VAN JAARSVELD, P. P., EDELHOCH, H., GOODMAN, D. S. and ROBBINS, J.: The interaction of human plasma retinolbinding protein with prealbumin. *J. Biol. Chem.*, **248** (1973) p. 4698.
MORGAN, F. J., CANFIELD, R. E. and GOODMAN, D. S.: The partial structure of human plasma prealbumin and retinol-binding protein. *Biochim. Biophys. Acta*, **236** (1971) p. 798.
PETERSON, P. A., RASK, L., ÖSTBERG, L., ANDERSSON, L., KAMWENDA, F. and PETROFT, H., Studies on the transport and cellular distribution of vitamin A in normal and vitamin A-deficient rats with

special reference to the vitamin A-binding plasma protein. *J. Biol. Chem.*, **248** (1973) p. 4009.
VAHLQUIST, A., PETERSON, P. A. and WIBELL, L.: Metabolism of the vitamin A transporting protein complex. I. Turnover studies in normal persons and in patients with chronic renal failure. *Eur. J. Clin. Invest.*, **3** (1973) p. 352.

GITTEN CEDERBLAD (113-115)

DUSSAULT, J. H., FISHER, D. A., NICOLOFF, J. T., ROW, V. V. and VOLPE, R.: The effect of alteration of thyroxine binding capacity on the dialyzable and absolute fractions of triiodothyronine in circulation. *Acta Endocrinol.*, **72** (1973) p. 265.
MARSHALL, J. S. and PENSKY, J.: Studies on thyroxine-binding globulin (TBG). III. Some physical characteristics of TBG and its interaction with thyroxine. *Arch. Biochem. Biophys.* **146** (1971) p. 76.
MARSHALL, J. S., PENSKY, J. and GREEN, A. M.: Studies on human thyroxine-binding globulin. VI. The nature of slow thyroxine-binding globulin. *J. Clin. Invest.*, **51** (1972) p. 3173.
NILSSON, S. F. and PETERSON, A.: Studies on thyroid hormone-binding proteins. *J. Biol. Chem.*, **250** (1975) p. 8543.
PAGES, R. A., ROBBINS, J. and EDELHOCH, H.: Binding of thyroxine and thyroxine analogs to human serum prealbumin. *Biochem.*, **12** (1973) p. 2773.
ROBBINS, J.: Inherited variations in thyroxine transport. *Mt. Sinai J. Med. New York*, **40** (1973) p. 511.
SCHUSSLER, G. C.: Thyroxine-binding globulin: specificity for the hormonally active conformation of triiodothyronine. *Science*, **178** (1972) p. 172.

GITTEN CEDERBLAD (115-117)

AMARAL, L., LIN, K., SAMUELS, A. J. and WERTHAMER, S.: Human liver nuclear transcortin. *Biochim. Biophys. Acta*, **362** (1974) p. 332.
BURTON, R. M. and WESTPHAL, U.: Steroid hormone-binding proteins in blood plasma. *Metab. Clin. Exp.*, **21** (1972) p. 253.
LE GAILLARD, F., HAN, K-K. and DAUTREVAUX, M.: Caractérisation et propriétés physicochimiques de la transcortine humaine. *Biochimie*, **57** (1975) p. 559.
PATERSON, J. Y. F.: The rate constants for the interaction of cortisol and transcortin, and the rate of dissociation of transcortin-bound cortisol in the liver. *J. Endocrinol.*, **56** (1973) p. 551.
ROSNER, W.: Recent studies on the binding of cortisol in serum. *J. Steroid Biochem.*, **3** (1972) p. 531.
UETE, T. and TSUCHIKURA, H.: Study of mechanism of autoregulatory system of corticosteroid metabolism in liver. *Metab. Clin. Exp.*, **21** (1972) p. 77.

HANS BENNICH (119-127)

Advances in Immunology. Ed. F. J. Dixon and H. G. Kunkel. Academic Press, New York, London.
Contemporary Topics in Molecular Immunology. Ed. F. P. Inman. Plenum Press, New York.
ROITT, I. M.: *Essential Immunology.* Blackwell Scientific Publications, Oxford (1974).

LARS Å. HANSON (127-187)

ALLISON, A. C.: Mechanisms of tolerance and autoimmunity. *Ann. Rheum. Dis.*, **32** (1973) p. 283.
BENNICH, A. and JOHANSSON, S. G. O.: Structure and function of human immunoglobulin E. *Adv. Immunol.*, **13** (1971) p. 1.

BRITISH MEDICAL RESEARCH COUNCIL: *Hypogammaglobulinaemia in the United Kingdom.* Her Majesty's Stationery Office, London (1971).
BRUTON, O. C.: Agammaglobulinemia. *Pediatrics,* **9** (1952) p. 722.
COHEN, I. R. and WEKERLE, H.: Regulation of autosensitization. The immune activation and specific inhibition of self-recognizing thymus-derived lymphocytes. *J. Exp. Med.,* **137** (1973) p. 224.
COOMBS, R. R. A. and GELL, P. G. H.: Classifications of allergic reactions responsible for clinical hypersensitivity and disease. In: *Clinical Aspects of Immunology.* Ed. P. G. H. Gell and R. R. A. COMBS. Blackwell, Oxford 2nd ed. (1968) p. 575.
GOOD, R. A.: Structure—function relations in the lymphoid system. In: *Clinical Immunobiology.* Ed. F. H. Bach and R. A. Good. Academic Press, New York **1** (1972) p. 1.
HANSON, L. Å. and BRANDITZAEG, P.: Secretory antibody systems. In: *Immunologic Disorders in Infants and Children* Ed. E. R. Steihm and V. A. Fulginiti. W. B. Saunders, Philadelphia (1973) p. 107.
HENSON, P. M. and BENVENISTE, J.: Antibody—leucocyte—platelet interactions. In: *Biochemistry of the Acute Allergic Reaction.* Ed. K. F. Austen and E. L. Becker. Blackwell, Oxford (1971) p. 111.
ISHIZAKA, K.: Biosynthesis of IgE antibodies. In: *The Role of Immunological Factors in Infectious, Allergic and Autoimmune Processes.* Miles International Symposium, Eds. R. F. Beers, Jr and E. G. Basset. Raven Press. New York 8 (1976).
LANDSTEINER, K.: *The Specificity of Serological Reactions.* Harvard Univ. Press, Cambridge, Mass. (1945).
LAURELL, C.-B.: Quantitative estimation of proteins by electrophoresis in agarose gel containing antibodies. *Anal. Biochem.,* **15** (1966) p. 45.
MANCINI, G., CARBONARA, A. O. and HEREMANS, J. F.: Immunochemical quantitation of antigens by single radial immunodiffusion. *Immunochemistry,* **2** (1965) p. 235.
METCHNIKOFF, E.: *Lectures on the Comparative Pathology of Inflammation.* Kegan, Paul, Trench, Trüber, London (1893).
MILLER, J. F. A. P.: Immunological function of the thymus, *Lancet,* **II** (1961) p. 748.
MÜLLER-EBERHARD, H. J.: Complement. *Ann. Rev. Biochem.,* **44** (1975) p. 697.
OGRA, P. L., MORAG, A. and BEUTNER, K. R.: Amplification of local immune systems with active immunization. In: *The Immune System and Infectious Diseases.* Ed. E. Neter and F. Milgrom. Fourth International Convocation of Immunology. Karger, Basel (1975).
OSLER, A. G. and SANDBERG, A. L.: Alternate complement pathways. *Prog. Allergy,* **17** (1973) p. 51.
OUCHTERLONY, Ö. and NILSSON, L.-Å.: Immunodiffusion and immunoelectrophoresis. In: *Handbook of Experimental Immunology.* Ed. D. M. Blackwell, Oxford, 2nd edn. (1973).
SISKIND, G. W. and BENACERRAF, B.: Cell selection by antigen in the immune response. *Adv. Immunol.* **10** (1969) p. 1.
WALDMAN, R. H. and GANGULY, R.: Cell-mediated immunity and the local immune system. In: *The Immune System and Infectious Diseases.* Ed. E. Neter and F. Milgrom. Fourth International Convocation of Immunology. Karger, Basel (1975).

GÖRAN MÖLLER (187-197)

PERLMANN, P. and HOLM, G.: Cytotoxic effect of lymphoid cells. *Advances in Immunology,* **2** (1969) p. 117.
Strong and weak histocompatibility antigens. *Transplantation Reviews,* **3** (1970).
Human transplantation antigens. *Transplantation Reviews,* **4** (1970).
Antigen recognition in cell-mediated immunity. *Transplantation Reviews,* **10** (1972).
Interaction between humoral antibodies and cell-mediated immunity. *Transplantation Reviews,* **13** (1972).
T and B lymphocytes in humans. *Transplantation Reviews,* **16** (1973).
Effector cells in cell-mediated immunity. *Transplantation Reviews,* **17** (1973).
SMITH, R. T.: Tumor specific immune mechanisms. *New England J. Med.,* **278** (1968) p. 12.
Immunological surveillance against neoplasia. *Transplantation Reviews,* **7** (1971).
Tumor associated embryonic antigens. *Transplantation Reviews,* **19** (1974).

BENGT GULLBRING (198–219)

ALLEN, F. H. and TIPPETT, P. A.: A new Rh blood type which reveals the Rh antigen G. *Vox Sang.* **3** (1958) p. 321.
COOMBS, R. R. A., MOURANT, A. E. and RACE, R. R.: A new test for the detection of weak and 'incomplete' Rh agglutinins. *Brit. Exp. Path.*, **26** (1945) p. 255.
EKLUND, J. and NEVANLINNA, H. R.: Rh prevention: a report and analysis of a national programme. *J. Med. Gen.*, **10** (1973) p. 1.
FOX, F.: The structure of cell membranes. *Scient. Am.*, **266** (1972) p. 30.
FREDA, V. J., GORMAN, J. G. and POLLACK, W.: Rh factor: prevention of immunization and clinical trial on mothers. *Science*, **151** (1966) p. 828.
HEIKEN, A. and RASMUSON, M.: Genetical studies on the Rh blood group system. *Hereditas*, **55** (1966) p. 192.
LEVINE, P., TRIPODI, D., STRUCK, J., ZMIJEWSKI, C. M. and POLLACK, W.: Hemolytic anemia associated with Rh but not with Bombay blood. *Vox Sang.*, **24** (1973) p. 417.
MOLLISON, P. L.: *Blood Transfusion in Clinical Medicine.* Blackwell Scientific Publ. 5th edn. (1972).
MORGAN, W. T. J. and WATKINS, W. M.: Genetic and biochemical aspects of human blood-group A-, B-, H-, Le^a- and Le^b-specificity. *Brit. Med. Bull.*, **25** (1969) p. 30.
NILSSON, S. B.: *Maternal A and B Antibodies in ABO Hemolytic Disease of the Newborn.* Thesis, Malmö (1967).
RACE, R. R. and SANGER, R.: *Blood Groups in Man.* Blackwell Scientific Publ. 6th edn. (1975).
ROSENFIELD, R. E.: A-B hemolytic disease of the newborn. Analysis of 1480 cord blood specimens, with special reference to the direct anti-globulin test and to the group 0 mother. *Blood*, **10** (1955) p. 17.

LARS-OLOV ANDERSSON and RAGNAR LUNDÉN (221–222)

DAVIE, E. W. and FUJIKAWA, K.: Basic mechanisms in blood coagulation. *Ann. Rev. Biochem.*, **44** (1975) p. 799.
NILSSON, I. M.: *Blödnings- och trombossjukdomar.* Kabi, Almqvist & Wiksell (1971).

BIRGER BLOMBÄCK (223–253)

BACHMANN, L., SCHMITT-FUMIAN, W. W., HAMMEL, R. and LEDERER, K.: Size and shape of fibrinogen. I. Electron microscopy of the hydrated molecule. *Macromol. Chemic.*, **176** (1975) p. 2603.
BANG, N. U.: A molecular structural model of fibrin based on electron microscopy of fibrin polymerization. *Thromb. Diath. Haemorrh.*, Suppl. **13** (1964) p. 73.
BLOMBÄCK, B.: Fibrinogen to fibrin transformation. In: *Blood Clotting Enzymology.* Ed. W. H. Seegers. Academic Press, New York (1967) p. 143.
BLOMBÄCK, B.: Carbohydrates in blood-clotting proteins. In: *Glycoproteins, their Composition, Structure and Function.* Ed. A. Gottschalk. 5 Part B. Elsevier, Amsterdam (1972) p. 1069.
BLOMBÄCK, B. and BLOMBÄCK, M.: The molecular structure of fibrinogen. *Ann. N.Y. Acad. Sci.*, **202** (1972) p. 77.
BLOMBÄCK, B., BLOMBÄCK, M., HENSCHEN, A., HESSEL, B., IWANAGA, S., and WOODS, K. R.: N-terminal disulphide knot of human fibrinogen. *Nature* **218** (1968a) p. 130.
BLOMBÄCK, M., BLOMBÄCK, B., MAMMEN, E. F. and PRASAD, A. S.: Fibrinogen Detroit—a molecular defect in the N-terminal disulphide knot of human fibrinogen? *Nature*, **218** (1968b) p. 134.
BLOMBÄCK, B., HESSEL, B., HOGG, D. and CLAESSON, G.: Substrate specificity of thrombin on proteins and synthetic substrates. In: *Chemistry and Biology of Thrombin.* Eds. R. L. Lundblad, J. W. Fenton and K. G. Mann. Ann Arbor Science Publishers, Inc. Michigan, USA (1977) p. 275.

BLOMBÄCK, B., HOGG, D. H., GÅRDLUND, B., HESSEL, B. and KUDRYK, B.: Fibrinogen and fibrin formation. *Thrombos Res. Suppl.*, II (1976) p. 329.

BUDZYNSKI, A. Z., STAHL, M., KOPEĆ, M., LATALLO, Z. S., WEGRZYNOWICZ, Z. and KOWALSKI, E.: High molecular weight products of the late stage of fibrinogen proteolysis by plasmin and their structure relation to the fibrinogen molecule. *Biochim. Biophys. Acta*, **147** (1967) p. 313.

CARTWRIGHT, T. and KEKWICK, R. G. O.: A comparative study of human, cow, pig and sheep fibrinogen. *Biochim. Biophys. Acta*, **236** (1971) p. 550.

CASPARY, E. A. and KEKWICK, R. A.: Some physicochemical properties of human fibrinogen. *Biochem. J.*, **67** (1957) p. 41.

COPLEY, A. L.: Bleeding time, other *in vivo* hemostasis tests and the arrest of hemorrhage. *Thrombos. Res.*, **7** (1974) p. 1.

DOOLITTLE, R. F.: Structural aspects of the fibrinogen to fibrin conversion. *Adv. Protein Chem.*, **27** (1973) p. 1.

DOOLITTLE, R, F., CASSMAN, K. G., COTTRELL, B. A., FRIEZNER, S. J., and TAKAGI, T.: Amino acid sequence studies on the α-chain of human fibrinogen. Covalent structure of the α-chain portion of fragment D. *Biochemistry*, **16** (1977a) p. 1710.

DOOLITTLE, R. F., CASSMAN, K. G., COTTRELL, B. A., FRIEZNER, S. J., HUCKO, J. T. and TAKAGI, T.: Amino-acid sequence studies on the α-chain of human fibrinogen. Characterization of 11 cyanogen bromide fragments. *Biochemistry*, **16** (1977b) p. 1703.

FERRY, J. D. and MORRISSON, P. R.: Preparation and properties of serum and plasma proteins. VIII. The conversion of human fibrinogen to fibrin under various conditions. *J. Am. Chem Soc.*, **69**, (1947) p. 388.

FINLAYSON, J. S. and MOSESSON, M. W.: Heterogeneity of human fibrinogen. *Biochemistry*, **2** (1963) p. 42.

GAFFNEY, P. J.: Heterogeneity of human fibrinogen. *Nature New Biol.*, **230** (1971) p. 54.

GAFFNEY, P. J.: Localisation of carbohydrate in the subunits of human fibrinogen and its plasmin induced fragments. *Biochim. Biophys. Acta*, **263** (1972) p. 453.

GAFFNEY, P. J.: Fibrin (-ogen) interactions with plasmin. *Haemostasis*, **6** (1977a) p. 2.

GAFFNEY, P. J.: Structure of fibrinogen and degradation products of fibrinogen and fibrin. *British Med. Bull.*, **33** (1977b) p. 245.

GAFFNEY, P. J. and DOBOS, P.: A structural aspect of human fibrinogen suggested by its plasmin degradation. *Febs lett.*, **15** (1971) p. 13.

GÅRDLUND, B.: Human fibrinogen- amino acid sequence of fragment E and of adjacent structures in the Aα- and Bβ-chains. *Thrombosis Research*, **10** (1977) p. 689.

GÅRDLUND, B., HESSEL, B., MARGUERIE, G., MURANO, G., and BLOMBÄCK, B.: Primary structure of human fibrinogen. Characterization of disulfide containing cyanogen bromide fragment *European J. Biochem.*, **77** (1977) p. 595.

HALL, C. E. SLAYTER, H. S.: The fibrinogen molecule: its size, shape and mode of polymerization *J. Biophys. Biochem. Cytol.*, **5** (1959) p. 11.

HENSCHEN, A.: Peptide chains in S-sulfo-fibrinogen and S-sulfo-fibrin: isolation methods and general properties. *Ark. Kemi*, **22** (1964) p. 375.

HENSCHEN, A. and EDMAN, P.: Large scale preparation of S-carboxymethylated chains of human fibrin and fibrinogen and the occurrence of γ-chain variants. *Biochim. Biophys. Acta*, **263** (1972) p. 351.

HESSEL, B.: On the structure of the COOH-terminal part of the αA-chain of human fibrinogen. *Thrombos. Res.*, **7** (1975) p. 75.

KÖPPEL, G.: Morphology of the fibrinogen molecule. *Thromb. Diath. Haemorrh. Suppl.*, **39** (1970) p. 71.

KRAJEWSKI, T., and BLOMBÄCK, B.: The location of tyrosine-0-sulphate in fibrinopeptides. *Acta Chem. Scand.*, **22**. (1968) p. 1339.

KUDRYK, B., BLOMBÄCK, B. and BLOMBÄCK, M.: Fibrinogen Detroit—an abnormal fibrinogen with non-functional amino-terminal polymerization domain. *Thromb. Res.*, **9** (1976) p. 25.

KUDRYK, B. J., COLLEN, D., WOODS, K. R. and BLOMBÄCK, B.: Evidence for localization of polymerization sites in fibrinogen. *J. Biol. Chem.*, **249** (1974) p. 3322.

LAHIRI, B. and SHAINOFF, J. R.: Fate of fibrinopeptides in the reaction between human plasmin and fibrinogen. *Biochim. Biophys. Acta*, **303** (1973) p. 161.

LAKI, K.: *Fibrinogen*. Academic Press, New York, London (1968).
LORAND, L.: Fibrinoligase: The fibrinstabilizing factor system of blood plasma. *Ann. N. Y. Acad. Sci.*, **202** (1972) p. 6.
LOTTSPEICH, F. and HENSCHEN, A.: Amino acid sequence of human fibrinogen. Preliminary note on the peptides obtained by cyanogen bromide cleavage of the β-chain. *Hoppe-Seyler's Z. Physiol. Chem.*, **358** (1977a) p. 1521.
LOTTSPEICH, F. and HENSCHEN, A.: Amino acid sequence of human fibrin. Preliminary note on the completion of the γ-chain sequence. *Hoppe-Seyler's Z. Physiol. Chem.*, **358** (1977b) p. 935.
LY, B. and GODAL, H. C. Denaturation of fibrogen, the protective effect of calcium. *Haemostasis*, **1** (1973) p. 204.
LY, B., KIERULF, P. and ARNESEN, H.: Molecular aspects of the clottable proteins of human plasma during fibrinogenolysis *Thrombos. Res.*, **5** (1974) p. 301.
MAMMEN, E. F., PRASAD, A. S., BARNHART, M. I. and AU, C. C.: Congenital dysfibrinogenemia: fibrinogen Detroit. *J. Clin. Invest.*, **48** (1969) p. 235.
MARDER, V. J., SHULMAN, N. R. and CARROLL, W. R.: High molecular weight derivatives of human fibrinogen produced by plasmin. 1. Physicochemical and immunological characterization, *J. Biol. Chem.*, **244** (1969) p. 2111.
MARGUERIE, G., CHAGNIEL, G. and SUSCILLON, M.: The binding of calcium to bovine fibrinogen. *Biochim. Biophys. Acta*, **490** (1977) p. 94.
MARGUERIE, G. and STUHRMANN, H. B.: A neutron small-angle scattering study of bovine fibrinogen. *J. Mol. Biol.*, **102** (1976) p. 143.
MIHALYI, E.: Physicochemical studies of bovine fibrinogen. III. Optical rotation of the native and denatured molecule. *Biochim. Biophys. Acta*, **102** (1965) p. 487.
MILLS, D. and KARPATKIN, S.: Heterogeneity of human fibrinogen: possible relation to proteolysis by thrombin and plasmin as studied by SDS-polyacrylamide gel electrophoresis. *Biochem. Biophys. Res. Commun.*, **40** (1970) p. 206.
MOSESSON, M. W., ALKJAERSIG, N., SWEET, B. and SHERRY, S.: Human fibrinogen of relatively high solubility. Comparative biophysical, biochemical and biological studies with fibrinogen of lower solubility. *Biochemistry*, **6** (1967) p. 3279.
MOSESSON, M. W. and FINLAYSON, J. S.: The search for the structure of fibrinogen. *Progr. in Hemostasis and Thrombosis*, **3** (1976) p. 61.
MOSESSON, M. W., GALANAKIS, D. K. and FINLAYSSON, J. S.: Comparison of human plasma fibrinogen subfractions and early plasmic fibrinogen derivatives. *J. Biol. Chem.*, **249** (1974) p. 4656.
MOSHER, D, F, and BLOUT, E. R.: Heterogeneity of bovine fibrinogen and fibrin. *J. Biol. Chem.*, **248** (1973) p. 6896.
MURANO, G.: The molecular structure of fibrinogen. *Semin. Thrombos. Haemostas*, **1**, July 1974.
NAKAMURA, S., TAKAGI, T., IWANAGA, S., NIWA, M. and TAKAHASHI, K.: Amino acid sequence studies on the fragments produced from horseshoe crab coagulogen during gel formation: homologies with primate fibrinopeptide B. *Biochem. Biophys. Res. Commun.*, **72** (1976) p. 902.
NOSSEL, H. L., YUDELMAN, L., CANFIELD, R. E., BUTLER, JR., W. P., SPANONDIS, K., WILNER, G. D. and QURESHI, G. D.: Measurement of fibrinopeptide A in human blood, *J. Clin. Invest.*, **54** (1974) p. 43.
PLOW, E. and EDGINGTON, T. S.: Immunobiology of fibrinogen. Emergence of neoantigenic expressions during physiologic cleavage *in vitro* and *in vivo*. *J. Clin. Invest.*, **52** (1973) p. 273.
PLOW, E. F. and EDGINGTON, T. S.: A cleavage-associated neoantigenic marker for a γ-chain site in the NH_2-terminal aspect of the fibrinogen molecule. *J. Biol. Chem.*, **250** (1975) p. 3386.
SCHERAGA, H. A.: Active site mapping of thrombin. In: *Chemistry and Biology of Thrombin*. Eds., R. L. Lundblad, J. W. Fenton, II and K. G. Mann. Ann Arbor Science Publishers, Michigan, USA (1977) p. 145.
SCHERAGA, H. A. and LASKOWSKI, M. Jr.: The fibrinogen-fibrin conversion. *Adv. Protein Chem.*, **12** (1957) p. 1.
SOLUM, N. O.: The coagulogen of *Limulus polyphemus* hemocytes. A comparison of the clotted and non-clotted forms of the molecule. *Thromb. Res.*, **2** (1973) p. 55.
STRYER, L., COHEN, C. and LANGRIDGE, R.: Axial period of fibrinogen and fibrin. *Nature*, **197** (1963) p. 793.
TOONEY, N. M. and COHEN, C.: Microcrystals of a modified fibrinogen. *Nature*, **237** (1972) p. 23.

STAFFAN MAGNUSSON (254–276)

CLAEYS, H., SOTTRUP-JENSEN, L., ZAJDEL, M., PETERSEN, T. E. and MAGNUSSON, S.: Multiple gene duplication in the evolution of plasminogen. Five regions of sequence homology with the two internally homologous structures in prothrombin. *FEBS Letters*, **61** (1976) p. 20.

DAVIE, E. W. and FUJIKAWA, K.: Basic mechanisms in blood coagulation. *Ann. Rev. Biochem.*, **44** (1975) p. 799.

DAYHOFF, M. O.: *Atlas of Protein Sequence and Structure.* Vol. 5. National Biomedical Research Foundation, Washington (1972). Plus Suppl.

ENFIELD, D. L., ERICSSON, L. H., WALSH, K. A., NEURATH, H. and TITANI, K.: Bovine factor X_1 (Stuart factor): Primary structure of the light chain. *Proc. Nat. Acad. Sci. USA*, **72** (1975) p. 16.

ESMON, C. T., SADOWSKI, J. A. and SUTTIE, J. W.: A new carboxylation reaction. The vitamin-K-dependent incorporation of $H^{14}CO_3$ into prothrombin. *J. Biol. Chem.*, **250** (1975) p. 4744.

HAUSCHKA, P. V., LIAN, J. B. and GALLOP, P. M.: Direct identification of the calcium-binding amino acid γ-carboxylglutamate in mineralized tissue. *Proc. Nat. Acad. Sci. USA*, **72** (1975) p. 3925.

HEMKER, H. C. and VELTKAMP, J. J.: *Prothrombin and Related Coagulation Factors.* Leiden University Press (1975).

MAGNUSSON, S., PETERSEN, T. E., SOTTRUP-JENSEN, L. and CLAEYS, H.: Complete primary structure of prothrombin: Isolation, structure and reactivity of ten carboxylated glutamic acid residues and regulation of prothrombin activation by thrombin. In: *Proteases and Biological Control.* Eds. E. Reich, D. B. Rifkin and E. Shaw. Cold Spring Harbor, N.Y. (1975) p. 123.

MAGNUSSON, S.: Thrombin and prothrombin. In: *The Enzymes*, 3rd, ed. Vol. 3. Ed. P. D. Boyer, Academic Press, New York (1971) p. 277.

MAGNUSSON, S., SOTTRUP-JENSEN, L., PETERSEN, T. E., DUDEK-WOJCIE-CHOWSKA, G. and CLAEYS, H.: Homologous 'kringle' structures common to plasminogen and prothrombin. Substrate specificity of enzymes activating prothrombin and plasminogen. In: *Proteolysis and Physiological Regulation.* Eighth Miami Winter Symposia. Eds.: K. Brew and D. W. Ribbons, Academic Press, New York (1976).

MAGNUSSON, S., SOTTRUP-JENSEN, L., PETERSEN, T. E., MORRIS, H. R. and DELL, A.: Primary structure of the vitamin-K-dependent part of prothrombin. *FEBS Letters*, **44** (1974) p. 189.

MARKWARDT, F.: Hirudin as an inhibitor of thrombin. In: *Methods in Enzymology.* Eds.: G. E. Perlmann and L. Lorand, Academic Press, New York, **17** (1970) p. 924.

MORRIS, H. R., DELL, A., PETERSEN, T. E., SOTTRUP-JENSEN, L. and MAGNUSSON, S.: Mass-spectrometric identification and sequence location of the ten residens of the new amino acid (γ-carboxyglutamic acid) in the N-terminal region of prothrombin. *Biochem. J.*, **153** (1976) p. 663.

OWEN, M. C., LORIER, M. and CARRELL, R. W.: $α_1$-Antitrypsin: Structural relationships of the substitutions of the S and Z variants. *FEBS Letters*, **88** (1978) pp. 234–6.

PETERSEN, T. E., DUDEK-WOJCIECHOWSKA, G., SOTTRUP-JENSEN, L. and MAGNUSSON, S.: Sequence of human antithrombin-III. In: *Atlas of Protein Sequence and Structure* Vol. 5, Suppl. 3., Ed. M. Dayhoff. (1979).

PETERSEN, T. E., ROBERTS, H. R., SOTTRUP-JENSEN, L., MAGNUSSON, S. and BAGDY, D.: Partial primary structure of hirudin, a thrombin-specific inhibitor. In: *Protides of the Biological Fluids.* Ed. H. Peeters, Pergamon, Oxford 23 (1976).

SOTTRUP-JENSEN, L., CLAEYS, H., ZAJDEL, M., PETERSEN, T. E. and MAGNUSSON, S.: The primary structure of human plasminogen: Isolation of two lysine-binding fragments and one 'mini'-plasminogen (MW 38 000) by elastase-catalyzed specific limited proteolysis. In: *Progress in Chemical Fibrinolysis and Thrombolysis*, Vol. 3. Eds, J. F. Davidson et al. Raven Press, New York (1978) p. 191.

SOTTRUP-JENSEN, L., ZAJDEL, M., CLAEYS, H., PETERSEN, T. E. and MAGNUSSON, S.: Amino-acid sequence of activation cleavage site in plasminogen: Homology with 'pro' part of prothrombin. *Proc. Nat. Acad. Sci. USA*, **72** (1975) p. 2577.

STENFLO, J., FERNLUND, P., EGAN, W. and ROEPSTORFF, P.: Vitamin-K-dependent modifications of glutamic acid residues in prothrombin. *Proc. Nat. Acad. Sci. USA*, **71** (1974) p. 2730.

STENFLO, J. and SUTTIE, J. W.: Vitamin-K-dependent formation of γ-carboxyglutamic acid. *Ann. Rev. Biochem.*, **46** (1977) p. 157.

Suttie, J. W. and Jackson, C. R.: Prothrombin structure, activation and biosynthesis. *Physiol. Rev.*, **57** (1977) p. 71.
Titani, K., Fujikawa, K., Enfield, D. L., Ericsson, L. H., Walsh, K. A. and Neurath, H.: Bovine factor X_1 (Stuart factor): Amino acid sequence of the heavy chain. *Proc. Nat. Acad. Sci. USA*, **72** (1975) p. 3802.

LARS HOLMBERG (276–281)

Bennett, B., Ratnoff, O. D. and Levin, J.: Immunologic studies in von Willebrand's disease. *J. Clin. Invest.*, **51** (1972) p. 2597.
Bloom, A. L., Giddings, J. C. and Wilke, C. J.: Factor VIII on the vascular intima: possible importance in haemostasis and thrombosis. *Nature (New Biol.)*, **241** (1973) p. 217.
Bouma, B. N., Herdijk-Hos, J. M., de Graaf, S. and Sixma, J. J.: Presence of factor VIII-related antigen in blood platelets of patients with von Willebrand's disease. *Nature*, **257** (1975) p. 510.
Bouma, B. N., Wiegerinck, Y., Sixma, J. J., van Mourik, J. A. and Mochtar, I. A.: Immunological characterization of purified anti-haemophilic factor A (Factor VIII) which corrects abnormal platelet retention in von Willebrand's disease. *Nature (New Biol.)*, **236** (1972) p. 104.
Cooper, H. A. and Wagner, R. H.: The defect of hemophilic and von Willebrand's disease plasmas studied by a recombination technique. *J. Clin. Invest.*, **54** (1974) p. 1093.
Holmberg, L., Jeppsson, J. O., Nilsson, I. M. and Stenflo, J.: Cyanogen bromide and tryptic fragments of normal and haemophilic factor VIII. *Thromb. Res.*, **6** (1975) p. 523.
Holmberg, L., Mannucci, P. M., Turesson, I., Ruggeri, Z. M. and Nilsson, I. M.: Factor VIII antigen in the vessel wall in von Willebrand's disease and haemophilia A. *Scand J. Haematol.*, **13** (1974) p. 33.
Holmberg, L. and Nilsson, I. M.: Von Willebrand's disease. *Ann. Rev. Med.*, **26** (1972) p. 33.
Howard, M. A., Sawers, R. J. and Firkin, B. G.: Ristocetin: a means of differentiating von Willebrand's disease into two groups. *Blood*, **41** (1973) p. 687.
Jaffe, E.: Endothelial cells and the biology of factor VIII. *New. Engl. J. Med.*, **296** (1977) p. 377.
Kernoff, P. B. A., Gruson, R. and Rizza, C. R.: A variant of factor VIII related antigen. *Br. J. Haematol.*, **26** (1974) p. 435.
Mannucci, P. M., Pareti, F. I., Holmberg, L., Nilsson, I. M. and Ruggeri, Z. M.: Studies on the prolonged bleeding time in von Willebrand's disease. *J. Lab. Clin. Med.*, **88** (1976) p. 662.
Meyer, D., Jenkins, C. S. P., Dreyfus, M. and Larrieu, M.-J.: Experimental model for von Willebrand's disease. *Nature*, **243** (1973) p. 293.
Nilsson, I. M., Blombäck, M., Jorpes, E., Blombäck, B. and Johansson, S.-A.: v. Willebrand's disease and its correction with human plasma fraction I-O. *Acta Med. Scand.*, **159** (1957) p. 179.
Peake, I. R., Bloom, A. L. and Giddings, J. C.: Inherited variants of factor VIII-related protein in von Willebrand's disease. *New Engl. J. Med.*, **291** (1974) p. 113.
Piovella, F., Ascari, E., Sitar, G. M., Malamani, G. D., Cattaneo, G., Magliulo, E. and Sterti, E.: Immunofluorescent detection of factor VIII-related antigen in human platelets and megakaryocytes. *Haemostasis* **3** (1974) p. 288.
Zimmerman, T. S., Ratnoff, O. D. and Powell, A. E.: Immunologic differentiation of classic haemophilia (factor VIII deficiency) and von Willebrand's disease. *J. Clin. Invest.*, **50** (1971) p. 244.
Zimmerman, T. S., Roberts, J. and Edgington, T. S.: Factor VIII related antigen: multiple molecular forms in human plasma. *Proc. Natl. Acad. Sci. USA*, **72** (1975) p. 5121.

LARS-OLOV ANDERSSON (281–285)

Andersson, L.-O., Borg, H. and Miller-Andersson, M.: Purification and characterization of human factor IX. *Thromb. Res.*, **7** (1975) p. 451.

FRYKLUND, L., BORG, H. and ANDERSSON, L.-O.: Aminoterminal sequence of human factor IX. Presence of γ-carboxyl glutamic acid residues. *FEBS Letters*, **65** (1976) p. 187.
FUJIKAWA, K., THOMPSON, A. R., LEGAZ, M. E., MEGER, R. G. and DAVIE, E. W.: Isolation and characterization of bovine factor IX. *Biochemistry*, **12** (1973) p. 4938.
MÉNACHÉ, D.: The turnover rate of the coagulation factors II, VII and IX under normal metabolic conditions. *Thromb. Diath. Haemorrh.* Suppl. **13** (1964) p. 187.
ÖRSTAVIK, K. H., ÖSTERUD, B., PRYDZ, H. and BERG, K.: Electroimmunoassay of factor IX in hemophilia B. *Thromb. Res.*, **7** (1975) p. 373.
ÖSTERUD, B. and FLENGSRUD, R.: Purification and some characteristics of the coagulation factor IX from human plasma. *Biochem. J.*, **145** (1975) p. 469.
SOULIER, J. P., BLATRIX, C. and STEINBUCH, M.: Fractions 'coagulantes' contenant les facteurs de coagulation absorbables par le phosphate tricalcique. *Press Me'd.*, **72** (1964) p. 1223.
SOULIER, J. P., MÉNACHÉ, D., STEINBUCH, M., BLATRIX, Ch. and Josso, F.: Preparation and clinical use of P.P.S.B. *Thromb. Diath. Haemorrh.* Suppl., **35** (1969) p. 61.
SUOMELA, H.: Multiple forms of human factor IX in chromatography and isoelectric focusing. *Thromb. Res.*, **7** (1975) p. 101.
TULLIS, J. L.: Clinical Experience with Factor IX Concentrates. Hemophilia and New Haemorrhagic States. International symposium, New York. Ed., K. M. Brinkhous. The University of North Carolina, Press, Chapel Hill (1970) p. 35.
TULLIS, J. L., MELIN, M. and JURGIAN, P.: Clinical use of human prothrombin complexes. *New. Engl. J. Med.*, **273** (1965) p. 667.
VELTKAMP, J. J., DRION, E. F. and LOELIGER, E. A.: Defection of the carrier state in hereditary coagulation disorders. I. *Thromb. Diath. Haemorrhag.* **19** (1975) p. 279.

RAGNAR LUNDÉN (285-288)

DAVIE, E. M. and FUJIKAWA, K.: Basic mechanisms in blood coagulation. *Ann. Rev. Biochem.*, **44** (1975) p. 799.
BAUGH, R. F. and HOUGIE, C.: Biochemistry of blood coagulation. In: *Recent Advances in Blood Coagulation*. Ed. L. Poller No. 2. Churchill Livingstone Edinburgh, London, New York (1977) p. 1.

PER WALLÉN (288-304)

ABIKO, Y., IWAMOTO, M. and TOMIKAWA, M.: Plasminogen-plasmin system. V. A stoichiometric equilibrium complex of plasminogen and a synthetic inhibitor. *Biochim. Biophys. Acta*, **185** (1969) p. 242.
AOKI, N.: Preparation of plasminogen activator from vascular trees of human cadavers. *J. Biochem.*, **75** (1974) p. 731.
ARNESEN, H. and FAGERHOL, M. K.: α_2-Macroglobulin, α_1-antitrypsin and antithrombin III in plasma and serum during fibrinolytic theraphy with urokinase. *Scand. J. Clin. Lab. Investig.*, **29** (1972) p. 259.
ASTRUP, T.: Tissue activators of plasminogen. *Fed. Proc.*, **25** (1966) p. 42.
ASTRUP, T.: The physiology of fibrinolysis. In: *Thrombosis and Urokinase*. Eds. R. Paoletti and S. Sherry. Academic Press, London (1977) p. 11.
ASTRUP, T.: Fibrinolysis an overview. The Prix Servier Lecture. In: *Progress in Chemical Fibrinolysis* Vol. III. Eds. J. F. Davidson, M. Samama and P. Desnoyers. Raven Press, N.Y. (1978) p. 1.
ASTRUP, T. and PERMIN, P. M.: Fibrinolysis in the animal organism. *Nature* **159** (1947) p. 681.
BARG, Jr, W. F., BOGGIANO, E. and DERENZO, E. C.: Interaction of streptokinase and human plasminogen. II. Starch gel electrophoretic demonstration of a reaction product with activator activity. *J. Biol. Chem.*, **240** (1965) p. 2944.

BROCKWAY, W. J. and CASTELLINO, F. J.: Measurement of the binding of antifibrinolytic amino acids to various plasminogen. *Arch. Biochem. Biophys.*, **151** (1972) p. 194.
CHRISTENSEN, L. R.: Streptococcal fibrinolysis: A proteolytic reaction due to a serum enzyme activated by streptococcal fibrinolysin. *J. Gen. Physiol.*, **28** (1945) p. 363.
COLE, E. R. and BACHMANN, F. W.: Purification and properties of a plasminogen activator from pig heart. *J. Biol. Chem.*, **252** (1977) p. 3729.
COLLEN, D. and DE MAEYER, L.: Molecular biology of human plasminogen. I. Physicochemical properties and microheterogeneity. *Thromb. Diath. Haemorrh.*, **34** (1975) p. 396.
COLLEN, D., TYTGAT, G., CLAYES, H., VERSTRAETE, M. and WALLÉN, P.: Metabolism of plasminogen in healthy subjects: Effect of tranexamic acid. *J. Clin. Investig.*, **51** (1972) p. 1310.
DASTRE, A.: Fibrinolyse dans le sang. *Arch. Physiol. Norm. Path.*, **5** (1893) p. 661.
DEUTSCH, D. G. and MERTZ, E. T.: Plasminogen purification from human plasma by affinity chromatography. *Science*, **170** (1970) p. 1095.
GROSKOPF, W. R., SUMMARIA, L. and ROBBINS, K. C.: Studies on the active center of human plasmin. Partial amino acid sequence of a peptide containing the active center serine residue. *J. Biol. Chem.*, **244** (1969) p. 3590.
HEBERLEIN, P. J. and BARNHART, M. The Purification of Profibrinolysin and Fibrinolysin. In *Thrombosis and Bleeding Disorders*. Academic Press, New York (1971) p. 336.
HEDNER, U.: Studies on an inhibitor of plasminogen activation in human serum. *Thromb. Diath. Haemorrh.*, **30** (1973) p. 414.
HEDNER, U. and MARTINSSON, G.: Inhibition of activated Hageman factor (factor XIIa) by an inhibitor of the plasminogen activation (PA inhibitor). *Thromb. Res.*, **12** p.1015. (1978).
HEIMBURGER, N., HAUPT, H. and SCHWICK, H. G.: Proteinase inhibitors of human plasma. *Proc. Internat. Res. Conf. on Proteinase Inhibitors*. Munich Nov. 1970. Walter de Gruyter, Berlin (1971) p. 1.
KJELLMAN, H.: Syntetiska antifibrinolytika. In I. M. Nilsson, Blödnings och trombossjukdomar. Kabi, Almqvist och Wiksell, Stockholm (1971) p. 142.
KLINE, D. L.: Purification and crystallization of plasminogen (profibrinolysin). *J. Biol. Chem.*, **204** (1953) p. 949.
KOK, P. and ASTRUP, T.: Isolation and purification of a tissue plasminogen activator and its comparison with urokinase. *Biochemistry*, **8** (1969) p. 79.
KUCINSKI, C. S., FLETCHER, A. P. and SHERRY, S.: Effect of urokinase antiserum on plasminogen activators: Demonstration of immunologic dissimilarity between plasma plasminogen activator and urokinase. *J. Clin. Investig.*, **47** (1968) p. 1238.
McCLINTOCK, D. K. and BELL, P. H.: The mechanism of activation of human plasminogen by streptokinase. *Biochem. Biophys. Res. Comm.*, **43** (1971) p. 694.
MÜLLERTZ, S.: Molecular forms of plasmin and protease inhibitors in human fibrinolytic postmortem plasma. *Scand. J. Clin. Lab. Invest.*, **30** (1972a) p. 369.
NILÉHN, J. E. and GANROTH, P. O.: Plasmin, plasmin inhibitors and degradation products of fibrinogen in human serum during and after intravenous infusion of streptokinase. *Scand. J. Clin. Lab. Investig.* **20** (1967) p. 113.
NILSSON, I. M.: Blödnings- och trombossjukdomar. Kabi, Almqvist and Wiksell, Stockholm (1971) p. 223.
NILSSON, I. M., KROOK, H., STERNBY, H. H., SÖDERBERG, E. and SÖDERSTRÖM, N.: Severe thrombotic disease in a young man with bone marrow and skeletal changes and with a high content of an inhibitor in the fibrinolytic system. *Acta Med. Scand.*, **169** (1961) p. 23323.
NILSSON, I. M. and PANDOLFI, M.: Fibrinolytic response of the vascular wall. *Thromb. Diath. Haemorrh. Suppl.*, **40** (1970) p. 232.
NORMAN, P. S.: Studies of the plasmin system. II. Inhibition of plasmin by serum or plasma. *J. Exp. Med.*, **108** (1958) p. 53.
PANDOLFI, M.: Histochemistry and assay of plasminogen activator(s). *Europ. J. Clin. Biol. Res.*, **17** (1972) p. 254.
RICKLI, E. E. and OTAVSKY, W. J.: A new method of isolation and some properties of the heavy chain of human plasmin. *Eur. J. Biochem.*, **59** (1975) p. 441.
ROBBINS, K. C., SUMMARIA, L., HSIEH, B. and SHAH, R. J.: The peptide chains of human plasmin. Mechanism of activation of human plasminogen to plasmin. *J. Biol. Chem.*, **242** (1967) p. 2333.

SAITO, H., RATNOFF, O. D. and DONALDSON, V. H.: Defective activation of clotting, fibrinolytic and permeability-enhancing systems in human Fletcher trait plasma. *Circulation Res.*, **34** (1974) p. 641.
SCHICK, L. A. and CASTELLINO, F. J.: Direct evidence for the generation of an active site in the plasminogen moiety of the streptokinase-human plasminogen activator complex. *Biochem. Biophys. Res. Comm.*, **57** (1974) p. 47.
SIEFRING, G. E. and CASTELLINO, F. J.: Metabolic turnover studies on the two major forms of rat and rabbit plasminogen. *J. Biol. Chem.*, **249** (1974) p. 1434.
SJÖHOLM, I., WIMAN, B. and WALLÉN, P.: Studies on the conformational changes of plasminogen induced during activation to plasmin and by 6-aminohexanoic acid. *Eur. J. Biochem.*, **39** (1973) p. 471.
SOBERANO, M. E., ONG, E. B., JOHNSON, A. J., LEVY, M. and SCHOELLMANN, G.: Purification and characterization of two forms of urokinase. *Biochim. Biophys. Acta*, **445** (1976) p. 763.
SOTTRUP-JENSEN, L., CLAEYS, H., ZAJDEL, M., PETERSEN, T. E. and MAGNUSSON, S.: The primary structure of human plasminogen. Isolation of two lysine-binding fragments and one 'mini' plasminogen (Miw. 38000) by elastase-catalyzed specific limited proteolysis. In: *Progress in Chemical Fibrinolysis* Vol. III. Eds. J. F. Davidson, M. Samama and P. Desnoyers. Raven Press, N.Y. (1978) p. 191.
THORSEN, S.: Differences in the binding to fibrin to native plasminogen and plasminogen modified by proteolytic degradation. Influence of ω-amino acids. *Biochim. Biophys. Acta*, **393** (1975) p. 55.
THORSEN, S. and ASTRUP, T.: Substrate composition and the effect of ε-aminocaproic acid on tissue plasminogen activator and urokinase-induced fibrinolysis. *Thromb. Diath. Haemorrh.*, **32** (1974) p. 306.
THORSEN, S., GLAS-GREENWALT, P., ASTRUP, T.: Difference in the binding to fibrin of urokinase and tissue plasminogen activator. *Thromb. Diath. Haemorrh.*, **28** (1972) p. 65.
TILLET, W. S. and GARNER, R. O.: The fibrinolytic activity of hemolytic streptococci. *J. Exp. Med.*, **58** (1933) p. 485.
TODD, A. S.: Histological localization of fibrinolysin activator. J. Path. Bact., 78 (1959) p. 281.
VIOLAND, B. N. and CASTELLINO, F. J.: Mechanism of the urokinase-catalyzed activation of human plasminogen. *J. Biol. Chem.*, **251** (1976) p. 3906.
WALLÉN, P.: Studies on the purification of human plasminogen. II. Further purification of human plasminogen on cellulose ion exchangers and by means of gel filtration on Sephadex. *Arkiv Kemi*, **19** (1962) p. 469.
WALLÉN, P.: Chemistry of plasminogen activation. In: *Progress in Chemical Fibrinolysis*. Vol. III. Eds. J. F. Davidson, M. Samama and P. Desnoyers. Raven Press, N.Y. (1978) p. 167.
WALLÉN,, P. and BERGSTRÖM, K.: Effect of lysine on the purification of human plasminogen on cellulose ion exchangers. *Acta Chem. Scand.*, **13** (1959) p. 1464.
WALLÉN, P., KOK, P. and RÅNBY, M.: The tissue activator of plasminogen. In: *Regulatory Proteolytic Enzymes and Their Inhibitors*. Proc. of the 11th FEBS Meeting Vol. 46. Pergamon Press, Oxford (1978) p. 127.
WALLÉN, P. and WIMAN, B.: Characterization of human plasminogen. I. On the relationship between different molecular forms of plasminogen demonstrated in plasma and found in purified preparations. *Biochim. Biophys. Acta*, **221** (1970) p. 20.
WALLÉN, P. and WIMAN, B.: On the generation of intermediate plasminogen and its significance for the activation. In: *Proteases and Biological Control*. Eds. E. Reich, D. B. Rifkin and E. Shaw. Cold Spring Harbor, N.Y. (1975) p. 291.
WIMAN, B.: Biochemistry of the plasminogen to plasmin conversion. In: *Fibrinolysis: Current Fundamental and Clinical Concepts*. Eds. P. J. Gaffney and S. Balkuv-Ulutin. Academic Press, London, New York, San Francisco (1978) p. 47.
WIMAN, B. and WALLÉN, P.: Structural relationship between 'Glutamic acid' and 'Lysine' forms of human plasminogen and their interaction with the NH_2-terminal activation peptide as studied by affinity chromatography. *Eur. J. Biochem.*, **50** (1975) p. 489.
WIMAN, B. and WALLÉN, P.: The specific interaction between plasminogen and fibrin. A physiological role of the lysine binding site in plasminogen. *Thromb. Res.*, **10** (1977) p. 213.
WIMAN, B. and WALLÉN, P.: Primary structure of the B-chain of human plasmin. *Eur. J. Biochem.* **76** (1977) p. 129.

LARS-OLOV ANDERSSON, MONICA EINARSSON, and RAGNAR LUNDÉN (305–308)

ABILDGAARD, U.: Purification of two progressive antithrombins of human plasma. *Scand. J. Clin. Lab. Invest.*, **19** (1967) p. 190.
ERIKSSON, S.: Antitrypsinbrist. *Läkart.* **69** (1972) p. 729.
MILLER-ANDERSSON, M., BORG, H. and ANDERSSON, L.-O.: Purification of antithrombin III by affinity chromatography. *Thromb. Res.*, **5** (1974) p. 439.
MOROI M. and AOKI, N.: Isolation and characterization of α_2-plasmin inhibitor from human plasma. *J. Biol. Chem.*, **251** (1976) p. 5956.
MÜLLERTZ, S. and CLEMMENSEN, I.: The primary inhibitor of plasma in human plasma. *Biochem. J.*, **159** (1976) p. 545.
OHLSSON, K.: *Interaction between Plasma Protease Inhibitors and Some Proteolytic Enzymes in vitro* and *in vivo*. Malmö (1971).
ROSENBERG, J., BEELER, D. and ROSENBERG, R. D.: Acitvation of human prothrombin by highly purified human factors V and X_a in the presence of human antithrombin. *J. Biol. Chem.*, **250** (1975) p. 1607
WIMAN, B. and COLLEN, D.: Purification and characterization of human antiplasmin, the fast-acting plasmin inhibitor in plasma. *Eur. J. Biochem.*, **78** (1977) p. 19.

BENGT G. JOHANSSON (309–370)

AXELSEN, N. H. (ed): *Quantitative Immunoelectrophoresis. New Developments and Applications*. Universitetsforlaget, Oslo (1975).
AXELSEN, N. H., KRÖLL, J. and WEEKE, B. (eds): *A Manual of Quantitative Immunoelectrophoresis. Methods and Applications*. Universitetsforlaget, Oslo (1973).
AXELSEN, N. H., KRÖLL, J. and WEEKE, B. (eds): *A Manual of Quantitative Immunoelectrophoresis. Methods and Applications*. Universitetsforlaget, Oslo (1973).
BJERRUM, O. J., INGILD, A., LÖWENSTEIN, H. and WEEKE, B.: Carbamylated antibodies used for quantitation of human IgG. A routine method. *Scand. J. Immunol. Suppl.*, **1** (1973) p. 145.
CLARKE, H. G. and FREEMAN, T.: A quantitative immuno-electrophoresis method (Laurell electrophoresis). In: *Protides of the Biological Fluids*. Ed. H. Peeters. Pergamon Press, Oxford (1971) p. 503.
CROWLE, A. J.: *Immunodiffusion*. Academic Press, New York, London (1973).
ENGVALL, E. and PERLMAN, P.: Enzymelinked immunosorbent assay (ELISA). Quantitative assay of immunoglobulin G. Immunochemistry, **8** (1971) p. 871.
FISCHER, L.: *An Introduction to Gel Chromatography*. North Holland Publ. Co., Amsterdam (1969).
FRIBERG, L.: Chronic cadmium poisoning. *Arch. Industr. Health.*, **20** (1959) p. 401.
GANROT, P. O.: Crossed immunolectrophoresis. *Scand. J. Clin. Lab. Invest.*, **29**, Suppl. 124 (1972) p. 39.
GANROT, P. O.: Variation of the concentration of some plasma proteins in normal adults, in pregnant women and in newborns. *Scand. J. Clin. Lab. Invest.*, **29**, Suppl. 124 (1972) p. 83.
GANROT, K. and LAURELL, C.-B.: Measurement of IgG and albumin content of cerebrospinal fluid, and its interpretation. *Clin. Chem.*, **20** (1974) p. 571.
GRUBB, A.: Crossed immunolectrophoresis and electroimmuno assay of IgM. *J. Immunol.*, **112** (1974) p. 1420.
HELLSING, K.: *Influence of Polymer on the Antigen-antibody Reaction in a Continuous Flow System: Automated Immunoprecipitation Reactions*. Ed. Technicon Instrument Corp., Tarrytown, N.Y. (1973).
HOBBS, J. R.: Immunoglobulins in clinical chemistry. *Adv. Clin. Chem.* **14** (1971) p. 219.
HÄLLÉN, J. and LAURELL, C.-B.: Plasma protein pattern in cirrhosis of the liver. *Scand. J. Clin. Lab. Invest.* **29**, Suppl. 124 (1972) p. 97.
JOHANSSON, B. G.: Agarose gel electrophoresis. *Scand. J. Clin. Lab. Invest.*, **29**, Suppl. 124 (1972) p. 7.
JOHANSSON, B. G. and RAVNSKOV, U.: The serum level and urinary excretion of α_2-microglobulin, β_2-microglobulin and lysozyme in renal disease. *Scand. J. Urol. Nephrol.*, **6** (1972) p. 249.

References

JOHANSSON, B. G., KINDMARK, C.-O., TRELL, E. and WOLLHEIM, F.: Sequential changes of plasma proteins after myocardial infarction. *Scand. J. Clin. Lab. Invest.*, **29**, Suppl. 124 (1972) p. 117.

JOHANSSON, S. G. O., BENNICH, H. and BERG, T.: The clinical significance of IgE. *Progr. Clin. Immunol.*, **1**, (1972).p. 192.

KINDMARK, C.-O. and LAURELL, C.-B.: Sequential changes of the plasma protein pattern in inoculation hepatitis. *Scand. J. Clin. Lab. Invest.* **29**, Suppl. 124 (1972) p. 105.

KINDMARK, C.-O. and THORELL, J.: Quantitative determination of individual serum proteins by radio-electroimmuno assay and use of ^{125}I-labelled antibodies (application to C-reactive protein). *Scand. J. Clin. Lab. Invest.*, **29**, Suppl. 124 (1972) p. 49.

KOLB, W. P. and MÜLLER-EBERHARD, H. J.: Neoantigens of the membranes attack complex of human complement. *Proc. Nat. Acad. Sci.*, **72** (1974) p. 1687.

LAURELL, C.-B.: Antigen-antibody crossed electrophoresis. *Analyt. Biochem.*, **10** (1965) p. 358.

LAURELL, C.-B.: Quantitative estimation of proteins by electrophoresis in agarose gel containing antibodies. *Analyt. Biochem.*, **15** (1966) p. 45.

LAURELL, C.-B.: Electroimmuno assay. *Scand. J. Clin. Lab. Invest.*, **29**, Suppl. 124 (1972) p. 21.

LAURELL, C.-B. (ed): *Electrophoretic and Electro-immunochemical Analysis of Proteins.* Universitetsforlaget, Oslo (1972).

LAURELL, C.-B.: Composition and variation of the gel electrophoretic fractions of plasma, cerebrospinal fluid and urine. *Scand. J. Clin. Lab. Invest.* **29**, Suppl. 124 (1972) p. 71.

LAURELL, C.-B., KULLANDER, S. and THORELL, J.: Effect of administration of a combined estrogen-progestin contraceptive on the level of individual plasma proteins. *Scand. J. Clin. Lab. Invest.*, **22** (1968) p. 337.

LAURELL, C.-B., LUNDH, B. and NOSSLIN, B.: *Klinisk kemi i praktisk medicin.* Studentlitteratur, Lund (1976).

LIPSCHITZ, D. A., COOK, J. D. and FINCH, C. A.: A clinical evaluation of serum ferritin as an index of iron stores. *New Engl. J. Med.*, **290** (1974) p. 1213.

MANCINI, G., CARBONARA, A. O. and HEREMANS, J. F.: Immunochemical quantitation of antigens by single radial immunodiffusion. *Immunochemistry*, **2** (1965) p. 235.

MANUEL, Y., RVILLARD, J. P. and BETUEL, H. (eds): *Proteins in Normal and Pathological Urine.* S. Karger, Basel (1970).

MAURER, H.: *Disc Electrophoresis and Related Techniques of Polyacrylamide Gel Electrophoresis.* Walter de Gruyter, Berlin, New York (1971).

MÜLLER-EBERHARD, U. and HENG-LIEM, H.: Hemopexin. I: Structure and Functions of Plasma Proteins. Ed. A. C. Allison, Plenum Press, London 1 (1974) p. 35.

NÖRGAARD-PEDERSEN, B.: A highly sensitive radioimmunoelectrophoretic quantitation of human alpha-fetoprotein. *Clin. Chim. Acta*, **48** (1973) p. 345.

NÖRGAARD-PEDERSEN, B.: Human alpha-fetoprotein. *Scand. J. Immunol. Suppl.*, **4** (1976).

PIERCE, J., JEPPSSON, J. O. and LAURELL, C.-B.: Alpha-1-antitrypsin phenotypes determined by isoelectric focusing of the cysteine-antitrypsin mixed disulphide in serum. *Analyt. Biochem.*, **74** (1976). In press.

PISCATOR, M.: *Proteinuria in Chronic Cadmium Poisoning.* Thesis, Stockholm (1966).

PUTNAM, F. W. (ed.).: *The Plasma Proteins.* Academic Press, New York (1975).

RAVNSKOV, U.: On renal handling of plasma proteins. *Scand. J. Urol. Nephrol. Suppl.*, **20** (1973).

SCHULZE, H. E. and HEREMANS, J. F.: *Molecular Biology of Human Proteins.* Elsevier, Amsterdam, London, New York (1969).

TEJLER, L. and GRUBB., A.: A complex-forming glycoprotein heterogeneous in charge present in human plasma, urine and cerebro-spinal fluid. *Biochim. Biophys. Acta*, (1976). In press.

TURNER, M. W. and HULME, B.: *The Plasma Proteins: An Introduction.* Pitman Medical & Scientific Publ. Co. Ltd., London (1971).

WADSWORTH, C. and HANSON, L. Å.: Comparative analysis of immune electrophoretic precipitates employing an amodified immune electrophoretic technique. *Int. Arch. Allergy*, **17** (1960) p. 165.

WEEKE, B.: Quantitative estimation of human immunoglobulins following carbamylation by electrophoresis in antibody-containing agarose. *Scand. J. Clin. Lab. Invest.*, **22** (1968) p. 351.

WEEKE, B.: *Humane serumproteiner identificert og kvantitert med Laurell's immunelektroforeser.* Disputats, Köbenhavn (1973).

Index

ABO incompatibility 207, 217
ABO system 205, 206, 208, 211, 217
Adrenaline 23
Affinity 136
Affinity chromatography 40
Afibrinogenaemia 250
Agammaglobulinaemia 69
Agar gel electrophoresis 316, 360
Agarose electrophoresis 316–17, 335, 366
Age variations 340
Agglutination 142, 200–2, 206
AHF (Factor VIII) 31, 32, 276–81
Albumin 1, 2, 4, 9, 11, 19, 36, 43–72, 335, 338, 342, 351, 364, 368, 370
   abnormal loss of 66
   amino acids 47
   binding 51–53, 54
   biochemistry 43–54
   bovine serum 48
   breakdown 56, 61
   chemical properties 47–50
   determination of 44, 311
   distribution of 55, 56, 60
   disulphide bridges 50
   functions of 54–55
   heterogeneity 46
   hydrodynamic properties 45
   important functions 54
   in illness 63–67
   loss of 67, 70
   metabolism regulation 56
   microheterogeneity 46
   nitrogen 47
   normal values 55
   organ storage with 71–72
   physicochemical properties 44–46
   physiology and clinical aspects 54–71
   purification 43
   redistribution of 66
   reduced synthesis 64
   residues in 48–50
   size and shape of molecule of 45
   solubility of 45
   structure and functional relations 53–54
   synthesis of 56–60
      colloid pressure 59
      hormone balance 58
      nutrition effects 58
      stress and trauma effects 59
      temperature effects 59
   therapy indications 69–71
   ultraviolet absorption spectrum 46
Alkaline phosphatase 317
Alkylsulphates 52
Alkylsulphonates 52
Allergens 174, 176, 180
Allergies
   atopic 176–80
   contact 182
   drug 181–82
Alloantigens 132
Allotypes 126
Amino acids 1–3, 13, 14, 47, 124, 125, 297
   albumin 47
   C-terminal 112, 113
ε-Aminocaproic acid 297, 299, 304
trans-4-Aminomethylcyclohexase acid (AMCHA) 297
Ammonium sulphate precipitation methods 37–38
Amylase 317
Analbuminaemia 55
Analytical methods 309–70
Anamnestic response 136
Anaphylatoxins 147
Androgens 89, 341
Angiotensin 260
Anilinonaphthalenesulphonic acid 53
Antibodies 14, 119, 126, 155, 182, 200
   ABO system 206
   blood group 200–3
   demonstration of 202
   formation of 132–37
   in defence against infection 156–63
Antibody deficiency syndromes 165, 168
Antibody-mediated immunity 172
Antichymotrypsin 336, 351, 357
Antigen–antibody complexes 184
Antigen–antibody reactions 140–46
Antigen suicide 193
Antigenic determinants 125
Antigens 14, 15, 119, 132, 182
   characteristics of 131–32
   erythrocyte 199
   tumour-associated 194, 197
   tumour-specific 194

Antiglobulin sera 202
Antihaemophilic factor 19
Antihaemophilic factor A (AHF) 276
Antilymphocyte globulin (ALG) 193
Antiplasmin 303, 306
Antiserum 15
Antithrombin 307–8
Antithrombin-III 276, 307–8
α_1-Antitrypsin 305–6, 311, 336, 339, 342–44, 351, 353, 357, 359
Apolipoproteins 72–73, 79–82, 84
Arginyl-156 273
Arterioles 23
Arteriosclerosis 27
Arthritis 184
Arthus's reaction 183
Asn-77 264
Asn-101 264
Asn-376 264
Asn-X-Ser 264
Asn-X-Thr 264
Asparagine 264
Association constant 136
Ataxia-telangiectasia 173
Atopic allergies 176–80
Autoantigenity 132
Autoimmune diseases 165, 184–87
Autoimmune disorders 169, 171
Autoimmune haemolytic anaemia 169
Avidity 136

Bassen–Kornzweig disease 94
B-cells 131, 132, 185, 189
BCG-vaccine 173, 197
Bence Jones proteinuria 345, 365, 366
Binding coefficient 136
Biospecific adsorption 40–41
Biuret method 309, 310
Blombäck's fraction I-O 31–32
Blood, microcirculation of 23–27
Blood activators 301
Blood–brain barrier 24, 368
Blood coagulation 17
Blood diseases 362–64
Blood group antibodies 200–3
Blood group genetics 204–5
Blood group serology 198–219
Blood group substances 210
Blood group systems of clinical interest 218–19
Blood plasma 1, 17
Blood transfusion and ABO incompatibility 207
Blood vessels 17
B-lymphocytes 129–33, 165, 169, 184, 185
Body fluids 364
Bone marrow 128

Bone marrow diseases 362–64
Botulinus 158
Bowel diseases 356
Brucella 164
Burns 70

C^w antigen 214
Ca^{2+} binding 264–68, 273
Calcium ions 335
Cancer of stomach 67
Candida infection 167
Capillary loop 24
Capillary membrane 23
Capillary networks 24
Capillary permeability 23
γ-Carboxyglutamic acid 264–68, 273
Carditis 184
Catabolism and hypoalbuminaemia 64
CEA 197
Cell-mediated immunity 131, 137–40, 158, 163–64, 171, 172, 174, 193, 196
Cell membrane 198
Cellulose acetate membranes 316
Cephalin 74
Cerebrospinal fluid 368–70
Ceruloplasmin 19, 36, 96, 336, 342, 351, 353
  assay of 327
  biochemistry 96
  biological function 97
  chemical structure 96
  determination of 311
  enzymic function 97
  synthesis 98
γ-Chain disease 346
Chediak–Higashi syndrome 167
Chemical methods 309–12
Cholestasis, protein and lipoprotein changes in 360
Cholesterol 72–75
Christmas factor 282
Chromatographic methods 12–14, 39–41
Chromatography 84, 302
Chromoproteins 5
Chylomicronaemia 91
Chylomicrons 76, 82–84, 86
Chymotrypsin 259
CM-Sephadex 36, 37
CNBr-fragments 230, 233
Coagulation 281, 301
Coagulation factors 221–22, 285–88
Coagulation fibrinolysis 20
Cohn fractionation 29
Cohn method 11–12
Cold ethanol method 11
Colloid osmosis 54, 59
Colloids 5
Complement binding reactions 145

Complement defects   168
Complement factors   17, 20, 351, 353
  assay of   151
  inhibitors of   149–50
Complement sequence   147, 151
Complement system   145, 147–51
  activation of   147–49
  components of   150
Contact allergies   182
Coombs's test   202
Copper
  administration to animals   98
  distribution of   97
  metabolism defects   99
  turnover of   97
Corticosteroids   116, 343
Counter immunoelectrophoresis   330–33
C-reactive protein (CRP)   339, 351, 353, 354, 357
Creatinine   368
Cross-reactions   140
Crossed immunoelectrophoresis   329–30, 335, 351
C-terminal amino acid   112, 113
Cyanogen bromide   230
Cyclic AMP   86, 177–78, 180
Cytotoxic (or cytolytic) reactions   137, 147, 176, 181, 182, 186

D antigen   213
DEAE-cellulose   282, 287, 302
DEAE-Sephadex gel   34, 36, 37
Defective parathyroid glands   171
Deficiency states   343–44
Dehydrogenase   317
Delayed hypersensitive reaction   139, 176
Determinant   131
Determination of individual plasma proteins   311
Determination of total protein   309–11
Dextran   14
Diabetes insipidus   183
Diabetes mellitus   89
Diagnostic use of plasma protein analyses   335
Diapedisis   27
Dicoumarol   265
Di George's syndrome   171
Diglyceride   86
Dinitrochlorbenzene (DNCB)   182
Diphtheria   158
Disopropylfluorophosphate (DFP)   255
DNA   183
DNA synthesis   192, 193
Double diffusion technique   15, 143, 323
Drug allergies   181–82
Drugs   53
Ductus thoracicus   86

Duffy system   219
Dyes   52, 311–12
Dysgammaglobulinaemia   171

EDTA plasma   335
Effector function   189
Electroimmunoassay   142, 311, 325–29, 351
Electron microscope   23, 27
Electrophoresis   7–9, 11, 14, 15, 314, 316–18, 335
Electrophoretic mobility   5–7, 17, 72
Electrophoretic plasma protein patterns
  normal variants of   337–38
  pathological variations in   338
Electrostatic bonds   141
Endocarditis lenta   362
Endothelial cells   23, 24, 27
Enzyme immunoassays   335
Erythrocyte antigens   199
Erythron   362
Erythropoiesis   362
Ether fractionation   38

Factor III   285
Factor V   267, 285
Factor VII   271, 286
Factor VIII   31, 32, 276–81
Factor IX   34, 271, 273, 281, 308
Factor IX$_a$ 273
Factor X$_a$ 273, 275, 277, 286, 308
Factor X$_a$ 259, 261, 267, 268, 273, 274
Factor XI   281, 287, 308
Factor XII   287
Factor XIII   287–88
Farmer's lung   183
Fatty acid anions   54
Fatty acids   73
Ferritin   363
Ferroxidase   97
a-Fetoprotein   333, 338, 360
Fibrin   237–47, 304
  types of   253
Fibrin polymer   247–49
Fibrin stabilizing factor (FSF)   287
Fibrinogen   2, 11, 19, 223–53, 339, 342, 351, 353, 357
  amino acid analysis of   229
  antigenic structure of   249
  heterogeneity of   229
  in health and disease   250
  molecular weight   224
  molecule   226, 237, 246
  occurrence and role   223
  physicochemical properties   224
  polypeptide chains of   227–28
  primary structure of   230–37

Fibrinogen—(contd)
  production 33
  prosthetic groups 228
  solubility 225
  subunits and prosthetic groups of 227–29
Fibrinogen Detroit 251
Fibrinogen–fibrin transformation 237
Fibrinogene 37
Fibrinolysis 225, 288, 303–4
Fibrinolytic system activation 293–99
Fibrinopeptides A and B 238–47
Fibrous proteins 9
Fluorescein-tagged antigens 335
Fluorescence methods 310
Fluram technique 310
Folic acid 362
Folin–Ciocalteau phenol reagent 310
Fraction III 41
Fraction IV 36
Fractionation methods 4, 11, 29–41
Free fatty acids 73, 74, 86

Gamma globulins 9, 11, 17, 19, 34–36
Gastroenteropathies with loss of protein 67
Gastrointestinal diseases 354–56
Gel filtration 39–40, 313–15
Gel immunoprecipitation techniques 330
Globular protein 9
Globulin 1, 2, 4, 9, 11, 17, 19, 34–36, 55, 357
Glomerular proteinuria 366, 367
Glomerulonephritis 146, 186, 361
Glu-plasminogen 291–93, 296, 297, 299, 304
Glycine 111
Glycolipids 208
Glycoproteins 37, 199
Golgi apparatus 85
Goodpasture's syndrome 186
Granulocytes 154
Granulocytopoenia 165
Granulomatosis 167
Group specific proteins (Gc) 336

Haem 17
Haem–haemopexin complex 107, 108
Haem metabolism 94
Haemoglobin 4
  catabolism of 108
  haptoglobin binding with 105, 108
Haemolysis 362, 363
Haemolytic diseases in new-born 207, 210
Haemopexin 106–9, 351
  binding of porphyrins to 107–8
  biochemistry 106
  biological function 107
  chemical structure 106
  determination in plasma 108
  functions of 107
Haemophilia A 276, 279
Haemophilia B 281–85
Haemophilia C 281
Haemophilus influenzae 168
Hageman factor 301
Hapten 132
Haptoglobin 19, 36, 95, 102–6, 258, 336, 338, 340, 342, 351, 353, 362
  binding with haemoglobin 105, 108
  biochemistry 102
  biological function 106
  carbohydrate portion of 105
  chemical structure 102
  determination of 311
  genetic variants 105
  synthesis 106
Haptoglobin–haemoglobin complex 105
Heart diseases 67
Heart disorders 362
Heavy chain disease 346
α-Helix 1
Heparin cofactor 276
Hepatic sinusoids 23
Hepatitis 159, 357–59
Hereditary angio-oedema 168
Heteroantigens 132
High speed cinemicrophotography 23
Hirudin 273
Histamine 24, 147
Histocompatibility antigens 187
HLA antigens 190, 192
HLA system 187–88
HLA typing 192
Hormone balance 58
Human plasma proteins 17–21
Humoral antibodies 190
Hydrogen bonds 141
Hydrophobic pocket 53
Hyperalbuminaemia 63
Hyperbilirubinaemia 338
Hypercholesterolaemia 89
Hyperlipidaemia 90
Hyperlipoproteinaemia 90–91
  clinical manifestations 91–92
  frequency of 93
  reference values 93
Hypersensitivity reactions 176, 181
Hypertension 27
Hypertrophic gastritis 67
Hypoalbuminaemia
  causes of 63–67
  special conditions of 67–69
Hypogammaglobulinaemia 168–70
Hypolipoproteinaemias 93–94
Hypoproteinaemia 356
Hyposensitization 180
Hypothyroidism 89

Idiotypes   126
IgA   121, 160–62, 168–71, 200, 312, 327, 337, 339, 344, 345, 348, 349, 356, 359–61
IgD   120, 350
IgE   120, 162, 173, 177, 350
IgG   70, 120, 124, 136, 147, 158, 160, 169, 170, 176, 177, 200–2, 206, 312, 327, 337, 339, 340, 343–45, 348–50, 359, 361, 368–70
IgG2   171
IgM   121, 136, 147, 160, 168–71, 174, 176, 200, 201, 206, 312, 327, 340, 344, 345, 348, 349, 358, 359
Immediate hypersensitivity reaction   174
Immune complex diseases   182–84
Immune complexes   176
Immune reactions
   against transplanted tissue   188–89
   in tumour immunology   195
Immune response   128, 140, 151
Immunization   159
Immunoadherence   148
Immunoadsorption   40
Immunochemical methods   318–35
Immunochemistry   15
Immunodiffusion   142
Immunoelectrophoresis   142, 323–24
Immunoelectrophoretic method   15, 367
Immunofixation   330
Immunofluorescence techniques   146
Immunogens   132.
Immunoglobulin alterations in disease   344–51
Immunoglobulin deficiency   344
Immunoglobulin levels   340
Immunoglobulins   17, 19, 20, 119–219
   antigenic properties of   125
   basic structure   119
   biosynthesis   126–27
   classes of   120–21, 123
   constant region   124
   decrease in level of   344
   hypervariable regions   124
   monoclonal increase of level of   345–48
   oligoclonal reactions   350
   polyclonal increase   348
   properties of   122
   structures of heavy chains of various classes   121–24
   subgroups   124
   sugar chains   127
   use of term   119
   variable region   124
   see also IgA, etc.
Immunological diseases, mechanisms of   174
Immunological mechanisms   127–51
Immunological memory   136
Immunological surveillance in tumour immunology   195–97
Immunonephelometry   311, 333
Immunoprecipitation reactions   330
Immunoradiometric assay (IRMA)   334
Immunosorbent assay   145
Immunosuppression   193–94
Infection defence mechanisms
   antibodies in   156–63
   defects in   164–74
   defence against   151–74
   non-specific   152, 165
   specific   168
Inflammatory conditions   312, 351–54
Inflammatory injuries   163
Inflammatory patterns   361
Inflammatory reaction   148, 154, 165, 364, 370
Insulin   86
Interferon   153
Inter-α-trypsin inhibitor   336
Ion exchange cellulose columns   14
Ion exchange chromatography   40
Iron
   and bacteria growth   102
   binding with transferrin   100
Iron deficiency   363
Iron haemostasis   101
Isoantigens   132
Isoelectric point (LP)   7
Isoenzymes, separation of   317
Isotypes   126

Jaundice   339

Kabi fractionation   30–37
K-antigen   218–19
Kazal's inhibitor   273
K-cells   138
Kell system   218
Kidd system   219
Kidney disease   361–62
Kidney storage   71
Kinin   301
Kininogens   301
Kjeldahl method   310
KSCN   300

Lactoferrin   102
Large intestine   69
Lecithin   74, 75
Lecithin-cholesterol-acyl-transferase (LCAT)   74, 81, 87, 93, 358
Leukaemia   165, 363–65, 368
Lewis system   208

Light absorption method 7
Light chain disease 345–46
Light microscope 23, 27
Linked gene theory 212
Lipid metabolism 74–76
Lipids 72, 73
Lipoprotein-A deficiency 93
Lipoprotein X 78, 360
A-β-Lipoproteinaemia 94
Lipoproteins 17, 72–94, 316
  abnormal 78
  density variation 72
  electrophoresis of 82, 91, 92
  factors influencing concentration in plasma 88–90
  families of 79, 83–84
  floating β-lipoproteins 79
  high density (HDL) 72, 77–78, 82–84, 88, 89, 336
  immunochemical methods 83
  in plasma 76–78
  low density (LDL) 72, 77, 82–84, 87, 89
  metabolism 84–88
  methods used in study of 82–83
  micellular or macromolecular 72
  nephelometry 83
  pathological 78
  precipitation methods 82
  quantification of 83
  sinking pre-β-LP 78
  structure 84
  terminology 72
  ultracentrifugation 82
  very low density (VLDL) 72, 76, 82–85, 87, 89, 315
α-Lipoproteins 338, 339, 358
β-Lipoproteins 336–37, 339, 340, 360
Listeria 163, 164
Liver 23
  synthesis of albumin in 57
Liver cancer 360
Liver cirrhosis 64, 69, 339, 360
Liver disease 359
Liver tumour 360
Lupus erythematosus 168, 183, 185, 186
Lupus erythematosus disseminatus 165, 169
Luteinizing hormone (LH) 260–61
Lymph glands 132
Lymphatic cells 151
Lymphatic leukaemia 344
Lymphoblasts 137
Lymphocytes 169; see also B-lymphocytes; T-lymphocytes
Lymphokines 137–40
Lymphoma 344
Lysine 297, 299
Lysine-agarose 41
Lysolecithin 74

Lysosomal disorders 167
Lysozyme, determination of 311
Lysozymuria 365
Lys-plasminogen 291–93, 297, 299

α_2-Macroglobulin 307, 336, 338, 340
Macroglobulinaemia 9
Macrophage arming factor 138–39
Malabsorption 165
Malnutrition and hypoalbuminaemia 64
M-components 345–48
Measles 163
Menlqs kinky hair syndrome 99
Metal transport 96
Microcirculation of blood 23–27
Micrococcus lysodeicticus 311
β_2-microglobulin 368
Micropolyspora faeni 183
Microvascular bed 27
Migration inhibitory factor (MIF) 138, 140
Mixed lymphocyte culture 192
Molecular biology 9
Molecular weights 5
Monoglyceride 86
Multiple sclerosis 163
Mycobacteria 155, 164
Myelomatosis 344

NADPH 109
d-Naphthyl acetate esterase (ANAE) 128
Neoprothrombin-S 261, 274
Neoprothrombin-T 261, 274
Nephelometry 83, 333
Nephrotic syndrome 351
Nitro-blue tetrazolium reduction test (NBT) 167
p-Nitrophenylguinidinobenzoate (NPGB) 302
Noradrenaline 23
N-terminal Ser- 261
Nutrition effects 58

Oestrogen 89, 338, 341
Oral contraceptives 341
Organ storage with albumin 71–72
Orosomucoid 327, 343, 351
Oxygen 23

Pancreas insufficiency 165
Parathyroid glands 171
Penicillin 181
Penicilloyl 181
Peptide bonds 1, 3, 254
Periarteritis nodosa 184
Periodic system 8

Petechiae 27
pH effects 7, 14
pH-mobility curve 8
Phagocytes 165
Phagocytosis 148, 153, 155, 156, 160, 167
Phagosomes 153
Phospho-di-esterase 180
Phosphoglycerides 74
Phospholipids 72–75, 198, 264
Physicochemical methods 312–18
Phythaemagglutinin (PHA) 169, 174, 199
Plasma protein patterns
  normal variations in 339–41
  steroid hormones influence on 341
Plasma proteins 1, 17
  biophilic 95
  classification 95
  distribution 95
  metabolism 95
  suicidal 95
Plasmin 230, 233, 288–90, 293
a_2-Plasmin inhibitor 306
Plasmin solution 34
Plasminogen 17, 19, 268, 275, 288
  activation kinetics 297
  activators 299–303
  activators in blood 301
  fibrin and activator interaction 304
  isolation 34
  purification and properties 289–93
  recovery 41
  structural changes during activation 293
  structure of 293
Platelet-aggregating factor (PAF) 184
Platelet aggregation 256
Pneumococcus 154, 155, 157
Pneumocystis carinii 173
Polyarcrylamide gel electrophoresis 316, 318
Polyethylene glycol (PEG) 39
Polypeptides 79–82, 87, 119, 124, 126, 127, 227, 258
Polysaccharide 154
Porphyrins, binding to haemopexin 107–8
Postgastrectomy syndrome 68
Prealbumin 111–12, 342, 351, 356
Precipitation 39, 141
Precipitin 15
Prekallikrein 301
Prerenal proteinuria 364
Primary reaction 141
Properdin 153
Protease inhibitors 17, 21, 305, 306
Proteases 258
Protein-losing enteropathy 355–56
Protein molecules 5
Protein solutions 4
Proteins
  importance of 1

preparation of 4
purity of 4
Proteinuria 364–68
  electrophoretic analysis 366
  glomerular 366, 367
  low molecular weight 366
  prerenal 364
  tubular 366
Proteolysis 254, 274, 305–8
Prothrombin 351
  activation by limited proteolysis 274
  activation by staphylocoagulase 275
  activation to thrombin 254–55
  biosynthesis 275–76
  internal sequence homology 264
  kringle structures 264, 268, 275
  nomenclature 261–75
  primary structure 262
  specific cleavage by Factor X_a and by thrombin 261
Provocation tests 178
Pulmonary emphysema 343

Quantitative gel immunodiffusion 324
Quantitative precipitation in solution 321–23

Radial immunodiffusion 324, 327, 368
Radio ImmunoSorbent Test 179
Radioelectroimmunoassay 328–29
Radioimmunoassay 145, 333–35
Radioimmunological techniques 335
RAST (Radio AllergoSorbent Test) 179
Reagins 174, 177
Red blood cells 142, 147, 200–2, 208, 212
Refractive index gradient 5
Renal disease 361–62
Respiratory proteins 5, 8
Reticuloendothelial system (RES) 87
Retinol-binding protein (RBP) 111–13, 356
  biochemistry 111
  biological function 112
  chemical structure 111
  prealbumin 112
Rh antibodies 213
Rh antigen 200, 215
Rh immunization 215–17
Rh_{null} 214–15
Rh prophylaxis 217–18
Rh system 210–18
  nomenclature 211
  special antigens within 214
Rh types, frequencies of 212
Rhesus monkey 211
Rheumatic arthritis 126, 165, 169, 184
Rivanol precipitation 38
mRNA 127

Index

Rocket electrophoresis 142
Rocket immunoelectrophoresis 325–29
Rubella 163

Salmonella 164
Scale method 5
Secondary manifestations 141
Secondary response 136
Sedimentation 4
Sedimentation coefficient 8
Sedimentation diagram 5
Sedimentation pattern 17
Sedimentation velocity method 5, 9
Separation methods 1, 309
Sephadex 14, 34, 36, 37, 84, 313, 315
Serotonin 24
Serum proteins 1
Serum sickness 183
Serve combined immunodeficiency (SCID) 172
Sex variations 339–40
Sickle-cell anaemia 167
Simple radial immunodiffusion 142
Skin tests 178, 179
Slow Reacting Substance-A (SRS-A) 178
Small intestine 68
Smooth muscle cells 23
Solubility behaviour 11
Sphingomyelin 74
Staphylocoagulase 275
Staphylococcus albus 154, 157
Staphylococcus aureus 155, 157
Staphylothrombin 275
Stem cells 128
Steroid hormones 115
   binding to protein 116
   influence on plasma protein patterns 341
Stomach cancer 67
Streptococci 155
Streptococcus haemolyticus 301
Streptokinase 301–3
Streptokinase-plasmin complex 302
Streptomyces griseus 275
Subacute sclerosing panencephalitis 163, 369
Svedberg (unit) 8
Synthetic polymers, precipitation with 39

Tangier's disease 93
T-cells 131, 132, 138, 164, 185, 189, 190, 196, 197
Technicon Auto Analyser 333
Termoactinomyces vulgaris 183
Testosterone 342
Thrombin
   A-chain 256, 259, 261
   B-chain 256–61
   catalytic activity 259
   function and specificity 255–56
   historical outline 254
   homology with serine proteases and haptoglobin 258
   inhibition by antithrombin-III 276
   partial homology/analogy with angiotensin and with luteinizing hormone (LH) 260–61
   primary structure 256
   prothrombin activation to 254–55
   tentative tertiary structure 259
Thrombokinase 255
Thromboplastin 255, 285
Thrombosis 251–53, 256
Thymus alymphoplasia 171
Thymus hypoplasia 171
Thyroglobulin 184
Thyroid hormones 113–15
   and protein 114
   biochemistry 113
   biological function 114
   chemical structure 113
   genetic variants 114
Thyroxine 113
Thyroxine-binding globulin 113, 114, 342
Thyroxine-binding prealbumin 111, 114, 335
T-independent antigens 193
Tiselius electrophoresis technique 9
Tissue activators 299
T-lymphocytes 128–31, 137, 139, 140, 145, 156, 157, 163, 164, 169, 172, 176, 177, 182, 184–87
Tosyl-L-arginine methyl ester (TAMe) 255
Total protein, determination of 309–11
Toxins 158, 160
Tranexamic acid (AMCA) 168
Transcobalamine 109–11
   biochemistry 109
   biological function 110
   chemical structure 109
   genetic variants 110
Transcobalamine I 109–10
Transcobalamine II 110–11
Transcortin 115–17, 342
   biochemistry 115
   biological function 116–17
   chemical structure 115
   synthesis 116
Transcortin-bound cortisol 116–17
Transfer factor 174
Transferrin 19, 36, 99–102, 339, 342, 351, 356, 363, 368
   binding with iron 100
   biochemistry 99
   biological function 100–2
   chemical structure 99
   determination of 311

Transferring—(contd)
  genetic variants 100
Transplantation immunology 187–94
Transplantation surgery 71
Transplanted tissue, immune reactions
    against 188–89
Transport proteins 17, 20, 43–117
Triglycerides 72–74, 87
Triiodothyronine 113
Trypsin 255, 293
Trypsin inhibitors 273
Tryptophan 368
Tubercle bacteria 157
Tuberculin test 163, 164
Tubular proteinuria 366
Tumour antigens 194, 197
Tumour immunology 194–97
  immune reactions in 195
  immunological surveillance in 195–97
  practical applications of 197
Turbidimetric determinations of
    immunoprecipitates 333
Type 1 reaction 174, 181, 182, 184
Type 2 reaction 176, 182, 186
Type 3 reaction 176, 182, 183, 186
Type 4 reaction 176, 182, 187

Ultracentrifugation 5, 7, 9, 11, 82, 312
Uraemia 361–62

Urinary proteins 364
Urokinase 299

Vaccination 159
Van der Waals's forces 141
Vasculitis 184
Vena jugularis 86
Venules 27
Viruses 158, 160
Vitamin A 111, 112, 167
Vitamin B_{12} 110, 362
Vitamin K 34, 264–73, 275, 276, 283
von Willebrand's disease 277–81

Wassermann reaction 145
White blood cells 154
Wilson's disease 99
Wiskott–Aldrich syndrome 173, 174

Xg system 205

Zeta potential 201
Zone electrophoresis 14
Zymogen activation mechanism 258
Zymogenenzyme systems 254